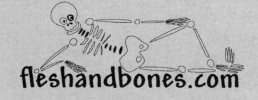

Oral Anatomy, Embryology and Histology

Commissioning Editor: Michael Parkinson
Project Development Manager: Siân Jarman
Project Manager: Frances Affleck
Designers: Judith Wright and George Ajayi

Oral Anatomy, Embryology and Histology THIRD EDITION

B. K. B. Berkovitz BDS, MSc, PhD

Reader, Division of Anatomy, Cell and Human Biology
Guy's, King's and St Thomas' School of Biomedical Sciences, London, UK

G. R. Holland BSc, BDS, PhD, CERT ENDO

Professor, Department of Cariology, Restorative Sciences and Endodontics, School of Dentistry and
Department of Cell and Developmental Biology, Faculty of Medicine, University of Michigan,
Ann Arbor, USA

B. J. Moxham BSc, BDS, PhD

Professor of Anatomy, Cardiff School of Biosciences, Cardiff University, Cardiff, UK

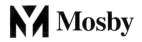 Mosby

EDINBURGH LONDON NEW YORK OXFORD PHILADELPHIA ST LOUIS SYDNEY TORONTO 2002

MOSBY
An imprint of Elsevier Limited

First published 2002

ISBN 0 7234 3181 7
  Reprinted 2002, 2003, 2005, 2006

International Student Edition 0 7234 3343 7

British Library Cataloguing in Publication Data
A catalogue record for this book is available from the British Library

Library of Congress Cataloguing in Publication Data
A catalogue record for this book is available from the Library of Congress Note Medical knowledge is constantly changing. As new information becomes available, changes in treatment, procedures, equipment and the use of drugs become necessary. The authors and the publishers have taken care to ensure that the information given in this text is accurate and up to date. However, readers are strongly advised to confirm that the information, especially with regard to drug usage, complies with the latest legislation and standards of practice.

ELSEVIER your source for books, journals and multimedia in the health sciences
www.elsevierhealth.com

Working together to grow
libraries in developing countries
www.elsevier.com | www.bookaid.org | www.sabre.org

ELSEVIER | BOOK AID International | Sabre Foundation

The publisher's policy is to use **paper manufactured from sustainable forests**

Printed in China
N/05

Contents

Preface

We are pleased to be invited by our publishers to produce a new edition of this book. In the 10 years that have elapsed since the previous edition, there have been significant advances in our knowledge of the microscopic anatomy (Chapters 7–16) and development (Chapters 17–26) of the orodental tissues, particularly in aspects of cellular and molecular biology. We were immediately faced with the decision of including this new information in the present volume and therefore making the book more detailed, or leaving much of it out to provide a simpler volume with a 'core-related' body of knowledge. Although it now seems fashionable to adopt the latter approach in many subjects to decongest what might otherwise be a crowded syllabus, we have decided to include this new information where it is likely to impinge on clinical practice, as illustrated by the following examples. Should a dental practitioner be undertaking orthodontic treatment or the placement of dental implants without basic knowledge of the bone biology underpinning successful treatment? Should a dental practitioner be undertaking periodontal therapy without understanding the principles underlying periodontal regeneration or tissue guided regeneration? Should a dental practitioner be undertaking endodontic treatment without an appreciation of how dentine-forming cells differentiate during normal tooth development and how they might arise following the formation of reparative dentine. If dental surgeons are not interested in the updating of knowledge of the structure and development of the teeth and surrounding tissues, who will be?

To improve the ease of correlating the text and illustrations, we have written this new edition more along the lines of a textbook, but without reducing the number of illustrations, as we still firmly believe that anatomical and histological textbooks must present information primarily in a visual form. Of nearly 900 illustrations, almost one-third are new. To incorporate the considerable amount of new material, while avoiding a significant increase in size, has meant deleting the section on comparative dental anatomy. In deleting this section, we are aware that comparative dental anatomy has been removed from the curriculum of most dental schools.

Although the text of Chapters 1–6, dealing with the macroscopic anatomy of the oral cavity and related areas, has changed least of all, we have been able to replace a number of illustrations and add new ones. The text for all other chapters has been thoroughly revised and updated. Many new illustrations have been included, in particular those related to the newer experimental techniques such as imunohistochemistry. We have also increased the space devoted to the clinical relevance of information related to basic science.

2002

B. K. B. B.
G. R. H.
B. J. M.

Acknowledgements

We are most grateful to the numerous colleagues who generously provided photographic material for our book and these have been acknowledged in the text. In addition, we owe a debt of thanks to the following researchers for their constructive criticisms of draft chapters: Dr T. Arnett, Dr A.E. Barrett, Dr J.H. Bennett, Professor M.C. Dean, Professor G. Embery, Professor J.R. Garrett, Dr A. Grigoriadis, Professor L. Hammarstrom, Professor S.J. Jones, Professor P. Morgan, Professor R.M. Palmer, Dr G.D. Procter, Professor P.T. Sharpe, Dr R.P. Shellis, Dr G.D. Singh, Professor M.M. Smith, Ms D. Symons, Professor T. Watson, Dr R. Wilson.

1 The *in vivo* appearance of the oral cavity

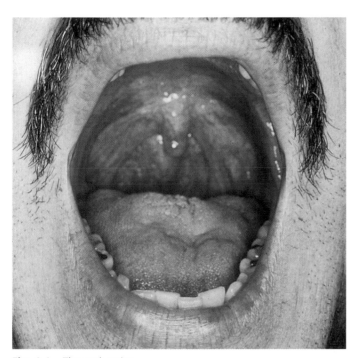

Fig. 1.1 The oral cavity.

The oral cavity (Fig. 1.1) extends from the lips and cheeks externally to the pillars of the fauces internally, where it continues into the oropharynx. It is subdivided into the vestibule external to the teeth and the oral cavity proper internal to the teeth. The palate forms the roof of the mouth and separates the oral and nasal cavities. The floor of the oral cavity consists of mucous membrane covering the mylohyoid muscle and is occupied mainly by the tongue. The lateral walls of the oral cavity are defined by the cheeks and retromolar regions. The primary functions of the mouth are concerned with the ingestion (and selection) of food, and with mastication and swallowing. Secondary functions include speech and ventilation (breathing).

THE LIPS

The lips (Fig. 1.2) are composed of a muscular skeleton (the orbicularis oris muscle) and connective tissue, and are covered externally by skin and internally by mucous membrane. The red portion of the lip (the vermilion) is a feature characteristic of humans. The sharp junction of the vermilion and the skin is termed the vermilion border. In the upper lip the vermilion protrudes in the midline to form the tubercle. The lower lip shows a slight depression in the midline corresponding to the tubercle. From the midline to the corners of the mouth the lips

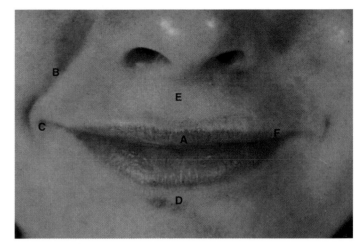

Fig. 1.2 The lips. A = tubercle; B = nasolabial groove; C = labiomarginal sulci; D = labiomental groove; E = philtrum, F = labial commissure.

widen and then narrow. Laterally, the upper lip is separated from the cheeks by nasolabial grooves. Similar grooves appear with age at the corners of the mouth to delineate the lower lip from the cheeks (the labiomarginal sulci). The labiomental groove separates the lower lip from the chin. In the midline of the upper lip runs the philtrum. The corners of the lips (the labial commissures) are usually located adjacent to the maxillary canine and mandibular first premolar teeth. The lips exhibit sexual dimorphism; as a general rule, the skin of the male is thicker, firmer, less mobile and hirsute. The lips illustrated are lightly closed at rest and are described as being 'competent'.

Incompetent lips (Fig. 1.3) describe a situation where, at rest and with the facial muscles relaxed, a lip seal is not

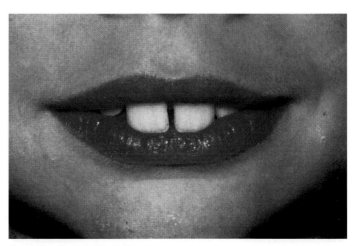

Fig. 1.3. Incompetent lips.

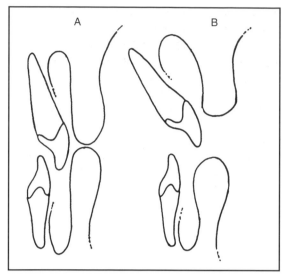

Fig. 1.4 A = Competent lips maintaining normal inclination of incisors. B = Incompetent lips resulting in proclination of upper incisors.

produced. It is of some importance that this is distinguished from conditions where the lips are merely held apart habitually (as often occurs with 'mouth breathers'). The lip posture illustrated in Fig. 1.3 can be described as being 'potentially competent' as the lips would be capable of producing a seal at rest if there were no interference caused by the protruding incisors. Where the lips are incompetent, the pattern of swallowing is often modified to produce an anterior oral seal. Accordingly, an oral seal may be formed by contact between the lower lip (or the tongue) and the palatal mucosa, and there may even be a forcible tongue thrust. It has been estimated that in the UK and the USA about 50% of children at the age of 11 years have some degree of lip incompetence.

The position and activity of the lips are important in controlling the degree of protrusion of the incisors. With competent lips (Fig. 1.4a) the tips of the maxillary incisors lie below the upper border of the lower lip, this arrangement helping to maintain the 'normal' inclination of the incisors. With incompetent lips (Fig. 1.4b) the maxillary incisors may not be so controlled and the lower lip may even lie behind them, thus producing an exaggerated proclination of these teeth. If there is tongue thrusting to provide an anterior oral seal, further forces that tend to protrude the incisors are generated. A tight, or overactive, lip musculature may be associated with retroclined incisors.

THE ORAL VESTIBULE

The oral vestibule (Fig. 1.5) is a slit-like space between the lips and cheeks and the teeth and alveolus. At rest, or with the mouth open, the vestibule and oral cavity proper directly communicate between the teeth. When the teeth bite together, the vestibule is a closed space that communicates with the oral cavity proper only behind the last molars (the retromolar regions). The mucosa covering the alveolus is reflected onto the lips and cheeks, forming a trough or sulcus called the vestibular fornix. In some regions of the sulcus, the mucosa may show distinct sickle-shaped folds running from the cheeks and lips to the alveolus. The upper and lower labial frena or frenula are such folds in the midline. Other folds of variable dimensions may traverse the sulcus in the regions of the canines or premolars. Such frena are said to be more pronounced in the lower sulcus. All folds contain loose connective tissue and are neither muscle attachments nor sites of large blood vessels.

The upper labial frenum should be attached well below the alveolar crest. A large frenum with an attachment near the crest may be associated with a midline diastema between the maxillary first incisors (Fig. 1.6). Prominent frena may also influence the stability of dentures.

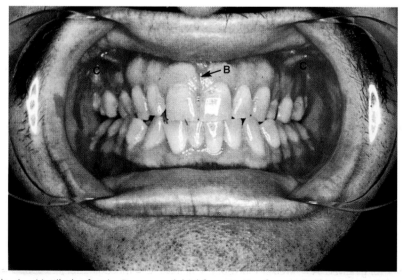

Fig. 1.5 The oral vestibule. A = Vestibular fornix; B = upper labial frenum; C = frenum in the region of the upper premolar teeth.

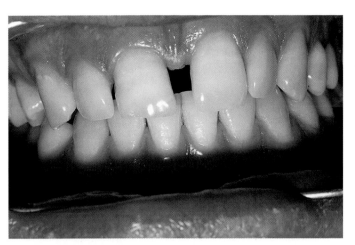

Fig. 1.6 Midline diastema between upper central incisor teeth, produced by an enlarged labial frenum.

THE GINGIVAE

The gums or gingivae, the oral mucosa covering the alveolar bone (which supports the roots of the teeth) and the necks (cervical region) of the teeth, are divided into two main components (Fig. 1.7). That portion lining the lower part of the alveolus is loosely attached to the periosteum via a diffuse submucosa and is termed the alveolar mucosa. It is delineated from the gingiva (which covers the upper part of the alveolar bone and the necks of the teeth) by a well defined junction, the mucogingival junction. The alveolar mucosa appears dark red, the gingiva pale pink. These colour differences relate to differences in the type of keratinisation and the proximity to the surface of underlying blood vessels. Indeed, small blood vessels may readily be seen coursing beneath the alveolar mucosa (Fig. 1.7b). The gingiva may be further subdivided into the attached gingiva and the free gingiva. The attached gingiva is firmly bound to the periosteum of the alveolus and to the teeth, and the free gingiva lies unattached around the cervical region of the tooth. A groove (the free gingival groove) may be seen between the free and attached gingiva. This groove corresponds roughly to the floor of the gingival sulcus, which separates the inner surface of the attached

gingiva from the enamel itself (see Fig. 14.34). The interdental papilla is that part of the gingiva which fills the space between adjacent teeth. A feature of the attached gingiva is its surface stippling. The degree of stippling varies from individual to individual and according to age, sex and health of the gingiva. The free gingiva is not stippled. On the lingual surface of the lower jaw the attached gingiva is sharply differentiated from the alveolar mucosa towards the floor of the mouth by a mucogingival line. On the palate, however, there is no obvious division between the attached gingiva and the rest of the palatal mucosa as this whole surface is keratinised masticatory mucosa.

THE CHEEKS

The cheeks extend intraorally from the labial commissures anteriorly to the ridge of mucosa overlying the ascending ramus of the mandible posteriorly. They are bounded superiorly and inferiorly by the upper and lower vestibular sulci (Fig. 1.5). The mucosa is non-keratinised and, being tightly adherent to the buccinator muscle, is stretched when the mouth is opened and wrinkled when closed. Ectopic sebaceous glands may be evident in the mucosa as yellowish patches called Fordyce's spots (Fig. 1.8). Few structural landmarks are visible in the cheeks. The parotid duct drains into the cheek opposite the maxillary second molar tooth and its opening may be covered by a small fold of mucosa termed the parotid papilla. A hyperkeratinised line called the linea alba may be seen at a position related to the occlusal plane. In the retromolar region, in front of the pillars of the fauces, a fold of mucosa containing the pterygomandibular raphe extends from the upper to the lower alveolus (Fig. 1.9). The pterygomandibular space, in which the lingual and inferior alveolar nerves run, lies lateral to this fold and medial to a ridge produced by the mandibular ramus. The groove lying between the ridges produced by the raphe and the ramus of the mandible is an important landmark for insertion of a needle for local anaesthesia of the lingual and inferior alveolar nerves.

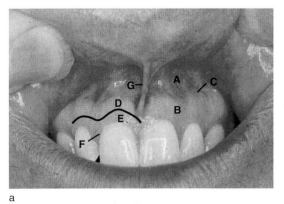

a

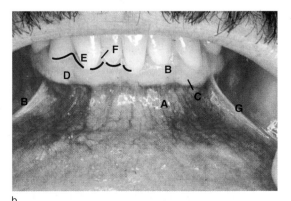

b

Fig. 1.7 Upper (a) and lower (b) gingivae. A = alveolar mucosa; B = gingiva; C = mucogingival junction, D = attached gingiva; E = free gingiva; F = interdental papilla; G = upper labial frenum.

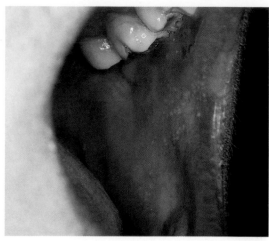

Fig. 1.8 Inner surface of the cheek, showing Fordyce spots as yellowish patches.

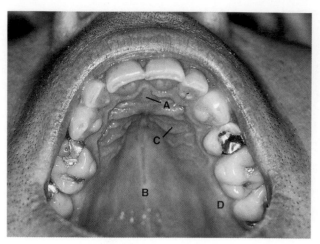

Fig. 1.10 The hard palate. A = Incisive papilla; B = palatine raphe; C = palatine rugae; D = alveolus.

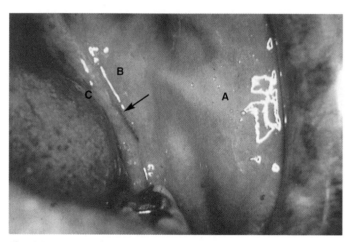

Fig. 1.9 Retromolar region. A = Inner surface of cheek; B = ridge overlying ramus of mandible; C = ridge overlying the pterygomandibular raphe. The arrow indicates a landmark for the insertion of needle for local anaesthesia of the lingual and inferior alveolar nerves.

When the upper (maxillary) and lower (mandibular) teeth are occluded, a small retromolar space is present behind the last molar tooth. This provides a pathway for the administration of nutrients in a patient whose jaws have been wired together following a fracture.

THE PALATE

The palate forms the roof of the mouth and separates the oral and nasal cavities. It is divided into the immovable hard palate anteriorly and the movable soft palate posteriorly. As their names suggest, the skeleton of the hard palate is bony while that of the soft palate is fibrous.

The hard palate is covered by a keratinised mucosa, which is firmly bound down to underlying bone and which also contains some taste buds. It shows a distinct prominence immediately behind the maxillary central incisors, the incisive

papilla (Fig. 1.10), which covers the nasopalatine nerves as they emerge from the incisive foramen. Extending posteriorly in the midline from the papilla runs a ridge termed the palatine raphe. Here, the oral mucosa is attached directly to bone without the presence of a submucous layer of tissue. Palatine rugae are elevated ridges in the anterior part of the hard palate that radiate somewhat transversely from the incisive papilla and the anterior part of the palatine raphe. Their pattern is unique to the individual and, like fingerprints, can be used for forensic purposes to help identify individuals. At the junction of the palate and the alveolus lies a mass of soft tissue (submucosa) in which run the greater palatine nerves and vessels. The shape and size of the dome of the palate varies considerably, being relatively shallow in some cases and having considerable depth in others.

The boundary between the soft palate and the hard palate is readily palpable and may be distinguished by a change in colour, the soft palate being a darker red with a yellowish tint. Extending laterally from the free border of the soft palate on each side are the palatoglossal and palatopharyngeal folds, the palatoglossal fold being more anterior (Fig. 1.11). These folds

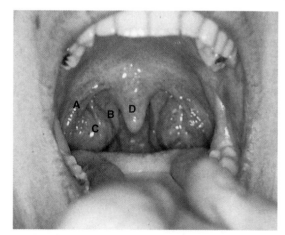

Fig. 1.11 The soft palate and oropharyngeal isthmus. A = Palatoglossal fold; B = palatopharyngeal fold; C = palatine tonsil; D = uvula.

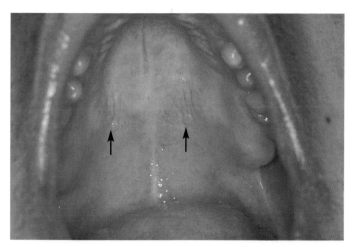

Fig. 1.12 Oral surface of the soft palate showing fovea palatini (arrows).

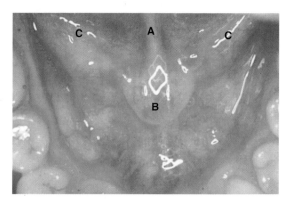

Fig. 1.13 Floor of the mouth. A = Lingual frenum; B = sublingual papilla; C = sublingual folds.

cover the palatoglossus and palatopharyngeus muscles and between them lies the tonsillar fossa, which in young individuals houses the palatine tonsil. The palatine tonsil is a collection of lymphoid material of variable size that is likely to atrophy in the adult. It exhibits several slit-like invaginations (the tonsillar crypts), one of which is particularly deep and named the intratonsillar cleft. The free edge of the soft palate in the midline is termed the palatal uvula. The oropharyngeal isthmus is where the oral cavity and the oropharynx meet. It is delineated by the palatoglossal and palatopharyngeal folds or arches (pillars of the fauces).

Knowledge of the anatomy of the palate has clinical relevance when siting the posterior border (postdam) of an upper denture. The denture needs to bed into the tissues at the anterior border of the soft palate (at a location sometimes referred to as the 'vibrating line' because the soft palate can be seen to move here on asking a patient to say 'ah'). In most individuals two small pits, the fovea palatini, may be seen (Fig. 1.12) one on each side of the midline; these represent the orifices of ducts from some of the minor mucous glands of the palate. The fovea palatini can also be seen on impressions of the palate and a postdam may usually be safely placed a couple of millimetres behind the pits.

THE FLOOR OF THE MOUTH

The floor of the mouth is a small horseshoe-shaped region above the mylohyoid muscle and beneath the movable part of the tongue (Fig. 1.13). It is covered by a lining of non-keratinised mucosa. In the midline, near the base of the tongue, a fold of tissue (called the lingual frenum) extends on to the inferior surface of the tongue. The sublingual papilla, onto which the submandibular salivary ducts open into the mouth, is a large centrally positioned protuberance at the base of the tongue. On either side of this papilla are the sublingual folds, beneath which lie the submandibular ducts and sublingual salivary glands.

THE TONGUE

The tongue is a muscular organ with its base attached to the floor of the mouth. It is attached to the inner surface of the mandible near the midline and gains support below from the hyoid bone. It functions in mastication, swallowing and speech and carries out important sensory functions, particularly those of taste. The lymphoid material contained in its posterior third has a protective role.

The inferior surface of the tongue, related to the floor of the mouth, is covered by a thin lining of non-keratinised mucous membrane that is tightly bound down to the underlying muscles. In the midline, extending onto the floor of the mouth, lies the lingual frenum (Fig. 1.14). Rarely, this extends across the floor of the mouth to be attached to the mandibular alveolus. Such an overdeveloped lingual frenum (ankyloglossa) may restrict movements of the tongue. Lateral to the frenum lie irregular, fringed folds: the fimbriated folds. Also visible through the mucosa are the deep lingual veins.

The dorsum of the tongue may be subdivided into the anterior two-thirds or palatal part and the posterior third or pharyngeal part. The junction of the palatal and pharyngeal parts is marked by a shallow V-shaped groove, the sulcus terminalis (Fig. 1.15). The angle (or 'V') of the sulcus terminalis is directed posteriorly. In the midline, near the angle, may be seen a small pit called the foramen caecum. This is the primordial site of development of the thyroid gland. The mucosa of the

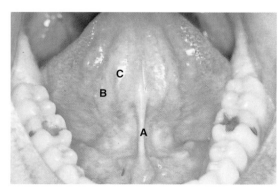

Fig. 1.14 Inferior surface of the tongue. A = Lingual frenum; B = fimbriated fold; C = deep lingual vein.

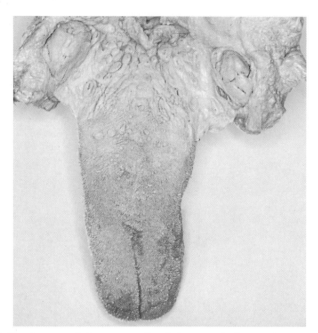

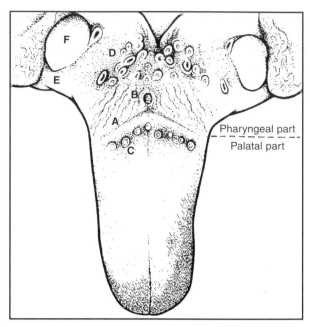

Fig. 1.15 Dorsum of the tongue. A = Sulcus terminalis; B = foramen caecum; C = circumvallate papillae; D = lingual follicles; E = palatoglossal arches; F = palatine tonsil.

palatal part of the tongue is partly keratinised and is characterised by the abundance of papillae. The most conspicuous papillae on the palatal surface of the tongue are the circumvallate papillae, which lie immediately in front of the sulcus terminalis. The pharyngeal surface of the tongue is covered with large rounded nodules termed the lingual follicles. These follicles are composed of lymphatic tissue, collectively forming the lingual tonsil. The posterior part of the tongue slopes towards the epiglottis, where three folds of mucous membrane are seen: the median and lateral glossoepiglottic folds. The anterior pillars of the fauces (the palatoglossal arches) extend from the soft palate to the sides of the tongue near the circumvallate papillae.

The dorsum of the tongue is covered with numerous whitish, conical elevations: the filiform papillae, which are keratinised (Fig. 1.16). Interspersed between the filiform papillae are isolated reddish prominences, the fungiform papillae. These are non-keratinised and contain taste buds. The fungiform papillae are most numerous at the tip of the tongue.

The 10–15 circumvallate papillae (Fig. 1.17) are considerably larger than either the filiform or fungiform papillae. They

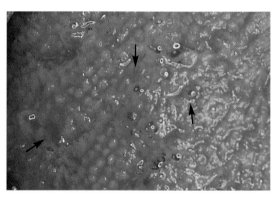

Fig. 1.17 Dorsum of the tongue, showing circumvallate papillae (A). B = Lingual follicles.

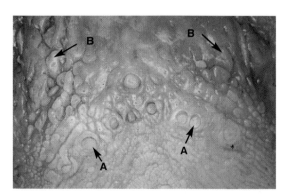

Fig. 1.16 Dorsum of the tongue, showing filiform and fungiform (arrows) papillae.

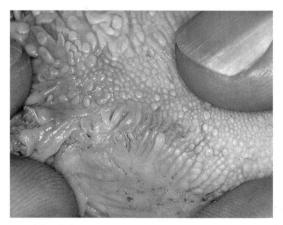

Fig. 1.18 Side of the tongue, showing slit-like appearance of foliate papillae.

lie immediately in front of the sulcus terminalis, do not project beyond the surface of the tongue and are surrounded by a circular 'trench'. The surface of the posterior third of the tongue lying behind the sulcus terminalis is non-keratinised and is covered by a number of smooth elevations produced by underlying lymphoid tissue.

Foliate papillae (Fig. 1.18) appear as a series of parallel, slit-like folds of mucosa on each lateral border of the tongue, near the attachment of the palatoglossal fold (anterior pillar of the fauces). The foliate papillae are of variable length in humans and are the vestige of large papillae found in many other mammals.

2 Dento-osseous structures

THE JAWS

The jaws are the tooth-bearing bones. They comprise three bones. The two maxillary bones form the upper jaw. The lower jaw is a single bone, the mandible (Fig. 2.1).

The skull is the most complex osseous structure in the body. It protects the brain, the organs of special sense and the cranial parts of the respiratory and digestive systems. The skull is divided into the neurocranium (which houses and protects the brain and the organs of special sense) and the viscerocranium (which surrounds the upper parts of the respiratory and digestive tracts). The jaws contribute the major part of the viscerocranium, comprising about 25% of the skull. The jaws have evolved from the gill arch elements of early agnathan vertebrates. It is probable that one or two anterior gill arches gradually disappeared with the expansion of the mouth cavity, so that the gill arch which developed phylogenetically into the jaws of ancestral gnathostomes was not the first of the series. Note that the upper jaw not only contains teeth but also contributes to the skeleton of the nose, orbit, cheek and palate.

The Maxilla

The maxilla consists of a body and four processes: the frontal, zygomatic, alveolar and palatine processes. Only the palatine process cannot be seen from the lateral aspect of the maxilla (Fig. 2.2). The anterolateral surface of the maxilla (the malar

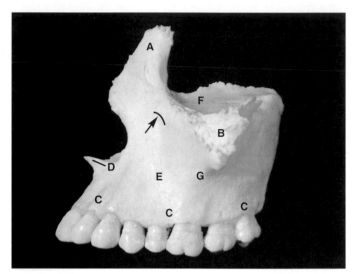

Fig. 2.2 Lateral aspect of the maxilla. A = Frontal process; B = zygomatic process; C = alveolar process; D = anterior nasal spine; E = canine fossa; F = orbital plate; G = jugal crest. The infraorbital foramen is arrowed.

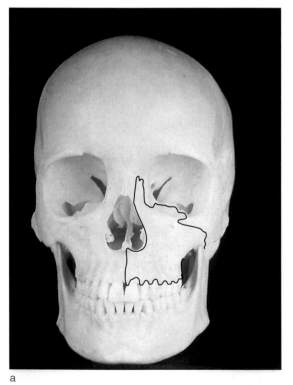

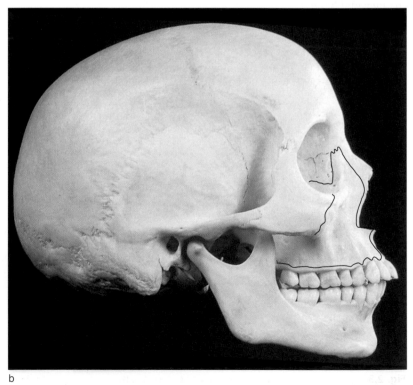

a   b

Fig. 2.1 Front (a) and side (b) views of the skull, showing the relationship between the jaws and the remainder of the skull. The black line describes the boundaries of a maxillary bone.

surface) forms the skeleton of the anterior part of the cheek. In the midline, the alveolar processes of the two maxillae meet at the intermaxillary suture whence they diverge laterally to form the opening into the nasal fossae (the piriform aperture). At the lower border of the piriform aperture, in the midline, lies the bony projection termed the anterior nasal spine. The malar surface of the body of the maxilla is concave, forming the canine fossa. Superiorly, the malar surface is continuous with the orbital plate of the maxilla and forms the floor of the orbit. Anterior to the orbital plate, the frontal process extends above the piriform aperture to meet the nasal and frontal bones. Below the infraorbital rim lies the infraorbital foramen through which the infraorbital branch of the maxillary nerve and the infraorbital artery from the maxillary artery emerge onto the face. The posterolateral surface of the maxilla (the infratemporal surface) forms the anterior wall of the infratemporal fossa. The malar and infratemporal surfaces meet at a bony ridge extending from the zygomatic process to the alveolus adjacent to the first molar tooth. This ridge is called the zygomaticoalveolar, or jugal, crest. The posterior convexity of the infratemporal surface is termed the maxillary tuberosity and presents several small foramina associated with the posterior superior dental nerves (which supply the posterior maxillary teeth). The zygomatic process extends both from the malar and the infratemporal surfaces of the maxilla. From the entire lower surface of the body arises the alveolar process, which supports the maxillary teeth.

The medial aspect of the maxilla is illustrated in Fig. 2.3. This part of the maxilla forms the lateral wall of the nose. In the specimen illustrated, the central hollow of the body of the maxilla (the maxillary air sinus or antrum) is divided by a bony septum. In front of the antrum lies a deep vertical groove called the lacrimal sulcus. This sulcus meets the lower edge of the lacrimal bone to form the nasolacrimal canal. Behind the antrum lies the palatine groove, which is converted into a canal carrying the greater palatine nerve and artery by the perpendicular plate of the palatine bone. The maxillary palatine process extends horizontally from the medial surface of the maxilla where the body meets the alveolar process.

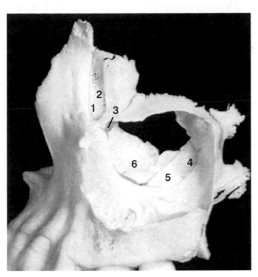

Fig. 2.4 Osteology of the maxillary air sinus showing adjacent bones reducing the size of the ostium. 1 = Lacrimal groove of maxilla; 2 = lacrimal groove; 3 = lacrimal bone; 4 = ethmoid bone; 5 = palatine bone; 6 = inferior nasal concha. Courtesy of Professor R.M.H. McMinn.

The lateral wall of the nasal fossa consists mainly of the medial surface of the maxilla. This surface of the isolated bone is occupied mainly by the large maxillary hiatus (Fig. 2.3). To reduce the size of this space *in vivo*, the hiatus is overlapped by the lacrimal bone and the ethmoid bone above, the palatine bone behind, and the inferior concha below (Fig. 2.4).

The Maxillary sinus

The maxillary sinus (antrum) is the largest of the paranasal sinuses, and is situated in the body of the maxilla. It is pyramidal in shape. The base (medial wall) forms part of the lateral wall of the nose. The apex extends into the zygomatic process of the maxilla. The roof of the sinus is part of the floor of the orbit, and the floor of the sinus is formed by the alveolar process and part of the palatine process of the maxilla. The anterior wall of the sinus is the facial surface of the maxilla, and the posterior wall is the infratemporal surface of the maxilla. Running in the roof of the sinus is the infraorbital nerve and vessels. The anterior superior alveolar nerve and vessels run in the anterior wall of the sinus. The posterior superior alveolar nerve and vessels pass through canals in the posterior surface of the sinus. The medial wall of the maxillary sinus contains the opening (ostium) of the sinus that leads into the middle meatus of the nose. As this opening lies well above the floor of the sinus, its position is unfavourable for drainage (see Fig. 5.5a). Infections of the maxillary sinus may therefore require surgical intervention, creating a more favourable drainage channel closer to the floor of the sinus.

The roots of the cheek teeth are related to the floor of the maxillary sinus (Fig. 2.5). The most closely related are the roots of the second permanent maxillary molar, especially the apex of its palatal root; the roots of the first and third molars and the second premolar are only slightly further away. Sometimes only mucosa separates the roots from the sinus. Care must be taken (particularly when extracting fractured roots in this region) to avoid creating an oroantral fistula,

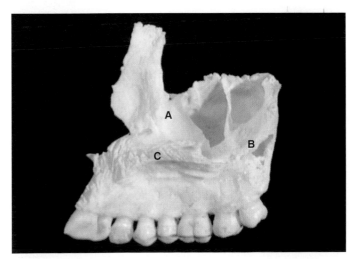

Fig. 2.3 Medial aspect of the maxilla. A = Lacrimal sulcus; B = palatine groove; C = palatine process of maxilla. Note the large opening into the maxillary sinus.

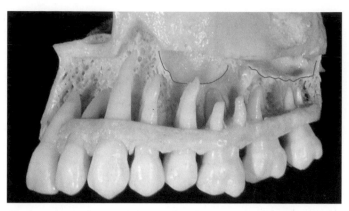

Fig. 2.5 Lateral view of the maxilla, showing close relationship of roots of the cheek teeth to the floor of the maxillary sinus (red outline).

when an epithelial-lined channel exists between the oral cavity and maxillary sinus.

The maxillary air sinus is lined by respiratory epithelium (a ciliated columnar epithelium), with numerous goblet cells. The sinus is innervated by the infraorbital nerve and superior alveolar branches of the maxillary nerve.

An inferior view of the maxillae shows their important contributions to the hard palate (Fig. 2.6). The four major bones contributing to the hard palate are the palatine processes of the maxillae and the horizontal plates of the palatine bones. The maxillary palatine processes arise as horizontal plates at the junction of the bodies and alveolar processes of the maxillae. The boundary between the palatine

and alveolar processes is well defined in its posterior aspect only; anteriorly, the angle between the two is less well defined. The junction between the palatine processes in the midline is termed the median palatine suture. Anteriorly, behind the central incisors, this junction is incomplete, thus forming the incisive fossa, through which pass the nasopalatine nerves. Unlike the nasal surface, the oral surface of the palatine process is rough and irregular. The posterior edges of the palatine processes articulate with the horizontal plates of the two palatine bones to form the transverse palatine suture. Laterally this junction is incomplete, forming the greater palatine foramina, through which pass the greater palatine nerves and vessels. Behind the greater palatine foramina lie the lesser palatine foramina, through which pass the lesser palatine nerves and vessels. The junction of the two palatine bones in the midline completes the median palatine suture. The posterior borders of the horizontal palatine plates are concave and in the midline form a sharp ridge of bone called the posterior nasal spine. To the posterior edge of the hard palate is attached the fibrous palatine aponeurosis of the soft palate, which is formed by the tendons of the tensor veli palatini muscles.

Maxillary alveolar processes

The maxillary alveolar processes extend inferiorly from the bodies of the maxillae and support the teeth within bony sockets (Fig. 2.7). Each maxilla can contain a full quadrant of eight permanent teeth or five deciduous teeth. The form of the

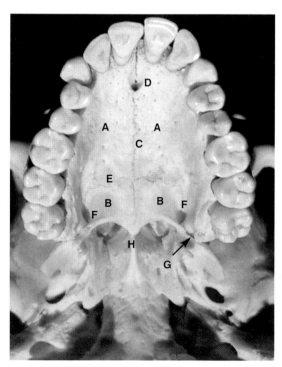

Fig. 2.6 Oral surface of the hard palate. A = Palatine processes of maxillae; B = horizontal plates of the palatine bones; C = median palatine suture; D = incisive fossa; E = transverse palatine suture; F = greater palatine foraminae; G = lesser palatine foramen; H = posterior nasal spine.

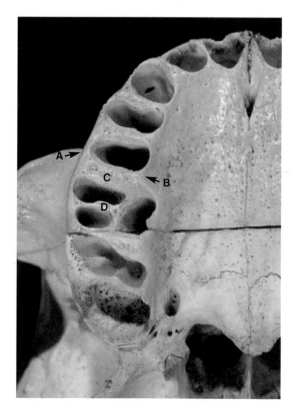

Fig. 2.7 View of the maxilla following removal of teeth to show the disposition of the roots in the alveolus. A = Buccal alveolar plate; B = palatal alveolar plate; C = interdental bony septa between the second premolar and first permanent molar; D = interradicular septum between buccal roots of first permanent molar.

alveolus is related to the functional demands put upon the teeth. When the teeth are removed the alveolus resorbs.

Essentially, the alveolar process consists of two parallel plates of cortical bone, the buccal and palatal alveolar plates, between which lie the sockets of individual teeth. Between each socket lie interalveolar or interdental septa. The floor of the socket has been termed the fundus, its rim the alveolar crest. The form and depth of each socket is defined by the form and length of the root it supports, and thus shows considerable variation. In multirooted teeth the sockets are divided by interradicular septa. The apical regions of the sockets of anterior teeth are closely related to the nasal fossae, while those of posterior teeth are closely related to the maxillary antra. The position of the sockets in relation to the buccal and palatal alveolar plates is shown in Fig. 2.12.

The Mandible

The mandible consists of a horizontal horseshoe-shaped component, the body of the mandible and two vertical components, the rami. The rami join the body posteriorly at obtuse angles. The body of the mandible carries the mandibular teeth and their associated alveolar processes. Before birth, the body consists of two lateral halves that meet in the midline at a symphysis. As viewed laterally (Fig. 2.8), on either side of the midline, close to the inferior margin of the body lies a distinct prominence called the mental tubercle. These tubercles constitute the mental protuberance or chin. Above the mental protuberance lies a shallow depression termed the incisive fossa. Behind this fossa, the canine eminence overlies the root of the mandibular canine. Midway in the height of the body of the mandible, related to the premolar teeth, is the mental foramen. The mental branches of the inferior alveolar nerve and artery pass onto the face through this foramen. The most common position for the mental foramen is on a vertical line passing through the mandibular second premolar. During the

first and second years of life, as the prominence of the chin develops the direction of the opening of the mental foramen alters from facing forwards to facing upwards and backwards. Rarely, there may be multiple mental foramina. The inferior margin of the body meets the posterior margin of the ramus at the angle of the mandible. This area is irregular, being the site of insertion of the masseter muscle and stylomandibular ligament. The alveolus forms the superior margin of the mandibular body. The junction of the alveolus and ramus is demarcated by a ridge of bone, the external oblique line, which continues downwards and forwards across the body of the mandible to terminate below the mental foramen. As this line progresses upwards, it becomes the anterior margin of the ramus and ends as the tip of the coronoid process. The coronoid and condylar processes form the two processes of the superior border of the ramus. The coronoid process provides attachment for the temporalis muscle. The condylar process has a neck supporting an articular surface, which fits into the mandibular fossa of the temporal bone to form a moveable synovial joint (the temporomandibular joint). The concavity between the coronoid and condylar processes is called the mandibular notch.

Several important features are seen on the internal (medial) surface of the mandible (Fig. 2.9). Close to the midline, on the inferior surface of the mandibular body, lie two shallow depressions called the digastric fossae, into which are inserted the anterior bellies of the digastric muscles. Above the fossae, in the midline, are the genial spines or tubercles. There are generally two inferior and two superior tubercles, which serve as attachments for the geniohyoid muscles and the genioglossus muscles respectively. Passing upwards and backwards across the medial surface of the body of the mandible is a prominent ridge. This is termed the mylohyoid or internal oblique ridge. From this ridge the mylohyoid muscle takes origin. The

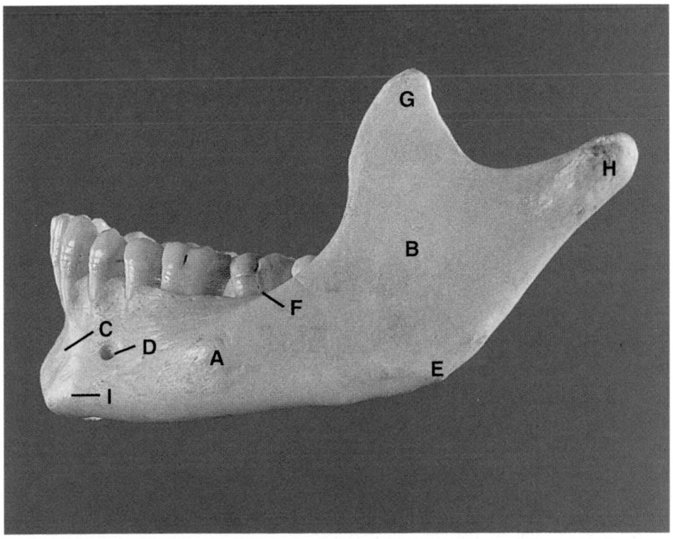

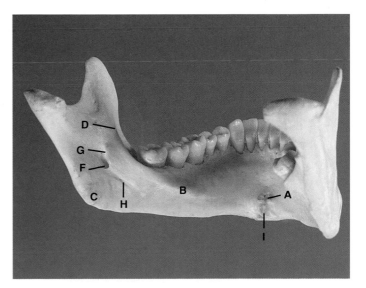

Fig. 2.8 Lateral aspect of the mandible. A = Body; B = ramus; C = incisive fossa; D = mental foramen; E = angle; F = external oblique line; G = coronoid process; H = condyle; I = mental protuberance.

Fig. 2.9 Inner (medial) surface of the mandible. A = Genial spines (tubercles); B = internal oblique ridge; C = attachment area for medial pterygoid muscle; D = temporal crest; E = retromolar triangle; F = mandibular foramen; G = lingula; H = mylohyoid groove; I = digastric fossa.

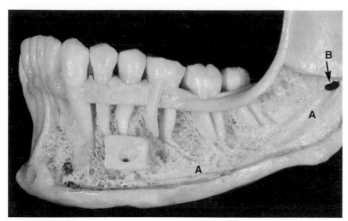

Fig. 2.10 Lateral view of the mandible, showing the roots of the teeth and the relationship of the mandibular canal (A). B = Mandibular foramen.

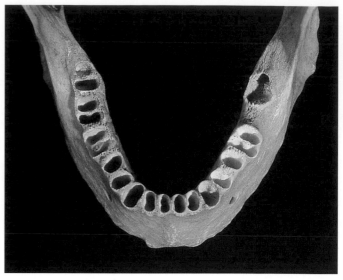

Fig. 2.11 The mandibular alveolus and the arrangement of the tooth sockets. Note that the left second permanent mandibular molar had previously been extracted and the socket had healed.

mylohyoid ridge arises between the genial tubercles and digastric fossa and increases in prominence as it passes backwards to end on the anterior surface of the ramus. Because the mylohyoid muscle forms the floor of the mouth the bone above the mylohyoid ridge forms the anterior wall of the oral cavity proper, while that below the ridge forms the lateral wall of the submandibular space. The following features may be seen on the medial surface of the ramus. Around the angle of the mandible, the bone is roughened for the attachment of the medial pterygoid muscle. Commencing at the tip of the coronoid process, a ridge of bone called the temporal crest runs down the anterior surface of the ramus to end behind the mandibular molars at the retromolar triangle. In the centre of the medial surface of the ramus lies the mandibular foramen, through which the inferior alveolar nerve and artery pass into the mandibular canal. A bony process, the lingula, extends

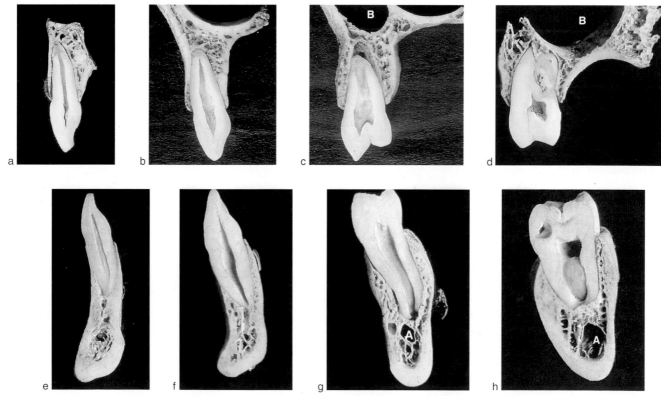

Fig. 2.12 Buccolingual sections through the maxilla and mandible demonstrating the distribution of alveolar bone in relation to the roots of the teeth. (a) maxillary incisor region; (b) maxillary canine region; (c) maxillary premolar region; (d) maxillary molar region; (e) mandibular incisor region; (f) mandibular canine region; (g) mandibular premolar region; (h) mandibular molar region. Note the relationship of the mandibular cheek teeth to the mandibular canal (A) and of the maxillary cheek teeth to the maxillary sinus (B). Courtesy of the Royal College of Surgeons of England.

from the anterosuperior surface of the foramen. The mylohyoid groove may be seen running down from the posteroinferior surface of the foramen.

The mandibular canal that transmits the inferior alveolar nerve, artery and veins, begins at the mandibular foramen and extends to the region of the premolar teeth, where it bifurcates into the mental and incisive canals (Fig. 2.10). The course of the mandibular canal and its relationship with the teeth is variable; this variation is illustrated in connection with the course of the inferior alveolar nerve on page 79.

The mandibular alveolus

As for the maxilla, the mandibular alveolus consists of buccal and lingual alveolar plates joined by interdental and inter-radicular septa (Fig. 2.11). In the region of the second and third molars the external oblique line is superimposed upon the buccal alveolar plate. The form and depth of the tooth sockets are related to the morphology of the roots of the mandibular teeth and the functional demands placed upon them.

Fig. 2.12 illustrates buccolingual sections through the teeth and jaws, demonstrating the directional axes and bony relationships of the teeth and their alveoli and the relative thickness of the buccal and lingual alveolar plates. The relationships of the mandibular teeth to the mandibular canal, and the maxillary teeth to the maxillary sinus have clinical significance. Thus, the thickness of bone may determine the direction in which teeth are levered during extractions and explain why local infiltration techniques can be used for anaesthetising anterior mandibular teeth, but not mandibular molar teeth. Care must be taken when exploring for fractured roots in this region in order to avoid an oroantral fistula due to the presence of the maxillary sinus in close relationship to the maxillary molar teeth, while the presence of the inferior alveolar nerve and its branches requires care when placing dental implants in the region.

TOOTH MORPHOLOGY

Humans have two generations of teeth: the deciduous (or primary) dentition and the permanent (or secondary) dentition. No teeth have erupted into the mouth at birth, but by the age of 3 years all the deciduous teeth have erupted. By 6 years, the first permanent teeth appear and thence the deciduous teeth are exfoliated one by one to be replaced by their permanent successors. A complete permanent dentition is present at or around the age of 18 years. Thus, given the average life of 75 years, the functional lifespan of the deciduous dentition is only 5% of this total, while with care and luck that of the permanent dentition can be over 90%. In the complete deciduous dentition there are 20 teeth – 10 in each jaw; in the complete permanent dentition there are 32 teeth – 16 in each jaw.

In both dentitions there are three basic tooth forms: incisiform, caniniform and molariform. Incisiform teeth (incisors) are cutting teeth, with thin, blade-like crowns. Caniniform teeth (canines) are piercing or tearing teeth, having a single, stout, pointed, cone-shaped crown. Molariform teeth (molars and premolars) are grinding teeth possessing a number of cusps on an otherwise flattened biting surface. Premolars are

bicuspid teeth; they are peculiar to the permanent dentition and replace the deciduous molars. Table 2.1 gives definitions of terms used for the descriptions of tooth form.

Dental notation

The types and numbers of teeth in any mammalian dentition can be expressed using dental formulae. The type of tooth is represented by its initial letter – I for incisors, C for canines,

Table 2.1 *Some terms used for the description of tooth form*

Crown	Clinical crown – that portion of a tooth visible in the oral cavity. Anatomical crown – that portion of a tooth covered with enamel.
Root	Clinical root – that portion of a tooth which lies within the alveolus. Anatomical root – that portion of a tooth covered by cementum.
Cervical margin	The junction of the anatomical crown and the anatomical root.
Occlusal surface	The biting surface of a posterior tooth (molar or premolar).
Cusp	A pronounced elevation on the occlusal surface of a tooth.
Incisal margin	The cutting edge of anterior teeth, analogous to the occlusal surface of the posterior teeth.
Tubercle	A small elevation on the crown.
Cingulum	A bulbous convexity near the cervical region of a tooth.
Ridge	A linear elevation on the surface of a tooth
Marginal ridge	A ridge at the mesial or distal edge of the occlusal surface of posterior teeth. Some anterior teeth have equivalent ridges.
Fissure	A long cleft between cusps or ridges.
Fossa	A rounded depression in a surface of a tooth.
Buccal	Towards or adjacent to the cheek. The term buccal surface is reserved for that surface of a premolar or molar which is positioned immediately adjacent to the cheek.
Labial	Towards or adjacent to the lips. The term labial surface is reserved for that surface of an incisor or canine which is positioned immediately adjacent to the lips.
Palatal	Towards or adjacent to the palate. The term palatal surface is reserved for that surface of a maxillary tooth which is positioned immediately adjacent to the palate.
Lingual	Towards or adjacent to the tongue. The term lingual surface is reserved for that surface of a mandibular tooth which lies immediately adjacent to the tongue.
Mesial	Towards the median. The mesial surface is that surface which faces towards the median line following the curve of the dental arch.
Distal	Away from the median. The distal surface is that surface which faces away from the median line following the curve of the dental arch.

P for premolars, M for molars. The deciduous dentition is indicated by the letter D. The formula for the deciduous human dentition is $DI\frac{2}{2} DC\frac{1}{1} DM\frac{2}{2} = 10$, and for the permanent dentition $I\frac{2}{2} C\frac{1}{1} PM\frac{2}{2} M\frac{3}{3} = 16$, where the numbers following each letter refer to the number of teeth of each type in the upper and lower jaws on one side only. Identification of teeth is made not only according to the dentition to which they belong and basic tooth form but also according to their anatomical location within the jaws. The tooth-bearing region of the jaws can be divided into four quadrants: the right and left maxillary and mandibular quadrants. A tooth may thus be identified according to the quadrant in which it is located – e.g. a right maxillary deciduous incisor or a left mandibular permanent molar. In both the permanent and deciduous dentitions the incisors may be distinguished according to their relationship to the midline. Thus, the incisor nearest the midline is the central (or first) incisor and the more laterally positioned incisor the lateral (or second) incisor. The permanent premolars and the permanent and deciduous molars can also be distinguished according to their mesiodistal relationships (see Fig. 2.13). The molar most mesially positioned is designated the first molar, the one behind it being the second molar. In the permanent dentition, the tooth most distally positioned is the third molar. The mesial premolar is the first premolar, the premolar behind it being the second premolar.

A dental shorthand may be used in the clinic to simplify tooth identification. The permanent teeth in each quadrant are numbered 1–8 and the deciduous teeth in each quadrant are lettered A–E. The symbols for the quadrants are derived from an imaginary cross, with the horizontal bar placed between the upper and lower jaws and the vertical bar running between the upper and lower central incisors. Thus, the maxillary right first permanent molar is allocated the symbol 6⌋ and the mandibular left deciduous canine c⌉. This system of dental shorthand is termed the Zsigmondy system. An alternative scheme has been devised by the *Federation Dentaire Internationale*, in which the quadrant is represented by a number:

1 = maxillary right quadrant
2 = maxillary left quadrant
3 = mandibular left quadrant   } Permanent
4 = mandibular right quadrant
5 = maxillary right quadrant
6 = maxillary left quadrant
7 = mandibular left quadrant   } Deciduous
8 = mandibular right quadrant

In this system the quadrant number prefixes a tooth number. Thus, the maxillary right first permanent molar is symbolised as 1,6 and the mandibular left deciduous canine as 7,3.

Fig. 2.13 summarises some of the terminology employed for the identification of teeth according to their location in the jaws.

Differences between teeth of the deciduous and permanent dentitions

1. The dental formula for the deciduous dentition is:
   $DI\frac{2}{2} DC\frac{1}{1} DM\frac{2}{2} = 10$

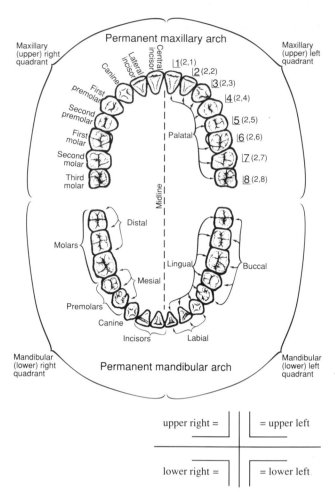

Fig. 2.13 Terminology employed for the identification of teeth according to their location in the jaws.

That of the permanent dentition is:
$I\frac{2}{2} C\frac{1}{1} PM\frac{2}{2} M\frac{3}{3} = 16$.

2. The deciduous teeth are smaller than their corresponding permanent successors although the mesiodistal dimensions of the permanent premolars are generally less than those for the deciduous molars.

3. Deciduous teeth have a greater constancy of shape than permanent teeth.

4. The crowns of deciduous teeth appear bulbous, often having pronounced labial or buccal cingula.

5. The cervical margins of deciduous teeth are more sharply demarcated and pronounced than those of the permanent teeth, the enamel bulging at the cervical margins rather than gently tapering.

6. The cusps of newly erupted deciduous teeth are more pointed than those of the corresponding permanent teeth.

7. The crowns of deciduous teeth have a thinner covering of enamel (average width 0.5–1.0 mm) than the crowns of permanent teeth (average width 2.5 mm).

8. The enamel of deciduous teeth, being more opaque than that of permanent teeth, gives the crown a whiter appearance.

9. The enamel of deciduous teeth is softer than that of permanent teeth and is more easily worn.

10. Enamel of deciduous teeth is more permeable than that of permanent teeth.

Fig. 2.14 Comparisons between models of deciduous (A) and permanent (B) dental arches and some examples of deciduous and permanent teeth. C = Deciduous canine; D = permanent canine; E = deciduous second molar; F = permanent first molar.

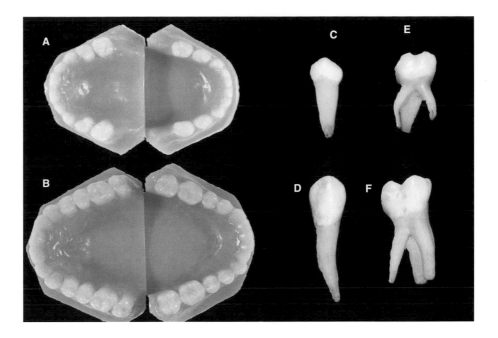

11. The aprismatic layer of surface enamel (see pages 107–108) is wider in deciduous teeth.
12. The enamel and dentine of *all* deciduous teeth exhibit neonatal lines (see page 112)
13. The roots of deciduous teeth are shorter and less robust than those of the permanent teeth.
14. The roots of the deciduous incisors and canines are longer in proportion to the crown than those of their permanent counterparts.
15. The roots of the deciduous molars are widely divergent, extending beyond the dimensions of the crown.
16. The pulp chambers of deciduous teeth are proportionally larger in relation to the crown than those of the permanent teeth. The pulp horns in deciduous teeth are more prominent.
17. The root canals of deciduous teeth are extremely fine.
18. The dental arches for the deciduous dentition are smaller.

Some of these differences are illustrated in Fig. 2.14.

The following descriptions of individual teeth will be considered according to tooth class (incisors, canines, premolars and molars) rather than by membership of either the permanent or deciduous dentitions. For each class, the permanent teeth will be described before the deciduous teeth. This arrangement allows emphasis of the basic features common to each class to be made.

To help visualise the tooth as a three-dimensional object, the illustrations of each tooth are arranged according to the 'third angle projection technique', which aligns each side of a tooth to its occlusal or incisal aspect. The morphology of the pulp is treated independently of the morphology of the external surfaces of the teeth on pages 28 to 33. For the chronology of the developing dentitions see pages 356–362, for the average dimensions of the teeth see Tables 2.2 and 2.3 (page 27), and for ethnic variations in tooth morphology see pages 27–28.

The incisors

Human incisors have thin, blade-like crowns that are adapted for the cutting and shearing of food preparatory to grinding. Viewed mesially or distally, the crowns of the incisors are roughly triangular in shape, with the apex of the triangle at the incisal margin of the tooth (Fig. 2.15). This shape is thought to facilitate the penetration and cutting of food. Viewed buccally or lingually, the incisors are trapezoidal, the shortest of the uneven sides being the base of the crown cervically.

The maxillary first (central) permanent incisor

This tooth (Fig. 2.16) is the widest mesiodistally of all the permanent incisors and canines, the crown being almost as wide as it is long. Like all incisors, it is basically wedge or chisel shaped and has a single conical root.

From the incisal view, the crown and incisal margin are centrally positioned over the root of the tooth. The incisal

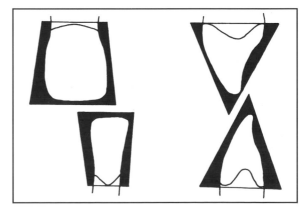

Fig. 2.15 Schematic drawings of incisor crown form, illustrating the relationship between anatomic and geometric form. Redrawn after Dr R.C. Wheeler.

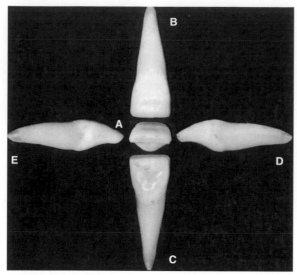

Fig. 2.16 Maxillary first (central) permanent incisor: A = incisal surface; B = labial surface; C = palatal surface; D = mesial surface; E = distal surface.

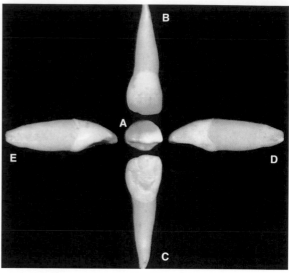

Fig. 2.17 Maxillary second (lateral) permanent incisor: A = incisal surface; B = labial surface; C = palatal surface; D = mesial surface; E = distal surface.

margin presents as a narrow, flattened ridge rather than as a fine, sharp edge. The incisal margin may be grooved by two troughs, the labial lobe grooves, which correspond to the divisions between three developmental lobes (or mammelons) seen on newly erupted incisors. The mammelons are lost by attrition soon after eruption. From the incisal aspect, the crown outline is bilaterally symmetrical, being triangular. However, the mesial profile may appear slightly larger than the distal profile. From the labial view the crown length can be seen to be almost as great as the root length. The crown has a smooth, convex labial surface. It may be marked by two faint grooves that run vertically towards the cervical margin and which are extensions of the labial lobe grooves. The convexity of the labial surface is especially marked cervically, the labial surface sometimes being flat at its middle and incisal regions. The mesial surface is straight and approximately at right angles to the incisal margin. The distoincisal angle, however, is more rounded and the distal outline more convex. A line drawn through the axial centre of the tooth lies roughly parallel to the mesial outline of the crown and root. Viewed palatally, the crown is more irregular, its middle and incisal regions being concave, giving a slightly shovel-shaped appearance to the incisor. The palatal surface of the crown is bordered by mesial and distal marginal ridges. Near the cervical margin lies a prominent cingulum. The cingulum may be single, divided or replaced by prominent portions of the marginal ridges. Occasionally, a slight ridge of enamel may run towards the incisal margin, dividing the palatal surface into two shallow depressions. The mesial and distal views of the crown illustrate the fundamental wedge-shaped or triangular crown form of the incisor.

The sinuous cervical margin is concave towards the crown on the palatal and labial surfaces and convex towards the crown on the mesial and distal surfaces, the curvature on the mesial surface being the most pronounced of any tooth in the dentition. The single root of the central incisor tapers towards the apex. The root is conical in cross section and appears narrower from the palatal than from the labial aspect.

The maxillary second (lateral) permanent incisor

Shown in Fig. 2.17, this is one of the most variable teeth in the dentition, although generally it is morphologically a diminutive form of the maxillary central incisor with slight modifications. The crown is much narrower and shorter than that of the central incisor, though the crown:root length ratio is considerably decreased.

From the incisal aspect, the crown has a more rounded outline than the adjacent central incisor. Viewed labially, the mesioincisal and distoincisal angles and the mesial and distal crown margins are more rounded than those of the central incisor. The palatal aspect of the crown is similar to that of the central incisor, though the marginal ridges and cingulum are often more pronounced. Consequently, the palatal concavity appears deeper. Lying in front of the cingulum is a pit (foramen caecum) that may extend some way into the root. The mesial and distal aspects of the lateral incisor differ little from those of the central incisor. A common morphological variation is the so-called 'peg-shaped' lateral incisor, which has a thin root surmounted by a small conical crown.

The course of the cervical margin and the shape of the root are similar to those of the central incisor. However, the root is often slightly compressed and grooved on the mesial and distal surfaces.

The mandibular incisors have the smallest mesiodistal dimensions of any teeth in the permanent dentition. They can be distinguished from the maxillary incisors not only by their size but also by the marked lingual inclination of the crowns over the roots, the mesiodistal compression of their roots and the poor development of the marginal ridges and cingula.

The mandibular first (central) permanent incisor

Viewed incisally this tooth has a bilaterally symmetrical triangular shape (Fig. 2.18). The incisal margin in the specimen shown in the figure has been worn and appears flat, although in the newly erupted tooth three mammelons are usually

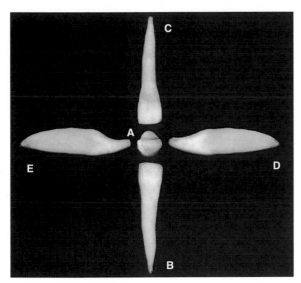

Fig. 2.18 Mandibular first (central) right permanent incisor: A = incisal surface; B = labial surface; C = lingual surface; D = mesial surface; E = distal surface.

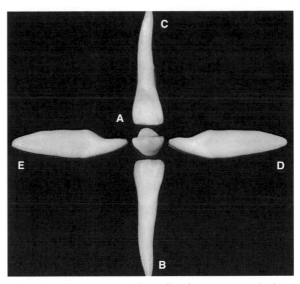

Fig. 2.19 Mandibular second (lateral) right permanent incisor: A = incisal surface; B = labial surface; C = lingual surface; D = mesial surface; E = distal surface.

present. The incisal margin is at right angles to a line bisecting the tooth labiolingually. Viewed labially the crown of the incisor is almost twice as long as it is wide. The unworn incisal margin is straight and approximately at right angles to the long axis of the tooth. The mesioincisal and distoincisal angles are sharp and the mesial and distal surfaces are approximately at right angles to the incisal margin. The profiles of the mesial and distal surfaces appear very similar, being convex in their incisal thirds and relatively flattened in the middle and cervical thirds. The lingual surface is smooth and slightly concave, the lingual cingulum and mesial and distal marginal ridges appearing less distinct than those of the maxillary incisors. The mesial and distal views show the characteristic wedge shape of the incisor and the inclination of the crown lingually over the root.

The cervical margins on the labial and lingual surfaces show their maximum convexities midway between the mesial and distal borders of the root. The cervical margin on the distal surface is said to be less curved than that on the mesial surface. The root is narrow and conical, though flattened mesiodistally. It is frequently grooved on the mesial and distal surfaces, the distal groove being more marked and deeper.

The mandibular second (lateral) permanent incisor

The mandibular second incisor (Fig. 2.19) closely resembles the mandibular central incisor. However, it is slightly wider mesiodistally and is more asymmetric in shape. The distal surface diverges at a greater angle from the long axis of the tooth, giving it a fan-shaped appearance, and the distoincisal angle is more acute and rounded. Another distinguishing characteristic is the angulation of the incisal margin relative to the labiolingual axis of the root: in the central incisor the incisal margin forms a right angle with the labiolingual axis, whereas that of the lateral incisor is 'twisted' distally in a lingual direction.

The maxillary first (central) deciduous incisor

This is similar morphologically to the corresponding permanent tooth (Fig. 2.20). However, because the width of the

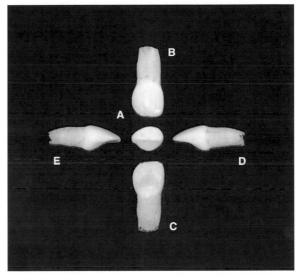

Fig. 2.20 Maxillary first (central) right deciduous incisor: A = incisal surface; B = labial surface; C = palatal surface; D = mesial surface; E = distal surface.

crown of the deciduous incisor nearly equals the length it appears plumper than its permanent successor. From the incisal view, the straight incisal margin appears to be centred over the bulk of the crown. Unlike the permanent teeth, no mammelons are seen on the incisal margin of the newly erupted deciduous incisor. The labial surface is slightly convex in all planes and unmarked by grooves, lobes or depressions. The mesioincisal angle is sharp and acute, while the distoincisal angle is more rounded and obtuse. On the palatal surface, the cingulum is a very prominent bulge that extends some way up the crown (sometimes to the incisal margin to form a ridge). Unlike those of its permanent successor, the marginal ridges are poorly defined and the concavity of the palatal surface is shallow. Mesial and distal views show the typical incisal form of the crown. There is a low, rounded cingulum at the margin of the labial surface.

As with all deciduous teeth, the cervical margins are more pronounced but less sinuous than those of their permanent successors. The fully formed root is conical in shape, tapering apically to a rather blunt apex. Compared with the corresponding permanent tooth, the root is longer in proportion to the crown. In the four deciduous incisors illustrated in this book, newly erupted teeth have been utilised as they show minimum wear of the crown. However, the roots are not yet fully formed.

The maxillary second (lateral) deciduous incisor

This is similar in shape to the maxillary first deciduous incisor, though smaller (Fig. 2.21). One obvious difference is the more acute mesioincisal angle and the more rounded distoincisal angle. The palatal surface is more concave and the marginal ridges more pronounced. Viewed incisally, the crown appears almost circular (in contrast to the central incisor, which appears diamond shaped). As with the first deciduous incisor, there is a rounded labial cingulum cervically. The palatal cingulum is generally lower than that of the first deciduous incisor.

The course of the cervical margin and the shape of the root are similar to those of the first deciduous incisor.

The mandibular first (central) deciduous incisor

The mandibular central incisor (Fig. 2.22) is morphologically similar to its permanent successor. However, it is much shorter and has a low labial cingulum. The mesioincisal and distoincisal angles are sharp right angles and the incisal margin is straight in the horizontal plane. Although there are generally no mammelons or grooves on the incisal margin, in the specimen illustrated three mammelons may be discerned. The lingual cingulum and the marginal ridges are poorly defined.

The single root is more rounded than that of the corresponding permanent tooth and, when complete, tapers and tends to incline distally.

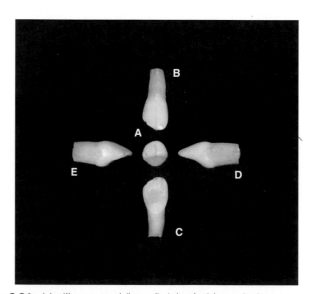

Fig. 2.21 Maxillary second (lateral) right deciduous incisor: A = incisal surface; B = labial surface; C = palatal surface; D = mesial surface; E = distal surface.

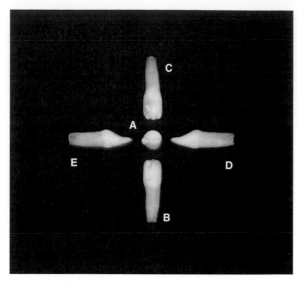

Fig. 2.22 Mandibular first (central) right deciduous incisor: A = incisal surface; B = labial surface; C = lingual surface; D = mesial surface; E = distal surface.

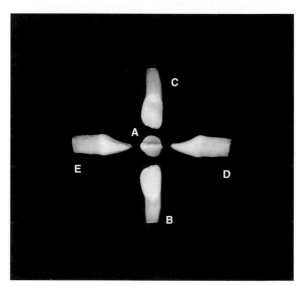

Fig. 2.23 Mandibular second (lateral) right deciduous incisor: A = incisal surface; B = labial surface; C = lingual surface; D = mesial surface; E = distal surface.

The mandibular second (lateral) deciduous incisor

This is a bulbous tooth (Fig. 2.23) that resembles its permanent successor. It is wider than the mandibular first deciduous incisor and is asymmetric. The mesioincisal angle is more obtuse and rounded than that of the mandibular first deciduous incisor and the incisal margin slopes downward distally. Should the distoincisal angle be markedly rounded then the tooth may be difficult to distinguish from a maxillary second deciduous incisor.

Unlike the permanent tooth, the root is rounded. When complete, it is longer than the root of the mandibular first deciduous incisor.

The canines

Canines are the only teeth in the dentition with a single cusp. Morphologically, they can be considered transitional between

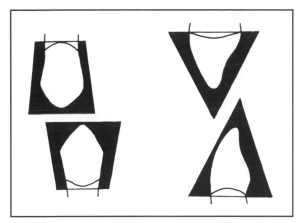

Fig. 2.24 Schematic drawings of canine crown form, illustrating the relationship between anatomic and geometric form. Redrawn after Dr R.C. Wheeler.

incisors and premolars. Like the incisors, the crowns of canines are roughly triangular in shape when viewed mesially or distally and trapezoidal buccally and lingually (Fig. 2.24).

The maxillary permanent canine

This is a stout tooth (Fig. 2.25) with a well developed cingulum and the longest root of any tooth. Viewed from its incisal aspect, it appears asymmetric. If a plane is envisaged passing through the apex of the cusp to the cingulum on the palatal surface, then the distal portion of the crown is much wider than the mesial portion. It is thought that the pointed shape of the canine tooth is related to an increase in size of a central mammelon at the expense of mesial and distal mammelons. Prominent longitudinal ridges pass from the cusp tip down both the labial and palatal surfaces. A relatively

frequent variation in the morphology of the incisal ridge is the development of an accessory cusp on its distal arm. The labial surface of the canine is marked by the longitudinal ridge, which extends from the cusp towards the cervical margin. The incisal part of the crown occupies at least one-third of the crown height. Note that, from this view, the mesial arm of the incisal margin is shorter than the distal arm, and the distoincisal angle is more rounded than the mesioincisal angle. The profiles of the mesial and distal surfaces converge markedly towards the cervix of the tooth. The mesial profile is slightly convex, the distal profile markedly convex. The mesial surface of the crown forms a straight line with the root, the distal surface meets the root at an obtuse angle. The palatal surface shows distinct mesial and distal marginal ridges and a well defined cingulum. The longitudinal ridge from the tip of the cusp meets the cingulum and is separated from the marginal ridges on either side by distinct grooves or fossae. Viewed mesially or distally the distinctive feature is the stout character of the crown and the great width of the cervical third of both the crown and root.

The cervical margin of this tooth follows a course similar to that of the incisors but the curves are less pronounced. The curvature of the cervical margin on the distal surface is less marked than that on the mesial surface. The root is the largest and stoutest in the dentition and is triangular in cross section (its labial surface being wider than its palatal surface). The mesial and distal surfaces of the root are often grooved longitudinally.

The mandibular permanent canine

This is similar to the maxillary canine, but smaller, more slender, and more symmetrical (Fig. 2.26). The cusp is generally less well developed: indeed, with attrition, the low cusp may be lost and the tooth may resemble a maxillary second permanent incisor.

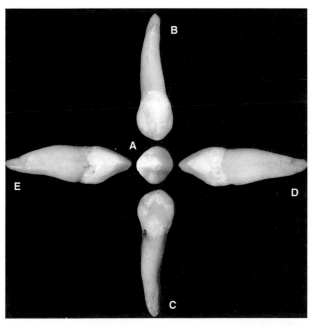

Fig. 2.25 Maxillary right permanent canine: A = incisal surface; B = labial surface; C = palatal surface; D = mesial surface; E = distal surface.

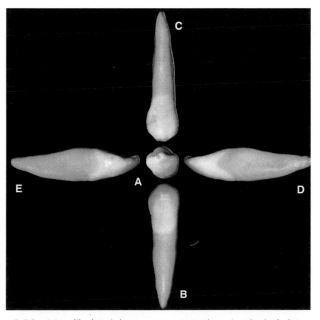

Fig. 2.26 Mandibular right permanent canine: A = incisal view; B = labial surface; C = lingual surface; D = mesial surface; E = distal surface.

From the incisal aspect, there are no distinct longitudinal ridges from the tip of the cusp onto the labial and lingual surfaces. Viewed labially, the incisal margin occupies only one-fifth of the crown height and the cusp is less pointed. The crown is narrower mesiodistally than that of the maxillary canine so it appears longer, narrower and more slender. The mesial and distal profiles tend to be parallel or only slightly convergent towards the cervix. The labial and mesial surfaces are clearly defined, being inclined acutely to each other, whereas the labial surface merges gradually into the distal surface. On the lingual surface the cingulum, marginal ridges and fossae are indistinct. The lingual surface is flatter than the corresponding palatal surface of the maxillary permanent canine and simulates the lingual surface of the mandibular incisors. Viewed mesially and distally, the wedge-shaped appearance of the canine is clear. These proximal surfaces are longer than those of the maxillary canine. The labiolingual diameter of the crown near the cervix is less than the corresponding labiopalatal diameter of the maxillary canine.

The cervical margin of this tooth follows a course similar to that of the incisors. The crownward convexity on the mesial surface is generally more marked than that on the distal surface. The root is normally single, though occasionally it may bifurcate. In cross section the root is oval, being flattened mesially and distally. The root is grooved longitudinally on both its mesial and distal surfaces.

The maxillary deciduous canine

This tooth has a fang-like appearance and is similar morphologically to its permanent successor, though more bulbous (Fig. 2.27). It is generally symmetrical but where there is asymmetry it is usual for the mesial slope of the cusp to be longer than the distal slope. Bulging of the tooth gives the crown a diamond-shaped appearance when viewed labially or palatally, with the crown margins overhanging the root profiles. The width of the crown is greater than its length. On the labial

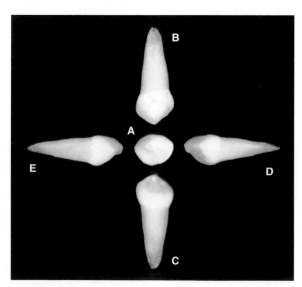

Fig. 2.27 Maxillary right deciduous canine: A = incisal view; B = labial surface; C = palatal surface; D = mesial surface; E = distal surface.

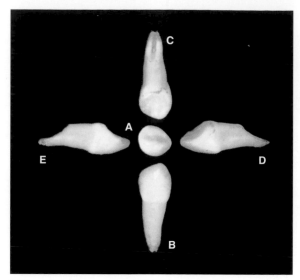

Fig. 2.28 Mandibular right deciduous canine: A = incisal view; B = labial surface; C = lingual surface; D = mesial surface; E = distal surface.

surface there is a low cingulum cervically, from which runs a longitudinal ridge up to the tip of the cusp. A similar longitudinal ridge also runs on the palatal surface. This ridge extends from the cusp apex to the palatal cingulum and divides the palatal surface into two shallow pits. The marginal ridges on the palatal surface are low and indistinct.

The root is long compared with the crown height and is triangular in cross section.

The mandibular deciduous canine

This is more slender than the maxillary deciduous canine (Fig. 2.28). The crown is asymmetrical and the cusp tip displaced mesially. Consequently, the mesial arm is shorter and more vertical than the distal arm. On the labial surface there is a low, labial cingulum. On the lingual surface the cingulum and marginal ridges are less pronounced than the corresponding structures on the palatal surface of the maxillary deciduous canine. The longitudinal ridges on both the labial and lingual surfaces are poorly developed. The width of the crown is less than the length.

The root is single and tends to be triangular in cross section. Note the root resorption seen in the specimen illustrated; this would be associated with the shedding of the tooth.

The premolars

Premolars are unique to the permanent dentition. They are sometimes referred to as 'bicuspids', because they have two main cusps – a buccal and a palatal (or lingual) cusp – that are separated by a mesiodistal occlusal fissure. The buccal surface of the buccal cusp is similar in shape to the cusp of a canine, to which it may be considered analogous, while the palatal or lingual cusp corresponds developmentally to the cingulum of the anterior teeth. Thus, premolars are considered to be transitional between canines and molars.

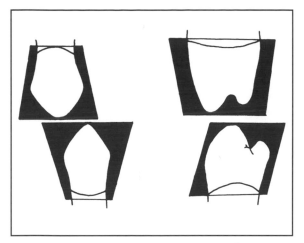

Fig. 2.29 Schematic drawings of premolar crown form, illustrating the relationship between anatomic and geometric form. Redrawn after Dr R.C. Wheeler.

Viewed mesially or distally the maxillary premolars are trapezoidal in shape, the longest side of the trapezoid being the base of the crown at the cervical margin (Fig. 2.29). It is thought that, because the occlusal surface is not as wide as the base of the crown, the tooth can penetrate the food more easily, while minimising the occlusal forces. The mandibular premolars, however, are roughly rhomboidal in shape. The rhomboidal outline is inclined lingually, thus allowing correct intercuspal contact with the maxillary antagonists. Viewed buccally or lingually, all the premolars are trapezoidal, the shortest of the uneven sides being the bases of the crowns cervically.

The maxillary first premolar

When viewed occlusally this tooth has a crown that appears ovoid, being broader buccally than palatally (Fig. 2.30). Thus, the profiles of the mesial and distal surfaces converge palatally. The mesiobuccal and distobuccal corners are less rounded than the mesiopalatal and distopalatal corners. The mesial and distal borders of the occlusal surface are marked by distinct ridges, the mesial and distal marginal ridges. The buccal and palatal cusps are separated by a central occlusal fissure that runs in a mesiodistal direction. The occlusal fissure crosses the mesial marginal ridge onto the mesial surface. On the distal side, the fissure terminates in a fossa before the distal marginal ridge. Supplementary grooves from the central fissure are rare.

Viewed buccally the first premolar bears a distinct resemblance to the adjacent canine. A longitudinal ridge may be seen passing down the buccal cusp. The mesial and distal ridges of the buccal cusp each form a 30° slope and the mesio- and disto-occlusal angles are prominent, giving the crown a 'bulging-shouldered' ovoid appearance. The mesial slope is generally longer than the distal slope.

Viewed palatally the buccal part of the crown appears larger in all dimensions than the palatal part so that the entire buccal profile of the crown is visible from the palatal aspect. The palatal cusp is lower, and its tip lies more mesially than the tip of the buccal cusp.

From the mesial aspect the unequal height of the cusps is clearly seen. Note the canine groove extending across the marginal ridge from the occlusal surface. The cervical third of the mesial surface is marked by a distinct concavity, the canine fossa.

The distal aspect of the crown differs from the mesial aspect in that it lacks a canine groove and canine fossa.

The cervical margin follows a fairly level course around the crown, deviating slightly towards the root on the buccal and palatal surfaces and away from the root on the mesial and distal surfaces. There are usually two roots, a buccal and palatal root, though sometimes there is only a single root. However, even a single root is deeply grooved on its mesial and distal surfaces.

The maxillary second premolar

This tooth (Fig. 2.31) is similar in shape to the maxillary first

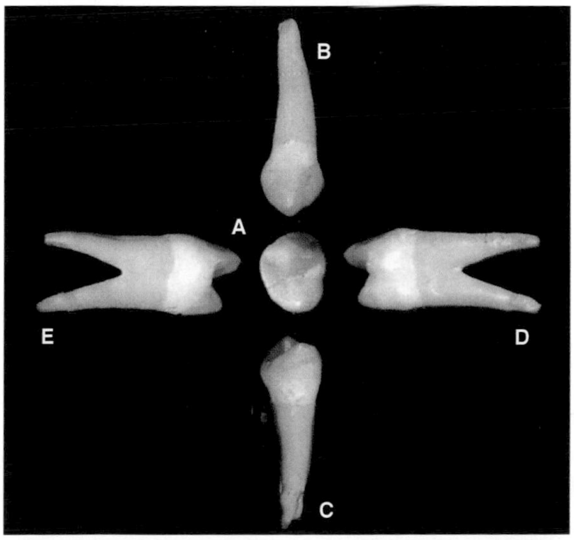

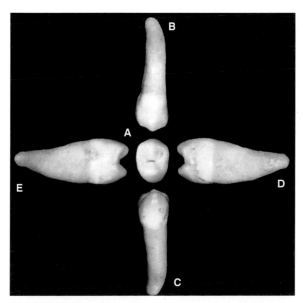

Fig. 2.30 Maxillary first right premolar: A = occlusal surface; B = buccal surface; C = palatal surface; D = mesial surface; E = distal surface.

Fig. 2.31 Maxillary second right premolar: A = occlusal surface; B = buccal surface; C = palatal surface; D = mesial surface; E = distal surface.

premolar, except for the following features. Viewed occlusally the mesiobuccal and distobuccal corners are more rounded and the mesial and distal profiles do not converge lingually, being nearly parallel. The occlusal surface appears more compressed, the mesiodistal dimension of the crown being smaller. The central fissure appears shorter and does not cross the mesial marginal ridge. From the buccal aspect, the mesio- and disto-occlusal angles are less prominent. These features give the crown a 'narrow-shouldered' appearance. The two cusps are smaller and more equal in size than those of the first premolar. The height of the buccal cusp is one-quarter of the height of the crown measured from the base of the occlusal fissure, while the height of the buccal cusp of the first premolar is up to one-half the height of the crown. Viewed palatally less of the buccal profile is visible. Mesially and distally the tooth appears similar to the first premolar but there is no canine fossa or canine groove on the mesial surface.

The cervical margin appears similar to that of the maxillary first premolar but is slightly less undulating. The root is single.

The mandibular premolars differ from the maxillary premolars in that occlusally the crowns appear rounder and the cusps are of unequal size, the buccal cusp being the most prominent. Furthermore, the first and second premolars differ more markedly from each other than do the maxillary premolars.

The mandibular first premolar

This is the smallest premolar (Fig. 2.32). As it comprises a dominant buccal cusp and a very small lingual cusp that appears not unlike a cingulum, some consider it to be a modified canine. From the occlusal aspect more than two-thirds of the buccal surface is visible, although only a small portion of the lingual surface can be seen. The occlusal outline is diamond shaped and the occlusal table, outlined by the cusps and marginal ridges, is triangular. The buccal cusp is broad, with its apex approximately overlying the midpoint of the crown. The lingual cusp is less than half the size of the buccal cusp. The buccal and lingual cusps are connected by a blunt, transverse ridge that divides the poorly developed mesiodistal occlusal fissure into mesial and distal fossae. The mesial fossa is generally smaller than the distal fossa. A canine groove often extends from the mesial fossa over the mesial marginal ridge onto the mesiolingual surface of the crown. Viewed buccally, the crown is nearly symmetrical, though the mesial profile is more curved than the distal. The buccal surface is markedly convex in all planes. From the lingual aspect the entire buccal profile and the occlusal surface are visible. Thus, the mandibular first premolar differs from other premolars in that the occlusal plane does not lie perpendicular to the long axis of the tooth but is included lingually. The tilt of the occlusal plane can also be appreciated from the mesial and distal aspects.

The cervical line follows an almost level course around the tooth. The root is single, conical, and oval to nearly round in cross section. The root is grooved longitudinally both mesially and distally, the mesial groove being the more prominent.

The mandibular second premolar

The mandibular second premolar (Fig. 2.33) differs from the mandibular first premolar in a number of respects. Its crown is generally larger. The lingual cusp is better developed, although it is not quite as large as the buccal cusp. From the occlusal aspect its outline appears round or square, the mesial and distal profiles being straight and parallel. The mesiodistal occlusal fissure between the cusps is well defined. However, like the first premolar, the fissure ends in mesial and distal fossae, the distal fossa being generally larger than the mesial. Unlike the first premolar, a transverse ridge does not usually join the apices of the cusps. Accessory cusplets are common on both buccal and lingual cusps. The lingual cusp is usually subdivided into mesiolingual and distolingual cusps, the mesio-lingual cusp being wider and higher than the distolingual. The

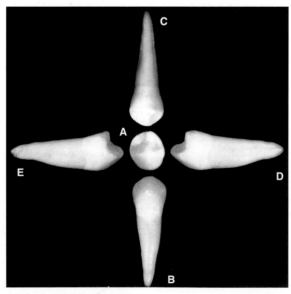

Fig. 2.32 Mandibular first right premolar: A = occlusal surface; B = buccal surface; C = lingual surface; D = mesial surface; E = distal surface.

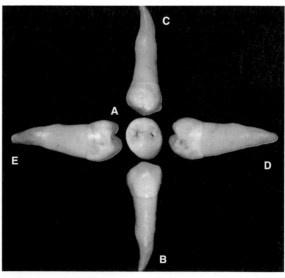

Fig. 2.33 Mandibular second right premolar: A = occlusal surface; B = buccal surface; C = lingual surface; D = mesial surface; E = distal surface.

groove separating the mesiolingual and distolingual cusps lies opposite the tip of the buccal cusp. From the buccal aspect the crown of the second premolar is symmetrical. From this view the buccal cusp generally appears shorter and more rounded than that of the mandibular first premolar. Lingually, little if any of the occlusal surface and buccal profile is visible. From the mesial and distal aspects the occlusal surface appears horizontal to the long axis of the tooth, unlike the mandibular first premolar. The crown is wider buccolingually than that of the first premolar and the buccal cusp does not incline as far over the root. The mesial marginal ridge is higher than the distal marginal ridge.

The cervical margin follows an almost level course around the tooth. The root is single, conical, and nearly round in cross section.

The molars

Molars present the largest occlusal surfaces of all teeth. They have three to five major cusps (although the maxillary first deciduous molar has only two). Molars are the only teeth that have more than one buccal cusp. Generally, the lower molars have two roots while the upper have three. The permanent molars do not have deciduous predecessors.

Like the premolars, the maxillary molars are roughly trapezoidal when viewed mesially and distally, while the mandibular molars are rhomboidal. Viewed buccally or lingually, the molars are trapezoidal (Fig. 2.34).

The maxillary first permanent molar

This is usually the largest molar in each quadrant (Fig. 2.35). Viewed occlusally, the crown is rhombic in outline. The mesiopalatal and distobuccal angles are obtuse. The longest diameter of the crown runs from the mesiobuccal to the distopalatal corners. It has four major cusps separated by an irregular H-shaped occlusal fissure. The occlusal table may be divided into two distinct components (the trigon and talon) by an oblique ridge, which passes diagonally across the occlusal

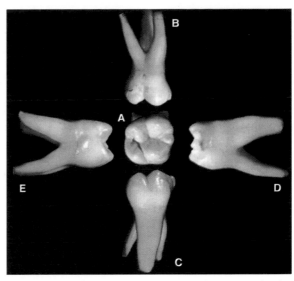

Fig. 2.35 Maxillary first right permanent molar; A = occlusal surface; B = buccal surface; C = palatal surface, D = mesial surface; E = distal surface.

table from the mesiopalatal cusp to the distobuccal cusp. The trigon bears the mesiobuccal, mesiopalatal and distobuccal cusps, and the talon bears the distopalatal cusp. The trigon is characteristically triangular in shape, the apex of the triangle being directed palatally. The mesiopalatal cusp is the largest, the buccal cusps being smaller and of approximately equal size. The buccal cusps form the base of the trigon. The mesial marginal ridge forms the mesial side of the trigon and its distal side is formed by the oblique ridge. An accessory cusplet of variable size may be seen on the palatal surface of the mesiopalatal cusp. This cusplet is termed the tubercle of Carabelli and is found on about 60% of maxillary first permanent molars. The trigon has a central fossa from which a fissure extends mesially to terminate in a mesial pit before the mesial marginal ridge. Another fissure extends buccally from the central fossa to pass onto the buccal surface of the crown between the two buccal cusps. The distopalatal cusp of the talon is generally the smallest cusp of the tooth and is separated from the mesiopalatal cusp by a distopalatal fissure, which curves distally to end in a distal pit before the distal marginal ridge. The oblique ridge may be crossed by a shallow fissure, which connects the central fossa of the trigon with the distopalatal fissure and distal pit of the talon, completing the H-shaped fissure pattern. That the tips of the palatal cusps are situated nearer the mid-mesiodistal diameter of the crown than those of the buccal cusps is characteristic of maxillary molars.

From the buccal aspect, the buccal cusps are seen to be approximately equal in height, though the mesiobuccal cusp is wider than the distobuccal cusp. The buccal surface is convex in its cervical third but relatively flat in its middle and occlusal thirds. The buccal groove extends from the occlusal table, passing between the cusps to end about halfway up the buccal surface. The mesial profile is convex in its occlusal and middle thirds but flat, or even concave, in the cervical third. The distal profile, on the other hand, is convex in all regions.

Viewed palatally, the disproportion in size between the mesiopalatal and distopalatal cusps is most evident. The

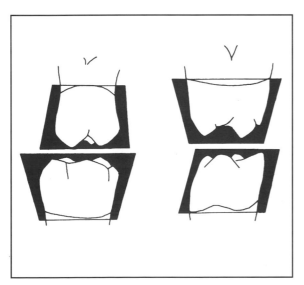

Fig. 2.34 Schematic drawings of molar crown form, illustrating the relationship between anatomic and geometric form. Redrawn after Dr R.C. Wheeler.

mesiopalatal cusp is blunt and occupies approximately three-fifths of the mesiodistal width of the palatal surface. The palatal surface is more or less uniformly convex in all regions. A palatal groove extends from the distal pit onto the occlusal surface between the palatal cusps to terminate approximately halfway up the palatal surface.

From the mesial and distal aspects, the maximum bucco-palatal dimension is at the cervical margin, from which the buccal and palatal profiles converge occlusally. The mesial marginal ridge is more prominent than the distal ridge and may have a number of distinct tubercles although such tubercles are rare on the distal marginal ridge.

The cervical margin follows a fairly even contour around the tooth. There are three roots, two buccal and one palatal, arising from a common root stalk. The palatal root is the longest and strongest and is circular in cross section. The buccal roots are more slender and are flattened mesiodistally; the mesio-buccal root is usually the larger and wider of the two. At the root stalk, the palatal root is more commonly related to the distobuccal root than to the mesiobuccal root.

The maxillary second permanent molar

This closely resembles the maxillary first permanent molar but shows some reduction in size and slightly different cusp relationships (Fig. 2.36). Viewed occlusally, the rhomboid form is more pronounced than in the first molar and the oblique ridge is smaller. The talon (distopalatal fissure cusp) is considerably reduced. The occlusal fissure pattern is similar to that of the first molar but is more variable, and supplemental grooves are more numerous. Two features of the buccal surface differentiate the second molar: the smaller size of the crown and the distobuccal cusp. From the palatal view, the reduction in size of the distopalatal cusp is more visible. A tubercle of Carabelli is not usually found on the mesiopalatal cusp. The mesial and distal surfaces differ little from those of the first molar, except that the tubercles on the mesial marginal ridge are less numerous and less pronounced.

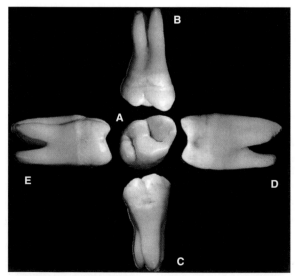

Fig. 2.36 Maxillary second right permanent molar: A = occlusal surface; B = buccal surface; C = palatal surface; D = mesial surface; E = distal surface.

Like the first molar, the second molar has three roots, two buccal and one palatal. However, they are shorter and less divergent than those of the first molar and may be partly fused. The apex of the mesiobuccal root is generally in line with the centre of the crown, unlike that of the first molar, which generally lies in line with the tip of the mesiobuccal cusp.

Variations in morphology of the maxillary second permanent molar are quite common. Total reduction of the distopalatal cusp such that only the trigon remains is frequent. Less frequently, the crown may appear compressed because of fusion of the mesiopalatal and distobuccal cusps, resulting in an oval crown possessing three cusps in a straight line.

The maxillary third permanent molar

Being the most variable in the dentition, this tooth is not illustrated. Its morphology may range from that characteristic of the adjacent maxillary permanent molars to a rounded, triangular crown with a deep central fossa from which numerous irregular fissures radiate outwards. Most commonly, the crown is triangular in shape, having the three cusps of the trigon but no talon. The roots are often fused and irregular in form. Third permanent molars are the teeth most often absent congenitally.

Differences between maxillary and mandibular molars

The mandibular molars differ from the maxillary molars in the following respects.

1. The mandibular molars have two roots, one mesial and one distal.
2. They are considered to be derived from a five-cusped form.
3. The crowns of the lower molars are oblong, being broader mesiodistally than buccolingually.
4. The fissure pattern is cross-shaped.
5. The lingual cusps are of more equal size.
6. The tips of the buccal cusps are shifted lingually so that, from the occlusal view, the whole of the buccal surface is visible.

The mandibular first permanent molar

The crown of this tooth, when viewed occlusally, is somewhat pentagonal in outline (Fig. 2.37). It is broader mesiodistally than buccolingually. The occlusal surface is divided into buccal and lingual parts by a mesiodistal occlusal fissure, which arises from a deep central fossa. The buccal side of the occlusal table has three distinct cusps: mesiobuccal, distobuccal and distal. Each cusp is separated by a groove, which joins the mesiodistal fissure. On the lingual side are two cusps: mesiolingual and distolingual. The fissure separating the lingual cusps joins the mesiodistal fissure in the region of the central fossa. The lingual cusps tend to be larger and more pointed, though they are not disproportionately larger than the mesiobuccal and distobuccal cusps. The tips of the buccal cusps are displaced lingually, are rounded and are lower than the lingual cusps. The smallest cusp is the distal cusp, which is displaced slightly towards the buccal surface. In 90% of cases, the mesiolingual cusp is joined to the distobuccal cusp across

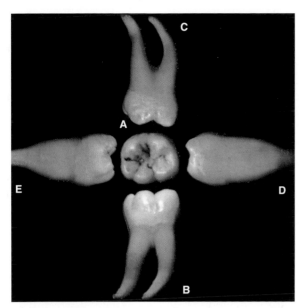

Fig. 2.37 Mandibular first right permanent molar: A = occlusal surface; B = buccal surface; C = lingual surface; D = mesial surface; E = distal surface.

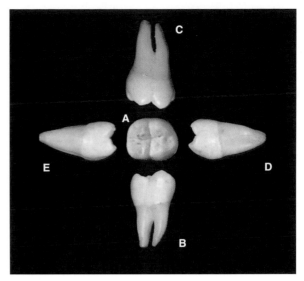

Fig. 2.38 Mandibular second right permanent molar: A = occlusal surface; B = buccal surface; C = lingual surface; D = mesial surface; E = distal surface.

the floor of the central fossa. This feature and the five-cusped pattern is termed the *Dryopithecus* pattern. This 'primitive' pattern is characteristic of all the lower molars of the anthropoid apes and their early ancestors, the dryopithecines. Because of the resulting Y-shaped tissue pattern and the five cusps, the *Dryopithecus* pattern is sometimes referred to as a 'Y5' pattern. In the 10% of cases where the mesiobuccal and distolingual cusps meet, a more cruciate system of fissures is produced: this is sometimes referred to as a '+5' pattern.

From the buccal aspect three cusps are seen, the distal cusp being the smallest. The fissure separating the mesiobuccal and distobuccal cusps arises from the central fossa on the occlusal surface and terminates halfway up the buccal surface in a buccal pit. The buccal surface appears markedly convex, especially at the cervical third of the crown. This convexity is associated with the characteristic lingual inclination of the buccal cusps.

From the lingual aspect, although the two lingual cusps are nearly equal in size, the mesiolingual cusp appears slightly larger. The fissure between the lingual cusps arises from the central fossa on the occlusal surface but does not extend a significant way down the lingual surface. The lingual surface is convex in its occlusal and middle thirds but is flat or concave cervically. Part of the buccal profiles and proximal surfaces may be seen.

Viewed mesially, the mesial marginal ridge joining the mesiobuccal and mesiolingual cusps is V-shaped, being notched at its midpoint. The mesial surface is flat or concave cervically and convex in its middle and occlusal thirds.

From the distal aspect the distal marginal ridge joining the distal and distolingual cusps also appears V-shaped. The cervical third of the distal surface is relatively flat, the middle and occlusal thirds highly convex. Thus, the distal surface is more convex than the mesial surface due to the distal cusp. The proximal views of the illustration highlight the highly convex slope of the buccal surface compared with the lingual surface.

The cervical margin follows a uniform contour around the tooth. The two roots, one mesial and one distal, arise from a common root stalk. They are both markedly flattened mesiodistally and the mesial root is usually deeply grooved. Both roots curve distally.

The mandibular second permanent molar

When viewed occlusally the crown exhibits a regular, rectangular shape (Fig. 2.38); the buccal profile is thus nearly equal in length to the lingual profile unlike the mandibular first permanent molar. There are four cusps, the mesiobuccal and mesiolingual cusps being slightly larger than the distobuccal and distolingual cusps. The cusps are separated by a cross-shaped occlusal fissure pattern, which may be complicated by numerous supplemental grooves. From the buccal aspect the crown appears smaller than that of the first molar. A fissure extends between the buccal cusps from the occlusal surface and terminates approximately halfway up the buccal surface. Like that of the mandibular first molar, the buccal surface is highly convex. From the lingual aspect the buccal profiles and proximal surfaces are not visible and the crown is noticeably shorter than the first molar. The mesial and distal aspects of the second molar resemble those of the first molar although, because there is no distal cusp, the proximal surfaces are more equal in terms of their convexity. The mesial and distal marginal ridges do not converge and are not as markedly notched at their midpoint.

The mesial and distal roots are flattened mesiodistally, and are smaller and less divergent than those of the first molar. They may be partly fused. The mesial root is not as broad as that of the first molar, and the distal inclination of the roots is usually more marked.

The mandibular third permanent molar

This has a variable morphology, though not as variable as that of the maxillary third permanent molar. Its clinical significance lies in the fact that it is commonly impacted. It is the smallest of the mandibular molars but can be as large as the mandibular first molar. The crown usually has four or five cusps. In shape, it is normally a rounded rectangle or circular. Its occlusal fissure pattern is generally very irregular. As a rule, the roots are greatly reduced in size and are fused. They show a marked distal inclination.

The maxillary first deciduous molar

This is the most atypical of all molars, deciduous or permanent (Fig. 2.39). In form it appears intermediate between a premolar and a molar. It is the smallest molar.

Viewed occlusally, the crown is an irregular quadrilateral with the buccal and palatal surfaces lying parallel to one another. However, the mesiobuccal corner is extended to produce a prominent bulge, the molar tubercle. If crowns are to be fitted this bulge may have to be smoothed over because of the undercut. The mesiopalatal angle is markedly obtuse. The tooth is generally bicuspid; the buccal (more pronounced) and palatal cusps are separated by an occlusal fissure that runs mesiodistally. A shallow buccal fissure may extend from the central mesiodistal fissure to divide the buccal cusp into two, the mesial part being the larger. The lingual cusp also may be sub-divided into two. The tips of the cusps converge towards the midline, reducing the occlusal surface of the tooth. From the buccal aspect the crown appears squat, its height being less than its width. On the mesial side lies the buccal cingulum, which extends to the molar tubercle. From the palatal aspect the palatal surface appears shorter mesiodistally than the buccal surface, the profile of which can be seen from this view. The mesial and distal views show the cervical bulbosity of the buccal and palatal surfaces. Note the prominent molar tubercle mesially. Marginal ridges link the buccal and palatal cusps. No fissure crosses the marginal ridges.

The tooth has three roots (two buccal and one palatal), which arise from a common root stalk. The mesiobuccal root is flattened mesiodistally; the distobuccal root is smaller and more circular; the palatal root is the largest and is round in cross section. The distobuccal and palatal roots may be partly fused.

The maxillary second deciduous molar

The maxillary second deciduous molar (Fig. 2.40) closely resembles the maxillary first permanent molar (see Fig. 2.35), though its size, whiteness, widely diverging roots and low buccal cingulum ought to distinguish it. A tubercle of Carabelli on the mesiopalatal cusp is often well developed.

The mandibular first deciduous molar

Unlike the maxillary first deciduous molar this is molariform, but has a number of unique features (Fig. 2.41). From the occlusal aspect the crown appears elongated mesiodistally and is an irregular quadrilateral with parallel buccal and lingual

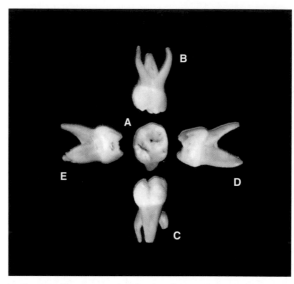

Fig. 2.40 Maxillary second right deciduous molar: A = occlusal surface; B = buccal surface; C = palatal surface; D = mesial surface; E = distal surface.

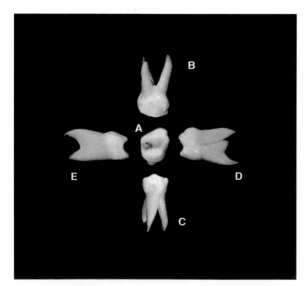

Fig. 2.39 Maxillary first right deciduous molar: A = occlusal surface; B = buccal surface; C = palatal surface; D = mesial surface; E = distal surface.

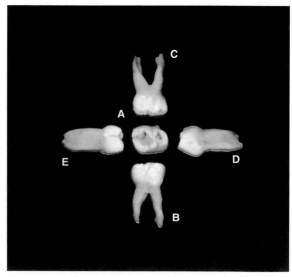

Fig. 2.41 Mandibular first right deciduous molar: A = occlusal surface; B = buccal surface; C = lingual surface; D = mesial surface; E = distal surface.

surfaces. The mesiobuccal corner is extended, forming a molar tubercle, and the mesiolingual angle markedly obtuse. The occlusal table can be divided into buccal and lingual parts by a mesiodistal fissure. The buccal part consists of two cusps, the mesiobuccal cusp being larger than the distobuccal cusp. The lingual part of the tooth is narrower than the buccal part and has two cusps separated by a lingual fissure, the mesiolingual cusp being larger than the distolingual cusp. The buccal cusps are larger than the lingual cusps. A transverse ridge may connect the mesial cusps, dividing the mesiodistal fissure into a distal fissure and a mesial pit. Often a distal pit is found just mesial to the distal marginal ridge. A supplemental groove from the mesial pit may extend over the mesial marginal ridge. From the buccal aspect the mesiobuccal cusp occupies at least two-thirds of the crown area and projects higher occlusally than the distobuccal cusp. The distal slopes of the buccal cusps are longer than the mesial. The profile of the mesial surface appears flat, that of the distal surface convex. The molar tubercle on the mesial corner of the buccal surface can be seen in this view. From the lingual aspect the cusps are conical in shape. The distolingual cusp appears only as a bulging protuberance on the distal margin. Mesially and distally the buccal and lingual aspects converge towards the midline of the crown. The mesial marginal ridge is more prominent than the distal marginal ridge. Note the bulge associated with the buccal cingulum near the cervical margin of the mesiobuccal cusp.

The mandibular first deciduous molar has two divergent roots, mesial and distal, which are flattened mesiodistally. The mesial root is often grooved.

The mandibular second deciduous molar

This is a smaller version of the mandibular first permanent molar (see Fig. 2.37), though it is narrower, whiter and has widely diverging roots (Fig. 2.42). Other distinguishing features are the cingulum on the mesiobuccal corner of the crown, the greater convexity of the mesial and distal surfaces and the more extensive central fossa on the occlusal surface. The mesiolingual and distobuccal cusps are not usually joined to give the *Dryopithecus* pattern.

The average dimensions of the permanent and deciduous teeth are listed in Tables 2.2 and 2.3.

Ethnic and racial differences in tooth morphology

The preceding description of the morphology of teeth is, of necessity, only generalised and is related to caucasians. Superimposed on the basic shapes of teeth are minor morphological variations affecting both deciduous and permanent teeth. Such variations are inherited, depend on many genes, and vary minimally in response to environmental factors. Their

Table 2.2 *Average dimensions of the permanent teeth*

Tooth	Crown height (mm)	Length of root (mm)	Mediodistal crown diameter (mm)	Labiolingual crown diameter (mm)
Maxillary				
1	10.5	13.0	8.5	7.0
2	9.0	13.0	6.5	6.0
3	10.0	17.0	7.5	8.0
4	8.5	14.5	7.0	9.0
5	8.5	14.0	7.0	9.0
6	7.5	12.5	10.5	11.0
7	7.0	11.5	9.5	11.0
8	6.5	11.0	8.5	10.0
Mandibular				
1	9.0	12.5	5.0	6.0
2	9.5	14.0	5.5	6.5
3	11.0	15.5	7.0	7.5
4	8.5	14.0	7.0	7.5
5	8.0	14.5	7.0	8.0
6	7.5	14.0	11.0	10.0
7	7.0	12.0	10.5	10.0
8	7.0	11.0	10.0	9.5

Table 2.3 *Average dimensions of deciduous teeth*

Tooth	Crown height (mm)	Length of root (mm)	Mediodistal crown diameter (mm)	Labiolingual crown diameter (mm)
Maxillary				
A	6.0	10.0	6.5	5.0
B	5.6	10.2	5.2	4.0
C	6.5`	13.0	6.8	7.0
D	5.1	10.0	7.1	8.5
E	5.7	11.7	8.4	10.0
Mandibular				
A	5.0	9.0	4.0	4.0
B	5.2	9.8	4.5	4.0
C	6.0	11.2	5.5	4.9
D	6.0	9.8	7.7	7.0
E	5.5	12.5	9.7	8.7

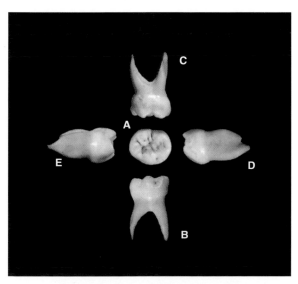

Fig. 2.42 Mandibular second right deciduous molar: A = occlusal surface; B = buccal surface; C = lingual surface; D = mesial surface; E = distal surface.

presence and degree of penetrance form the foundation of dental anthropology and have been utilised in distinguishing human races on a dental basis. The results of such studies enable us to trace the relationships between races and the racial affinity between human populations. A race may be defined as a subdivision of a species containing members sharing common biological and cultural characteristics. Thus, if the same highly heritable dental variants occur with a similar frequency in two populations, then the populations are likely to have a high degree of affinity. These anthropological studies generally use complex statistical analysis of groups of traits rather than a single feature. Where frequencies of the features are low, a large sample size is necessary. The following is a list of the more common secondary dental traits encountered in dental anthropology, although many more are reported in the literature.

1. Winging of maxillary central incisors. Instead of the central incisors being straight and arranged along the dental arch, they are inclined mesially and their incisal edges form a V shape.
2. Shovel-shaped maxillary central incisors. Exaggerated and extensive marginal ridges give the tooth a shovel appearance. The palatal concavity is thus exaggerated. Indeed, the depth of the palatal fossa is the best indicator of the degree of shovelling. This may vary and at its most pronounced also involves the labial surface, giving rise to a 'double-shovelled' appearance. While predominantly found in the maxillary incisors, it can affect the mandibular incisors. This trait is particularly common in Chinese, Japanese and Eskimos, and low in Negroes and Europeans.
3. The frequency of peg-shaped maxillary second (lateral) permanent incisors.
4. The presence of only a single root on the maxillary first permanent premolar.
5. The presence of accessory cusps on the maxillary first permanent molar. Accessory cusps regularly occur on the buccal and palatal surfaces. As mentioned on page 23, there is often a cusplet on the palatal surface of the mesio-palatal cusp known as the tubercle of Carabelli, which may vary from a large elevation to a mere groove. It has a low incidence in Negroes. When present on the buccal surface, accessory cusps are known as paramolar cusps.
6. The reduced size or absence of a distopalatal cusp on the maxillary second permanent molar.
7. The presence of a reduced, peg-shaped maxillary third permanent molar.
8. The presence of an additional cusp on the mandibular second premolar. Although the lingual cusp on this tooth is generally subdivided into two, an additional cusp may be present, giving a total of four for the tooth.
9. The pattern of fissures on the mandibular first permanent molar. The fissure pattern may have a 'Y' or '+' configuration (see page 25 and Fig. 2.43). Further subdivisions are 'X' or 'C' (crenulated – where the occlusal surface does not exhibit a clear groove pattern but is covered with fine dendritic crenulations as in third molars).

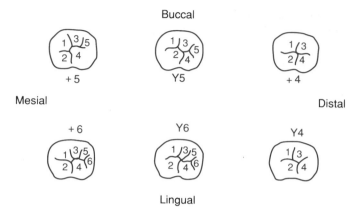

Fig. 2.43 Mandibular molars showing variation in fissure pattern and number of cusps.

10. The number of cusps on the mandibular molars: there may be six, five, or four. The additional sixth cusp is known as the protostylid and is associated with the mesiobuccal cusp. Where four cusps are present, the distal cusp has been lost (see Fig. 2.43).
11. The presence of three roots on the mandibular first permanent molar.
12. The number of cusps present on the mandibular permanent second molar. This tooth may exhibit four or five cusps.

Two additional features are often incorporated into anthropological investigations of dental variation, even though they are not strictly morphological features. These are hypodontia (the frequency of missing teeth) and hyperdontia (the frequency of supernumerary teeth).

PULP MORPHOLOGY

The dental pulp occupies the pulp chamber in the crown of the tooth and the root canal(s) in the root(s). The pulp chamber conforms, in basic shape, to the external form of the crown (Fig. 2.44). Root canal anatomy varies with tooth type and

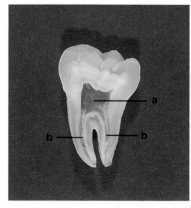

Fig. 2.44 Ground section of a molar tooth showing the pulp chamber (a) and root canals (b).

root morphology. At the apex of the root, the root canal becomes continuous with the periapical periodontal tissues through an apical foramen. Knowledge of the morphology of the pulp chamber and root canal is clinically significant: for example, when removing caries and restoring teeth, it is important to avoid exposing the pulp. Furthermore, when the pulp is diseased and must be removed and replaced with a filling material (root canal therapy), it is essential to remove and replace all the pulp tissue and avoid injuring the periapical supporting tissues.

In the general descriptions of the pulp morphology in teeth of the permanent dentition that follow, each tooth is illustrated from the labial (buccal) and distal surfaces. The red outline shows the pulp cavity in the young tooth, the blue outline shows the pulp in the old tooth. In anterior teeth, the pulp chambers merge almost imperceptibly into the root canals. In the premolar and molar teeth, the pulp chambers and root canals are distinct. Pulp horns (or cornua) extend from the pulp chambers to the mesial and distal angles of the incisor tooth crowns and towards the cusps of posterior teeth. Each root most often contains one root canal, but two are not unusual (mandibular molars, for example, commonly have two root canals in their mesial roots). When roots are fused, the tooth still maintains the usual number of root canals. The size of the pulp chamber and the diameter of the root canals decrease significantly with age and in response to caries, attrition or other external stimuli due to the deposition of secondary (and sometimes tertiary) dentine (see pages 138–143). When the tooth first erupts into the oral cavity, root development is incomplete and the apical foramen is wide (see Fig. 25.2). The apical foramen narrows with subsequent development of the root and a constriction formed from cementum develops. This constriction marks the boundary between pulpal and periapical tissue (see Fig. 26.6).

Incisors

Maxillary first (central) permanent incisor

Viewed from the labial aspect, the pulp chamber of the maxillary first permanent incisor (Figs 2.45, 2.46) follows the outline of the crown, being widest towards the incisal edge. In a young tooth the pulp chamber has three pulp horns that correspond to the mammelons present during development. Viewed distally, the pulp tapers towards the incisal edge and widens cervically. A constriction (the cervical bulge) separates the single and centrally placed root canal from the pulp chamber. The root canal tapers towards the apical foramen, where it

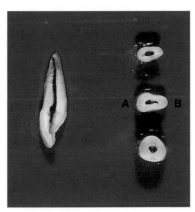

Fig. 2.46   Sectioned maxillary first permanent incisor demonstrating pulp morphology. A = Labial; B = palatal.

may curve slightly either distally or labially. In cross section, the root canal is ovoid for much of its extent but, in common with canals in other teeth, becomes round as it nears the apex. With age, the dimensions of the pulp chamber and root canal are reduced as secondary dentine is laid down. The pulp chamber recedes and may disappear completely. In conducting root canal therapy on older teeth, locating the root canal in the absence of a pulp chamber may be the major clinical challenge.

Maxillary second (lateral) permanent incisor

The pulp chamber of this incisor (Fig. 2.47) is similar to, but smaller than, that of the maxillary central incisor. The root canal is single, slightly ovoid and commonly curves both distally and palatally.

Mandibular first (central) permanent incisor

The pulp chamber of the mandibular central permanent incisor (Figs 2.48, 2.49) is similar to that described for the maxillary first incisor although, being in a much smaller tooth, it is smaller. The pulp chamber is oval in cross section, being wider labiolingually than mesiodistally, and is constricted at the cervical margin. The root canal is ovoid, becoming round in the apical third. As many as 30% of lower central incisors have two root canals, although most of these fuse near the apex and exit by a single foramen.

Mandibular second (lateral) permanent incisor

Both tooth and root canal system are larger than those of the

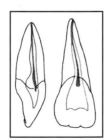

Fig. 2.45   Schematic representation of the pulp morphology of the maxillary first permanent incisor.

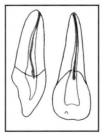

Fig. 2.47   Schematic representation of the pulp morphology of the maxillary second permanent incisor.

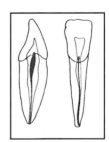

Fig. 2.48   Schematic representation of the pulp morphology of the mandibular first permanent incisor.

mandibular central incisor (Fig. 2.50). Two root canals are somewhat more common (43%). Most of these root canals exit by separate foramina.

Canines

Maxillary permanent canine

The pulp chamber of the maxillary permanent canine (Figs 2.51, 2.52) is narrow with a single pulp horn that points cuspally. Both the pulp chamber and the single root canal are wider labiopalatally than mesiodistally. The root canal does not constrict markedly until the apical third of the root is reached. The root canal, which is always single, is oval or triangular in cross section except in its apical third, where it is round.

Mandibular permanent canine

The pulp cavity of the mandibular permanent canine (Figs 2.53, 2.54) resembles that of the maxillary permanent canine, although it is smaller in all dimensions. The root canal is oval in cross section, being wider buccopalatally, but becomes round apically. About 6% of these teeth have two root canals, usually with separate foramina.

Premolars

Maxillary first premolar

The maxillary first premolar (Figs 2.55, 2.56) usually has two roots (85% of cases), although they are sometimes fused. The two canals generally exit by separate foramina. A single root and single canal is present in less than 10% of cases. A small number (5%) have three canals (sometimes in three roots). The pulp chamber is wide buccopalatally with two distinct pulp horns pointing towards the cusps. From the buccal view, the pulp chamber is much narrower. The floor of the pulp chamber is rounded with the highest point in the centre. It usually lies within the root just apical to the cervix. Where the root canals arise from the pulp chamber the orifices are funnel shaped. The pulp chamber is closest to the surface mesially, where the shape of the crown is indented by the canine fossa. The dental pulp is commonly exposed in this area by caries or restorative cavities that are extended interproximally. The root canals diverge but are usually straight individually and taper evenly from their origin to the apical foramina. In cross section the root canals are generally round. With age, the general shape of the pulp cavity remains the same but its dimensions, particularly the height of the pulp chamber, are reduced.

Maxillary second premolar

The maxillary second premolar (Figs 2.57, 2.58) has in most instances (75%) a single root with a single root canal. Its pulp chamber extends apically well below the cervical margin. The appearance of the pulp cavity viewed from the buccal aspect is similar to that in the first premolar. When two canals are present, they most commonly have separate apical foramina. In cross section the root canal is oval until the apical third of the root, where it becomes round.

Mandibular first premolar

The pulp chamber in the mandibular first premolar (Figs 2.59, 2.60), like that of the maxillary premolars, is wider buccolingually than mesiodistally. Unlike the maxillary premolars, there is usually only one pulp horn, which extends into the buccal cusp. Occasionally, a small pulp horn may pass to the reduced lingual cusp. There is usually a single root canal (in 75% of cases) that becomes constricted towards the middle third of the root. Most teeth that have two canals have two apical foramina.

Mandibular second premolar

The pulp morphology of the mandibular second premolar (Fig. 2.61) differs little from that described for the mandibular first premolar, although a higher proportion (85%) have single canals and there are usually two well developed pulp horns projecting towards its cusps.

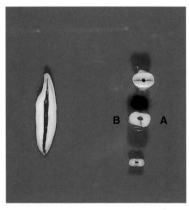

Fig. 2.49 Sectioned mandibular first permanent incisor demonstrating pulp morphology. A = Labial; B = lingual.

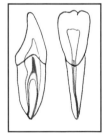

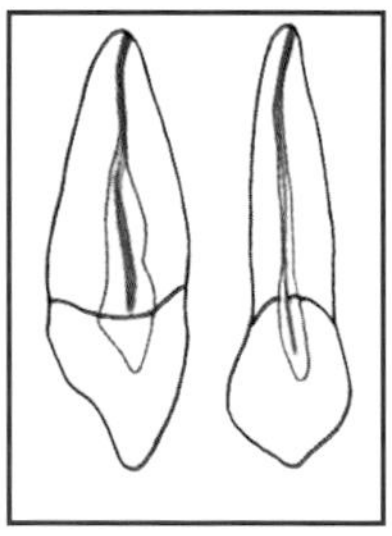

Fig. 2.50 (*Left*) Schematic representation of the pulp morphology of the mandibular second permanent incisor.

Fig. 2.51 (*Right*) Schematic representation of the pulp morphology of the maxillary permanent canine.

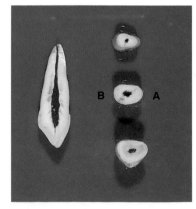

Fig. 2.52 Sectioned maxillary permanent canine demonstrating pulp morphology. A = Labial; B = palatal.

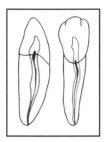

Fig. 2.53 Schematic representation of the pulp morphology of the mandibular permanent canine.

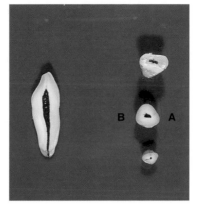

Fig. 2.54 Sectioned mandibular permanent canine tooth demonstrating pulp morphology. A = Labial; B = lingual.

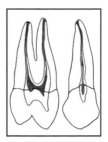

Fig. 2.55 Schematic representation of the pulp morphology of the maxillary first premolar.

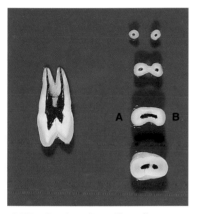

Fig. 2.56 Sectioned maxillary first premolar demonstrating pulp morphology. A = Buccal; B = palatal.

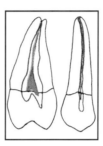

Fig. 2.57 Schematic representation of the pulp morphology of the maxillary second premolar.

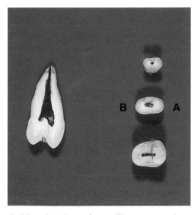

Fig. 2.58 Sectioned maxillary second premolar demonstrating pulp morphology. A = Buccal; B = palatal.

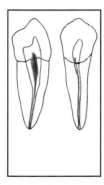

Fig. 2.59 Schematic representation of the pulp morphology of the mandibular first premolar.

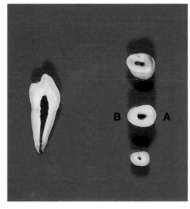

Fig. 2.60 Sectioned mandibular first premolar demonstrating pulp morphology. A = Buccal; B = lingual.

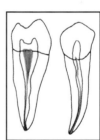

Fig. 2.61 Schematic representation of the pulp morphology of the mandibular second premolar.

Molars

Maxillary first permanent molar

The pulp chamber of the maxillary first permanent molar (Figs 2.62, 2.63) is rhomboidal in shape, being wider bucco-palatally than mesiodistally. Four pulp horns arise from the roof, one to each of the major cusps. The pulp horn to the mesiobuccal cusp is the longest. The floor of the pulp chamber generally lies below the cervical margin. Three root canals are present (or four in 60% of cases), their orifices being funnel shaped. The root canal of the mesiobuccal root leaves the pulp chamber in a mesial direction and is often significantly curved. In cross section it appears as a narrow slit, being wider buccopalatally. Its anatomy may be complicated by irregular branching or bifurcation near the apical foramen. When a fourth canal is present, it is in the mesiobuccal root. Two-thirds of the fourth canals rejoin the main canal of the mesio-buccal root near the root apex. The palatal root canal is the widest and longest of the three root canals. The floor of the pulp chamber is marked by a series of developmental grooves that join the orifices of the root canals.

Maxillary second permanent molar

The pulp cavity of the maxillary second permanent molar (Fig. 2.64) is similar to that of the first molar, but smaller with the rhomboidal shape more compressed. The roots of this tooth are more convergent, bringing the root canal orifices closer together on the pulpal floor. The roots are commonly fused. A second mesiobuccal canal is less common than in the first molar (40% of cases).

Mandibular first permanent molar

The pulp chamber in the mandibular first permanent molar (Figs 2.65, 2.66) is wider mesiodistally than buccolingually. It is also wider mesially than distally. There are five pulp horns projecting to the cusps, the lingual pulp horns being longer and more pointed. The floor of the pulp chamber lies at, or just below, the level of the cervical margin. The root canals leave

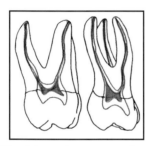

Fig. 2.62 Schematic representation of the pulp morphology of the maxillary first permanent molar.

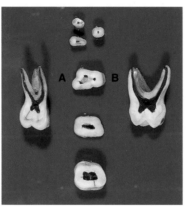

Fig. 2.63 Sectioned maxillary first permanent molar demonstrating pulp morphology. The tooth on the left shows the root canals of the mesiobuccal and palatal roots, while that on the right shows the two buccal root canals. A = Buccal; B = palatal.

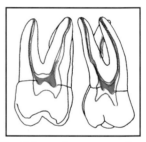

Fig. 2.64 Schematic representation of the pulp morphology of the maxillary second permanent molar.

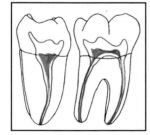

Fig. 2.65 Schematic representation of the pulp morphology of the mandibular first permanent molar.

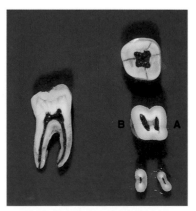

Fig. 2.66 Sectioned mandibular first permanent molar demonstrating pulp morphology. A = Buccal; B = lingual.

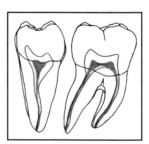

Fig. 2.67 Schematic representation of the pulp morphology of the mandibular second permanent molar.

the pulp chamber through funnel-shaped orifices, of which the mesial are finer than the distal. The mesial root has two root canals, mesiobuccal and mesiolingual. The mesiobuccal root canal follows a curved path, the mesiolingual canal is straighter; both are circular in cross section. In 30% of teeth the distal root has two canals. The distal canal, especially when single, is considerably larger and more oval in cross section than the mesial root canals and follows a straighter course.

Mandibular second permanent molar

The pulp morphology of the mandibular second permanent molar (Fig. 2.67) closely resembles that of the adjacent first molar, although there are only four pulp horns and only rarely (8% of cases) two canals in the distal root.

Shape of the pulp chamber in deciduous teeth

As in permanent teeth, the shape of the deciduous pulp chamber reflects the shape of the crown but in the deciduous teeth the chamber is relatively larger and the pulp horns longer and closer to the surface of the tooth. All incisors and canines have single canals that are either round or oval (being compressed mesiodistally). In 10% of deciduous mandibular incisors there are two root canals. The pulp chambers of deciduous mandibular molars are proportionately larger than those of the deciduous maxillary molars. The mesiobuccal pulp horn in deciduous molars is particularly near to the occlusal surface and thus highly vulnerable to exposure by dental caries, trauma or cavity preparation. Small canals running from the pulp chamber to the furcation region are common in deciduous molars. In the slender roots of deciduous molars, the root canals are narrower mesiodistally and more ribbon-shaped than those in permanent teeth. This, and the severe curvature of deciduous roots, makes complete debridement and obturation of the root canal system difficult. Although pulpotomy is the more common treatment for the diseased deciduous pulp, pulpectomy and canal obturation is feasible. When resorption of the deciduous root begins, it commences on the lingual surfaces of the anterior teeth and furcal surfaces of molars; this complicates root canal therapy as the exit to the canal system becomes very wide and may be some distance from the root end as visualised radiographically. Other features to bear in mind are:

- The maxillary first deciduous molar has two to four root canals, with two canals in the mesiobuccal root in 75% of cases. The palatal and distobuccal roots are often fused (one-third of cases), but contain distinct canals.
- The maxillary second deciduous molar has two to five root canals (Fig. 2.68). The mesiobuccal root usually bifurcates or contains two canals (90% of cases). Palatal and distobuccal roots sometimes fuse and contain a single, common canal.
- The mandibular first deciduous molar may have two to four canals (Fig. 2.69). Most mesial roots (75%) have two canals, 25% of distal.
- The mandibular second deciduous molar usually has three canals, but can vary from two to five. Two canals are seen in 85% of mesial roots but only 25% of distal roots have two canals.

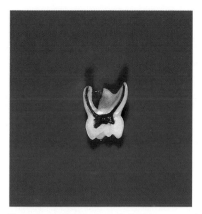

Fig. 2.68 Sectioned maxillary second deciduous molar demonstrating pulp morphology.

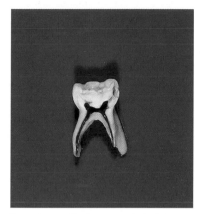

Fig. 2.69 Sectioned mandibular second deciduous molar demonstrating pulp morphology.

THE ALIGNMENT AND OCCLUSION OF THE PERMANENT TEETH

The relationships of the teeth, both within and between the dental arches, are of fundamental importance to an understanding of mastication and for such clinical disciplines as orthodontics and prosthetics. Tooth alignment is the term that refers to the arrangement of the teeth within the dental arches; occlusion refers to the relationship of the dental arches when tooth contact is made.

Traditionally, textbooks describe a standard set of tooth relationships that is called 'normal' (i.e. normal alignment and normal occlusion). Normal is a term that is generally used to describe situations that are the ordinary or most frequent; alternatively, normal may define an authoritative standard or ideal which, in medical terms, is the healthy state. In these terms, malocclusions could be regarded as normal for they are more commonly found in the population than 'normal' occlusion (approximately 75% of the population of the USA have some degree of occlusal 'disharmony'). Malocclusions do not always predispose to dental disease and, in most cases, are not associated with masticatory dysfunction, speech defects, bruxism, or pain in and around the temporomandibular joint. Furthermore, our knowledge of the association between the structure and function of the dental arches during mastication is not yet sufficient to provide an authoritative standard for tooth relationships; in structural terms, the ideal occlusion is a rather subjective concept. If there is an ideal occlusion, it can presently be defined only in broad functional terms. We believe therefore that the occlusion is 'ideal' when:

- the teeth are aligned such that the masticatory loads are within physiological range and act through the long axes of as many teeth in the arch as possible;
- mastication involves alternating bilateral jaw movements (and not habitual, unilateral biting preferences as a result of adaptation to occlusal interference);
- lateral jaw movements occur without undue mechanical interference;
- in the rest position of the jaw, the gap between teeth (the freeway space; see page 42) is correct for the individual concerned;
- the tooth alignment is aesthetically pleasing to its possessor.

Despite our reservations, the traditional descriptions of 'normal' tooth relationships provide a convenient model for the classification of malocclusions in clinical situations. However, we have chosen to use the terms 'anatomical alignment' and 'anatomical occlusion' instead of 'normal alignment' and 'normal occlusion' in order to avoid the difficulties of defining normality with respect to tooth relationships. The occlusion of the deciduous dentition and the development of occlusion is considered in a later part of this book (Chapter 26).

The anatomical alignment of teeth

Each dental arch (maxillary/upper and mandibular/lower) generally takes the form of a catenary curve (Fig. 2.70). Such a curve is described when a rope or chain is hung at both ends. There are no spacings or rotations of teeth within the arch, and therefore all teeth are in contact with neighbouring teeth along the arch.

Superimposed on the occlusal surfaces of the teeth shown in Figure 2.70 are Angle's 'lines of occlusion'. Because the maxillary arch is broader than the mandibular arch, the line of occlusion for the maxillary arch passes through the cingulae of the anterior teeth and through the central fossae of the posterior teeth. However, the line of occlusion for the mandibular arch runs along the incisal edges of the anterior teeth and along the buccal cusps of the posterior teeth.

The well aligned dental arch may be divided into different segments. A curved line in the coronal plane describes the anterior segment. This segment extends across the midline from canine to canine. The middle segments are described by straight lines extending from the distal edge of the canines to the mesiobuccal cusps of the first molars. The posterior segments extend from the mesiobuccal cusps of the first molars backwards. Both the middle and posterior segments lie in the sagittal plane, the posterior segments being more nearly parallel to this plane than the middle segments.

The positions of the teeth within the dental arch are determined by numerous factors and forces. Indeed, the spatial configuration of the arches is dependent upon an interaction

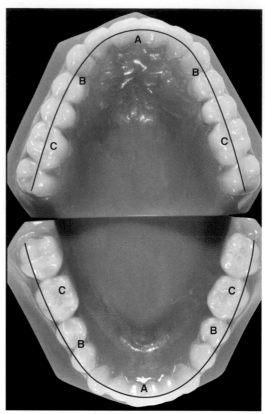

Fig. 2.70 The form of the maxillary and mandibular dental arches showing the anatomical alignment of the teeth and Angle's lines of occlusion.

between the eruptive movements carrying the teeth into their functional positions and, once erupted, the forces brought to bear upon each tooth. The term 'neutral zone' (Fig. 2.71) is used to describe that space in which there is an equilibrium of forces so that the teeth attain a position of relative stability. A change in balance in this system, such as that produced by

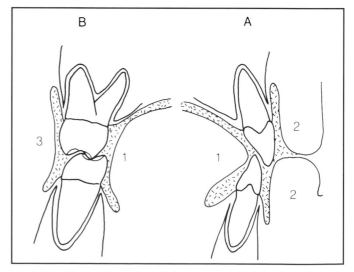

Fig. 2.71 The configuration of the neutral zone (the stippled area) in the incisor region (A) and the molar region (B). The tongue is labelled 1, the lips 2, and the cheek 3. Redrawn after Professors B.J. Kraus, R.E. Jordan and L. Abrams.

abnormal tongue-thrusting behaviour during swallowing and abnormal lip posture, can result in malalignment of the teeth.

The size of the dental arches varies considerably between individuals. Table 2.4 provides the average widths of the dental arches for the completed deciduous dentition (6 years) and the completed permanent dentition (18 years) for males. Averages for females are usually 1 mm less.

Figures 2.72–2.79 describe the angulation or axial positioning of individual teeth within the alveolus relative to perpendiculars dropped from a hypothetically flat occlusal plane. In these diagrams the angles quoted are average figures, though variation is considerable.

Viewed labially, the maxillary incisors have slight distal inclinations whereas the canine has a distinct mesial angulation.

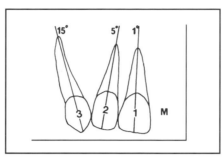

Fig. 2.72 The alignment of the maxillary incisors and canine viewed labially. The teeth are not drawn to scale and the numerical dental shorthand is used to identify the tooth. All angles quoted are average figures. M = Mesial.

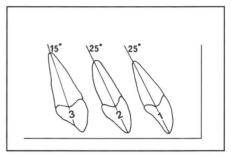

Fig. 2.73 The alignment of the maxillary incisors and canine viewed distally. The teeth are not drawn to scale and the numerical dental shorthand is used to identify the tooth. All angles quoted are average figures.

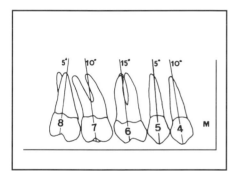

Fig. 2.74 The alignment of the maxillary premolars and molars viewed buccally. The teeth are not drawn to scale and the numerical dental shorthand is used to identify the tooth. All angles quoted are average figures. M = Mesial.

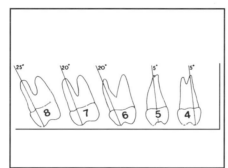

Fig. 2.75 The alignment of the maxillary premolars and molars viewed distally. The teeth are not drawn to scale and the numerical dental shorthand is used to identify the tooth. All angles quoted are average figures.

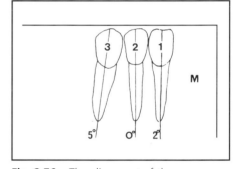

Fig. 2.76 The alignment of the mandibular incisors and canine viewed labially. The teeth are not drawn to scale and the numerical dental shorthand is used to identify the tooth. All angles quoted are average figures. M = Mesial.

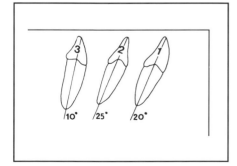

Fig. 2.77 The alignment of the mandibular incisors and canine viewed distally. The teeth are not drawn to scale and the numerical dental shorthand is used to identify the tooth. All angles quoted are average figures.

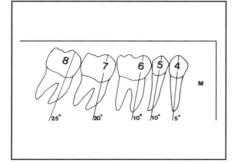

Fig. 2.78 The alignment of the mandibular premolars and molars viewed buccally. The teeth are not drawn to scale and the numerical dental shorthand is used to identify the tooth. All angles quoted are average figures. M = Mesial.

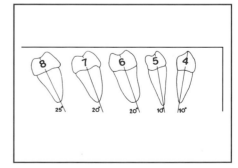

Fig. 2.79 The alignment of the mandibular premolars and molars viewed distally. The teeth are not drawn to scale and the numerical dental shorthand is used to identify the tooth. All angles quoted are average figures.

Table 2.4 *Average widths of the dental arches (males)*

Age (years)	Between maxillary canines (mm)	Between mandibular canines (mm)	Between maxillary first molars (mm)	Between mandibular first molars (mm)
6	28	23	42	40
18	32	25	47	43

When these teeth are viewed distally all show pronounced proclinations into the lip (although the canine is slightly more vertical). For the mandibular incisors and canine, when viewed labially, the incisors are more or less vertical and the canine has a slight mesial inclination. When viewed distally, these anterior mandibular teeth, like the anterior maxillary teeth, are proclined.

When viewed buccally, the maxillary premolars and molars change from a slight mesial angulation (premolars) to a distal inclination (the third molar). This contrasts with the mandibular posterior teeth, which show increasing mesial inclination moving back through the arch. When the maxillary premolars and molars are viewed distally, the teeth change from being essentially vertical in the premolar region to being distinctly buccally inclined in the molars. This again contrasts with the mandibular premolars and molars, where the teeth become more lingually inclined moving through the arch.

The curvatures of the teeth and arches

The impression could readily be gained from Figs 2.72–2.79 that the axes of the teeth are straight and run perpendicular to a horizontal, flat, occlusal plane. However, neither the axes of the teeth nor the occlusal planes are straight but are curved in all directions (Figs 2.80, 2.81). The curved axes of the teeth have a tendency to parallelism and are inclined mesially. It is often thought, mistakenly so, that the forces of mastication are at right angles to the occlusal surfaces of the teeth. If this were so, and if the occlusal planes and axes of the teeth were not curved, the arches might not be stable and the masticatory loads might be at an unfavourable angle to the teeth. Indeed, it is thought that, during mastication, the loads strike the teeth such that there is a mesial component of force (see page 362). The occlusal plane shows two types of curvature – the curve of Spee and the curve of Wilson.

The teeth align themselves such that the occlusal plane is not flat but describes a relatively linear curve in the antero-posterior direction, the **curves of Spee** (Fig. 2.82). The mandibular curve of Spee is concave whereas the maxillary curve is convex. An appreciation of the contribution of each tooth to the curve of Spee may be gained from analysis of the alignment of the long axes of the posterior teeth viewed buccally (see Figs 2.74, 2.78) and from the axes of the anterior teeth viewed distally (Figs 2.73, 2.77). Although the maxillary and mandibular curves of Spee are different they are nevertheless complementary and thereby may help achieve occlusal balance during mastication by encouraging simultaneous contact in more than one area of the dental arches. If the curves are exaggerated, however, there will be

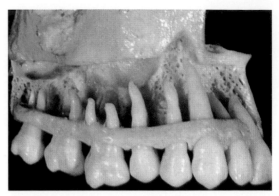

Fig. 2.80 The curvatures of the maxillary teeth within the alveolar bone of the maxilla.

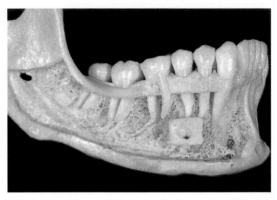

Fig. 2.81 The curvatures of the mandibular teeth within the alveolar bone of the mandible.

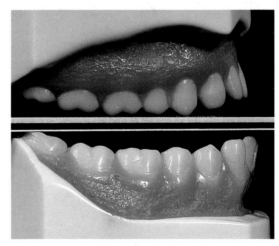

Fig. 2.82 Curvatures of the occlusal plane – the curve of Spee.

crowding in the mandibular arch and increased spacing in the maxillary arch.

The occlusal **curves of Wilson** (Fig. 2.83) are aligned in the transverse plane. Analysis of the alignment of the long axes of the posterior teeth (Figs 2.75, 2.79) shows that the curves of Wilson are such that the occlusal surfaces of the mandibular molars are directed lingually, while those of the maxillary molars are directed buccally. As for the curves of Spee, the curves of Wilson for the maxillary and mandibular posterior teeth are opposite but complementary. The curves of Spee and Wilson were once thought to be related three-

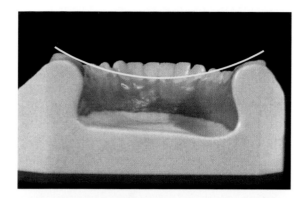

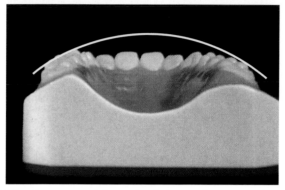

Fig. 2.83 Curvatures of the occlusal plane – the curves of Wilson.

The anatomical occlusion of teeth

The relationships of the jaws in function are so variable that our understanding of the functional articulation of teeth remains poor. To simplify analysis, several occlusal positions have been strictly defined. These positions may be classified into those which are symmetric and those which are asymmetric. This corresponds with the classification of mandibular movements into symmetric and asymmetric movements (see pages 93–94). The symmetric occlusal positions include centric occlusion and bilaterally protrusive position. The asymmetric occlusal positions are those associated with lateral (side-to-side) movements. Within the clinic, centric occlusal position is regarded as the 'standard' or 'model' for orthodontic and prosthetic diagnoses and treatments. While it is important in the dental clinic to be confident that oral examinations are based upon an accurate recording of tooth relationships in centric occlusion, the consistent attainment of centric occlusal position for some patients is notoriously difficult. Clinicians have consequently developed a variety of strategies to attain this position, including palpating the mandibular condyles within the mandibular fossae, pronouncing certain sounds, words or phrases, fatiguing the mandible by making the patient make rapid movements of the lower jaw, and even hypnosis!

Centric occlusal position

The centric occlusal position (Fig. 2.85) is defined as the terminal position of physiological jaw movements. It is the relationship between the two arches when the teeth are brought into contact with the mandibular condyles centrally positioned, at rest, in the mandibular fossae.

According to the pioneer orthodontist Edward Angle, the key to the intercuspal relationships between the teeth in the centric occlusal position is to be found in the relative positions of the maxillary and mandibular first permanent molars. In the 'normal' or anatomical condition, each arch is bilaterally symmetrical. Because the anterior maxillary segment is

dimensionally, the occlusal surfaces of the teeth being aligned on the curved surface of a segment of a sphere having a radius of about 10 cm. However, attempts to demonstrate, and then measure, the spherical curves (of Monson) have been unsuccessful.

With age, and as a result of wear (attrition), the cusps of the teeth are worn away so that the curvatures of the occlusal plane are lost and the plane becomes flat (Fig. 2.84). In addition, wear will affect the overjet and overbite for the anterior teeth (see page 38) and the nature of the tooth contacts (see centric stops, page 39).

Fig. 2.84 Effects of wear on the curvatures of the occlusal plane, which becomes flat.

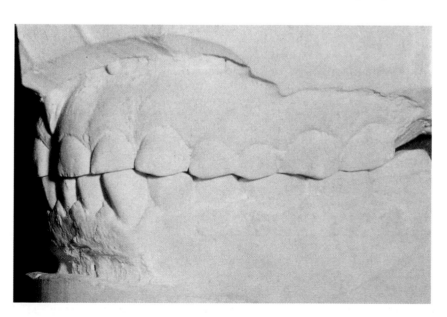

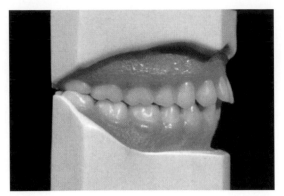

Fig. 2.85 Lateral view of the arrangement of teeth in anatomical centric occlusion.

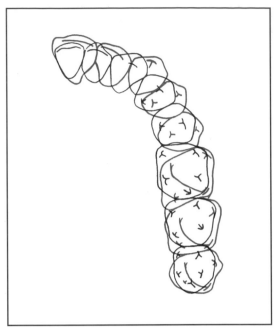

Fig. 2.87 The relationships between the occlusal surfaces of the maxillary (red) and mandibular (black) permanent teeth in anatomical centric occlusion.

slightly larger than the corresponding mandibular segment (due to the unequal sizes of the maxillary and mandibular central incisors), each maxillary tooth will contact its corresponding mandibular antagonist and its distal neighbour. Thus, the maxillary first permanent molar will contact the distal part of the mandibular first permanent molar and the mesial part of the mandibular second permanent molar. The only exceptions are the mandibular central incisor and the maxillary third molar. The relationships between maxillary and mandibular permanent teeth in anatomical centric occlusal position are shown in Fig. 2.86.

Fig. 2.87 illustrates the relationships between the maxillary and mandibular permanent teeth in anatomical centric occlusion by superimposing the occlusal surfaces of the teeth in the maxillary arch on those of the mandibular arch. This diagram shows not only the general anteroposterior relationships of the maxillary teeth and their antagonists but also the buccolingual relationships of the arches. As the maxillary arch is a little larger and broader than the mandibular arch, there is a slight overlap of the mandibular arch by the maxillary arch such that the buccal cusps of the maxillary teeth extend a few millimetres beyond the buccal occlusal edge of the mandibular teeth. This overlap is termed overjet.

When the buccolingual incisor relationships in anatomical centric occlusion are considered (Figs 2.88, 2.89), two types of 'overlap' of the mandibular incisors by the maxillary incisors

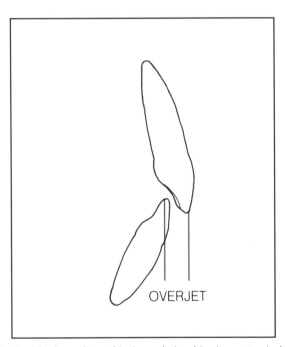

Fig. 2.88 The buccolingual incisor relationships in anatomical centric occlusion – overjet.

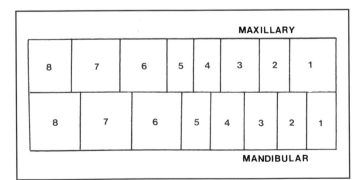

Fig. 2.86 Diagram illustrating the relationships between maxillary and mandibular permanent teeth in anatomical centric occlusal position. The teeth are identified according to the Zsigmondy system.

can be discerned. The overlap in the horizontal plane (overjet) is approximately 2–3 mm. The vertical overlap, specific to the incisors and canines, is termed overbite. The overbite in anatomical centric occlusion is such that the palatal surfaces of the maxillary incisors on average overlap the incisal third of the labial surfaces of the mandibular incisors. Fig. 2.90 provides a classification of overbite used in the orthodontic clinic.

With age, and as a result of attrition, the dimensions of the overjet and overbite decrease.

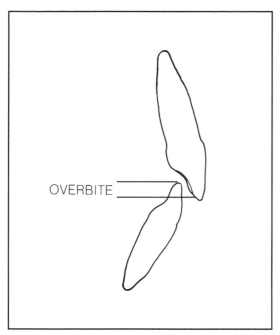

Fig. 2.89 The buccolingual incisor relationships in anatomical centric occlusion – overbite.

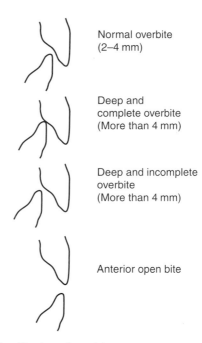

Normal overbite
(2–4 mm)

Deep and
complete overbite
(More than 4 mm)

Deep and incomplete
overbite
(More than 4 mm)

Anterior open bite

Fig. 2.90 Classification of overbite.

Fig. 2.91 shows the occlusal surfaces of the permanent dentition marked with the positions of hard contact in anatomical centric occlusion. These contacts are termed 'centric stops' (also sometimes referred to as 'holding contacts') and

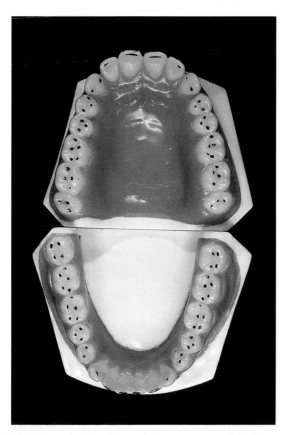

Fig. 2.91 The occlusal surfaces of the permanent dentition marked to show the position of centric stops in anatomical centric occlusion.

represent the intercuspal contact positions. When the 32 teeth within the permanent dentition occlude there are 138 centric stops, although this is seldom achieved during the normal bite. The major markings register on the occlusal surfaces of the posterior teeth (Fig. 2.91). The slopes of the maxillary palatal cusps make stops coincident with the stops within the central fossae of the mandibular posterior teeth. The stops in the central fossae of the maxillary teeth coincide with the stops on the slopes of the buccal cusps of the mandibular posterior teeth. The cusps seated in the central fossae are sometimes referred to as 'supporting cusps'. As befits the anatomical overjet relationships, the tips of the maxillary buccal cusps and the mandibular lingual cusps remain relatively unmarked. For the anterior teeth, the mandibular incisors have the centric stops on the incisal edges whereas the stops on the maxillary incisors are positioned down the palatal surface.

Similar marks to centric stops can be made in the clinic by interposing articulating paper between the teeth and then instructing the patient to go into centric occlusal position. With age, and with attrition, the occlusal surfaces become flattened as the cusps are worn and consequently the centric stops are significantly altered.

Variations in the relationships of the dental arches in centric position

Malocclusions should be regarded as anatomical variations rather than abnormalities for, although they may be aesthetically displeasing, they are rarely involved in masticatory dysfunction. Our lack of understanding of the relationships between masticatory efficiency and tooth and arch form is responsible for the classification of malocclusion in terms of variations in the anatomical centric position and not in more functional terms.

Malocclusions result from malposition of individual teeth, malrelationship of the dental arches and/or variation in skeletal morphology of the jaws. Techniques for determining the skeletal relationships of the jaws are described on pages 44–45. Two classifications describing malposition of teeth and mal-relationship of the arches are in general use – Angle's classification and a classification based upon the relationships of the incisors. A classification of malocclusion based upon canine relationships is also available for clinical use. However, this is much less employed than Angle's classification and the incisor relationship classification.

Angle's classification

Angle's classification of malocclusion was derived in 1899. It relies upon the relationship of the arches in the antero-posterior plane using the maxillary and mandibular first permanent molars as key teeth.

Angle's class I malocclusion. Although one or more of the teeth are malpositioned, this does not affect the 'standard' anatomical relationship of the first permanent molars. In the models shown in Fig. 2.92 the maxillary canine is missing and the premolars are malaligned but the upper first molar occludes correctly with the lower first and second molars.

Angle's class II malocclusion (division 1). Angle's Class II malocclusion is characterised by a 'prenormal' maxillary arch relationship, the maxillary first permanent molars occluding at least half a cusp more mesial to the mandibular first permanent molars than the standard anatomical position. 'Division 1' indicates that the maxillary incisors are proclined (Fig. 2.93).

Angle's class II malocclusion (division 2). The molar relationship is 'prenormal'; 'division 2' indicates that the maxillary incisors are retroclined (Fig. 2.94). Frequently only the central incisors are retroclined, the lateral incisors being proclined. For this malocclusion it is not uncommon to see increased overbite in the incisor region.

Angle's class III malocclusion. This malocclusion is characterised by a 'postnormal' maxillary arch relationship, the maxillary first permanent molars occluding at least half a cusp more distal to the mandibular first permanent molars than the 'standard' anatomical position. The incisor relationship varies from 'normal' overjet to an 'edge-to-edge' bite to reverse overjet (where the mandibular incisors lie labially to the maxillary incisors – as shown in Fig. 2.95).

Classification based on incisor relationships

As the permanent molars do not have a fixed relationship in the arch, and may migrate following early loss of deciduous teeth, the classification of malocclusion based upon incisor relationships (Fig. 2.96) is often preferred to Angle's classification. Furthermore, a classification of malocclusion related to the incisors is seen by many clinicians as being more appropriate because a major objective of orthodontic treatment is to establish an anatomical incisor relationship (patients being more concerned and aware of the aesthetics of the incisor relationship than they are of the molar relationship).

As for Angle's classification, the classification of malocclusions based upon incisor relationships uses the categories class I, class II (division 1), class II (division 2) and class III. However,

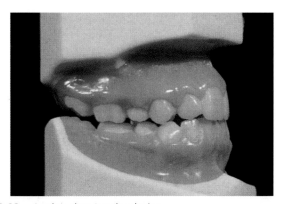

Fig. 2.92 Angle's class I malocclusion.

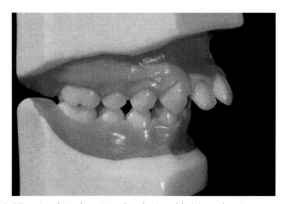

Fig. 2.93 Angle's class II malocclusion (division 1).

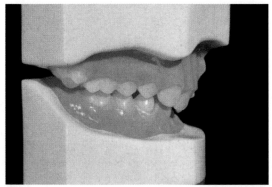

Fig. 2.94 Angle's class II malocclusion (division 2).

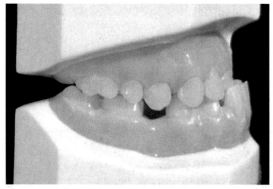

Fig. 2.95 Angle's class III malocclusion.

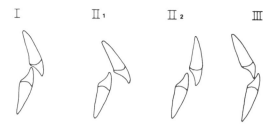

Fig. 2.96 Classification of malocclusion using incisor relationships.

care must be taken not to confuse these classifications – for example, an Angle's class I molar relationship might exist alongside an incisor class III relationship in the same person!

The incisor relationship classification was devised by Ballard and Wayman in the 1960s and has the full title of 'The British Standard Classification of Incisor relationships'. Studies have shown that there is remarkably poor agreement between examiners using this system of classification, apparently because the classification relies upon the relationship of incisors relative to a specific landmark – the cingulum plateau on the maxillary central incisor – and insufficient attention could be paid to the palatal anatomy of this tooth.

Class I incisor relationship. This represents the relationship where the incisors do not show any malposition. The incisal margins of the mandibular incisors occlude with, or lie directly below, the middle of the palatal surfaces of the maxillary incisors (i.e. on the cingulum plateau).

Class II incisor relationship. The incisal margins of the mandibular incisors lie behind the cingulum plateau on the palatal surfaces of the maxillary incisors. Division 1 indicates that the maxillary central incisors are proclined; division 2 indicates that the maxillary central incisors are retroclined.

Class III incisor relationship. The incisal margins of the mandibular incisors lie in front of the cingulum plateau on the palatal surfaces of the maxillary incisors, providing reduced overjet, edge-to-edge bite, or a reverse overjet.

Forms of malocclusion

Three common forms of malocclusion are: crowding, anterior open bite, and crossbite.

Crowding is the term used to describe the condition where teeth are markedly out of the line of the dental arch because there is disproportion between the size of the arch and the size of the teeth. The severe crowding illustrated in Fig. 2.97 reflects the developmental positions of the teeth before eruption (note that the second incisors develop inside the dental arch and the canines develop outside the arch). Spacing within an arch occurs where the teeth are small in relation to the size of the arch (or where there are missing teeth).

Anterior open bite (Fig. 2.98) occurs where there is no incisor contact and no incisor overbite. It may be caused by thumb sucking habits, by abnormal swallowing patterns or because of skeletal deformities. Skeletal anterior open bites sometimes result from lack of development of the anterior alveolar region, but more often are associated with an increase

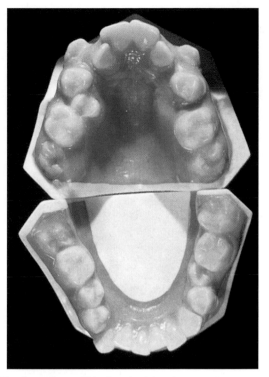

Fig. 2.97 Crowding within the dental arches.

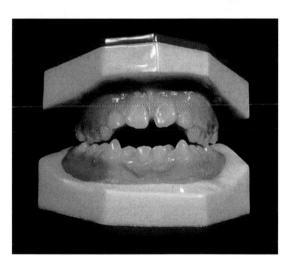

Fig. 2.98 Anterior open bite.

in anterior intermaxillary height (i.e. the distance between the maxillary and mandibular dental bases; see Fig. 2.111.

Crossbite (Fig. 2.99) is a transverse abnormality of the dental arches where there is an asymmetrical bite. It may be unilateral or, as illustrated in Fig. 2.99, bilateral. Crossbites are frequently related to discrepancies in the widths of the dental bases and may involve the displacement of the mandible to one side to obtain maximal intercuspation.

Table 2.5 provides data indicating the severity and type of malocclusions in the population of the USA. Approximately 80% of children and adolescents in the USA thus show some degree of malocclusion. Most commonly there are problems of crowding (for about 40% of children and 80% of adolescents). The second most common type of malocclusion is excessive overjet of the maxillary incisors (about 15% of children and of adolescents).

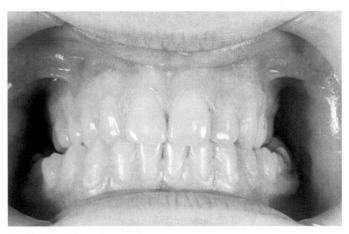

Fig. 2.99 Bilateral crossbite.

Table 2.5 *Severity and types of malocclusions in the general population of the USA*

	Distribution (%)	
	Age 6–11 years	Age 12–17 years
Severity		
Near-ideal occlusion	23	10
Mild malocclusion	40	35
Moderate malocclusion	23	26
Severe or very severe malocclusion	14	29
Type		
Crowding/malalignment problems		
Ideal	57	13
Moderate	39	44
Severe	4	43
Anteroposterior problems		
Overjet (6 mm or more)	17	15
Reverse overjet (1 mm or more)	1	
Vertical problems		
Open bite (2 mm or more)	1	1
Overbite (6 mm or more)	8	12
Transverse problems		
Lingual crossbite (two or more teeth)	5	6
Buccal crossbite (two or more teeth)	1	2

MANDIBULAR POSTURE

When the mandible is at rest, a gap of a few millimetres remains between the occlusal surfaces of the teeth – the so-called 'freeway space'. The opinion has long been held that the position of rest is innate and unalterable throughout life. However, the concept of a fixed mandibular resting posture is an oversimplification. Indeed, psychological state, body posture and fatigue are well known short-term influences that can change the resting interocclusal distance. Furthermore, research shows that, following speech, mastication or swallowing, the mandible appears to return to whatever position of rest it can find. In the long term, ageing and the removal of occlusal

contacts affect the resting position. Although the physiological mechanisms responsible for maintaining a rest position are not fully understood, evidence suggests that the physical properties of the soft tissues are responsible for the rest position, not tonic activity of the elevator muscles of the jaw.

Several instruments and techniques have been devised to measure freeway space – some elaborate, some relatively simple. All suffer from inaccuracies produced by examiner bias and misconceptions about the nature of the mandibular resting posture. The use of measuring techniques relies upon the concept that the mandibular resting position is innate and unalterable. Consequently, the removal of teeth is deemed not to affect the rest position. Thus, when a patient has lost all natural occlusal contacts, it is considered necessary only to put a prosthesis into the mouth at a level which reproduces the freeway space to restore the original occlusal vertical dimension.

Although most clinicians would prefer objective criteria for determining vertical jaw relationships many realise that, because of the relative instability of such relationships, at best one has to rely upon such subjective assessments as overall facial appearance, mandibular position during deglutition, jaw posture giving greatest comfort, position allowing the development of maximum biting force, and lip and tongue posture. Nevertheless, however one gauges the mandibular resting position, if prosthetic appliances are to be placed in the mouth, it is necessary to ensure that the vertical dimensions of the jaws are not adversely affected. Fig. 2.100 shows the appearance produced as a result of over-opening and Fig. 2.101 the appearance produced by over-closure. The result of over-opening is an elongation of the face, a parting of the lips at rest, and a 'strained' facial appearance. The general effect of over-closure on facial appearance is to produce features of increased age. There is a closer approximation of the nose and chin than normal. The greater the degree of over-closure, the more the soft tissues of the face appear to sag and fall in, and the more pronounced are the lines on the face.

THE RADIOGRAPHIC APPEARANCE OF JAWS AND TEETH

Dental radiography and radiology are concerned with the techniques of producing and interpreting photographic images of orodental tissues taken with X-rays. X-rays, being part of the spectrum of electromagnetic radiation, have a wavelength of approximately 10^{-8} cm (compared with wavelengths of around 10^{-4} cm for visible light). It is the short wavelength that allow X-rays to penetrate materials that would otherwise absorb or reflect light. However, X-rays do not pass through all matter with similar ease: materials composed of elements with low atomic numbers are readily penetrated and are described as being radiolucent, whereas elements with high atomic numbers absorb X-rays and are termed radio-opaque. Thus, gases and soft tissues are radiolucent while calcified materials such as bone and teeth are radio-opaque. X-rays produce a photosensitisation reaction when they strike a silver–salt emulsion. When a radio-opaque structure is placed between a beam of X-rays and a

Fig. 2.100 The appearance produced as a result of over-opening. A. Normal resting position and facial profile for a patient without dentures; B. Over-opened appearance produced typically by wearing dentures without provision of adequate freeway space. Courtesy of Professor D.C. Berry.

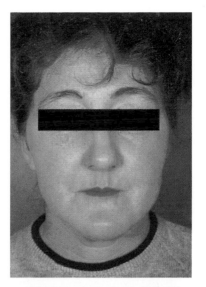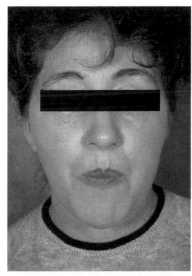

Fig. 2.101 The appearance produced by over-closure. (a) Normal resting position and facial profile of a patient who displays over-closure with an ill-fitting denture (b). Courtesy of Professor D.C. Berry.

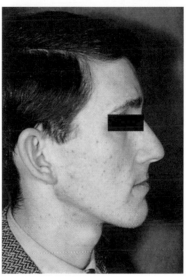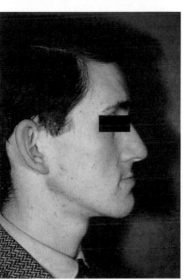

Table 2.6 *Extraoral radiographic projections describing jaws and teeth*

Projection/technique	Purpose
Posteroanterior skull (PA) (Fig. 2.102)	Survey of facial bones and mandible
Anteroposterior skull (AP) (Fig. 2.103)	Survey of posterior part of cranium, mandible and temporomandibular articulation
Reverse Towne's (Fig. 2.104)	Anatomy of mandibular condyles and temporomandibular articulation
Occipitomental skull (Fig. 2.105)	Survey of facial bones and air sinuses
Lateral skull (Fig. 2.106) (Fig. 2.106)	Survey of lateral regions of face, cranium and mandible. View of facial profile and covering soft tissues
Lateral skull with cephalostat (Fig. 2.110)	Recording of relationships between teeth, jaws and cranial base
Lateral oblique view of mandible (Fig. 2.107)	Survey of posterior regions of body and ramus of mandible
Orthopantomogram (Fig. 2.108)	A tomogram to display the whole of maxilla, mandible and the dentition on a single film
Transcranial temporomandibular joint (Fig. 2.109)	Movement of mandibular condyles in mandibular fossae
Sialography (Figs 2.120, 2.121)	Infusion of radio-opaque material into the main salivary ducts to study their structure and distribution
Tomography (Fig. 2.122)	Technique for the radiography of selected areas that under standard radiographic technique are obscured by superimposition of other structures (e.g. temporomandibular joint and air sinuses)

photographic plate which is subsequently developed, the radio-opaque structure is 'mapped out' as a white area on the negative. It is because of the properties of tissue penetration and photosensitisation that X-rays can be used in dentistry to provide valuable information concerning underlying hard tissue structures not otherwise visible.

X-rays produce a shadow picture without a focus; therefore the features of a large object such as a skull are not shown equally distinctly on a radiograph. As a general rule, structures nearest the photographic plate appear clearer than those some distance from it. Superimposition may also make interpretation of radiographs difficult, because most radiographs are two-dimensional representations of three-dimensional objects. Care must be taken not to overinterpret radiographs by diagnosing pathological conditions without recourse to other diagnostic aids or clinical findings. The prime use of a radiograph is therefore to describe gross topographic features.

Extraoral radiographic projections of jaws and teeth

Table 2.6 outlines the major extraoral radiographic projections used to view the human jaws and dentition. In this context, 'extraoral' indicates that the radiographic plate is positioned outside the mouth.

Among the specialised techniques worthy of fuller description here are Figs 2.102–2.109 concerned with cephalometric radiography, sialography and tomography.

Cephalometric analysis of lateral skull radiographs

Lateral skull radiographs (Fig. 2.110) are often used in dentistry to assess by measurement general skeletal morphology, particularly for recording relationships between the jaws and the cranial base. They are also of value for the evaluation of the direction and the amount of growth, for determining dentoskeletal relationships, and even for soft tissue analysis. In order to provide the most meaningful

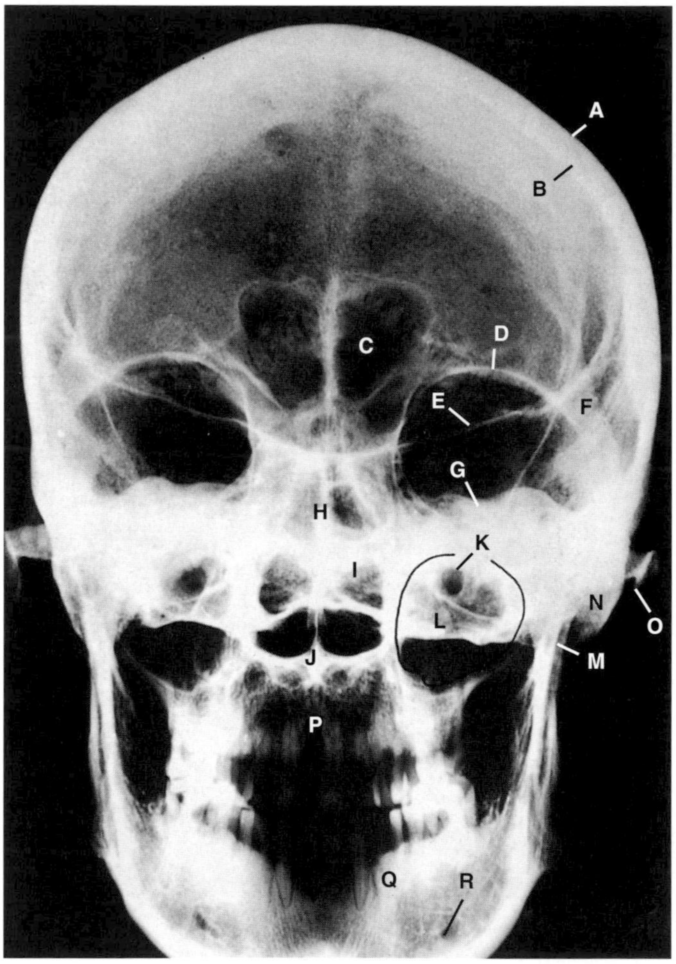

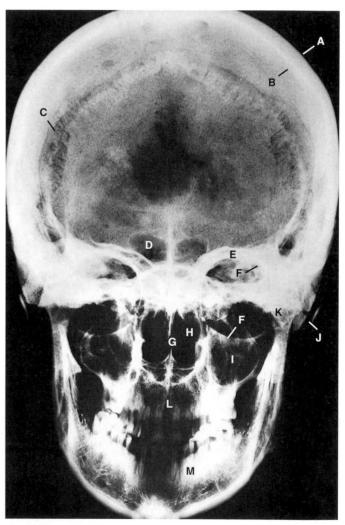

Fig. 2.102 Posterior (PA) view of skull. A = Outer table of cranium; B = inner table of cranium; C = frontal air sinus; D = superior rim of orbit; E = sphenoid ridge in middle cranial fossa; F = zygomatic process of frontal bone; G = petrous ridge; H = nasal septum; I = nasal fossa; J = anterior nasal spine; K = infraorbital foramen; L = maxillary air sinus; M = neck of mandibular condyle; N = mastoid process of temporal bone; O = zygomatic arch; P = maxilla and teeth; Q = body of mandible and teeth; R = mental foramen.

Fig. 2.103 Anteroposterior (AP) view of skull. A = Outer table of cranium; B = inner table of cranium; C = lambdoid suture; D = frontal air sinus; E = superimposed sphenoid, petrous and supraorbital ridges; F = rim of orbit; G = nasal septum; H = nasal fossa; I = maxillary air sinus; J = zygoma; K = condyle of mandible; L = maxilla and teeth; M = body of mandible and teeth.

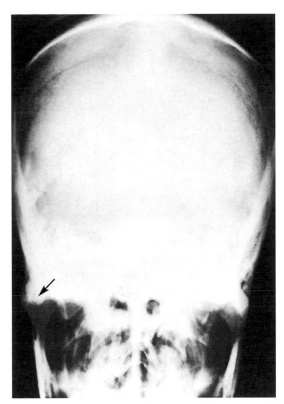

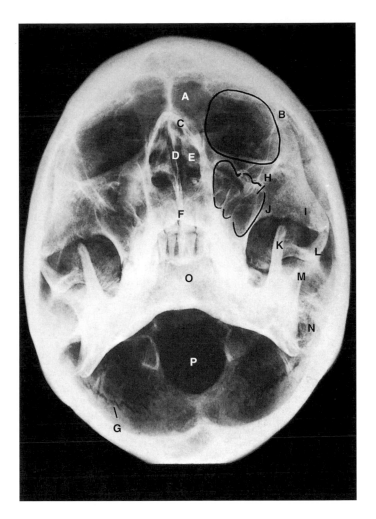

Fig. 2.104 Reverse Towne's view showing position of mandibular condyle (arrowed).

Fig. 2.105 (*Right*) Occipitomental view of skull (OM 30°).
A = Frontal air sinus; B = outline of orbit; C = nasal bones; D = nasal septum; E = nasal fossa with superimposed shadows of ethmoidal air cells; F = maxilla and teeth; G = lambdoid suture; H = malar (zygomatic) extension of maxillary sinus; I = zygoma; J = outline of maxillary air sinus; K = coronoid process of mandible; L = zygomatic process of temporal bone; M = condyle of mandible; N = mastoid air cells; O = body of mandible and teeth; P = foramen magnum.

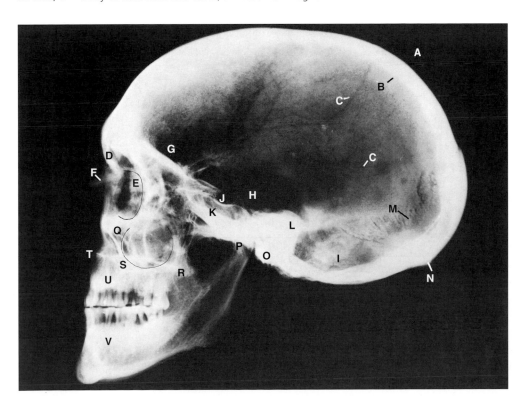

Fig. 2.106 Lateral skull radiograph. A = Outer table of cranium; B = inner table of cranium; C = depressions in cranium related to middle meningeal vessels; D = frontal air sinus; E = margins of orbit; F = nasal bone; G = anterior cranial fossa; H = middle cranial fossa; I = posterior cranial fossa; J = hypophyseal (pituitary) fossa; K = sphenoid air sinus; L = petrous ridge; M = lambdoid suture; N = external occipital protuberance; O = mastoid process; P = condyle of mandible; Q = margin of maxillary air sinus; R = coronoid process of mandible; S = hard palate; T = anterior nasal spine; U = maxilla and teeth; V = body of mandible and teeth.

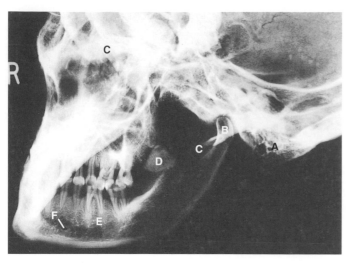

Fig. 2.107 Lateral oblique view of mandible. A = Mastoid process of temporal bone; B = condyle of mandible lying in mandibular fossa of temporomandibular joint; C = zygomatic arch; D = shadow of mandibular coronoid process on maxillary tuberosity; E = body of mandible showing teeth posterior to premolars; F = mental foramen.

common cephalometric landmarks used in dentistry (see also Table. 2.8).

Cephalometric analysis of jaw relationships and facial form

The mandibular plane passes through the menton and gonion (Fig. 2.112). It is used in conjunction with the Frankfort,

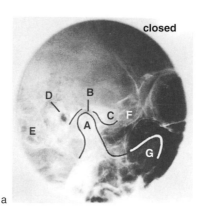

a

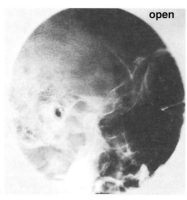

b

Fig. 2.109 Transcranial temporomandibular articulation (a, mouth closed; b, mouth open). A = Mandibular condyle; B = temporomandibular joint cavity space; C = articular tubercle; D = external acoustic meatus; E = mastoid air cells; F = zygomatic arch; G = coronoid process.

measurements, cephalometric radiographs are taken under standard conditions to enable comparisons between patients and for the same patient at different times. Thus, the position of the head must be standardised using a cephalostat (head holder) such that the beam of X-rays is shot in a predetermined plane to the head from a standard distance. This necessitates that the Frankfort plane (between the ear and orbit; see Fig. 2.112) is horizontal, that the dentition is in centric occlusion (see page 37) and that the lips are in their habitual position. Lateral skull radiographs are preferred for dental cephalometry primarily because the facial variations of greatest importance are located in the sagittal plane. Normal values for cephalometric measurements are given in Table 2.7.

Fig. 2.111 shows a lateral view of skull and tracing taken from a lateral skull radiograph and illustrates the most

Fig. 2.108 Orthopantomogram (OPG). A panoramic radiographic survey of the jaws and teeth. Dentition is radiographed at 6 years of age. A = External acoustic meatus; B = mandibular condyle; C = coronoid process of mandible; D = maxillary air sinus; E = nasal cavity; F = vertebral column.

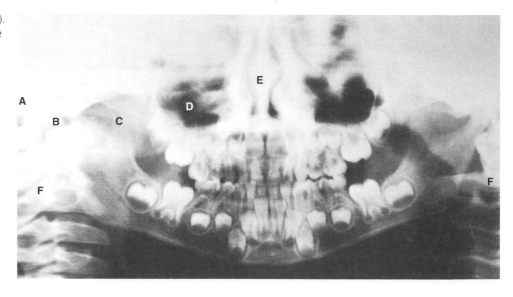

Fig. 2.110 Lateral skull radiograph taken using a cephalostat.

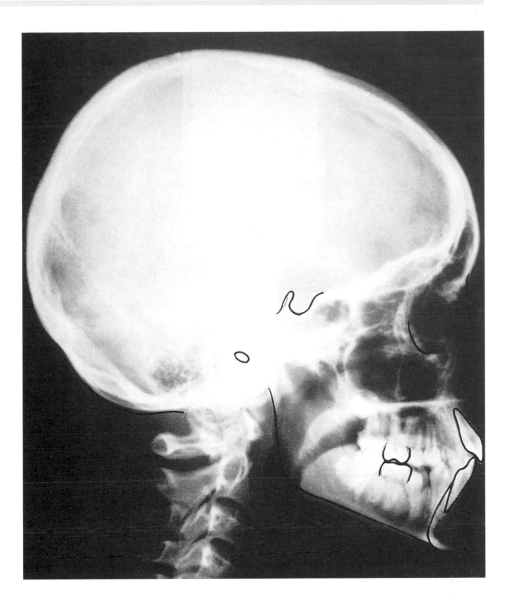

Table 2.7 *Normal values for cephalometric measurements*

Maxillary–mandibular plane angle	27 (± 5)°
SNA angle	82 (±) 3°
ANB angle	3 (± 1)°
Maxillary incisor/maxillary plane angle	109 (± 5)°
Mandibular incisor/mandibular plane angle	90 (±5)°
Maxillary incisor/mandibular incisor angle	135 (± 9)°
N–S–Ba angle	130° (150° at birth)

For abbreviations see Table 2.8

maxillary and Ba–N (see Table 2.8) planes to assess the vertical development of the anterior part of the face. The Frankfort plane extends from the orbitale to the portion. The Frankfort–mandibular angle in 'normal' subjects is said to be approximately 27°. The maxillary plane extends through the anterior and posterior nasal spines (ANS, PNS) and is easier to identify on a lateral skull radiograph than the Frankfort plane. Both the maxillary–mandibular plane angle

and the mandibular–cranial base (Ba–N) angle are of the same order as the Frankfort–mandibular plane angle. A plane termed the facial line can be drawn between the nasion and the pogonion. This plane aids the assessment of facial profile, and the angle it makes with the Frankfort plane indicates whether the profile is orthognathic, prognathic or retrognathic.

Fig. 2.113 describes the use of SNA and SNB angles to record maxillary–mandibular skeletal relationships. SNA measures the degree of prognathism of the maxillary alveolar base: its average value is 82°; SNB assesses the degree of prognathism of the mandibular alveolar base. The angle SNA–SNB (i.e. ANB) is frequently used to determine the skeletal pattern for the jaws because the cranial base (SN plane) is thought to undergo very little change from the later years of childhood. Where ANB is 2–5° the skeletal pattern is designated to be class I. Where ANB is greater than 5°, the jaws show a class II relationship with maxillary prognathism. Where ANB is less than 2°, the jaws show a class III relationship with mandibular prognathism. Should SNA be significantly different from its normal value, a correction must be made before assigning an ANB value to a specific skeletal class.

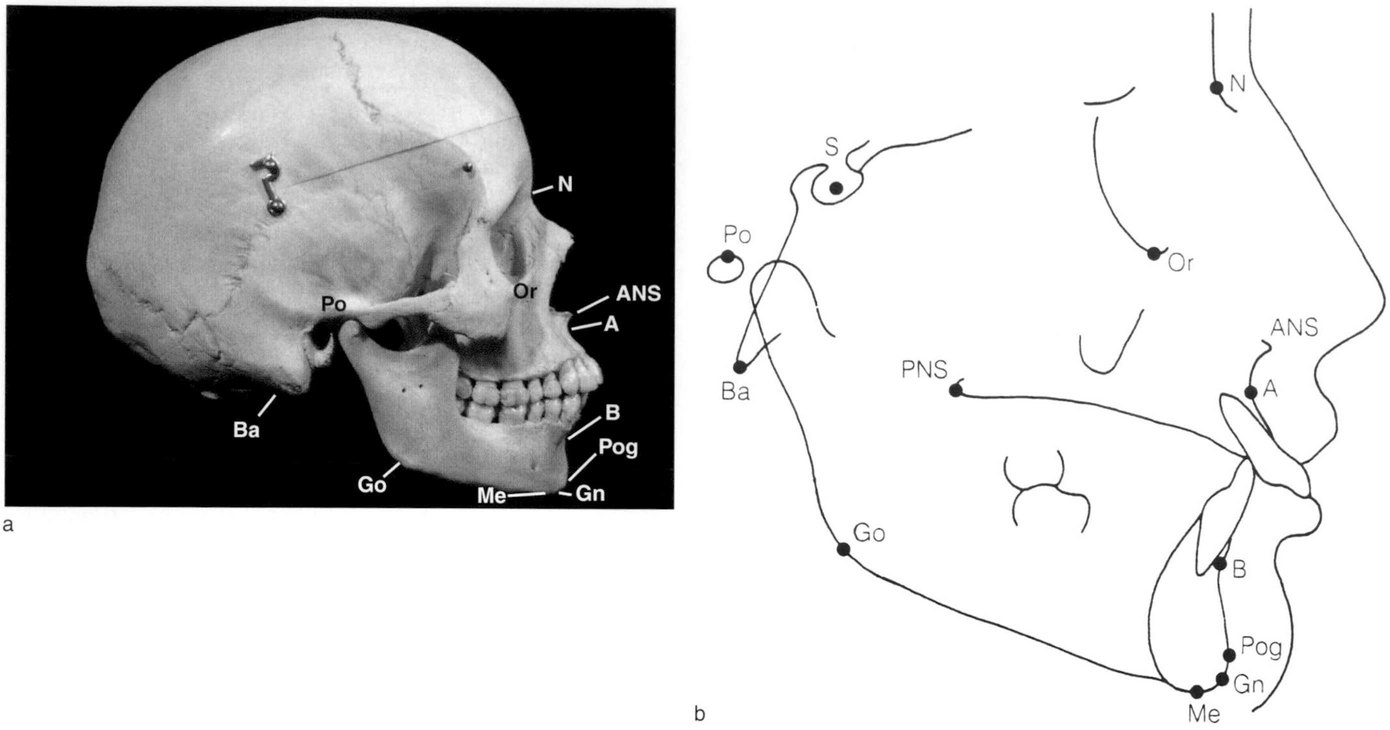

Fig. 2.111 Lateral view of skull (a) and tracing taken from a lateral skull radiograph (b), illustrating the most common cephalometric landmarks used in dentistry. Ba = Basion (the most inferior and posterior point on the basiocciput, lying on the anterior margin of the foramen magnum); S = sella point (centre of shadow of sella turcica (pituitary fossa)); N = nasion (junction between frontal and nasal bones in midline on the frontonasal suture); Po = porion (highest bony point of margin of external acoustic meatus); Or = orbitale (lowest point of the infraorbital margin); ANS = anterior nasal spine; PNS = posterior nasal spine; A = subspinale (A point: position of greatest concavity of maxillary alveolus in the midline); B = supramentale (B point: position of greatest concavity of mandibular alveolus in the midline); Pog = pogonion (most anterior point on the chin); Me = menton (lowest point of the chin); Gn = gnathion (point between the most anterior and inferior points of chin, established by bisecting the angle formed beween the N–Pog and mandibular planes); Go = gonion (most inferior and posterior point at the angle of the mandible, established by bisecting the angle formed between the planes through the lower border of the mandible and posterior border of ramus).

Table 2.8 *The most common cephalometric landmarks used in dentistry*

Basion (Ba)	The most inferior and posterior point on the basiocciput, lying on the anterior margin of the foramen magnum
Sella point (S)	Centre of shadow of sella turcica (pituitary fossa)
Nasion (N)	Junction between frontal and nasal bones in the midline on the frontonasal suture
Porion (Po)	Highest bony point of the margin of the external acoustic meatus
Orbitale (Or)	Lowest point of the infraorbital margin
Anterior nasal spine (ANS)	
Posterior nasal spine (PNS)	
Subspinale (A point)	Position of greatest concavity of the maxillary alveolus in the midline
Supramentale (B point)	Position of greatest concavity of the mandibular alveolus in the midline
Pogonion (Pog)	Most anterior point on the chin
Menton (Me)	Lowest point of the chin
Gnathion (Gn)	Point between the most anterior and inferior points of chin established by bisecting the angle formed between the N–Pog and mandibular planes
Gonion (Go)	Most inferior and posterior point at the angle of the mandible established by bisecting the angle formed between the planes through the lower border of the mandible and posterior border of ramus

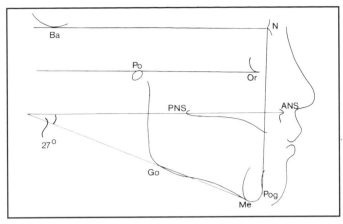

Fig. 2.112 Cephalometric analysis of jaw relationships and facial form. Ba = Basion; N = nasion; Po = porion; Or = orbitale; PNS = posterior nasal spine; ANS = anterior nasal spine; Go = gonion; Me = menton; Pog = pogonion. Frankfort plane = Po to Or.

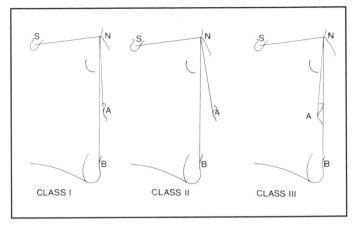

Fig. 2.113 The use of SNA and SNB angles to record maxillary–mandibular skeletal relationships. S = Sella point; N = nasion; A = subspinale (A point); B = supramentale (B point).

Fig. 2.114 and Table 2.9 provide the cephalometric landmarks used for assessing dentoskeletal relationships.

The inclinations of the incisors to the planes of the jaws are illustrated in Fig. 2.115. The inclination of the maxillary incisor can be determined by measuring the angle between a line drawn through its root axis and the Frankfort (or maxillary) plane. On average, this angle is 109°. The inclination of the mandibular incisor is assessed by the angle formed between its

Table 2.9 *Cephalometric landmarks for assessing dentoskeletal relationships*

Centroid of the maxillary incisor root (C)	The midpoint along the root axis of the most prominent maxillary incisor
Incision superius (IS)	The incisal tip of the most prominent maxillary incisor
Incision inferius (II)	The incisal tip of the most prominent mandibular incisor
Infradentale (Id)	The junction of alveolar crest with the outline of the most prominent mandibular incisor

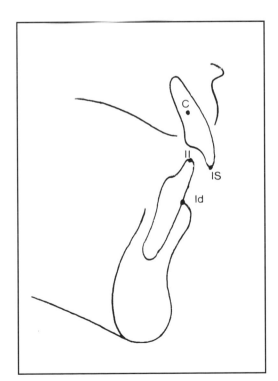

Fig. 2.114 Cephalometric landmarks used for assessing dentoskeletal relationships. C = Centroid of the maxillary incisor root (the midpoint along the root axis of the most prominent maxillary incisor); IS = incision superius (the incisal tip of the most prominent maxillary incisor); II = incision inferius (the incisal tip of the most prominent mandibular incisor); Id = infradentale (the junction of alveolar crest with the outline of the most prominent mandibular incisor).

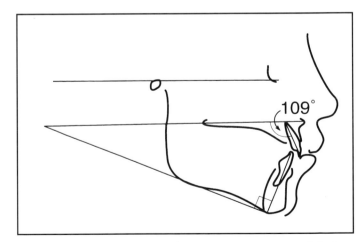

Fig. 2.115 The inclinations of the incisors to the planes of the jaws.

root axis and the mandibular plane: it is approximately a right angle. Interincisor relationships are described in Fig. 2.116. The angle formed by the junction of the longitudinal axes of the maxillary and mandibular central incisors is of the order of 135°; however, its clinical usefulness is limited because the anteroposterior relationship of the incisal edges is of greater importance. This is assessed by analysing the distance

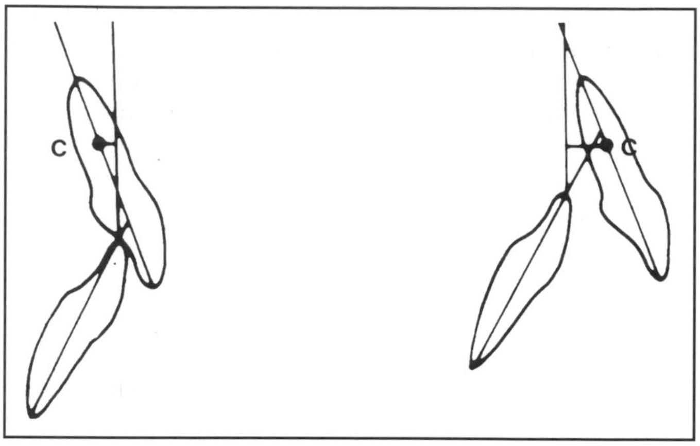

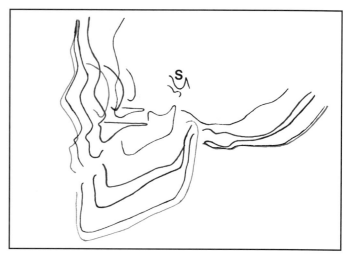

Fig. 2.116 Interincisor relationships. C = Centroid of the maxillary incisor root. Redrawn after Professors N.J.B. Houston and W.S. Tulley.

between the mandibular incisal edge and the centroid of the maxillary incisor root. Two examples are shown in Fig. 2.116. In both, the maxillary and mandibular incisors meet at the same angle of approximately 135°. However, they differ markedly in terms of the distances between the mandibular incisal edges and the centroids.

Cephalometric growth studies

Every bone of the skull in the growing child shows some degree of growth and consequently no point can be considered 'fixed'. For analytical convenience, however, several landmarks and strategies are defined and adopted to study the degree and direction of cranial growth. The Y-axis is a line from the sella point to the gnathion, and is used to describe the general direc-

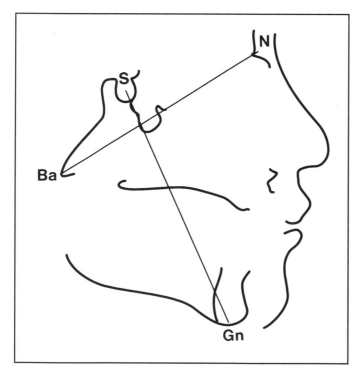

Fig. 2.117 Cephalometric growth studies – the Y-axis. Ba = Basion; S = sella point; N = nasion; Gn = gnathion.

tion of facial growth relative to the cranial base (Fig. 2.117). The angle between the Y-axis and the Ba–N plane is used to assess changes in growth direction.

A frequently employed strategy to assess growth relies upon the superimposition of successive cephalometric tracings of the same individual at different ages (Fig. 2.118). A reasonably reliable picture of growth of the facial skeleton can be obtained by superimposition at the S–N planes with registration of the sella point. Growth at the maxillary region is notoriously difficult to assess but can be analysed by superimposition at the maxillary plane with registration of the anterior surface of the zygomatic process of the maxilla. For the mandibular region, it is necessary to superimpose at the mandibular canal and at the inner surface of the mandible behind the chin.

Soft-tissue analysis

Soft-tissue analysis (Fig. 2.119) is possible from cephalometric

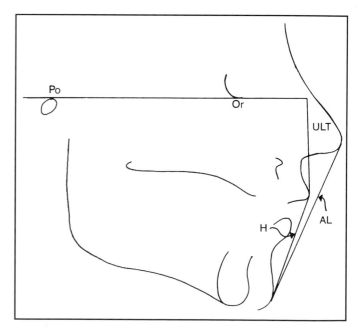

Fig. 2.118 Cephalometric growth studies – superimposition of tracings at different ages. S = Sella point.

Fig. 2.119 Soft tissue analysis from cephalometric radiographs. Po = Porion; Or = orbitale; H = the harmony line of Holdaway (H line); ULT = the upper lip tangent; AL = the aesthetic line.

radiographs provided that the soft-tissue outlines are sufficiently clear and that the lips are in their habitual posture. To undertake such analysis, reference is often made to the following three planes:

- The H line (the Harmony line of Holdaway) is drawn between the chin and the vermilion border of the upper lip. It can be used to assess the degree of lower lip pout. The vermilion border of the lower lip should be within 1 mm of the H line.

- The upper lip tangent (ULT) describes the plane perpendicular to the Frankfort plane and tangential to the vermilion border of the upper lip. It is used to assess the amount of upper lip curl, the concavity of the upper lip profile normally being 1–4 mm behind the upper lip tangent.
- The aesthetic line (AL) extends from the tip of the nose to the chin. The vermilion borders of both upper and lower lips usually lie close to the aesthetic line.

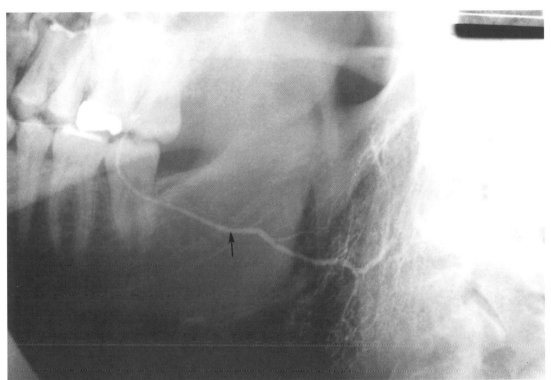

Fig. 2.120 Sialogram showing a normal parotid gland (arrow). Courtesy of Dr N. Drage.

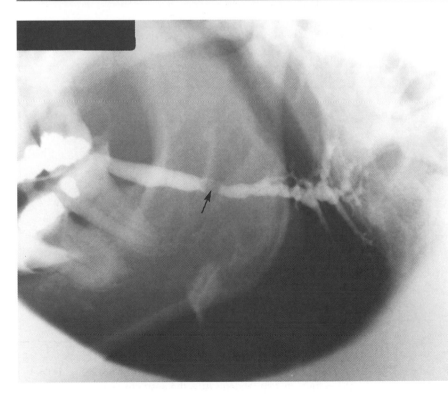

Fig. 2.121 Sialogram showing an obstruction in a dilated parotid duct (arrow). Courtesy of Dr N. Drage.

Sialography

Sialography is the technique whereby the duct systems of the major salivary glands are visualised by injecting an iodine-based contrast medium into the duct orifice (Fig. 2.120). This technique is used to identify obstructions (Fig. 2.121).

Tomographic examination of the temporomandibular articulation

Tomography is a radiographic technique used to study layers within a volume of tissue, in a way analogous to the examination of a single portion of bread within a whole loaf without physically slicing it. The two pictures of the temporomandibular joint illustrated here (Fig. 2.122) represent two layers in this region approximately 0.5 cm apart.

Intraoral radiographic projections of jaws and teeth

Table 2.10 outlines the major intra-oral radiographic projections used to view the human jaws and dentition. In this

Table 2.10 *Intraoral radiographic projections describing jaws and teeth*

Projection/technique	Purpose
Maxillary and mandibular occlusal views of teeth (Fig 2.123–2.125)	Relationship of structures in buccolingual plane
Periapical view of teeth (Fig. 2.126)	Examination of apices of teeth. Relationships of structures in mesiodistal plane
Bitewing examination of teeth (Fig. 2.127)	Survey of crowns of the teeth and the alveolar crests

context, 'intraoral' indicates that the radiographic plate is positioned inside the mouth.

Note that there are two maxillary occlusal views – the vertex approach (Fig. 2.123) and the nasal approach (Fig. 2.124). As the names suggest, these views of the maxilla essentially differ in the positioning of the X-ray tube, which is either to the vertex of the skull or to the nasion. Differences in the radiographic pictures obtained relate to the degree of superimposition (greater in the vertex occlusal) and the direction and proportions of the longitudinal axes of the teeth (more vertical and less distorted roots with the vertex occlusal). In addition to surveying the maxillary dentition, the maxillary occlusal views may also be used to define the nasal fossae and maxillary air sinuses.

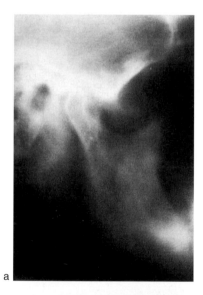
a

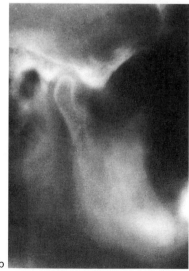
b

Fig. 2.122 Tomographic examination of the temporomandibular articulation. The two images (a and b) are about 0.5 cm apart.

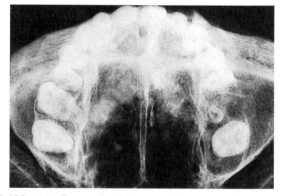

Fig. 2.123 Maxillary occlusal view – vertex approach.

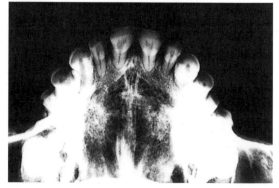

Fig. 2.124 Maxillary occlusal view – nasal approach.

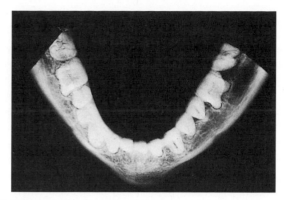

Fig. 2.125 Mandibular occlusal view.

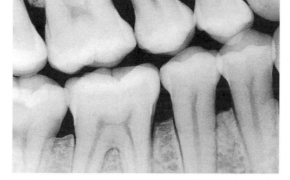

Fig. 2.127 Examination of the crowns of the permanent molars and associated alveolar crests using bitewing radiographs.

Anatomical features seen on intraoral radiographs

The importance of appreciating the radiographic appearance of the teeth and their supporting tissues needs hardly be emphasised. However, equally essential for the interpretation of an apparent divergence from the normal is an awareness of non-dental anatomical structures, which, to the unwary, may simulate pathological lesions on intraoral radiographs. The radio-opacities of normal anatomical structures seen on intraoral radiographs are given in Table 2.11.

The radiographic image of a tooth is illustrated in Fig. 2.128. Tooth substance absorbs more X-rays than any other tissue of comparable size and thickness. Enamel is the most radio-opaque and is easily distinguished covering the anatomical crown of the tooth. In normal teeth, the enamel is of uniform density, though in some areas where the enamel is thin (e.g. the cervical regions) it may appear relatively radiolucent. Such

an appearance may easily be misinterpreted as dental caries. Dentine and cementum cannot be readily distinguished from each other radiographically because of their similar capacity to absorb X-rays. Owing to the lower radio-opacity of dentine, it appears comparatively 'greyer' than the enamel and thus the enamel–dentine junction is clearly demarcated. The pulp of a tooth, being soft tissue, is readily penetrated by X-rays and consequently on a radiograph the pulp cavity is clearly defined as the central radiolucent region of the tooth. However, because of distortion, foreshortening and superimposition, care should be taken in assessing the pulpal anatomy from radiographs. The tooth is supported in the bony alveolus. In this text, the alveolus refers to the whole of the bony supporting tissue of the tooth, and the lamina dura refers to the compact bone lining the tooth socket. The morphology of the

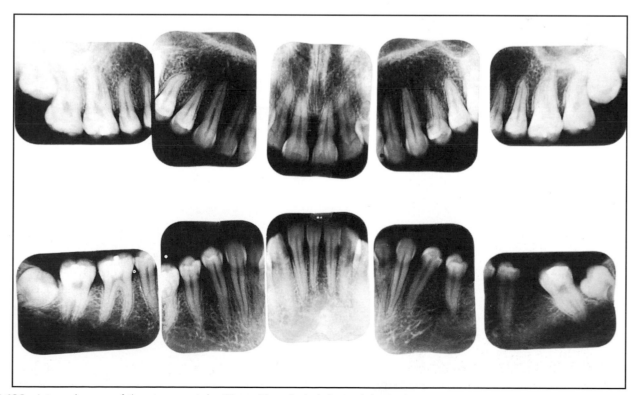

Fig. 2.126 Intraoral survey of the permanent dentition with periapical views of the teeth.

Table 2.11 *Radio-opacity of normal anatomical structures seen on intraoral radiographs*

Radiolucent	Radio-opaque
Dental pulp	Enamel
Gingiva and periodontal ligament	Dentine
Bone marrow	Cementum
	Cortical bony plates
	Lamina dura
Maxillary sinus	Bony walls of maxillary sinus
Nasal cavity	Bony walls of nasal cavity
Incisive foramen	Nasal septum
Median palatine suture	Anterior nasal spine
Intermaxillary suture	Maxillary tuberosity
Nasolacrimal canal	Zygomatic arch
	Coronoid process
Mandibular canal	Pterygoid hamulus
	Internal and external oblique lines of mandible
Mental foramen	Borders of mandibular canal
Mandibular symphysis	Mental and canine prominences
	Genial tubercles
Bony depressions (e.g. mental and submandibular fossa)	
Nutrient canals	

considered to be a very important structure in the radiographic interpretation of periodontal and periapical pathologies. It appears as a continuous radio-opaque lining of the socket and usually is continuous over the alveolar crests. However, the radio-opacity of the lamina dura does not indicate any hypermineralisation, being a consequence of superimposition. Discontinuity of the lamina dura in the root region is usually indicative of abnormality or disease. Between the root of the tooth and the lamina dura of the socket is the connective tissue of the periodontal ligament, which appears as a thin radiolucent region. Fig. 2.129 shows the appearance of developing and erupting teeth (molars and premolars) where there are radiolucent regions around the emerging crowns and around the developing root apices.

With respect to anatomical structures that appear in association with the maxillary dentition, Fig. 2.130 describes some radiolucent, anatomical features seen on an intraoral maxillary occlusal oblique view – i.e. the maxillary air sinus, the incisive foramen, the nasolacrimal canal and the nasal fossae. Fig. 2.131 shows how the incisive foramen and the nasal fossae can be seen on an intraoral periapical view of the maxillary central incisors. The medial palatine suture seen on an intraoral periapical view of the maxillary central incisors is

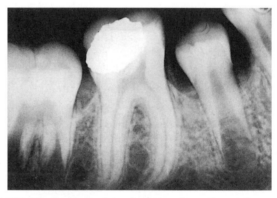

Fig. 2.129 Radiograph of developing and erupting molars and premolars.

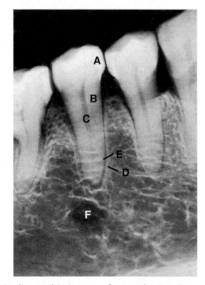

Fig. 2.128 Radiographic image of a tooth. A = Enamel; B = dentine; C = dental pulp; D = lamina dura; E = periodontal space; F = mental foramen.

margins of the alveolus (alveolar crest) is important in the diagnosis of periodontal disease. As a general rule, the width of the crest depends upon the distance the teeth are separated. Consequently, between the molars the crests are flat and horizontal, while between the incisors the crests rise only as points or spines. In the healthy situation, the crest rises to the level of the cemento-enamel junction. The lamina dura is

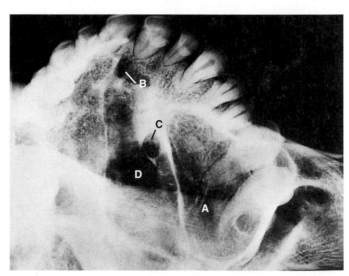

Fig. 2.130 Radiolucent, anatomical features seen on an intraoral maxillary occlusal oblique view. A = Maxillary antrum; B = incisive foramen; C = nasolacrimal canal; D = nasal fossa.

illustrated in Fig. 2.132. The malar (zygomatic) shadow viewed on an intraoral periapical view of the maxillary molars is seen in Fig. 2.133, and Fig. 2.134 shows the radio-opaque shadow cast by a coronoid process of the mandible superimposed on a maxillary tuberosity. In Fig. 2.135 the shadows of the pterygoid plates and pterygoid hamulus of the sphenoid bone near the maxillary tuberosity are shown.

Of particular importance in the upper jaw is the appearance of the maxillary air sinus or antrum. The floor of the sinus viewed on an intraoral periapical view of the maxillary pre-molars and molars is shown in Fig. 2.136. The maxillary antrum or sinus is an air-filled cavity of varying dimensions; it appears radiographically as a dark, radiolucent shadow bounded by radio-opaque lines representing the lining layers of cortical bone. The radiolucency is not usually uniform because of superimposition of the zygomatic process and the soft tissues of the cheek. The antrum often presents not as a single sinus but as several compartments due to bony septation. It is said that the cortical lining of the antrum is not continuous but exhibits numerous, small, linear interruptions associated with nutrient canals (Fig. 2.137). This radiographic charac-teristic may be important in avoiding misinterpretation of the sinus as a pathological lesion. The floor of the antrum is closely related to the root apices of the maxillary teeth. Generally, the sinus extends from the premolars to the tuberosity, though variations are frequent. Because of the close relationship of the teeth to the antrum, communication between the antrum and the oral cavity (oroantral fistula) following tooth extrac-tions is unfortunately all too frequent. Because of the problems of interpreting three-dimensional situations on a two-dimensional radiograph, care must be taken to avoid misreading the relation-ship of the teeth to the antrum. Fig. 2.138 shows the maxillary antrum seen on an intraoral view of an edentulous maxillary tuberosity and Fig. 2.139 illustrates the configuration termed the 'Y of Ennis' that is formed by the abutment of the anterior wall of the antrum and the floor of the nasal fossa.

With respect to anatomical structures that appear in associ-ation with the mandibular dentition, of particular importance is the radiographic appearance of the mandibular canal. The mandibular canal in the region of the mandibular third molar tooth is shown in Fig. 2.140. The mandibular canal com-mences at the mandibular foramen and passes downwards and forwards from the ramus into the body of the mandible where, near the root apices of the premolars, it terminates by dividing into the mental and incisive canals. The radiographic appearance of the mandibular canal is generally that of a radiolucent shadow bounded superiorly and inferiorly by radio-opaque lines. The width and position of the canal varies considerably. Most commonly, it is closely related to the roots of the molars, though it lies some distance from the roots of the premolars. Generally, the canal lies buccal to the root apices, a feature that should be remembered when inter-preting the relationship of the root apices to the canal. The precise relationship of the teeth to the canal is difficult to determine from radiographs, although some hint of a very close relationship can be obtained by reference to the densities of shadows cast by the roots and canal, the position and densities of the lamina dura and the radio-opaque margins of the canal, and the dimensions of the lumen of the canal. The appearance of the mental foramen near the apices of the mandibular premolars is shown in Fig. 2.141.

The mandibular symphysis at birth is shown on an intraoral mandibular occlusal radiograph in Fig. 2.142. This symphysis closes by the age of 3 years. Fig. 2.143 illustrates the genial tubercles (mental spines) seen on an intraoral peri-apical view of the mandibular central incisors. Note the characteristic radiographic appearance of the tubercles (i.e. a radiolucent dot surrounded by a distinct radio-opaque region). The internal and external oblique lines of the mandible are seen in Fig. 2.144, where an occlusal view of an edentulous man-dible demonstrates the prominent radio-opacities associated with these lines.

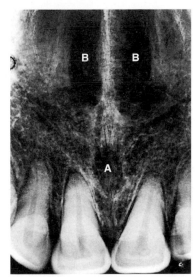

Fig. 2.131 The incisive foramen (A) and nasal fossae (B) seen on an intraoral periapical view of the maxillary central incisors.

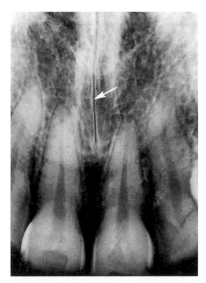

Fig. 2.132 The median palatine suture (arrowed) seen on an intraoral periapical view of the maxillary central incisors.

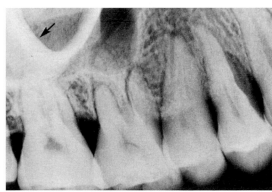

Fig. 2.133 Malar (zygomatic) shadow (arrowed).

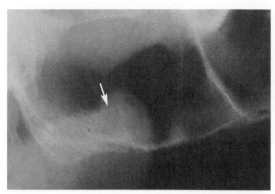

Fig. 2.134 Radio-opaque shadow cast by a coronoid process (arrowed).

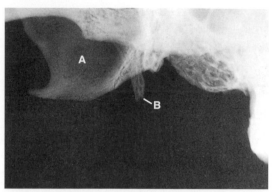

Fig. 2.135 Shadows of the pterygoid plates (A) and pterygoid hamulus (B) near the maxillary tuberosity.

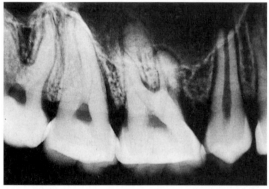

Fig. 2.136 The floor of the maxillary antrum seen on an intraoral periapical view of the maxillary premolars and molars.

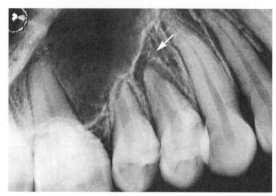

Fig. 2.137 Nutrient canals (arrowed) in the walls of the maxillary antrum.

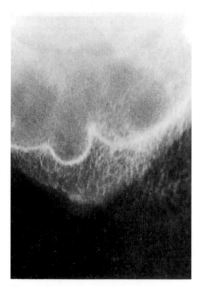

Fig. 2.138 The maxillary antrum seen on an intraoral view of an edentulous maxillary tuberosity.

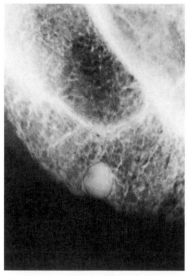

Fig. 2.139 The configuration termed the Y of Ennis.

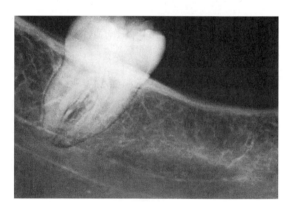

Fig. 2.140 Mandibular canal.

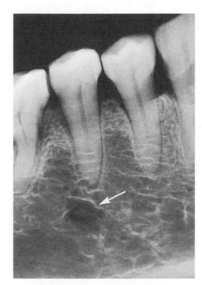

Fig. 2.141   Mental foramen (arrowed).

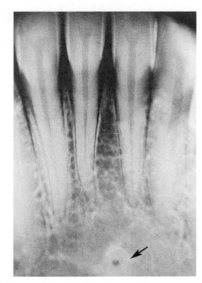

Fig. 2.143   The genial tubercles (arrowed).

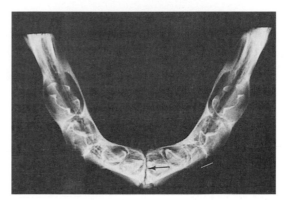

Fig. 2.142   The mandibular symphysis (arrowed) at birth.

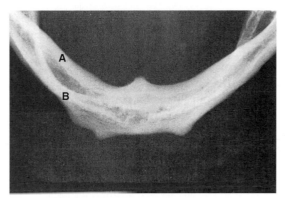

Fig. 2.144   Internal (A) and external (B) oblique lines of the mandible.

3 The regional topography of the mouth and related areas

This chapter considers aspects of the gross anatomy of orodental regions, principally the temporomandibular joint, the muscles, innervation and blood vessels of the mouth, jaws, face and oral cavity, the glands of the oral cavity, the tissue spaces around the jaws and the sectional anatomy of the oral cavity. In addition, aspects of the functional anatomy of mastication, swallowing and speech will be introduced.

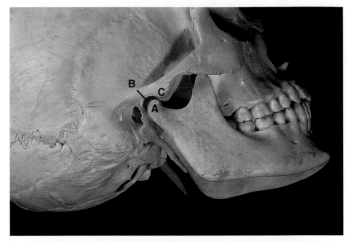

Fig. 3.1 The osteology of the temporomandibular joint. A = Mandibular condyle; B = mandibular fossa of temporal bone; C = articular eminence of temporal bone.

THE TEMPOROMANDIBULAR JOINT

The temporomandibular joint (TMJ) is the synovial articulation between the mandible and the cranium. For this reason, the joint is sometimes referred to as the craniomandibular joint. It is formed by the condylar process of the mandible articulating in the mandibular (glenoid) fossa of the temporal bone (Fig. 3.1). The TMJ, although basically a hinge joint, also allows for some gliding movements. Movement of the condylar head occurs within the mandibular fossa and down a bony prominence immediately anterior to the mandibular fossa, the articular tubercle (eminence) of the temporal bone. That there are two TMJs associated with a single mandible has considerable functional significance in that movement at one joint is accompanied by movement at the other.

As a synovial joint, the TMJ has two unusual features. First, the articular surfaces of the joint are covered with fibrous tissue (instead of the usual hyaline cartilage), which relates to the fact that the bony parts forming the joint develop

intramembranously (rather than endochondrally). Second, the joint cavity is divided into two joint spaces by an intra-articular disc. The histology of the TMJ is considered in Chapter 15.

The mandibular fossa

The mandibular fossa (Fig. 3.2) is an oval depression in the temporal bone, lying immediately anterior to the external

Fig. 3.2 The osteology of the mandibular fossa. A = Mandibular fossa; B = external acoustic meatus; C = articular eminence; D = zygomatic process of temporal bone; E = tympanic plate; F = petrosquamous fissure; G = petrotympanic fissure; H = squamotympanic fissure.

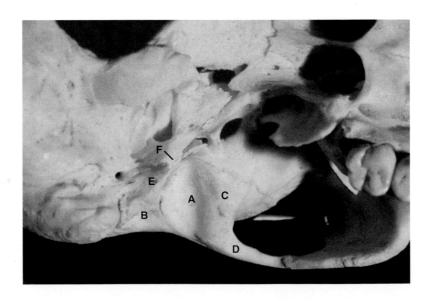

acoustic meatus. Its mediolateral dimension is greater than its anteroposterior one in order to accommodate the mandibular condyle, and it is wider laterally than medially. The curvature of the mandibular fossa varies and may show some relationship to the nature of the occlusion. The mandibular fossa is bounded anteriorly by the articular tubercle, laterally by the zygomatic process, and posteriorly by the tympanic plate. The posterior margin is elevated to form the posterior auricular ridge, which may be enlarged laterally as the postglenoid tubercle just anterior to the external auditory meatus. Medially, the mandibular fossa may be defined by a ridge, the medial glenoid plane. The squamous and tympanic parts of the temporal bone are delineated laterally by the squamotympanic fissure. This fissure bifurcates medially due to the presence of a small component of the petrous portion, the tegmen tympani, giving rise to the petrosquamous fissure anteriorly and the petrotympanic fissure immediately behind. The petrotympanic fissure is the site at which the chorda tympani nerve exits from the cranium into the infratemporal fossa.

The shape of the mandibular fossa does not exactly conform to the shape of the mandibular condyle, the intra-articular disc moulding together the joint surfaces. The bone of the central part of the fossa is thin. This indicates that masticatory loads are not dissipated through the mandibular fossa but through the teeth and thence the facial bones and base of the cranium.

The mandibular condyle

The size and shape of the mandibular condyle varies considerably in both size and shape (Figs 3.3, 3.4). When viewed from above, the condyle is roughly ovoid in outline, the anteroposterior dimension (approximately 1 cm) being about half the mediolateral dimension. The medial aspect is wider than the lateral. The long axis of the condyle is not, however, at right angles to the ramus, but diverges posteriorly from a strictly coronal plane. Thus the lateral pole of the condyle lies slightly anterior to the medial pole – if the long axes of the two condyles were extended, they would meet at an obtuse angle of approximately 145° at the anterior border of the foramen magnum. The convex anterior and superior surfaces of the head of the condyle are the articular surfaces. The articular surface area of the condyle is of the order of 200 mm², which is about half that of the mandibular fossa. The non-articular posterior surface of the condyle is broad and flat. The articular surface may be separated from the non-articular surface by a slight ridge, indicating the site of attachment of the joint capsule. The broad articular head of the condyle joins the ramus through a thin bony projection termed the neck of the condyle. A small depression, the pterygoid fovea, marks part of the attachment of the inferior head of the lateral pterygoid muscle and is situated on the anterior part of the neck below the articular surface of the condyle.

Capsule

The capsule of the TMJ is a thin, slack cuff that does not limit mandibular movements and is too weak to provide much

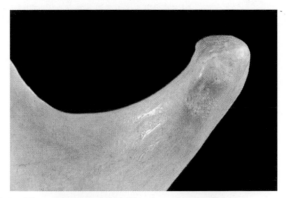

Fig. 3.3   The mandibular condyle viewed laterally.

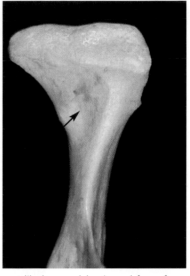

Fig. 3.4   The mandibular condyle viewed from from above. The pterygoid fovea is arrowed.

support for the joint (Fig. 3.5). Above, it is attached to the mandibular fossa, extending anteriorly to just in front of the crest of the articular eminence, posteriorly to the squamotympanic and petrotympanic fissures, medially to the medial glenoid plane and laterally between the lateral margin of the articular eminence and the postglenoid process. Below, it is attached to the neck of the condyle of the mandible. Posteriorly, the capsule is associated with the thick, vascular, but loosely arranged connective tissue of the bilaminar zone of the intra-articular disc (the retrodiscal pad). Internally, it is attached to the intra-articular disc and is lined by synovial membrane. The collagen fibres of the capsule run predominantly in a vertical direction. The capsule is richly innervated.

The synovial membrane lines the inner surface of the fibrous capsule and the margins of the intra-articular disc, but does not cover the articular surfaces of the joint. The synovial membrane secretes the synovial fluid that occupies the joint cavities, lubricates the joint and presumably also has nutritive functions. Important components of the synovial fluid are the proteoglycans, which aid the lubrication. At rest, the hydrostatic pressure of the synovial fluid has been reported as being subatmospheric, but this is greatly elevated during mastication.

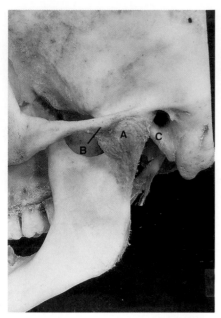

Fig. 3.5 The capsule of the temporomandibular joint (A). B = articular eminence; C = tympanic plate. Courtesy of Professor C. Dean.

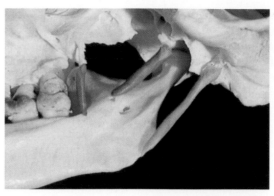

Fig. 3.6 Model showing accessory ligaments associated with the temporomandibular joint. Yellow = stylomandibular ligament; red = pterygomandibular raphe; green = spenomandibular ligament.

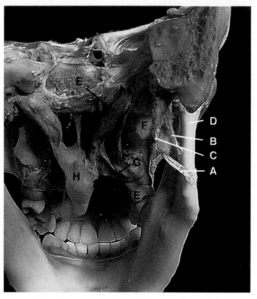

Fig. 3.7 Posterior view of the jaw apparatus showing the stylomandibular (A) and sphenomandibular (B) ligaments. C = Styloid process; D = posterior border of ramus of mandible; E = levator palati muscle; F = tensor palati muscle; G = pterygoid hamulus; H = soft palate. Courtesy of the Museums of the Royal College of Surgeons of England.

Temporomandibular ligament

The joint capsule is strengthened by the temporomandibular (lateral) ligament (Fig. 3.6). This ligament cannot be readily separated from the capsule. It takes origin from the lateral surface of the articular eminence of the temporal bone and inserts onto the posterior surface of the condyle. This ligament provides the main means of support for the joint, restricting distal and inferior movements of the mandible and resisting dislocation during functional movements. The temporomandibular ligament is reinforced by a horizontal band of fibres running from the articular eminence to the lateral surface of the condyle. These horizontal fibres restrict posterior movement of the condyle. The temporomandibular ligament is believed also to convert the potentially separating forces generated by the muscles opening the jaws into a force that compresses the condyle of the mandible onto the articular eminence. There is little evidence of any comparable ligament on the medial aspect of the joint capsule, so medial displacement is likely to be prevented by the lateral ligament of the opposite side.

Accessory ligaments

The accessory ligaments of the temporomandibular joint traditionally described are the stylomandibular ligament, the sphenomandibular ligament and the pterygomandibular raphe (Figs 3.6, 3.7). However, only the sphenomandibular ligament is likely to have any significant influence upon mandibular movements.

The sphenomandibular ligament is a remnant of the perichondrium of Meckel's cartilage (the cartilage of the embryonic first branchial arch; see page 284) and extends from the spine of the sphenoid bone to the lingula near the mandibular foramen. The sphenomandibular ligament is slack when the jaws are closed, but becomes tense at about the time when the condyle has passed in front of the temporomandibular ligament.

The stylomandibular ligament is a reinforced lamina of the deep cervical fascia as it passes medially to the parotid salivary gland. It extends from the top of the styloid process of the temporal bone and from the stylohyoid ligament to the angle of the mandible.

The pterygomandibular raphe (from which the buccinator and superior constrictor muscles arise) extends from the pterygoid hamulus to the posterior end of the mylohyoid line in the retromolar region of the mandible.

Recently, a new ligament has been described in association with the temporomandibular joint. This is the retinacular ligament. This arises from the articular eminence, descends along the ramus of the mandible and inserts into the fascia overlying the masseter muscle at the angle of the mandible. As this ligament is connected with the posterolateral aspect of the retrodiscal tissues, and contains an accompanying vein, it may function in maintaining blood circulation during masticatory movements.

Intra-articular disc

The intra-articular disc (meniscus) is of a dense, fibrous consistency and is moulded to the bony joint surfaces above and below (Figs 3.8–3.10). Blood vessels are evident only at the periphery of the intra-articular disc, the bulk of it being avascular. Above, the disc covers the slope of the articular eminence in front while below it covers the condyle. When viewed in sagittal section the upper surface of the disc is concavo-convex from front to back and the lower surface is concave. Viewed superiorly, the disc is somewhat rectangular or oval in outline. The disc is of variable thickness, being thinnest centrally over the articular surface of the mandibular condyle and thickest posteriorly in the region above and behind the mandibular condyle. The lateral half of the disc is thinner than the medial half. The medial and lateral margins of the disc are slightly thickened.

The intra-articular disc has been subdivided into three portions: anterior, intermediate and posterior (Fig. 3.8). The intermediate zone is the thinnest and is the area in contact with the intra-articular surface of the condyle. In the intermediate part the collagen bundles have been described as running preferentially in an anteroposterior direction, while in the anterior and posterior bands they run both anteroposterior and mediolaterally. The overall shape of the intraarticular disc is thought to provide a self-centering mechanism, which automatically acts to maintain its correct relationship to the articular surface of the mandibular condyle during mandibular movements.

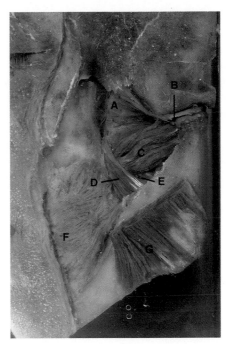

Fig. 3.9 Dissection showing the fibres of the upper head of the lateral pterygoid muscle (A) attaching to the intra-articular disc (B) of the temporomandibular joint. C = fibres of the lower head of the lateral pterygoid muscle inserting into the pterygoid fovea of the mandibular condyle; D = superficial head of medial pterygoid muscle; E = deep head of medial pterygoid muscle; F = buccinator muscle; G = cut edge of masseter muscle. Courtesy of Professor L. Garey.

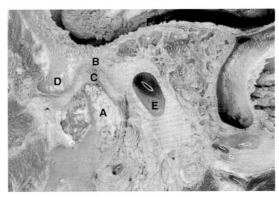

Fig. 3.10 Sagittal section of head showing the intra-articular disc (C). A = Mandibular condyle; B = mandibular fossa; D = articular eminence; E = external acoustic meatus; F = floor of middle cranial fossa.

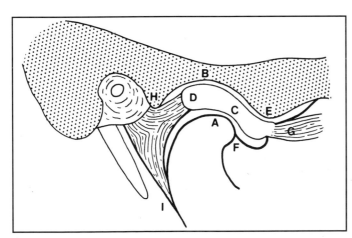

Fig. 3.8 Diagrammatic representation of the intra-articular disc. A = Mandibular condyle; B = mandibular fossa; C = central part of intra-articular disc; D = posterior part of intra-articular disc; E = articular eminence; F = attachment of anterior part of intra-articular disc to anterior margin of mandibular condyle; G = lateral pterygoid muscle; H = attachment of upper part of bilaminar zone; I = attachment of the lower part of the bilaminar zone.

The margin of the intra-articular disc merges peripherally with the joint capsule. Anteriorly, fibrous bands connect the disc to the anterior margin of the articular eminence above and to the anterior margin of the condyle below. Medially and laterally the disc is attached to the joint capsule and just below the medial and lateral poles of the condyle by triangular zones of connective tissue. Posteriorly, it is attached to the capsule by a bilaminar zone (retrodiscal tissue/pad – also page 252). The superior lamina is loose and possesses numerous vascular elements and elastin fibres. It attaches to the anterior margin of the squamotympanic fissure. The inferior lamina is relatively avascular, less extensible (as it has few elastin fibres) and is attached to the posterior margin of the condyle). The volume of the retrodiscal tissue appears to increase about five times as a result of venous engorgement, due to their continuity with the pterygoid venous plexus lying medial to the condyle. This activity fills the vacated space in the mandibular fossa and rapidly equilibrates any changes in intracapsular pressures that may hinder jaw movement. Changes in tissue fluid pressure during mandibular movements could also help regulate the flow of blood in the retrodiscal pad. As the mandibular condyle moves backwards during jaw closure, blood leaves the retrodiscal tissues. The close relationship of elastin fibres to the walls of blood vessels in the retrodiscal tissues has led to the view that the fibres function as a pump, facilitating blood flow during venous dilatation and compression.

The return of the intra-articular disc to its original position may be aided by the elastic recoil of the superior lamella. The return could be passive, due to the shape of the disc and its firm insertion to the lateral and medial poles of the condyle of the mandible; there is also evidence that the superior head of the lateral pterygoid is active only on final closure.

The intra-articular disc divides the temporomandibular joint cavity into superior and inferior joint cavities. About 1 ml of synovial fluid occupies the inferior joint cavity, while a little more occupies the superior joint cavity.

Although some regard the functions of the intra-articular disc as helping to spread the joint forces and stabilising the condyle, others see it as primarily destabilising the condyle and permitting it to move more freely.

Apart from being prone to disorders affecting other synovial joints, such as arthritis, the temporomandibular joint is the site for the condition referred to as internal derangement. In internal derangement the intra-articular disc is displaced usually in an anteromedial direction (Fig. 3.11). This may result in pain and/clicking of the joint and restrictions of jaw movements.

Nerves of the TMJ

The temporomandibular joint is richly innervated. Of particular importance in this context are the proprioceptive nerve endings important in the reflex control of mastication. Free nerve endings associated with nociception are also present. Innervation for the joint is provided by the auriculotemporal, masseteric and deep temporal nerves of the mandibular division of the trigeminal nerve.

THE MUSCLES OF MASTICATION

Although many muscles, both in the head and the neck, are involved in mastication, the 'muscles of mastication' is a collective term reserved for the masseter, temporalis and medial and lateral pterygoid muscles. All the muscles of mastication develop from the mesenchyme of the first branchial arch. They therefore receive their innervation from the mandibular branch of the trigeminal nerve. Closely associated

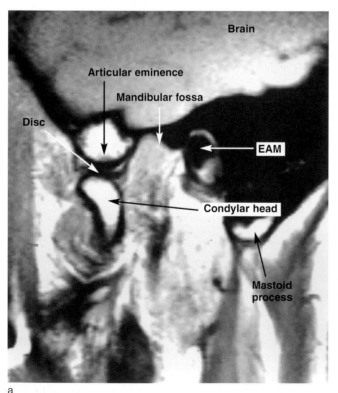
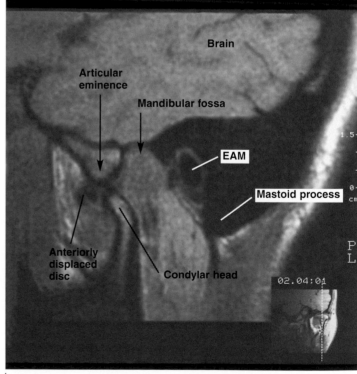

a   b

Fig. 3.11 (a) MRI showing normal position of intra-articular disc with the jaw in the open position; (b) MRI showing anterior displacement of disc (internal derangement) with the jaw in the open position. EAM = External acoustic meatus. Courtesy of Dr N. Drage.

functionally and developmentally with the muscles of mastication is the digastric muscle. The masseter and temporalis muscles lie on the superficial face, while the lateral and medial pterygoid muscles lie deeper within the infratemporal fossa.

Masseter

The masseter muscle consists of two overlapping heads (Fig. 3.12). The superficial head arises from the zygomatic process of the maxilla and from the anterior two-thirds of the lower border of the zygomatic arch. The deep head arises from the deep surface of the zygomatic arch. Internally, the muscle has many tendinous septa that greatly increase the area for muscle attachment and which provide a multipennate arrangement, thereby increasing its power. The superficial head passes downwards and backwards to insert into the lower half of the lateral surface of the ramus. The deep head, whose posterior fibres are more vertically oriented, inserts into the upper half of the lateral surface of the ramus, particularly over the coronoid process. The muscle elevates the mandible and is primarily active when grinding tough food. Indeed, the muscle exerts considerable power when the mandible is close to the centric occlusal position. On the basis of its fibre orientation, the posterior fibres of the deep head may have some retrusive capability for the mandible.

Temporalis

The temporalis muscle is the largest muscle of mastication. It takes origin from the floor of the temporal fossa of the lateral surface of the skull and from the overlying temporal fascia, and should thus be regarded as a bipennate muscle. The attachment is limited above by the inferior temporal line. From this wide origin, the fibres converge towards their insertion on the apex, the anterior and posterior borders, and the medial surface of the coronoid process (Fig. 3.13). Indeed, the insertion extends down the anterior border of the ramus almost as far as

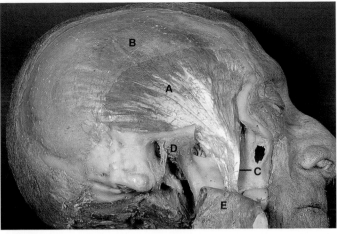

Fig. 3.13 The temporalis muscle (A) arising in part from the overlying temporal fascia (B) and inserting into the coronoid process (C) of the mandible. D = Mandibular condyle; E = deep surface of masseter muscle revealed following refection of the zygomatic arch.

the third molar tooth. The posterior fibres of the muscle pass horizontally forwards while the anterior fibres pass vertically downwards onto the coronoid process. To reach the coronoid process, the muscle runs beneath the zygomatic arch. The anterior (vertical) part elevates the mandible, while the posterior horizontal part retracts the protruded mandible. In certain sites, the masseter and temporalis muscles are joined. This is particularly so for the deep fibres of the deep head of the masseter and the overlying temporalis muscle. The functional significance of this 'zygomatico-mandibular mass' is unclear.

Both the masseter and the temporalis muscles are innervated by branches of the anterior division of the mandibular nerve (see page 84). Both receive their blood supply from the maxillary artery (masseteric and deep temporal branches), the superficial temporal artery (transverse facial and middle temporal branches) and, for the masseter muscle, the facial artery.

Pterygoids

In order to fully appreciate the anatomy of the pterygoid muscles, an understanding of the osteology of the infratemporal fossa is required as both muscles arise from bony landmarks within this fossa. The reader is therefore referred to page 71 and Fig. 3.30.

Lateral pterygoid

The lateral pterygoid muscle lies in the roof of the infratemporal fossa and has essentially a horizontal alignment. It has two heads, superior and inferior (Figs 3.14–3.16). The superior (upper) head is the smaller and arises from the infratemporal surface of the greater wing of the sphenoid bone (see page 71). The inferior (lower) head forms the bulk of the muscle and takes origin from the lateral surface of the lateral pterygoid plate of the sphenoid bone (see page 71). Both heads pass backwards and outwards and appear to merge before their areas of insertion. The fibres of the superior head insert into the capsule and possibly the medial aspect of

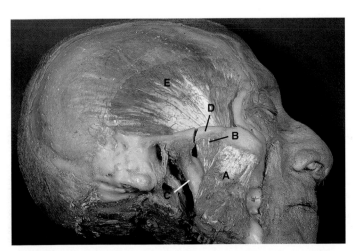

Fig. 3.12 The masseter muscle showing superficial (A) and deep (B) heads. C = Posterior border of ramus of mandible; D = zygomatic arch; E = temporalis muscle.

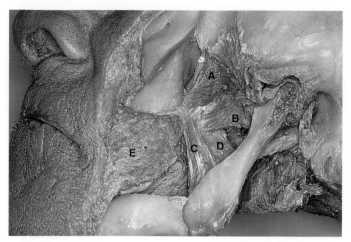

Fig. 3.14 Lateral view of the pterygoid muscles. A = Upper head of lateral pterygoid; B = lower head of lateral pterygoid; C = superficial head of medial pterygoid; D = deep head of lateral pterygoid; E = buccinator muscle.

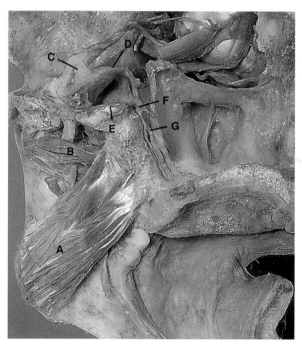

Fig. 3.15 Medial view of pterygoid muscles (A) in the infratemporal fossa. B = Lateral pterygoid muscle; C = trigeminal ganglion; D = maxillary nerve; E = nerve of pterygoid canal; F = pterygopalatine ganglion; G = greater and lesser palatine nerves. Courtesy of Professor L. Garey.

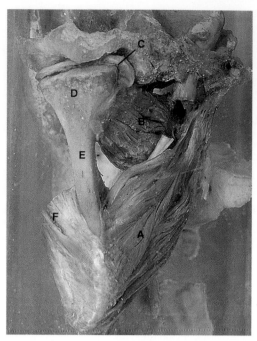

Fig. 3.16 Posterior view of the medial (A) and lateral (B) pterygoid muscles. C = Intra-articular disc of TMJ; D = mandibular condyle; E = posterior border of ramus of mandible; F = cut edge of masseter muscle. Courtesy of Professor L. Garey.

the anterior border of the intra-articular disc of the TMJ. The fibres of the inferior head of the lateral pterygoid muscle insert into the pterygoid fovea of the mandibular condyle. However, the precise insertions of the muscle are still controversial and have clinical relevance with regard to TMJ disorders, particularly internal derangement, where the disc is displaced usually in an anteromedial position and the jaw may become locked (Fig. 3.11). Such conditions may be associated with clicking joints, limited jaw movements and pain and some have attributed variations in the attachment, and therefore function, of the superior head as an aetiological factor in the

disease. Functionally, the superior and inferior heads should be considered as two separate muscles. The inferior head is concerned with mandibular protrusion, depression and lateral excursions. The superior head is activated during mandibular retrusion (providing controlled movements) and during clenching of the mandible.

Medial pterygoid

The medial pterygoid muscle consists of two heads (Figs 3.14–3.16). The bulk of the muscle arises as a deep head from the medial surface of the lateral pterygoid plate of the sphenoid bone (see page 71). The smaller superficial head arises from the maxillary tuberosity and the neighbouring part of the palatine bone (pyramidal process). From these sites of origin, the fibres of the medial pterygoid pass downwards, backwards and laterally to insert into the roughened surface of the medial aspect of the angle of the mandible. Tendinous septa within the muscle increase the surface area for muscle attachment, providing a multipennate arrangement and therefore increasing the power the muscle can exert. The main action of the muscle is to elevate the mandible but it also assists in lateral and protrusive movements. An accessory medial pterygoid muscle has been described as a separate slip of muscle close to the deep surface of the medial pterygoid. This takes origin from the base of the skull close to the foramen ovale and merges with the deep head of the medial pterygoid. Its function is unknown. The masseter and medial pterygoid muscles together form a muscular sling that supports the mandible on the cranium.

The medial pterygoid muscle is innervated by a branch of the mandibular nerve that arises proximal to the division of the mandibular nerve into anterior and posterior trunks

Fig. 3.17 The digastic muscle.
A = Posterior belly; B = tendon of digastric;
C = stylohyoid muscle splitting around
digastric tendon; D = anterior belly of
digastric; E = mylohyoid muscle.

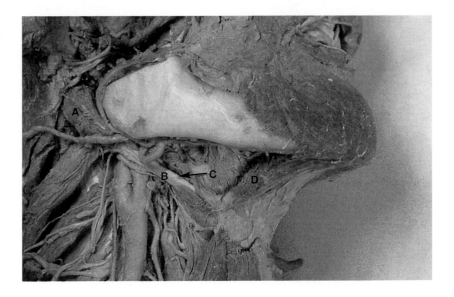

(see Fig. 4.17). The lateral pterygoid receives its nerve supply from the anterior trunk. Both muscles receive their blood supply as muscular branches from the maxillary artery.

Digastric

Because of its functional associations, the digastric muscle is described here although it usually is not strictly classified as a 'muscle of mastication'. This muscle is located below the inferior border of the mandible and consists of an anterior and a posterior belly connected by an intermediate tendon (Fig. 3.17). The posterior belly arises from the mastoid notch immediately behind the mastoid process of the temporal bone; it passes downwards and forwards towards the hyoid bone, where it becomes the digastric tendon. The digastric muscle passes through the insertion of the stylohyoid muscle and is attached to the greater horn of the hyoid bone by a fibrous loop. The anterior belly of the digastric muscle is attached to the digastric fossa on the inferior border of the mandible and runs downwards and backwards to the digastric tendon. The digastric muscle depresses and retrudes the mandible, and is involved in stabilising the position of the hyoid bone and in elevation of the hyoid during swallowing.

The anterior belly of the digastric muscle is innervated by the mylohyoid branch of the mandibular division of the trigeminal nerve, the posterior belly by the digastric branch of the facial nerve. This reflects different embryological origins, from first and second branchial arch mesenchyme respectively. The anterior belly receives its blood supply from the facial artery, the posterior belly from the posterior auricular and occipital arteries.

THE MUSCLES OF THE SOFT PALATE

The soft palate is supported by the fibrous palatine aponeurosis whose shape and position is altered by the activity of four pairs of muscles: the tensor veli palatini, the levator veli palatini, the

palatoglossus and the palatopharyngeus muscles. In addition, there is the musculus uvulae.

Tensor veli palatini

The tensor veli palatini muscle (Figs 3.18, 3.19) arises from the scaphoid fossa of the sphenoid bone at the root of the pterygoid plates and from the lateral side of the cartilaginous part of the auditory (pharyngotympanic) tube. From its origin, the fibres converge towards the pterygoid hamulus, whence the muscle becomes tendinous, the tendon bending at right angles around the hamulus to become the palatine aponeurosis. The anterior border of the aponeurosis is attached to the posterior border of the hard palate. Medially, it merges with the aponeurosis of the other side. Posteriorly, it becomes indistinct, merging with submucosa at the posterior edge of the soft palate. When the tensor veli palatini muscle contracts, the aponeurosis

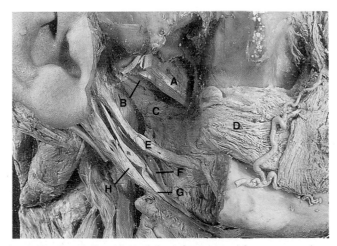

Fig. 3.18 Deep dissection of the infratemporal fossa to reveal tensor veli palatini muscle (A). B = Partially obscured levator palati muscle; C = superior constrictor muscle; D = buccinator muscle; E = styloglossus muscle; F = stylopharyngeus muscle; G = stylohyoid muscle; H = posterior belly of digastric muscle. Courtesy of Professor C. Dean.

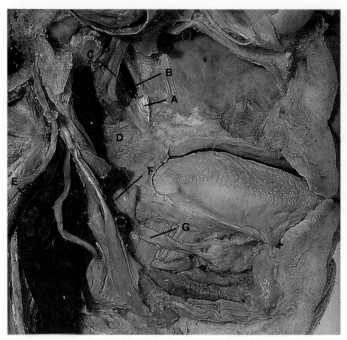

Fig. 3.19 Deep dissection of the infratemporal fossa with the tensor palati muscle (A) cut to reveal the levator palati muscle (B). C = Mandibular nerve; D = superior constrictor; E = internal carotid artery; F = styloglossus muscle; G = lingual nerve on hyoglossus muscle; H = sublingual gland. Courtesy of Professor L. Garey.

becomes a taut, horizontal plate of tissue upon which other palatine muscles may act to change its position.

The motor innervation of the tensor veli palatini is derived from the mandibular branch of the trigeminal nerve (via the nerve to the medial pterygoid muscle and the otic ganglion).

Levator veli palatini

The levator veli palatini muscle (Figs 3.18, 3.19; see also Fig.

3.24) originates from the base of the skull at the apex of the petrous part of the temporal bone, anterior to the opening of the carotid canal, and from the medial side of the cartilaginous part of the auditory tube. The muscle curves downwards, medially and forwards to enter the palate immediately below the opening of the auditory tube.

The levator muscles of the palate form a U-shaped muscular sling. When the palatine aponeurosis is stiffened by the tensor muscles, contraction of the levator muscles produces an upwards and backwards movement of the soft palate. In this way, the nasopharynx is shut off from the oropharynx by the apposition of the soft palate onto the posterior wall of the pharynx.

Palatopharyngeus

The palatopharyngeus muscle arises from two heads: one from the posterior border of the hard palate, the other from the upper surface of the palatine aponeurosis (Fig. 3.20). The two heads unite after arching over the lateral edge of the palatine aponeurosis, where the muscle passes downwards beneath the mucous membrane of the lateral wall of the oropharynx as the posterior pillar of the fauces (palatopharyngeal arch; see page 4). The muscle is inserted into the posterior border of the thyroid cartilage of the larynx. The main action of the palatopharyngeus muscle is to elevate the larynx and pharynx, but it may also arch the relaxed palate and depress the tensed palate.

Palatoglossus

The palatoglossus muscle arises from the aponeurosis of the soft palate and descends to the tongue in the anterior pillar of the fauces (see page 4), whence its fibres intercalate with the transverse fibres of the tongue (Fig. 3.20). The action of the palatoglossus is to raise the tongue in order to narrow the transverse diameter of the oropharyngeal isthmus.

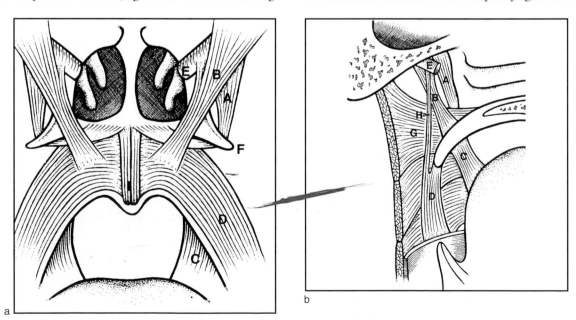

Fig. 3.20 Diagrammatic representation of palatal and pharyngeal muscles. (a) Posterior view; (b) medial view. A = Tensor veli palatini; B = levator veli palatini; C = palatoglossus; D = palatopharyngeus; E = auditory (pharyngotympanic or Eustachian) tube; F = pterygoid hamulus; G = superior constrictor muscle; H = salpingopharyngeus muscle; I = musculus uvulae.

Musculus uvulae

The musculus uvulae (Fig. 3.20) arises from the posterior nasal spine at the back of the hard palate and from the palatine aponeurosis. It passes backwards and downwards to insert into the mucosa of the uvula. It moves the uvula upwards and laterally and helps to complete the seal between the soft palate and pharynx in the midline region when the palate is elevated.

Nerve and blood supply

With the exception of the tensor veli palatini muscle, the nerve supply to the muscles of the palate is derived from the cranial part of the accessory nerve via the pharyngeal plexus.

The arterial supply to the muscles of the soft palate is derived from the facial artery (ascending palatine branch), the ascending pharyngeal artery and the maxillary artery (palatine branches).

Passavant's muscle

Passavant's muscle is a sphincter-like muscle that encircles the pharynx at the level of the palate, inside the fibres of the superior constrictor muscles. It is formed by fibres arising from the anterior and lateral part of the upper surface of the palatine aponeurosis. Contraction of this muscle forms a ridge (Passavant's ridge), against which the soft palate is elevated.

THE MUSCLES OF THE TONGUE

The tongue is composed of intrinsic and extrinsic muscles. The intrinsic muscles are restricted to the substance of the tongue and change its shape, while the extrinsic muscles arise outside the tongue and are responsible for bodily movement of the tongue.

Intrinsic muscles

The intrinsic muscles of the tongue can be divided into three fibre groups: transverse, longitudinal and vertical. Rarely can these three groups be distinguished in dissections, but their interlacing gives the tongue its characteristic appearance in cross section (Fig. 3.21). The transverse fibres arise from a sheet of connective tissue called the lingual septum, running longitudinally through the midline of the tongue. These transverse fibres pass laterally from the septum to intercalate with fibres of the other groups of intrinsic muscles. The longitudinal fibres may be subdivided into upper and lower groups, the superior and inferior longitudinal muscles of the tongue. The vertical fibres pass directly between the upper and lower surfaces, particularly at the lateral borders of the tongue. Contraction of the vertical fibres would make the tongue thinner (and wider). Contraction of the longitudinal fibres would shorten (and thicken) the tongue. Contraction of the transverse fibres would narrow (and widen) the tongue. The intrinsic muscles receive their motor innervation from the hypoglossal cranial nerve.

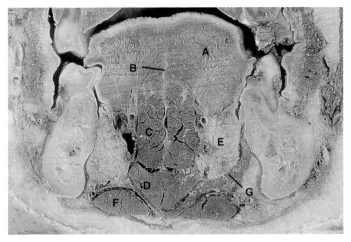

Fig. 3.21 Coronal section through the tongue and floor of the mouth. Note the interlacing of the intrinsic muscles in the body of the tongue (A). B = Lingual septum; C = genioglossus muscle; D = geniohyoid muscle; E = sublingual gland above mylohyoid; F = anterior belly of digastric muscle; G = mylohyoid muscle.

Extrinsic muscles

The extrinsic muscles of the tongue arise from the skull and hyoid bone and thence spread into the body of the tongue. The extrinsic musculature is composed of four groups of muscles: genioglossus, hyoglossus, styloglossus, and palatoglossus.

The genioglossus muscle (Figs 3.21–3.24) arises from the superior genial tubercle on the medial surface of the body of the mandible. At this level, the two genioglossus muscles cannot be readily separated. As the muscles enter the tongue, a thin strip of connective tissue intervenes between the right and left genioglossus muscles. The bulk of the fibres fan out into the body of the tongue but the superior fibres pass upwards and anteriorly to the tip of the tongue, and some of its inferior fibres insert onto the body of the hyoid bone. The genioglossus muscle is mainly a protractor and depressor of the tongue.

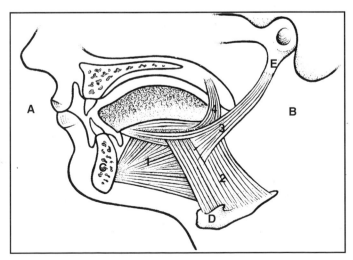

Fig. 3.22 Diagrammatic representation of the extrinsic muscles of the tongue. A = Anterior; B = posterior; C = mandible; D = hyoid bone; E = styloid process; 1 = genioglossus; 2 = hyoglossus; 3 = styloglossus; 4 = palatoglossus.

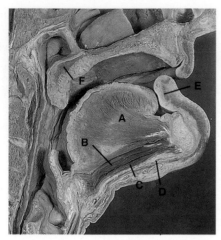

Fig. 3.23 Sagittal section of head showing genioglossus muscle (A). B = Geniohyoid muscle; C = mylohyoid muscle; D = platysma muscle; E = orbicularis oris muscle; F = levator palati muscle.

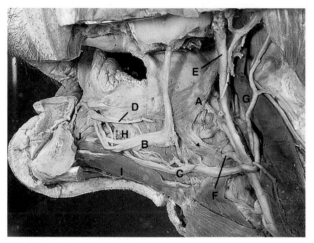

Fig. 3.24 Lateral view of tongue showing styloglossus muscle (A). B = Lingual nerve; C = hypoglossal nerve; D = submandibular duct (cut); E = external carotid artery; F = lingual artery; G = glossopharyngeal nerve; H = hyoglossus muscle; I = geniohyoid muscle; J = genioglossus muscle. Courtesy of Professor C. Dean.

The hyoglossus muscle (Figs 3.22, 3.24) originates from the superior border of the greater horn of the hyoid bone and passes vertically upwards into the tongue. Its function is to depress the tongue. At its origin, the hyoglossus muscle is separated from the attachment of the middle constrictor muscle of the pharynx beneath by the lingual artery.

Each styloglossus muscle (Figs 3.18, 3.22, 3.24) arises from the anterior surface of the styloid process of the temporal bone, from which the muscle runs downwards and forwards to enter the tongue below the insertion of the palatoglossus muscle. At this point, its fibres intercalate with the fibres of the hyoglossus before continuing forwards towards the tip of the tongue. The styloglossus muscle is a retractor of the tongue.

Each palatoglossus muscle (Fig. 3.22) arises from the aponeurosis of the soft palate and descends to the tongue in the anterior pillar of the fauces, whence its fibres intercalate with the transverse fibres of the tongue. The action of the palatoglossus muscles is to raise the tongue in order to narrow the transverse diameter of the oropharyngeal isthmus.

The extrinsic muscles of the tongue are innervated by the hypoglossal nerve (except for the palatoglossus, which is innervated by the cranial part of the accessory nerve via the pharyngeal plexus). The main source of the blood supply to the tongue is the lingual artery.

THE MUSCLES IN THE FLOOR OF THE MOUTH

The floor of the mouth is the region located between the medial surface of the mandible, the inferior surface of the tongue and the mylohyoid muscles. The mylohyoid muscles are attached to the mylohyoid lines of the mandible and consequently structures above these lines are related to the floor of the mouth, whereas structures below the lines are related to the upper part of the neck. This concept is of considerable clinical importance with respect to the spread of inflammation from infected teeth within the mandible (see page 74). The two mylohyoid muscles form a muscular diaphragm for the floor of the mouth (Figs 3.17, 3.21, 3.23). Above this diaphragm are found the genioglossus and geniohyoid muscles medially and the hyoglossus laterally. Below the diaphragm lie the digastric and stylohyoid muscles.

Mylohyoid

The mylohyoid muscle (Figs 3.21, 3.23, 3.24) arises from the mylohyoid line on the medial surface of the body of the mandible. Its fibres slope downwards, forwards and inwards. The anterior fibres of the mylohyoid muscle interdigitate with the corresponding fibres on the opposite side to form a median raphe. This raphe is attached above to the chin and below to the hyoid bone. The posterior fibres are inserted onto the anterior surface of the body of the hyoid bone. The muscle raises the floor of the mouth during the early stages of swallowing. It also helps to depress the mandible when the hyoid bone is fixed. The mylohyoid muscle is supplied by the mylohyoid branch of the inferior alveolar branch of the mandibular division of the trigeminal nerve. Its blood supply is derived from the lingual artery (sublingual branch), the maxillary artery (mylohyoid branch of the inferior alveolar artery) and the facial artery (submental branch).

Geniohyoid

The geniohyoid muscle originates from the inferior genial tubercle (mental spine). It passes backwards and slightly downwards to insert on to the anterior surface of the body of the hyoid bone (Figs 3.21, 3.23, 3.24). The geniohyoid muscle elevates the hyoid bone and is a weak depressor of the mandible. Its innervation is from the first cervical spinal nerve travelling with the hypoglossal nerve. Its blood supply is derived from the lingual artery (sublingual branch).

THE SUPERFICIAL MUSCLES OF THE FACE

The muscles of facial expression (Figs 3.25, 3.26) are characterised by their superficial arrangement in the face, by their activities on the skin (brought about directly by their attach-

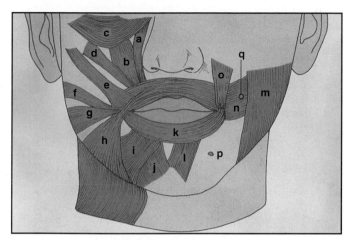

Fig. 3.25   Schematic diagram of the muscles of facial expression. a = Levator labia superioris alaeque nasi; b = levator labii superioris; c = orbicularis oculi; d = zygomaticus minor; e = zygomaticus major; f = risorius; g = platysma; h = depressor anguli oris; i = depressor labii inferioris; j = mentalis; k = orbicularis oris; m = masseter; n = buccinator; o = levator anguli oris; p = mental foramen; q = position of parotid duct piercing buccinator.

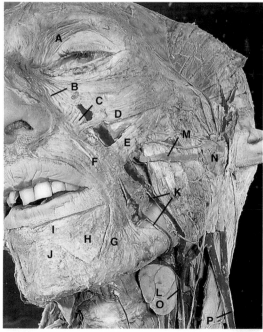

Fig. 3.26   The muscles of facial expression. A = Orbicularis oculi; B = levator labii superioris alaeque nasi; C = levator labii superioris; D = zygomaticus minor; E = zygomaticus major; F = levator anguli oris; G = depressor anguli oris; H = depressor labii inferioris; I = orbicularis oris; J = mentalis; K = facial vessels; L = submandibular gland; M = parotid duct; N = parotid gland with facial nerve branches; O = common facial vein formed by union of the facial vein and the anterior branch of the retromandibular vein; P = external jugular vein formed by the anterior branch of the retromandibular and the posterior auricular vein. Courtesy of Professor C. Dean.

ment to the facial integument) and by their common motor innervation, the facial nerve. They are all derived embryologically from mesenchyme of the second branchial arch. Functionally, the muscles of facial expression are grouped around the orifices of the face (the orbit, nose, ear and mouth) and should be considered primarily as muscles controlling the degree of opening and closing of these apertures: the expressive functions of the muscles have developed secondarily. The muscles of facial expression vary considerably between individuals in terms of size, shape and strength.

The superficial muscles around the lips and cheeks may be subdivided into two groups: the various parts of the orbicularis oris muscle, and muscles that are radially arranged from the orbicularis oris muscle. The fibres of orbicularis oris pass around the lips. The muscle is divided into four parts, each part corresponding to a quadrant of the lips. Its muscle fibres do not gain attachment directly to bone but occupy a central part of the lip. Muscle fibres in the philtrum insert onto the nasal septum. The range of movement produced by orbicularis oris includes lip closure, protrusion and pursing. The radial muscles can be divided into superficial and deep muscles of the upper and lower lips. The levator labii superioris, levator labii superioris alaeque nasi and zygomaticus major and minor are superficial muscles of the upper lip. The levator anguli oris is a deep muscle of the upper lip. The depressor anguli oris is a superficial muscle of the lower lip, and the depressor labii inferioris, and mentalis muscle are deep muscles of the lower lip. As their names suggest, the levator labii superioris elevates the upper lip, the depressor labii inferioris depresses the lower lip, and the corners of the mouth are raised and lowered by the levator and depressor anguli oris muscles.

Two muscles extend to the corner of the mouth: the risorius and buccinator muscles, risorius lying superficial to the buccinator. The risorius muscle stretches the angles of the mouth laterally. The buccinator muscle (see Fig. 3.9) arises from the pterygomandibular raphe and from the buccal side of the maxillary and mandibular alveoli above the molar teeth. Most of its fibres insert into mucous membrane covering the cheek; other fibres intercalate with orbicularis oris in the lips. As the fibres of the buccinator converge towards the angle of the mouth, the central fibres decussate. The main function of the buccinator muscle is to maintain the tension of the cheek against the teeth during mastication.

THE SALIVARY GLANDS

The parotid gland

The parotid gland (Fig. 3.27) is the largest of the major salivary glands and secretes a serous saliva. It occupies the region between the ramus of the mandible and the mastoid process. The parotid is pyramidal in shape; its apex extends beyond the angle of the mandible and the base is closely related to the external acoustic meatus. A deep surface of the gland rests anteriorly on the ramus and masseter muscle and extends around the posterior border of the mandible where it

Fig. 3.27 The shape and relations of the parotid gland (A). B = External acoustic meatus; C = parotid duct; D = masseter muscle; E = branches of facial nerve; F = great auricular nerve; G = facial vessels coursing through muscles of facial expression; H = superficial part of submandibular gland; I = superficial temporal vessels and auriculotemporal nerve.

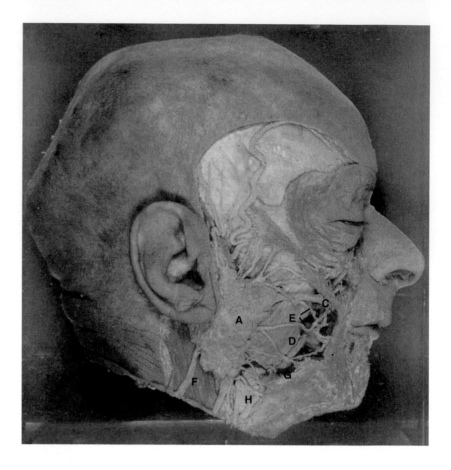

can reach the pharynx. The gland is surrounded by an un-yielding tough fibrous capsule, the parotid capsule. The parotid duct (Stensen's duct) appears at the anterior border of the gland and passes horizontally across the masseter muscle before piercing the buccinator to terminate in the oral cavity opposite the maxillary second molar. Lying with the duct on the masseter may be an accessory parotid gland.

Within the parotid gland are found the external carotid artery, the retromandibular vein and the facial nerve. Branches of the facial nerve are seen emerging from the anterior and inferior margins of the gland. Appearing at the superior border of the gland are the superficial temporal vessels and the auriculo-temporal nerve. From the inferior border of the gland may be seen the anterior and posterior branches of the posterior facial (retromandibular) vein. The former joins the facial vein to form the common facial vein, the latter joining the posterior auricular to form the external jugular vein (Fig. 3.26). Lymph nodes are also associated with the parotid gland.

The parasympathetic innnervation of the parotid gland is from the lesser petrosal branch of the glossopharyngeal nerve (see Fig. 4.13). The preganglionic fibres synapse in the otic ganglion and postganglionic fibres reach the gland by travelling with the auriculotemporal branch of the mandibular nerve. The sensory innervation of the parotid capsule is by the great auricular nerve, a branch of the cervical plexus (Fig. 3.27). The roots of this nerve are formed from the anterior primary rami of the second and third cervical nerves. The sensation of pain in mumps caused by enlargement of the gland (with subsequent tension on the unyielding parotid capsule) is mediated by the great auricular nerve.

The submandibular gland

The submandibular gland produces both serous and mucous saliva (in a 3:2 ratio). It is found in the floor of the mouth and in the suprahyoid region of the neck. A large part of the gland (the superficial part) is visible just beneath the inferior border of the mandible (Figs 3.26, 3.28). The gland has an important relationship with the mylohyoid muscle, wrapping around the free posterior border (not unlike the letter C). This gives rise to the smaller deep portion of the gland (Fig. 3.29). Posteriorly, the submandibular gland comes close to the apex of the parotid gland, with only the stylomandibular ligament inter-vening. The submandibular duct (Wharton's duct) appears from the deep part of the gland and wraps around the lingual nerve as it crosses the hyoglossus muscle to terminate on the sublingual papilla in the floor of the mouth (Figs 1.13, 3.29).

The sublingual gland

The sublingual gland, the smallest of the three major pairs of salivary glands, produces serous and mucous saliva in the approximate ratio of 1:3. It is located on the hyoglossus muscle in the floor of the mouth (Fig 3.19), adjacent to the sublingual fossa of the mandible. The gland is associated with the sublingual folds beneath the tongue. In coronal section the gland rests on the mylohyoid muscle (Fig. 3.21). The sublingual gland may be joined to the deep part of the submandibular gland to form a single sublingual–submandibular complex. The sublingual gland is subdivided into anterior and posterior parts. The ducts of the anterior part may unite to form a large

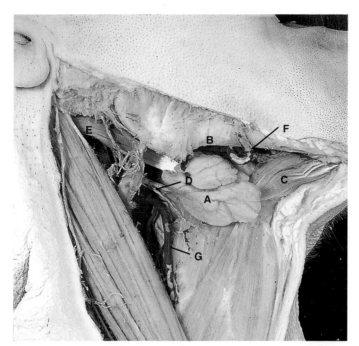

Fig. 3.28 The superficial part of the submandibular gland (A) seen in the upper part of the neck; B = Inferior border of mandible; C = anterior belly of the digastic muscle; D = hypoglossal nerve; E = posterior belly of the digastric muscle; F = facial artery on mylohyoid muscle; G = superior thyroid artery; Courtesy of Professor C. Dean.

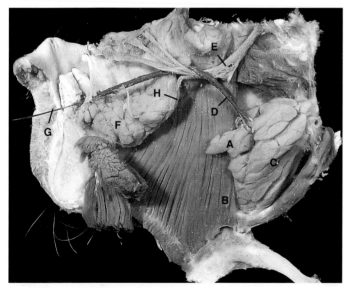

Fig. 3.29 Medial view of the floor of mouth showing deep part of the submandibular gland (A) passing around the free posterior border of the mylohyoid muscle (B); C = Superficial part of submandibular gland; D = submandibular duct wrapping around lingual nerve (E); F = sublingual gland; G = bristle in opening of the submandibular duct at the sublingual papilla; H = branches of the lingual nerve to the sublingual gland carrying parasympathetic fibres. Courtesy of Professor C. Dean.

main duct (Bartholin's duct), which either joins the submandibular duct or drains directly onto the sublingual papilla. The ducts from the posterior part of the sublingual gland drain through the sublingual fold.

The parasympathetic innervation of both the submandibular and sublingual glands is the chorda tympani branch of the facial nerve. Preganglionic fibres are carried via the lingual nerve to the submandibular ganglion. Postganglionic fibres pass from this ganglion to the submandibuar and sublingual glands (Fig. 3.14).

THE INFRATEMPORAL FOSSA

The infratemporal fossa is the space located deep to the ramus of the mandible. Together with the temporal fossa, pterygoid processes and maxillary tuberosity, the infratemporal fossa has been thought of by some anatomists as part of a 'masticatory muscle compartment' or 'masticatory space'.

The infratemporal fossa (Fig 3.30) is bounded anteriorly by the posterior surface of the maxilla, posteriorly by the styloid apparatus, carotid sheath and deep part of the parotid gland. Medially lie the lateral pterygoid plate and the superior constrictor of the pharynx. The roof is formed by the infratemporal surface of the greater wing of the sphenoid. The infratemporal fossa has no floor, being continuous with the neck. It communicates with the temporal fossa deep to the zygomatic arch; also with the pterygopalatine fossa through the pterygomaxillary fissure. At the base of the cranium, the foramen ovale and foramen spinosum enter the fossa through the sphenoid bone. The foramen lacerum and the petrotympanic, squamotympanic and petrosquamous fissures are also found close to the infratemporal fossa. On the medial surface of the ramus of the mandible is the mandibular foramen.

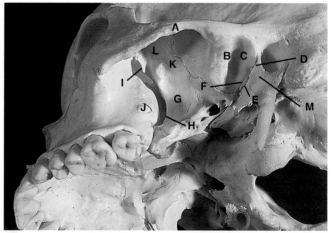

Fig. 3.30 The osteology of the infratemporal fossa. A = Zygomatic arch; B = articular eminence; C = mandibular fossa; D = squamotympanic fissure; E = petrotympanic fissure; F = petrosquamous fissure; G = lateral pterygoid plate; H = pterygomaxillary fissure leading into the pterygopalatine fossa; I = inferior orbital fissure; J = posterior border of maxilla; K = infratemporal crest of sphenoid bone; L = infratemporal surface of greater wing of sphenoid bone; M = tympanic plate.

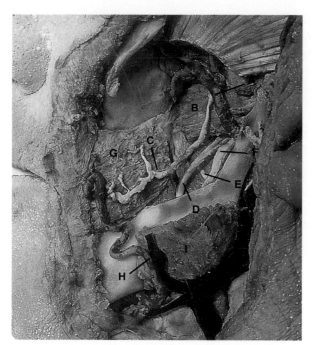

Fig. 3.31 Contents of the infratemporal fossa. A = Maxillary artery; B = lateral pterygoid (lower head); C = buccal branch of mandibular division of trigeminal nerve; D = lingual nerve; E = medial pterygoid muscle; F = inferior alveolar nerve; G = buccinator muscle; H = facial blood vessels; I = masseter muscle; Courtesy of Professor L. Garey.

The major structures within the infratemporal fossa (Fig. 3.31) are the lateral pterygoid and medial pterygoid muscles (see pages 63–64 for details), branches of the mandibular nerve (including the inferior alveolar, buccal and lingual nerves; see page 84), the chorda tympani branch of the facial nerve, the otic ganglion, the maxillary artery and the pterygoid venous plexus.

TISSUE SPACES AROUND THE JAWS

Knowledge of the tissue spaces around the jaws is necessary to understand the possible spread of infections (including oedema and pus) from a dental site into the rest of the head and neck.

Most structures in the body are ensheathed by a connective tissue covering of varying thickness. If thin and delicate, this connective tissue presents little resistance to the spread of infection; if the connective tissue layer is thick, tendinous or membranous, it resists the spread of infection (particularly over certain muscles). Such thick connective tissues, capable of holding surgical sutures, are sometimes referred to as 'true fascia'. From clinical experience it is evident that certain predictable pathways exist along which infection may spread. The loose connective tissue uniting fascial planes may be destroyed and the potential space delineated by adjacent structures considerably enlarged as inflammatory exudate accumulates. Such potential spaces are referred to as 'tissue spaces'.

The dissemination of infection in soft tissues is influenced by the natural barriers presented by bone, muscle and fascia.

Table 3.1 *The most important tissue spaces around the jaws*

Lower jaw	Upper jaw
1. Submental	10. Palatal
2. Submandibular	11. Canine fossa
3. Sublingual	12. Infratemporal
4. Buccal	
5. Submasseteric	
6. Parotid	
7. Pterygomandibular	
8. Parapharyngeal	
9. Peritonsillar	

Around the jaws are body compartments, the so-called tissue spaces, the boundaries of which are primarily defined by the mylohyoid, buccinator, masseter, medial pterygoid, superior constrictor and orbicularis oris muscles. The fascial layers of the neck are less important in influencing the spread of infection around the jaws. None of the 'spaces' are actually empty; they are potential spaces normally occupied by loose connective tissue. It is only when inflammatory products (or bleeding or tumours) destroy the loose connective tissue that an anatomically defined space is produced.

Infection may spread from one tissue space to another where the spaces are in direct communication or along the side of structures which pass from one tissue space to another (such as blood vessels or nerves). Infection can also invade tissue spaces by directly eroding the intervening fascia. In addition to such direct pathways, infection may also spread through the lymphatics and the blood vessels.

The most important potential tissue spaces around the jaws are shown in Table 3.1. With the exception of the submental, submandibular and palatal spaces, all the tissue spaces listed in the table are paired.

Fig. 3.32 shows the relationships of tissue spaces around the mandibular ramus. Because of the occurrence of inflammation in the soft tissues associated with partially impacted mandibular third molars (pericoronitis) and, less commonly, of dental abscesses of these teeth, the infratemporal fossa region is significant in terms of tissue spaces. This is due to the fact that the infratemporal fossa lies in a pivotal position, being intermediate between the tissue spaces of the face above and the tissue spaces of the neck below. The term **masticator tissue space** is sometimes used to describe the space enclosed by the investing layer of fascia ensheathing the muscles of mastication and the ramus of the mandible. The submasseteric, pterygomandibular, infratemporal and temporal tissue spaces are all part of this masticator tissue space.

The **submasseteric space(s)** may take the form of a series of spaces between the lateral surface of the ramus of the mandible and the masseter muscle. These spaces may form because the fibres of the masseter muscle have multiple insertions onto most of the lateral surface of the ramus and spaces may be found between the attachment of the superficial and deep parts of the muscle. Alternatively, they may relate to the passage of the neurovascular bundles. Whatever the true explanation,

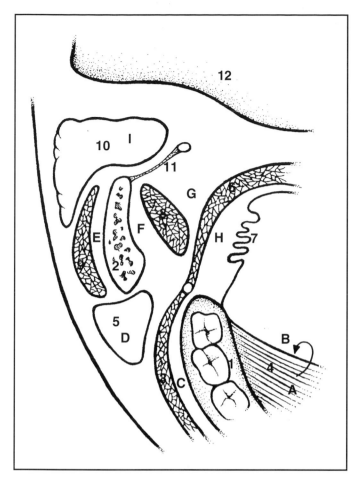

Fig. 3.32 The relationships of tissue spaces around the mandibular ramus. 1 = Body of mandible bearing the molar teeth; 2 = ramus of mandible; 3 = buccinator muscle; 4 = mylohyoid muscle; 5 = Buccal pad of fat; 6 = superior constrictor muscle; 7 = mucosa overlying palatal tonsil; 8 = medial pterygoid muscle; 9 = Masseter muscle; 10 = parotid gland; 11 = stylomandibular ligament; 12 = base of skull; A = sublingual space in the floor of the mouth above the mylohyoid muscle which, over its posterior margin, leads to B = submandibular space; C = buccal vestibule, delineated by the buccinator from D = buccal space; E = submasseteric spaces formed by the multiple insertion of the masseter muscle on the lateral surface of the ramus; F = pterygomandibular space bounded by the lateral surface of the medial pterygoid muscle and the medial surface of the ramus; G = parapharyngeal space bounded by the superior constrictor of the pharynx and the medial surface of the medial pterygoid muscle; H = peritonsillar space bounded by the medial surface of the superior constrictor of the pharynx and its mucosa; I = parotid space (in and around the parotid gland).

abscesses may develop between the masseter and the ramus of the mandible.

The **pterygomandibular space** lies between the ramus of the mandible laterally and the medial pterygoid muscle medially. Above lies the inferior head of the lateral pterygoid muscle. Anteriorly, beneath the overlying oral mucosa, lie fibres of the buccinator muscle, which arise from the pterygomandibular raphe. Immediately beneath the buccinator lies the tendon of the temporalis muscle. Posteriorly, the investing layer of deep cervical fascia covering the masseter and medial pterygoid muscles merges with the posterior border of the ramus, behind which lies the parotid gland. The pterygomandibular space is a prominent component of the infratemporal fossa. Between the ramus of the mandible and the medial pterygoid muscle lie the inferior alveolar and lingual nerves: the pterygomandibular space is therefore the site of injection for an inferior alveolar nerve block. It also contains the maxillary artery and pterygoid venous plexus.

The **infratemporal space** is the upper extremity of the pterygomandibular space. It lies behind the maxilla and is bounded medially by the lateral pterygoid plate and above by the base of the skull. It is in continuity with the deep temporal space laterally.

The **temporal space** consists of superficial and deep components that are found in relation to the temporalis muscle. The superficial temporal space lies on the lateral surface of the muscle, beneath the skin and the superficial (temporal) fascia. The deep temporal space lies between the medial (deep) surface of the muscle and the adjacent temporal bone.

Unlike infections involving odontogenic tissues that drain directly into the oral cavity (via the buccal or lingual sulci), those involving the tissue spaces around the infratemporal fossa do not drain directly into the oral cavity and have the potential to spread some distance through the head and neck. Of particular relevance in this regard are the tissue spaces around the pharynx, as involvement of these spaces may affect the larynx and thus compromise the airway. Symptoms associated with such conditions may include trismus, fever, dysphagia and dyspnoea and patients must be treated quickly because of the potential development of life-threatening situations. In the most extreme situation, inflammation will eventually spread to involve the thorax.

The parapharyngeal space is particularly prone to infections from the jaws and teeth. This space is restricted to the suprahyoid region of the neck and the infratemporal region. For infection to spread inferiorly from the parapharyngeal space, it must first pass into the retropharyngeal region because suprahyoid structures (particularly the sheath around the submandibular gland formed by the investing layer of deep cervical fascia) provide a restrictive inferior boundary.

The **pharyngeal tissue spaces** can be subdivided into the peripharyngeal spaces around, and external to, the pharynx and the intrapharyngeal space within it. With regard to the peripharyngeal spaces there is the parapharyngeal space laterally and the retropharyngeal space posteriorly. Some anatomists also include the submental and submandibular spaces as pharyngeal tissue spaces because they lie immediately anteriorly.

Each **parapharyngeal space** (or **lateral pharyngeal space**) passes laterally around the pharynx and is continuous posteriorly with the retropharyngeal space. Unlike the retropharyngeal space, however, it is a space that is restricted to the suprahyoid region. It contains loose connective tissue and is bounded medially by the pharynx (superior constrictor muscle) and laterally by the pterygoid muscles and the parotid gland. Superiorly, it is bounded by the base of the skull. Inferiorly, it does not extend right down the neck but is limited by the suprahyoid structures, such as the fascia associated with the styloid group of muscles and the submandibular gland. Behind is situated the carotid sheath. The lateral pharyngeal space is partly divided by the styloid process and associated group of muscles into an anterior compartment containing muscle and a posterior compartment containing the carotid sheath and cranial nerves IX–XII.

The **retropharyngeal space** is the area of loose connective tissue lying behind the pharynx and in front of the prevertebral fascia. It extends upwards to the base of the skull and downwards to the retrovisceral space in the infrahyoid part of the neck.

An **intrapharyngeal space** potentially exists between the inner surface of the constrictor muscles of the pharynx and the pharyngeal mucosa. Infections at this site are either restricted locally or spread through the pharynx into the retropharyngeal or parapharyngeal spaces. An important part of the intrapharyngeal space is the peritonsillar space. This lies around the palatine tonsil, between the pillars of the fauces. Infections here (quinsy) usually spread up or down the intrapharyngeal space, or through the pharynx into the parapharyngeal space.

The tissue spaces below the inferior border of the mandible and in the supra-hyoid region of the neck (i.e. the submental and submandibular tissue spaces) are illustrated in Fig. 3.33.

The **submental space** lies beneath the chin in the midline, between the mylohyoid muscles below and the investing layer of deep cervical fascia and platysma muscle superficially. It is bounded laterally by the two anterior bellies of the digastric muscles. The submental space communicates posteriorly over the anterior bellies of the digastric muscles with the two submandibular spaces.

The **submandibular space** is situated between the anterior and posterior bellies of the digastric muscle and is bounded above and laterally by the body of the mandible. It lies superficial to (below) the mylohyoid muscle (and more posteriorly the hyoglossus and styloglossus muscles) and is covered by the platysma muscle and by the investing layer of deep cervical fascia, which explains why abscesses in this region do not readily drain through the skin. The submandibular space communicates with the sublingual space around the posterior free border of the mylohyoid muscle and via small deficiencies within the muscular tissue of the mylohyoid muscle. The submandibular space contains the submandibular gland, facial vessels and submandibular lymph nodes. A submandibular abscess is commonly caused by spread of infection from the second or third mandibular molar tooth (Fig. 3.34).

The suprahyoid spaces (submental and submandibular spaces) are bounded inferiorly by the attachment of the investing layer of deep cervical fascia to the hyoid bone. Consequently, if oedema or pus accumulates in the suprahyoid region there will be a restriction in the spread into the rest of the neck. This is potentially very dangerous because the suprahyoid region will swell markedly and restrict the airway (Ludwig's angina).

Fig. 3.35 illustrates the relationships of tissue spaces to the tongue. The **sublingual space** lies in the floor of the mouth, above the mylohyoid muscles and below the oral mucosa. It is delineated in front, and at the sides, by the body of the mandible and behind (and below) by the attachment of the mylohyoid muscle to the hyoid bone. The sublingual space contains the sublingual gland and the submandibular duct.

In the anterior region of both the upper and lower jaws, the orbicularis oris muscle presents a barrier to pus between the vestibule on the oral side and the skin of the lip on the facial side. In the upper jaw, pus may accumulate between the muscles of facial expression, particularly in the canine fossa between the levator labii superioris and zygomaticus muscles.

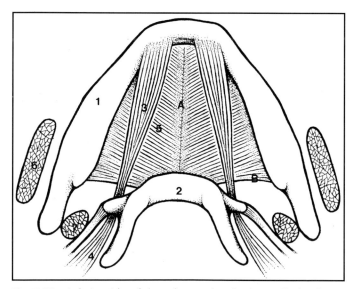

Fig. 3.33 Inferior view of the submental and submandibular tissue spaces. 1 = Body of mandible; 2 = hyoid bone; 3 = anterior belly of digastric muscle; 4 = posterior belly of digastric muscle; 5 = mylohyoid muscle; 6 = masseter muscle; 7 = medial pterygoid muscle; A = the submental space lying between the mylohyoid muscle and the investing layer of deep cervical fascia. Laterally, it is bounded by the two anterior bellies of the digastric muscles. The submental space communicates posteriorly with the submandibular space (B).

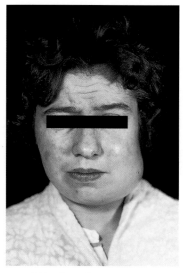

Fig. 3.34· Abscess within the submandibular tissue space. Courtesy of Professor J. Langdon.

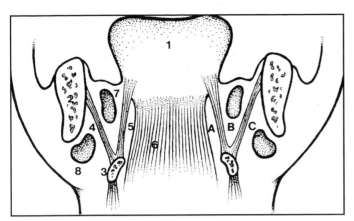

Fig. 3.35 The relationships of a number of tissue spaces to the tongue. 1 = Tongue; 2 = body of mandible; 3 = hyoid bone; 4 = mylohyoid muscle; 5 = hyoglossus; 6 = genioglossus; 7 = sublingual salivary gland; 8 = submandibular salivary gland; A = cleft between genioglossus and hyoglossus muscles that communicates directly with the parapharyngeal space; B = sublingual space between the mylohyoid and hyoglossus muscles; C = submandibular space below the mylohyoid muscle.

Other spaces around the mouth

Other spaces around the mouth that need to be described are the buccal, parotid and palatal tissue spaces.

The **buccal space** is located in the cheek. It has the buccinator muscle (covered by a delicate connective tissue layer called the buccopharyngeal fascia) medially, the skin of the cheek laterally, the pterygomandibular raphe (giving origin to the buccinator muscle) posteriorly, and some muscles of orbicularis oris anteriorly. The buccal space contains the parotid duct accompanied by blood vessels and branches of the facial nerve as well as the buccal pad of fat.

The **parotid space** surrounds the parotid gland and its contents. It is defined by the parotid capsule. The superficial layer of the parotid capsule is of variable thickness and is not a typical fascia as it contains muscle fibres that parallel those of the platysma muscle. It appears to be continuous with the fascia associated with the platysma muscle. The deep surface of the parotid capsule is derived from the investing layer of deep cervical fascia. Above the level of the stylomandibular ligament, the deep surface of the parotid capsule may be thin and may serve as a communicating pathway into the lateral pharyngeal space.

The **palatal space** in the hard palate exists only when pus strips the mucoperiosteum from the underlying bone of the hard palate.

The way in which infections of dental origin spread through the bone of the jaws into the tissue spaces naturally depends upon the site at which the pus escapes the bone. Thus, pus from a periapical abscess in a mandibular incisor that escapes inferior to the mylohyoid muscle will enter the submental space, while pus escaping superior to this muscle will enter the sublingual space. It should also be borne in mind that the tissue spaces are not discrete regions; they intercommunicate. Thus, a sublingual abscess may spread from the sublingual space over the posterior margin of the mylohyoid muscle into the submandibular space (see Figs 3.32, 3.33). Furthermore, none of the muscle or fascial barriers defining the spaces is impenetrable.

4 The vasculature and innervation of the mouth

BLOOD SUPPLY TO ORODENTAL TISSUES

The face is supplied mainly through the facial artery (Figs 4.1, 4.2; see also Fig. 3.27), a branch of the external carotid artery in the neck. The facial artery first appears on the face as it hooks round the lower border of the mandible, at the anterior edge of the masseter. It then runs a tortuous course between the facial muscles towards the medial angle of the eye. There is a rich anastomosis with the artery of the opposite side and with additional vessels supplying the face (transverse facial branch of the superficial temporal artery; infraorbital and mental branches of the maxillary artery; dorsal nasal branch of the ophthalmic artery).

The main arteries to the teeth and jaws are derived from the maxillary artery, a terminal branch of the external carotid, and running in the infratemporal fossa (Figs 3.31, 4.2). The

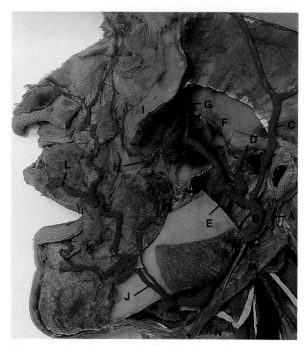

Fig. 4.2 Dissection showing the facial and maxillary arteries. A = Posterior auricular artery; B = external carotid artery; C = superficial temporal artery; D = middle meningeal artery; E = inferior alveolar artery; F = maxillary artery; G = deep temporal artery; H = posterior superior alveolar artery; I = third part of maxillary artery entering the pterygopalatine fossa; J = facial artery; K = inferior labial artery; L = superior labial artery; M = posterior belly of the digastric muscle; N = hypoglossal nerve. Courtesy of Professor L. Garey.

alveolar arteries follow roughly the same course as the alveolar nerves.

Mandibular teeth and periodontium

The inferior alveolar artery, which supplies the mandibular teeth, is derived from the maxillary artery before it crosses the lateral pterygoid muscle in the infratemporal fossa (see Fig. 4.2). A mylohyoid branch is given off before the inferior alveolar artery enters the mandibular foramen in the ramus of the mandible. The inferior alveolar artery passes through the mandibular foramen to enter the mandibular canal and terminates as the mental and incisive arteries.

Posteriorly, the buccal gingiva is supplied by the buccal artery (a branch of the maxillary artery as it crosses the lateral pterygoid muscle) and by perforating branches from the inferior alveolar artery. Anteriorly, the labial gingiva is

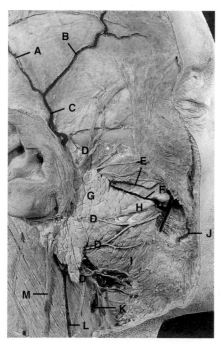

Fig. 4.1 Blood supply to the face. A = Parietal branch of superficial temporal artery; B = frontal branch of superficial temporal artery; C = superficial temporal artery; D = branches of facial nerve; E = transverse facial branch of superficial temporal artery; F = transverse facial vein; G = parotid gland; H = parotid duct; I = masseter muscle; J = facial artery; K = common facial vein formed by anterior branch of the retromandibular vein and facial veins; L = external jugular vein formed by posterior branch of the retromandibular and posterior auricular veins; M = great auricular nerve on sternocleidomastoid muscle. Courtesy of Professor C. Dean.

supplied by the mental artery and by perforating branches of the incisive artery. The lingual gingiva is supplied by perforating branches from the inferior alveolar artery and by the lingual artery, a branch of the external carotid artery.

Maxillary teeth and periodontium

The posterior superior alveolar artery arises from the maxillary artery in the pterygopalatine fossa. Occasionally, the posterior superior alveolar artery is derived from the buccal artery. It courses tortuously over the maxillary tuberosity before entering bony canals to supply molar and premolar teeth. The artery also gives off branches to the adjacent buccal gingiva, maxillary sinus and cheek.

The middle superior alveolar artery, when present, arises from the infraorbital artery (which is itself a branch of the third part of the maxillary artery in the pterygopalatine fossa). The middle superior alveolar artery runs in the lateral wall of the maxillary sinus, terminating near the canine tooth where it anastomoses with the anterior and posterior superior alveolar arteries. The anterior superior alveolar artery also arises from the infraorbital artery and runs downwards in the anterior wall of the maxillary sinus to supply the anterior teeth. Like the superior alveolar nerves, the superior alveolar arteries form plexuses.

The buccal gingiva around the posterior maxillary teeth is supplied by gingival and perforating branches from the posterior superior alveolar artery and by the buccal artery. The labial gingiva of anterior teeth is supplied by labial branches of the infraorbital artery and by perforating branches of the anterior superior alveolar artery.

The palatal gingiva around the maxillary teeth is supplied primarily by branches of the greater palatine artery, a branch of the third part of the maxillary artery in the pterygopalatine fossa.

The palate, cheek, tongue and lips

The palate derives its blood supply from the greater and lesser palatine branches of the maxillary artery. The greater palatine artery passes through the incisive foramen, where it anastomoses with the nasopalatine artery. The cheek is supplied by the buccal branch of the maxillary artery, and the floor of the mouth and the tongue by the lingual arteries. The lips are mainly supplied by the superior and inferior labial branches of the facial arteries.

VENOUS DRAINAGE OF ORODENTAL TISSUES

The venous drainage of this region is extremely variable. The facial vein is the main vein draining the face (see Figs 3.27, 4.1). It begins at the medial corner of the eye by confluence of the supraorbital and supratrochlear veins and passes across the face behind the facial artery. Below the mandible, it joins with the anterior branch of the retromandibular vein to form the common facial vein.

Teeth and periodontium

Small veins from the teeth and alveolar bone pass into larger veins surrounding the apex of each tooth, or into veins running in the interdental septa. In the mandible, the veins are then collected into one or more inferior alveolar veins, which themselves may drain anteriorly through the mental foramen to join the facial veins or posteriorly through the mandibular foramen to join the pterygoid plexus of veins in the infratemporal fossa. In the maxilla, the veins may drain anteriorly into the facial vein or posteriorly into the pterygoid plexus. No accurate description is available concerning the venous drainage of the gingiva, though it may be assumed that the buccal, lingual, greater palatine and nasopalatine veins are involved; apart from the lingual veins which pass directly into the internal jugular veins, these veins run into the pterygoid plexuses.

The palate, cheek, tongue and lips

The veins of the palate are rather diffuse and variable. However, those of the hard palate generally pass into the pterygoid venous plexus, those of the soft palate into the pharyngeal venous plexus. The buccal vein of the cheek drains into the pterygoid plexus. Venous blood from the lips drains into the facial veins via the superior and inferior labial veins. The veins of the tongue follow two different routes: those of the dorsum and sides of the tongue form the lingual veins, which, accompanying the lingual arteries, empty into the internal jugular veins; those of the ventral surface form the deep lingual veins (see Fig 1.14), which ultimately join the facial, internal jugular or lingual veins.

LYMPHATIC DRAINAGE OF ORODENTAL TISSUES

As with the venous system, the lymphatic drainage is extremely variable: Fig. 4.3 provides a 'consensus' view of the lymphatic drainage of the oral structures.

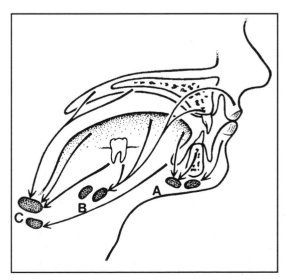

Fig. 4.3 Lymphatic drainage of oral structures. A = Submental nodes; B = submandibular nodes; C = jugulodigastric nodes.

Lymphatics from the lower part of the face generally pass through, or around, the buccal lymph nodes to reach the submandibular lymph nodes. However, lymphatics from the medial portion of the lower lip drain into the submental nodes.

The lymph vessels from the teeth usually run directly into the submandibular nodes on the same side. However, lymph from the mandibular incisors drains into the submental nodes. Occasionally, lymph from the molars passes directly into the jugulodigastric group of nodes.

The lymph vessels of the labial and buccal gingivae of the maxillary and mandibular teeth unite to drain into the submandibular nodes, although in the labial region of the mandibular incisors they may drain into the submental nodes. The lingual and palatal gingivae drain into the jugulodigastric group of nodes, either directly or indirectly through the submandibular nodes.

Lymphatics from most areas of the palate terminate in the jugulodigastric group of nodes. Vessels from the posterior part of the soft palate terminate in pharyngeal lymph nodes. Lymph from the floor of the mouth region can drain directly to the jugulodigastric nodes.

Lymphatics from the anterior two-thirds of the tongue may be subdivided into two groups: marginal and central vessels. The marginal lymphatic vessels drain the lateral third of the dorsal surface of the tongue and the lateral margin of its ventral surface. The remaining regions drain into the central vessels. The marginal vessels pass to the submandibular lymph nodes of the same side. The central vessels at the tip of the tongue pass to the submental lymph nodes. Central vessels behind the tip drain into ipsilateral and contralateral submandibular lymph nodes. Some marginal and central lymph vessels pass directly to the jugulodigastric group of nodes (or even the jugulo-omohyoid nodes). Lymphatics from the posterior third of the tongue drain into the deep cervical group of nodes, vessels centrally draining both ipsilaterally and contralaterally. Knowledge of the ipsilateral and contralateral drainage from the tongue is important clinically where, for example, a tumour near the central part of the tongue may be associated with spread into lymph nodes on both sides.

At the oropharyngeal isthmus lie the palatine tonsils between the pillars of the fauces (see Fig. 1.11) and the lingual tonsils on the pharyngeal surface of the tongue (see Fig. 1.15). These tonsils form part of a ring of lymphoid tissue known as Waldeyer's tonsillar ring. The other components are the tubal tonsils and adenoid tissue (pharyngeal tonsils) located in the nasopharynx.

INNERVATION OF ORODENTAL TISSUES

Excepting regions around the oropharyngeal isthmus, the oral mucosa receives sensory innervation from the maxillary and mandibular divisions of the trigeminal nerve. The trigeminal nerve also supplies the teeth and their supporting tissues (Table 4.1). Both the major and minor salivary glands are supplied by secretomotor parasympathetic fibres from the facial and glossopharyngeal nerves. The motor innervation of the muscles of the jaws and oral cavity is from the trigeminal, facial, accessory and hypoglossal nerves.

Table 4.1 *Nerve supply to the teeth and gingivae*

	Nasopalatine nerve	Greater palatine nerve		Palatal gingiva
Maxilla	Anterior superior alveolar nerve	Middle superior alveolar nerve	Posterior superior alveolar nerve	Teeth
	Infraorbital nerve	Posterior superior alveolar nerve and buccal nerve		Buccal gingiva
	1 2 3	4 5 6 7 8		Tooth position (Zsigmondy system)
	Mental nerve	Buccal nerve and perforating branches of inferior alveolar nerve		Buccal gingiva
Mandible	Incisive nerve	Inferior alveolar nerve		Teeth
	Lingual nerve and perforating branches of inferior alveolar nerve			Lingual gingiva

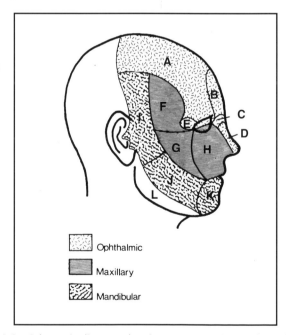

Fig. 4.4 Schematic diagram showing cutaneous innervation of the face. A = supraorbital nerve; B = supratrochlear nerve; C = infratrochlear nerve; D = external nasal nerve; E = lacrimal nerve; F = zygomaticotemporal nerve; G = zygomaticofacial nerve; H = infraorbital nerve; I = auriculotemporal nerve; J = buccal nerve; K = mental nerve; L = great auricular nerve.

Fig. 4.4 illustrates the cutaneous innervation of the face. All three divisions of the trigeminal nerve are involved, the ophthalmic division supplying the upper part of the face, forehead and scalp, the maxillary and mandibular divisions essentially supplying the upper and lower jaw regions respectively. Knowledge of these areas, and of the specific branches involved, is important clinically for assessing the effects of nerve damage and for an understanding of the successful anaesthetisation of the buccal, infraorbital and inferior alveolar (mental) nerves during dental treatment. The areas supplied by the three divisions of the trigeminal nerve also relate to aspects of the development of the face (see pages 270–271).

Dental operations on the teeth often require the injection of a local anaesthetic solution. Where only the teeth are to be operated upon then clearly only the nerves supplying the specific teeth need be anaesthetised. However, anaesthesia of the supporting tissues (including the gingivae) may be required for more extensive clinical procedures, including tooth extraction. Of particular importance are the inferior alveolar nerve (from the mandibular division of the trigeminal) supplying the mandibular dentition and the posterior, middle and anterior superior alveolar nerves (from the maxillary division of the trigeminal) innervating the maxillary dentition.

Inferior alveolar nerve

The course of the inferior alveolar nerve through the mandible is illustrated in Figs 4.5 and 4.6. The distribution of nerves to the mandibular premolars and molars is variable, dental branches coming either directly from the inferior alveolar nerve by short (Fig. 4.6a) or long (Fig. 4.6b) branches or indirectly through several alveolar branches (Fig. 4.6c). In

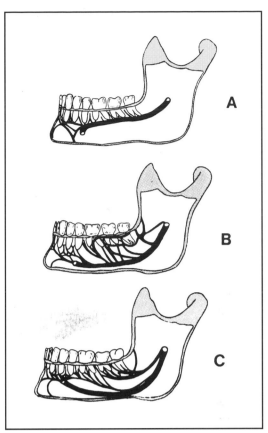

Fig. 4.6 Schematic diagram showing variation in the course of the inferior alveolar nerve through the mandible. Redrawn after Drs R.B. Carter and E.N. Keen.

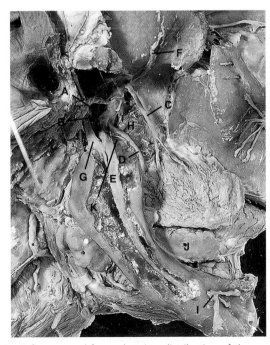

Fig. 4.5 Infratemporal fossa showing distribution of the mandibular nerve and the course of its inferior alveolar branch. A = Auriculotemporal nerve; B = middle meningeal artery; C = buccal branch; D = lingual nerve; E = inferior alveolar nerve with mylohyoid branch; F = deep temporal nerve; G = sphenomandibular ligament; H = medial pterygoid muscle; I = mental nerve; J = sublingual gland; K = chorda tympani. Courtesy of Professor C. Dean.

rare instances, the nerve to the mandibular third molar may arise from the inferior alveolar nerve before it enters the mandibular canal. Communications between the inferior alveolar nerve and nerves from the temporalis and lateral pterygoid muscles have been described, the nerves penetrating the mandible through foramina in the region of muscle attachments. It has been suggested that such nerve connections might explain why, in approximately 5% of patients, the teeth may not be anaesthetised after the main trunk of the inferior alveolar nerve has been blocked at the mandibular foramen by the injection of local anaesthetic solution.

It is said that, in any one individual, the mandibular canal remains in a relatively fixed position with respect to the lower border of the mandible. The canal is often closely related to the roots of the mandibular molars. Indeed, the roots of lower third molars may even be perforated by the mandibular canal.

In the premolar region the main trunk of the inferior alveolar nerve divides into mental and incisive nerves. The mental nerve runs for a short distance in a mental canal before leaving the body of the mandible at the mental foramen to emerge onto the face. In about 50% of cases, the mental foramen lies on a vertical line passing through the mandibular second premolar. However, in negroid ethnic groups, the mental foramen may be situated slightly more posteriorly, midway between the roots of the second premolar and first permanent molar. In an adult with a full dentition, the mental foramen usually lies midway between the upper and lower borders of the mandible. During the first and second years of life, as the prominence of the chin develops, the opening of the mental foramen alters in direction, from facing forwards to facing upwards and backwards. As well as supplying the skin of the lower lip, the mental nerve provides fibres to an incisor plexus, which innervates the labial periodontium of the mandibular incisors. The incisive nerve runs forwards in an intraosseous incisive canal. This nerve primarily supplies the incisors and canines but may also supply the first premolar. In some instances, the canine may be supplied directly from the inferior alveolar nerve.

Superior alveolar nerves

The superior alveolar nerves and associated dental plexuses are shown in Fig. 4.7. The posterior superior alveolar nerve arises from the maxillary nerve in the pterygopalatine fossa, whence it passes through the pterygomaxillary fissure to descend on the posterior wall (tuberosity) of the maxilla (see Fig. 4.8). The dental branches of the nerve enter the maxilla and run in narrow posterior superior alveolar canals above the roots of the molar teeth. A gingival branch does not enter

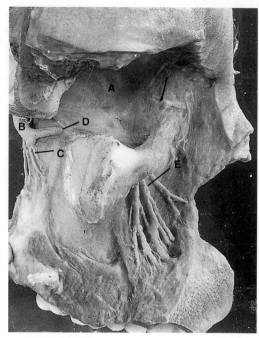

Fig. 4.8 Frontal aspect of face showing the maxillary nerve; A = Orbit; B = maxillary nerve; C = posterior superior alveolar nerve; D = infraorbital nerve in floor of orbit; E = infraorbital nerve entering face at infraorbital foramen.

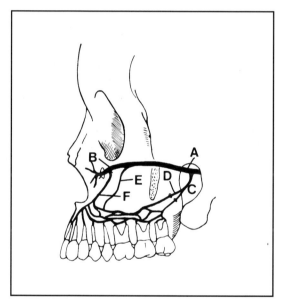

Fig. 4.7 The superior alveolar nerves and associated dental plexuses. A = Trunk of maxillary division of the trigeminal nerve; B = infraorbital nerve; C = pterygopalatine fossa; D = posterior superior alveolar nerves; E = middle superior alveolar nerve; F = anterior superior alveolar nerve.

the bone, however, but runs downwards and forwards along the outer surface of the maxillary tuberosity. The dental branches of the posterior superior alveolar nerve may arise from a common nerve trunk within the bone (Fig. 4.9b) or on the tuberosity before entering bone (Fig. 4.9a), or alternatively may appear as separate nerve trunks from the main trunk of the maxillary nerve in the pterygopalatine fossa (Fig. 4.9c). The middle superior alveolar nerve is found in about 70% of subjects. The nerve generally arises from the infraorbital nerve in the floor of the orbit/roof of the maxillary air sinus, although it may arise from the maxillary nerve in the pterygopalatine fossa. The nerve may run in the posterior, lateral or anterior walls of the maxillary sinus. It terminates above the roots of the premolar teeth. The anterior superior alveolar nerve arises from the infraorbital nerve within the infraorbital canal, generally as a single nerve but occasionally as two or three small branches. The nerve leaves the infraorbital canal near its termination and then, diverging laterally from the

Fig. 4.9 Three different patterns for the posterior superior alveolar nerves on the tuberosity of the maxilla.

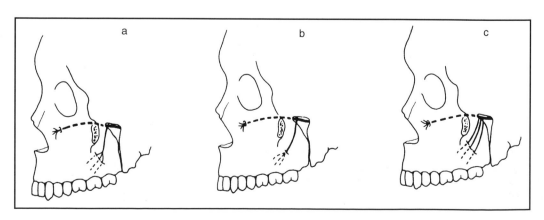

infraorbital nerve, runs in the anterior wall of the maxillary sinus. It terminates near the anterior nasal spine after giving off a small nasal branch. Note that the posterior superior alveolar nerve has an extrabony course that permits anaesthesia of the nerve trunk(s) as it passes across the maxillary tuberosity, whereas the middle and anterior superior alveolar nerves are entirely intrabony in their course and cannot be 'blocked' with an anaesthetic injection.

The superior alveolar nerve forms a plexus above the root apices of the maxillary teeth (Fig. 4.7). From this plexus nerves pass to the teeth, although it is difficult to trace the precise innervation of the teeth from specific superior alveolar nerves. As a general rule, however, the incisors and canines are supplied by the anterior nerve, the molars by the posterior nerve and intermediate areas by the middle nerve.

Sensory nerves to oral cavity

The sensory nerve supply to the palate is described in Figs 4.10

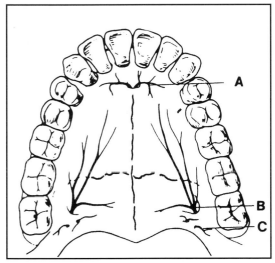

Fig. 4.10 The sensory nerve supply to the palate. A = Nasopalatine nerves; B = greater palatine nerve; C = lesser palatine nerve.

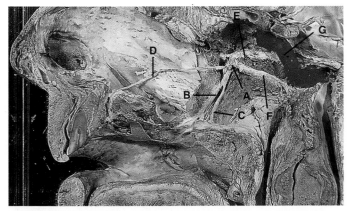

Fig. 4.11 The pterygopalatine ganglion (A) giving rise to the greater (B) and lesser (C) palatine nerves and the nasopalatine nerve (D). E = Maxillary nerve; F = nerve of pterygoid canal; G = internal carotid artery.

and 4.11. The nerve supply is derived from the maxillary division of the trigeminal nerve via branches of the pterygopalatine ganglion. A small area behind the incisor teeth is supplied by terminal branches of the nasopalatine nerves. These nerves emerge onto the palate at the incisive foramen. The remainder of the hard palate is supplied by the greater palatine nerves emerging onto the palate at the greater palatine foramina. The soft palate is supplied by the lesser palatine nerves emerging onto the palate via the lesser palatine foramina. Although the maxillary division of the trigeminal nerve supplies most of the palate, there is evidence to suggest that some areas supplied by the lesser palatine nerves may also be innervated by fibres from the facial nerve. The posterior part of the soft palate and the uvula may be supplied by the glossopharyngeal nerve.

The sensory innervation of the tongue is illustrated in Fig. 4.12. Three distinct nerve fields can be recognised on the dorsum of the tongue. The anterior part of the tongue, in front of the circumvallate papillae, is supplied by the lingual branch of the mandibular division of the trigeminal nerve (see Fig. 4.5). However, its accompanying chorda tympani fibres from the nervus intermedius part of the facial nerve are those associated with the perception of taste. Figure 4.5 shows the chorda tympani joining the lingual nerve in the infratemporal fossa. Behind, and including the circumvallate papillae, the tongue is supplied primarily by the glossopharyngeal nerve (providing both general sensation and taste). A small area on the posterior part of the tongue around the epiglottis is supplied by the vagus nerve (via its superior laryngeal branch). The mucosa on the ventral surface of the tongue is supplied by the lingual nerve.

The mucosa of the upper lip is supplied by the infraorbital branch of the maxillary division of the trigeminal nerve. That

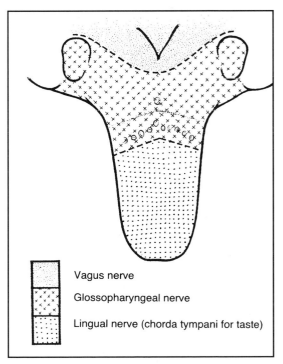

Fig. 4.12 Schematic representation of the sensory innervation of the tongue.

of the lower lip is supplied by the mental branch of the mandibular division of the trigeminal nerve (see Fig. 4.5). The mucosa of the cheeks is supplied by the buccal branch of the mandibular division of the trigeminal. The mucosa on the floor of the mouth is innervated by the lingual branch of the mandibular division of the trigeminal nerve. The mucosa over the pillars of the fauces (the oropharyngeal isthmus) is supplied by the glossopharyngeal nerve.

THE SECRETOMOTOR INNERVATION OF THE SALIVARY GLANDS

Parotid gland

The secretomotor supply of the parotid gland (Fig. 4.13) is derived through the otic parasympathetic ganglion. This ganglion is situated in the roof of the infratemporal fossa, close to the foramen ovale and the mandibular division of the trigeminal nerve. Like other parasympathetic ganglia in the head, three types of nerve fibre are associated with it: parasympathetic, sympathetic and sensory. However, only the parasympathetic fibres synapse in the ganglion. The preganglionic parasympathetic fibres to the otic ganglion originate from the inferior salivatory nucleus in the brainstem and pass with the glossopharyngeal nerve via its lesser petrosal branch. The sympathetic root of the otic ganglion is derived from postganglionic fibres from the superior cervical ganglion and reaches the otic ganglion via the plexus around the middle

meningeal artery in the infratemporal fossa. The sensory root is derived from the auriculotemporal branch of the mandibular division of the trigeminal nerve. The postganglionic parasympathetic fibres (with sensory and sympathetic fibres) reach the parotid gland through the auriculotemporal branch of the mandibular nerve.

Submandibular and sublingual glands

The secretomotor supply of the submandibular and sublingual glands (Fig. 4.14) is derived through the submandibular parasympathetic ganglion. This ganglion is situated, with the lingual nerve, on the hyoglossus muscle in the floor of the mouth above the deep part of the submandibular gland. The preganglionic parasympathetic fibres to the ganglion originate from the superior salivatory nucleus in the brainstem and pass with the nervus intermedius of the facial nerve, and subsequently its chorda tympani branch, to reach the lingual nerve in the infratemporal fossa (Fig. 4.5). It is via the lingual nerve that the preganglionic fibres are conveyed to the submandibular ganglion. The sympathetic root of the ganglion is derived from postganglionic fibres from the superior cervical ganglion and reaches the submandibular ganglion via the plexus around the facial artery. The sensory root is derived from the lingual nerve. The postganglionic parasympathetic fibres (with sensory and sympathetic fibres) pass directly to the adjacent submandibular gland but reach the sublingual gland after re-entering the lingual nerve.

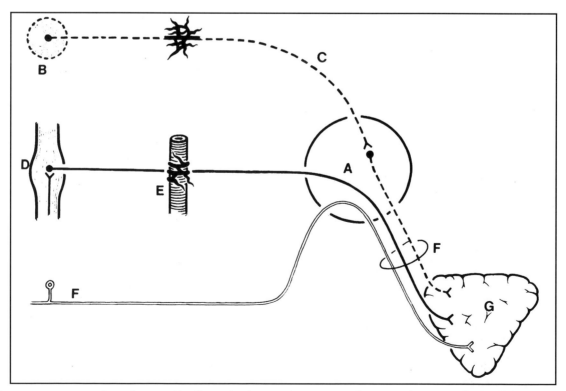

Fig. 4.13 The secretomotor supply to the parotid salivary gland. A = Otic parasympathetic ganglion; B = inferior salivatory nucleus; C = lesser petrosal branch of the glossopharyngeal nerve; D = postganglionic fibres from the superior cervical ganglion; E = sympathetic plexus around the middle meningeal artery; F = auriculotemporal branch of mandibular division of trigeminal nerve; G = parotid gland.

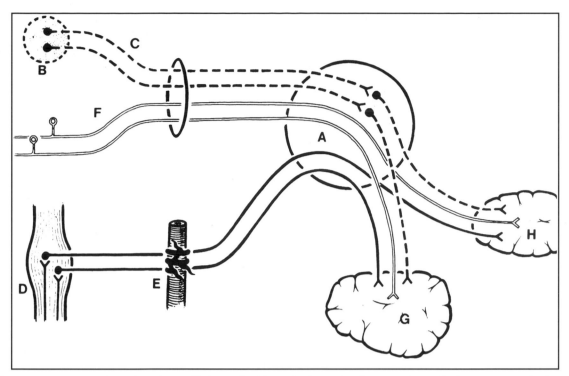

Fig. 4.14 The secretomotor supply to the submandibular and sublingual salivary glands. A = Submandibular parasympathetic ganglion; B = superior salivatory nucleus; C = chorda tympani branch of facial nerve; D = postganglionic fibres from the superior cervical ganglion; E = sympathetic plexus around the facial artery; F = lingual nerve; G = submandibular gland; H = sublingual gland.

THE INNERVATION OF THE ORAL MUSCULATURE

The functions of mastication, swallowing and speech are amongst the most complex in the body. This is reflected in the number and variety of muscles found around the mouth and by the range of cranial nerves that innervate them. Table 4.2 summarises the innervation of the oral musculature.

THE TRIGEMINAL NERVE (MAXILLARY AND MANDIBULAR DIVISIONS)

Maxillary division

The maxillary division of the trigeminal nerve (Figs 4.15, 4.16; see also Figs 4.8 and 4.11) contains only sensory fibres. It supplies the maxillary teeth and their supporting structures, the palate, the maxillary air sinus, much of the nasal cavity, and the skin overlying the middle part of the face. The nerve emerges into the pterygopalatine fossa through the foramen rotundum of the sphenoid bone. Its subsequent branches can be subdivided into branches from the main nerve trunk (Fig. 4.15) and branches from the pterygopalatine ganglion (see Fig. 4.16). From the main trunk are the meningeal, ganglionic, zygomatic, posterior superior alveolar and infraorbital nerves. The infraorbital nerve gives rise to the middle and anterior superior alveolar nerves. The branches of the maxillary nerve that arise via the pterygopalatine ganglion contain a mixture of sensory, parasympathetic (secretomotor) and sympathetic (vasomotor) fibres. The branches arising from the ganglion are the orbital, nasopalatine, posterior superior nasal, greater and lesser palatine, and pharyngeal nerves. Thus, the branches supplying the teeth and their supporting structures and the palate and the upper lip are the posterior, middle and anterior superior alveolar nerves, the nasopalatine and the greater and lesser palatine nerves, and the infraorbital nerve.

Table 4.2 *Innervation of the oral musculature*

Region	Muscle	Nerve
Lips	Orbicularis oris	Facial
Cheeks	Buccinator	Facial
Tongue (intrinsic musculature)	Transverse Longitudinal Vertical	Hypoglossal
Tongue (extrinsic musculature)	Genioglossus Hyoglossus Stylogossus	Hypoglossal
	Palatoglossus	Accessory (cranial part)
Floor of mouth	Mylohyoid	Mandibular division of trigeminal
	Geniohyoid	Hypoglossal (CI fibres)
Palate	Tensor veli palatini	Mandibular division of trigeminal
	Levator veli palatini Palatoglossus Palatopharyngeus Musculus uvulae	Accessory (cranial part)

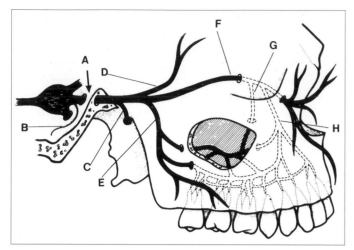

Fig. 4.15 Diagrammatic representation of the maxillary division of the trigeminal nerve and the branches that are derived directly from the nerve trunk. A = Maxillary nerve trunk passing through the foramen rotundum into the pterygopalatine fossa; B = meningeal branch; C = ganglionic branch; D = main zygomatic nerve; E = posterior superior alveolar nerve; F = infraorbital nerve; G = middle superior alveolar nerve; H = anterior superior alveolar nerve.

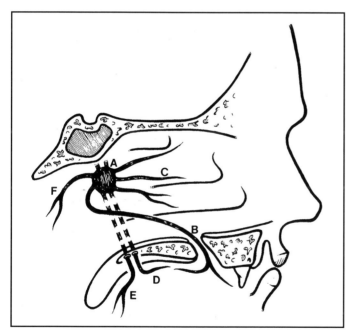

Fig. 4.16 Diagrammatic representation of the maxillary division of the trigeminal nerve and the branches that are derived via the pterygopalatine ganglion. A = Pterygopalatine ganglion; B = nasopalatine nerve; C = posterior superior nasal nerve; D = greater palatine nerve; E = lesser palatine nerve; F = pharyngeal nerve.

Mandibular division

The mandibular division of the trigeminal nerve (Fig. 4.17; see also Figs 3.31 and 4.5) is the largest division of the trigeminal nerve. It is the only division that contains motor fibres as well as sensory fibres. Its sensory fibres supply the mandibular teeth (and their supporting structures), the mucosa of the anterior two-thirds of the tongue and the floor

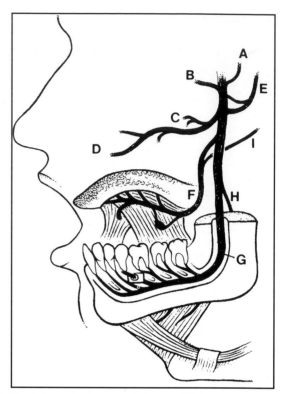

Fig. 4.17 Schematic diagram of the mandibular division of the trigeminal nerve. A = Meningeal branch; B = nerve to medial pterygoid; C = anterior trunk giving motor branches to masseter, temporalis and lateral pterygoid muscles; D = buccal nerve; E = auriculotemporal nerve; F = lingual nerve; G = inferior alveolar nerve; H = mylohyoid nerve; I = chorda tympani branch of facial nerve joining the lingual nerve.

of the mouth, the skin of the lower part of the face, and parts of the temple and auricle. Its motor fibres supply the muscles of mastication, the mylohyoid, anterior belly of the digastric, and the tensor veli palatini and tensor tympani muscles. The mandibular nerve emerges into the infratemporal fossa through the foramen ovale of the sphenoid bone. It lies deep to the lateral pterygoid muscle, where it gives off all its branches, dividing into anterior (mainly motor) and posterior (mainly sensory) trunks. Proximal to this division, it gives off the meningeal branch and the nerve to the medial pterygoid. The meningeal branch passes back into the middle cranial fossa through the foramen spinosum of the sphenoid bone (accompanied by the middle meningeal artery). The nerve to the medial pterygoid muscle passes through the otic ganglion (without synapsing) and, after supplying the muscle, continues on to supply the tensor veli palatini and tensor tympani muscles. The anterior trunk gives motor branches to the masseter, temporalis and lateral pterygoid, and the sensory buccal nerve. The posterior trunk gives off the sensory auriculotemporal, lingual and inferior alveolar nerves, and the motor mylohyoid nerve. Note that the chorda tympani branch of the facial nerve joins the lingual nerve and that postganglionic fibres from the otic parasympathetic ganglion run with the auriculotemporal nerve to provide secretomotor fibres to the parotid gland.

Central connections

Central connections of the trigeminal nerve are summarised in Fig. 4.18. The trigeminal nerve conveys discriminative tactile information from the ipsilateral half of the face and the top of the head; the axons of the trigeminal ganglion cells pass to the principal sensory nucleus and to the pars oralis of the spinal tract of the trigeminal nerve. Proprioceptive information from the ipsilateral muscles of mastication and the temporomandibular joint reach the mesencephalic nucleus of the trigeminal. However, recent evidence suggests that proprioceptive information from the teeth also pass to the principal sensory nucleus. Direct and indirect connections of these nuclei form the basis of cranial nerve reflexes. Signals from the principal sensory and mesencephalic nuclei are transmitted mainly via the contralateral ventral trigemino-thalamic tract (trigeminal lemniscus) and the ipsilateral dorsal trigeminothalamic tract to the nucleus ventralis posterior medialis of the thalamus. Axons from this nucleus pass through the posterior limb of the internal capsule to the inferior part of the postcentral gyrus and frontoparietal operculum. The nucleus of the spinal tract of the trigeminal nerve is subdivided into the pars oralis, pars interpolaris and pars caudalis. The pars oralis deals mainly with tactile signals. The pars interpolaris receives cutaneous and proprioceptive information and sends fibres to the cerebellum. The pars caudalis deals particularly with nociceptive signals (but also with tactile and thermal information). Fibres from the nucleus of the spinal tract pass to the reticular formation (for cranial nerve reflexes). Some fibres run near the medial lemniscus in the contralateral ventral trigeminothalamic tract to reach the various thalamic nuclei. The motor nucleus of the trigeminal nerve lies close to the principal central nucleus in the central part of the pons. It receives fibres from the other sensory trigeminal nuclei, the reticular formation, the cerebellum and the cerebral cortex via bilateral corticonuclear fibres.

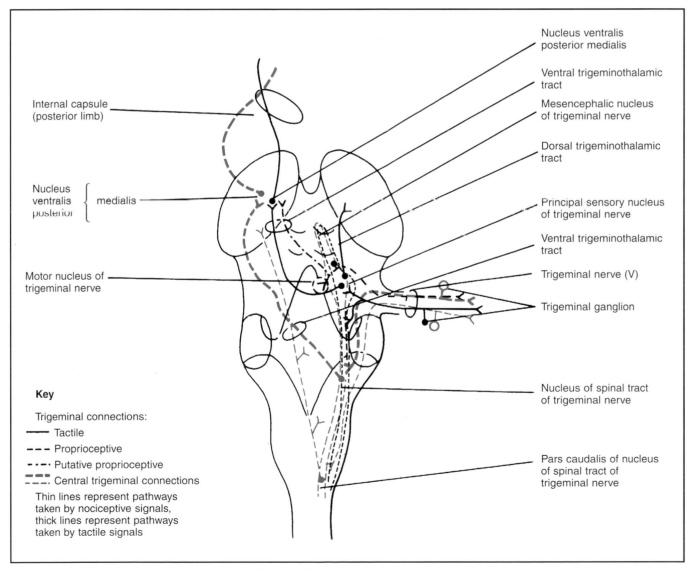

Fig. 4.18 The central connections of the trigeminal nerve.

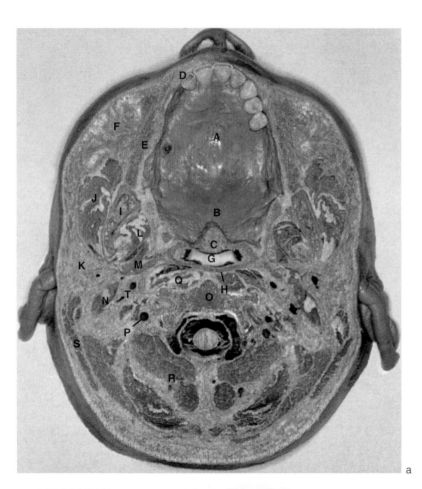

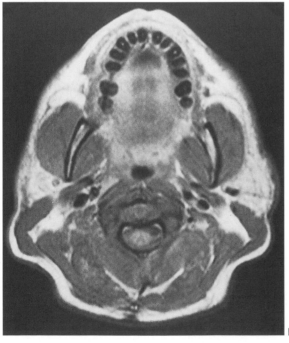

Fig. 5.1 (a) Transverse section through the head to show the palate and its topographic relationships. A = Hard palate; B = soft palate; C = uvula; D = upper lip; E = buccinator muscle; F = buccal pad of fat; G = nasopharynx; H = superior constrictor muscle of pharynx; I = ramus of mandible; J = masseter muscle; K = parotid gland; L = medial pterygoid muscle; M = styloid group of muscles: stylopharyngeus, stylohyoid, styloglossus; N = posterior belly of digastric muscle; O = axis (second cervical vertebra); P = vertebral artery; Q = prevertebral muscles; R = postvertebral muscles; S = sternocleidomastoid muscle; T = internal carotid artery and internal jugular vein. (b) MRI scan of the head at the level of the palate. Courtesy of Squadron Leader S.C.P. Blease.

The study of anatomical sections has become increasingly important in medicine with the advent of special imaging techniques such as computed tomography (CT) imaging and magnetic resonance imaging (MRI). Although these specialised techniques are available for some disciplines in dentistry, knowledge of sectional anatomy is important for all dentists because many of the procedures (surgical and anaesthetic) require a good knowledge of the relationships of structures around the mouth. Thus, the illustrations in this chapter provide transverse sections through the head at various levels relative to the oral cavity and alongside corresponding MRI images.

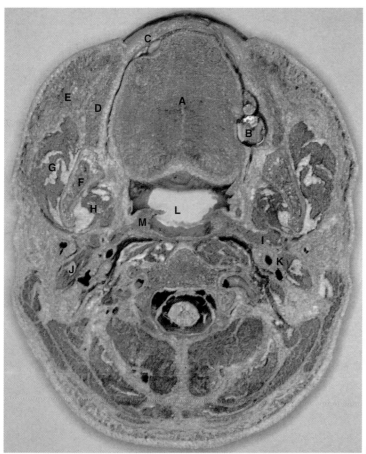

a

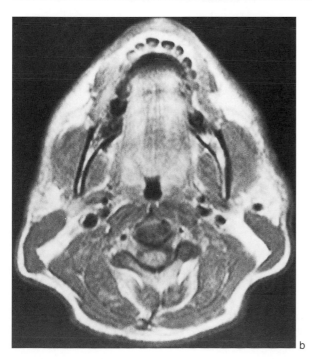

b

Fig. 5.2 (a) Transverse section through the head at the level of the palatine tonsil to show the tongue and its topographic relationships. A = Tongue; B = mandibular molar; C = lower lip; D = buccinator muscle; E = buccal pad of fat; F = ramus of mandible; G = masseter muscle; H = medial pterygoid muscle; I = styloid group of muscles; J = posterior belly of digastric muscle; K = carotid sheath containing internal carotid artery, internal jugular vein and vagus nerve; L = oropharynx; M = palatopharyngeus muscle. (b) MRI scan of the head at the level of the tongue and palatine tonsil. Courtesy of Squadron Leader S.C.P. Blease.

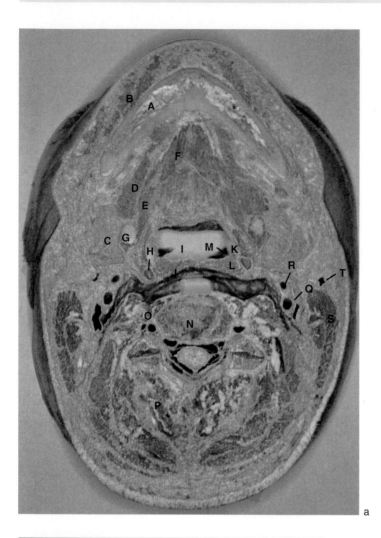

a

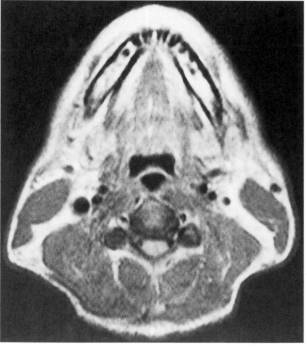

b

Fig. 5.3 (a) Transverse section through the head to show the floor of the mouth and its topographic relationships. A = Body of mandible; B = depressor labii superioris and depressor anguli oris muscles; C = submandibular gland; D = mylohyoid muscle; E = hyoglossus muscle; F = genioglossus muscle; G = tendon of digastric muscle; H = tip of greater horn of hyoid bone; I = oropharynx; J = middle constrictor muscle of pharynx; K = palatoglossal fold – anterior pillar of the fauces; L = palatopharyngeal fold – posterior pillars of the fauces; M = tonsillar crypt; N = cervical vertebra; O = prevertebral group of muscles; Q = carotid sheath containing internal carotid artery, internal jugular vein and vagus nerve; R = external carotid artery; S = sternocleidomastoid muscle; T = external jugular vein. (b) MRI scan of the head at the level of the floor of the mouth. Courtesy of Squadron Leader S.C.P. Blease.

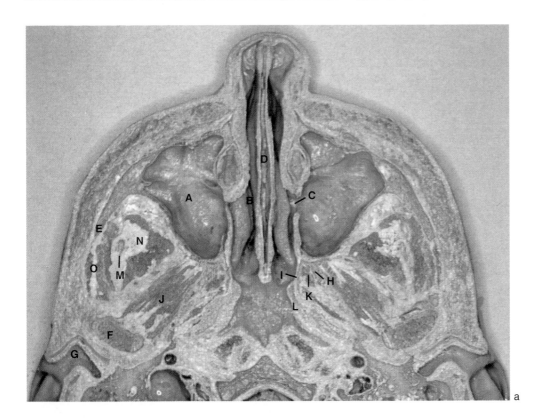

a

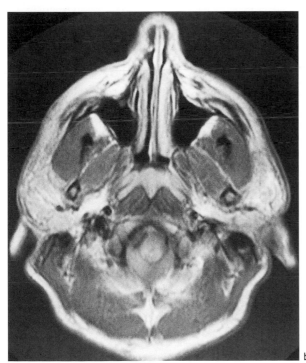

b

Fig. 5.4 (a) Transverse section through head to show the maxillary air sinuses and their topographic relationships.

A = Floor of maxillary air sinus; B = nasal fossa; C = ostium – opening of maxillary sinus into middle meatus on the lateral wall of the nose; D = nasal septum; E = zygomatic arch; F = condyle of mandible; G = external acoustic meatus; H = lateral pterygoid plate of sphenoid bone; I = medial pterygoid plate of sphenoid bone; J = lateral pterygoid muscle; K = medial pterygoid muscle; L = superior constrictor of pharynx; M = coronoid process of mandible; N = temporalis muscle; O = masseter muscle. (b) MRI scan of the head to show maxillary air sinuses. Courtesy of Squadron Leader S.C.P. Blease.

6 Functional anatomy

MASTICATION

Mastication is the process whereby ingested food is cut or crushed into small pieces, mixed with saliva, and formed into a bolus in preparation for swallowing. It is characteristic of mammals, which possess teeth of different forms (heterodonty) adapted to the comminution of food. In non-mammalians, the teeth are used mainly for prehension, the prey generally being seized head first and swallowed whole.

Various functions have been ascribed to mastication in humans. It:

1. enables the food bolus to be easily swallowed.
2. enhances the digestibility of food by:
   (a) decreasing the size of particles to increase the surface area for enzyme activity;
   (b) reflexively stimulating the secretion of digestive juices (e.g. saliva and gastric juice).
3. mixes the food with saliva, initiating digestion by the activity of salivary amylase.
4. prevents irritation of the gastrointestinal system by large food masses.
5. ensures healthy growth and development of the oral tissues.

Of all these, the increase in digestive efficiency is usually considered to be the primary purpose of mastication. Indeed, it has been suggested that there is an enormous gain in digestive efficiency without which the high rate of metabolism associated with homeothermy in mammals could not be sustained. However, some experimental evidence indicates that mastication produces little gain in digestive efficiency in humans. Table 6.1 classifies different foods according to the value of mastication in their digestion. The information in the table was obtained by research in which 1 g of either premasticated or unmasticated

food was placed in cotton net bags, swallowed and subsequently collected from the faeces. Category 1 foods were those that left some large residues if swallowed with or without mastication. Category 2 foods left some residues when unchewed but were usually completely digested when chewed. Category 3 foods were likely to be fully digested, with or without mastication. Thus, it is only for the few types of food in Category 2 that mastication improves digestion. That these results suggest that mastication produces little gain in digestive efficiency may simply be a reflection of the Western ability to select, grow and prepare foods so that all socially acceptable items of diet are inherently easily digestible.

Mastication occurs by the convergent movements of maxillary and mandibular teeth. In humans, most foods are first crushed by vertical movements of the mandible before being sheared by lateral to medial movements of the mandible to make a bolus. The initial crushing of the food does not require full occlusion of the teeth. Indeed, it is often only after the food has been well softened that the maxillary and mandibular teeth eventually contact. Once the cusps can interdigitate, the ridges on the slopes of the cusps shear the food as the mandibular teeth move across the maxillary teeth. As the cusps cross the depressions within the opposing occlusal surfaces, there is grinding of food, which has been likened to the action of a pestle and mortar.

Fig. 6.1 relates the morphology of the cheek teeth to the displacement of food during mastication. Several features, common to all the cheek teeth, provide protection for the adjacent gingiva during chewing. The marginal ridges bounding the interproximal edges of the occlusal surfaces of the teeth are important protective features. These ridges deflect most of the food, potentially driven between adjacent teeth by their opponents, onto the occlusal surfaces. The contact points beneath the marginal ridges should abut firmly to prevent food being wedged between the teeth and above the interdental papillae. These contacts are maintained by the process of mesial drift (see Chapter 26, page 362), despite the constant attrition of interproximal dental tissue. The buccal cusps of the mandibular cheek teeth bite between the buccal and palatal cusps of the maxillary cheek teeth, with the result that food trapped between them is forced up over the palatal sides of the maxillary teeth and down over the buccal sides of the mandibular teeth. The palatal gingiva for the maxillary teeth is thus protected by the marked curvature of these teeth. In addition, it is the buccal surfaces of the mandibular cheek teeth that are the most curved.

Mastication is not simply a result of rhythmically closing teeth of a particular form on a piece of food. This would simply produce random breakage of food. Two other functions are essential. Firstly, the placement of food between the occluding

Table 6.1	(Modified after J.H. Farrell)	
Category 1	*Category 2*	*Category 3*
Roast and fried pork	Roast chicken	Fried and stewed beef fat
Fried bacon	Stewed lamb	Fried and boiled cod
Roast, fried and stewed beef		Fried kipper
Roast and stewed mutton		Hard-boiled egg
Roast and fried lamb		Boiled rice
Fried and boiled potatoes		White and wholemeal bread
Boiled garden peas		
Boiled carrots		Cheddar cheese

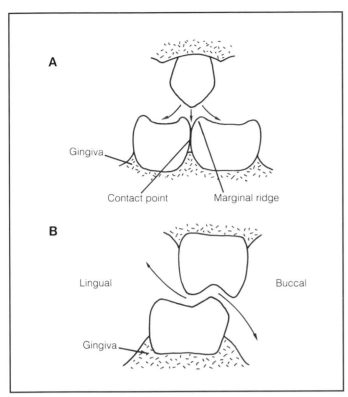

Fig. 6.1 Morphology of the cheek teeth in relation to the displacement of food (arrows). (a) Buccal view; (b) interproximal view.

surfaces of the teeth by the tongue. Secondly, the selection by the tongue of those pieces of food in the mouth that require further physical reduction. Other structural features associated with mastication that are peculiar to mammals include:

- temporomandibular jaw articulation
- serous salivary glands
- prismatic enamel
- secondary palate
- significant muscle development associated with lips, cheeks, tongue and muscles of mastication
- diphyodonty
- gomphosis type of tooth attachment.

The development of a temporomandibular articulation and increased mass of the muscles of mastication allow the force of the bite and the range of movement for chewing to be increased. Saliva adds to the moistening and lubrication of food during mastication and its enzymes allow some carbohydrate digestion to commence at an early stage in the mouth. The prismatic arrangement of dental enamel (see Chapter 7, page 104) and its greater thickness in mammals are said to be more efficient in resisting both masticatory loads and attrition than non-prismatic enamel. The development of a secondary palate is thought to be related to the necessity of maintaining ventilation during prolonged masticatory periods. The development of muscles within the lips, cheeks and tongue is associated with manipulation of the bolus within the mouth. The change from polyphyodonty (i.e. multiple tooth succession) to diphyodonty (two dentitions: deciduous and permanent) may be related to two factors, i) a 'grinding-in' period

necessary to produce an efficient cutting or grinding tooth surface or possibly ii) to the formation of a particular pattern of jaw movement by conditioned reflexes originating from stimulation of the periodontal receptors; it seems inefficient to replace such teeth too frequently. The gomphosis type of attachment (with a periodontal ligament; see Chapter 12, page 201) may be associated with the increased stresses and strains brought to bear on the tooth during mastication; it also allows for tooth movement. Such movement stimulates sensory receptors in the periodontal ligament, so providing information on the loading and movement of individual teeth.

Mastication is dependent upon a complex chain of events, that produce rhythmic opening and closing movements of the jaws and correlated tongue movements. The forces that are exerted on the teeth and jaws are very large and physiologically significant. Experiments involving the implantation of force transducers into the occlusal surfaces of teeth have shown that the bite force exerted on the food during mastication is of the order of 5–15 kg. This force varies according to the texture of the food. When bite pressure is measured with a gnathodynamometer, maximum pressures of the order of 50 kg can be readily recorded.

Rhythmic jaw movements (Fig. 6.2) are now generally accepted as being generated by a centre within the brainstem. This is referred to as an oral rhythm/pattern generator and is activated both by drive from the higher centres and by peripheral sensory input. The pattern of activity is distributed to the motor neuron pools, which also receive excitatory or

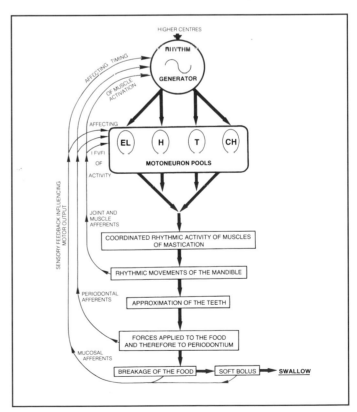

Fig. 6.2 A diagrammatic representation of the way jaw movements are thought to operate. EL = Jaw elevator musculature; H = hyoid and associated musculature; T = tongue and associated musculature; CH = cheek and associated musculature.

inhibitory sensory inputs from a variety of peripheral structures. The hypothesis is that the sensory input generated by closing on hard food supports the generation of rhythmic jaw activity, whereas closure on a softened bolus promotes tongue movement and food transport, eliciting a swallow: the effect is to terminate the rhythmic jaw activity.

The chewing cycle

Mammals generally chew on one side at a time. Two methods of chewing have been distinguished, depending upon the texture of the food:

1. Puncture/crushing. Hard food is first crushed and pierced between the teeth without direct tooth-to-tooth contact. This results in wear (attrition) of the teeth, especially at the tips of the cusps.
2. Shearing stroke. This method involves tooth contacts that take place only after the food has been sufficiently reduced. This type of movement produces attrition facets with characteristic directional scratch lines on the faces of the cusps.

The action of the teeth during mastication depends on their morphology, the movements of the mandible, and the nature of the forces generated by the muscles of mastication. The chewing cycle involves three basic phases (or strokes) of the mandible in relation to the maxilla. From a position in which the jaw is open, the closing stroke results in the teeth being brought into initial contact with the food; the work done in this phase is really against gravity. This is followed by the power stroke, when the food undergoes reduction. Movement of the mandible in this phase is slower than in the closing stroke because of the resistance caused by the food, even though there may be vastly greater masseter and temporalis muscle activity during this time. Finally, there is the opening stroke, when the mandible is lowered, with an initial slower stage followed by a faster stage.

Fig. 6.3 shows the occlusal relationships of the cheek teeth during chewing on the left side. From an open position the mandible is moved upwards and outwards, bringing the buccal cusps of the maxillary and mandibular teeth on the working (left) side in contact (Fig. 6.3a). As mentioned previously, the teeth may not contact each other during the initial masticatory cycles. In the power stroke the mandibular teeth then slide upwards and medially against the maxillary teeth to momentarily attain intercuspal position (Fig. 6.3b). Following attainment of the intercuspal position, the mandibular teeth continue downwards and inwards against the maxillary teeth (the lingual phase, Fig. 6.3c). The opening stroke then follows and the cycle is repeated. The relationships of the teeth on the balancing side are also illustrated in Fig. 6.3. Note that, while the teeth on the working side are moving through the buccal phase (Fig. 6.3a), those on the balancing (right) side are in the lingual phase, but in the reverse direction. Although the diagrams in Fig. 6.3 show tooth contact, it is probable that any contact on the balancing side is only transient.

In primates (including humans), the chewing cycle differs depending upon whether the food is solid or soft (Fig. 6.4). Note that the vertical component of condylar movement is due to its

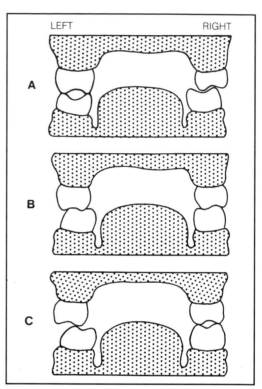

Fig. 6.3 Occlusal relationships of the cheek teeth during chewing on the left side. (a) Buccal phase on working (left) side; (b) intercuspal position; (c) lingual phase. Note the positions of the teeth on the balancing side (right).

movement up and down the slope of the articular eminence (see Chapter 3, page 59). The first cycle has a profile that is commonly found when solid food is chewed. After a previous opening, the jaw accelerates into relatively fast closing (phase labelled 'FC'). At this stage, the food is being accelerated only against gravity, and the electromyographic activity in the jaw-closing muscles is of low amplitude. As tooth–food–tooth contact is made ('TFT'), activity in the jaw-closing muscles increases and force is exerted on the food. The food resistance slows the jaw closing ('SC'). As the cusps continue to interdigitate, closing velocity slows to zero. The duration of this stationary phase is a matter of dispute. Because of uncertainty, the intercuspal phase ('ICP') is shown as a dashed line. The jaw subsequently opens with a relatively constant velocity. There is relatively little movement of the tongue producing food transport towards the pharynx. The second cycle shown in the figure is characteristic of the ingestion of soft food. The closing phase consists largely of fast closing because the food offers little resistance to jaw closure. Opening now consists of two phases – slow opening followed by fast opening. The duration of the first phase of opening (slow opening) correlates with the amplitude of tongue movement and with food transport towards the pharynx.

The main point being made here is that cycle form is variable, depending upon the sensory feedback (see page 94).

The envelope of motion

The pathway followed by the mandible during chewing is termed 'the envelope of motion' (Fig. 6.5). This demonstrates

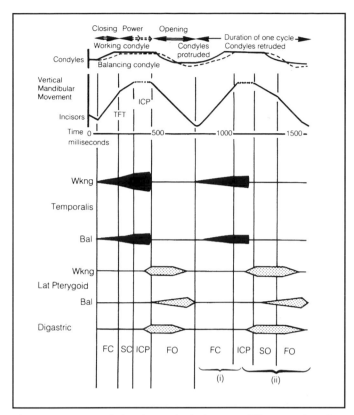

Fig. 6.4 Patterns of chewing cycle during two different cycles of jaw movement (cycle 1 for solid food; cycle 2 for soft food). FC = Fast-closing phase; SC = slow-closing phase; ICP = intercuspal phase; FO = fast-opening phase; TFT = tooth–food–tooth contact. Courtesy of Dr A. Thexton.

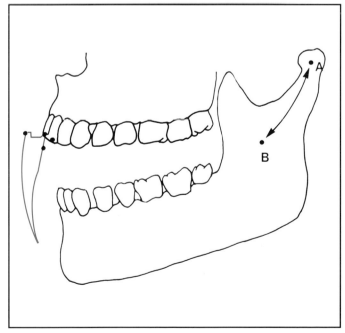

Fig. 6.5 The envelope of motion of the contact point between the mandibular incisors when viewed from the side (laterally and in the sagittal plane). See text for explanation of coloured trajectories and for the change in the fulcrum of movements from Point A to Point B.

the symmetrical mandibular movements produced during opening and closing of the jaw.

The envelope of motion is the volume of space within which all movements of a specified point on the mandible occur. The envelope is limited by anatomical considerations such as ligaments and tooth contacts. Most natural movements do not utilise this maximum volume but occur well within the 'envelope'. The yellow trajectory shown in Fig. 6.5 depicts a two-phased, conscious movement from the rest position to the fully opened position. The first phase is a hinge-like movement during which the condyles remain retruded within the mandibular fossae. When the teeth become separated by approximately 25 mm, the second phase of opening occurs and involves anterior movement or protrusion of the condyles down the articular eminences. The blue and red trajectories shown in the figure describe a biphasic path of closure from the fully opened mandibular position, which can be performed only with conscious effort. The first phase (the blue trajectory) takes the mandible up to a protruded closed position, while the second phase (the red trajectory) takes the mandible from this protruded contact position to a retruded contact position. The green trajectory describes the free, habitual, unconscious movement during both mandibular opening and closing. The points on the ramus of the mandible in the figure represent the centres of rotation during opening and closure. Point A is the fulcrum associated with simple hinge movements. The path described between points A and B represents the shift of the centre of rotation of the mandible; this shift occurs because of the transition from a pure hinge movement at the condyle to protrusion and rotation during opening (with the reverse during closing). Point B has been described as representing the point of rotation around the attachment of the sphenomandibular ligament at the lingula.

A 'profile' or 'envelope of motion' showing the average incisal movements in the frontal plane during a masticatory cycle is shown in Fig. 6.6. In the coronal plane (i.e. viewed from in front) the opening movement rarely goes straight down but deviates to one side. There is a wide variation in profiles between individuals and also continuous variation between consecutive

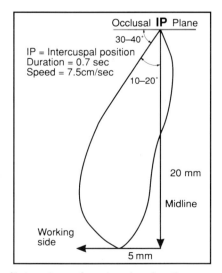

Fig. 6.6 Profile/envelope of motion showing the average incisal movements in the frontal plane during a masticatory cycle. Redrawn after Professor J. Ahlgren.

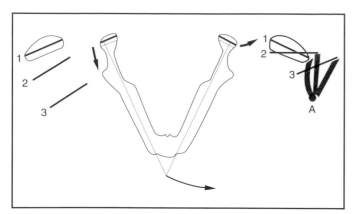

Fig. 6.7 Transverse movements of the lower jaw (lateral excursions or side-to-side movements). The thick lines represent the horizontal band of the temporomandibular ligament. A = articular eminence. Redrawn after Professors H. Sicher and E.L. Dubrul.

chewing cycles in the same individual: for example, the initial deviation may be towards the chewing side or away from it (as shown in Fig. 6.6). Furthermore, the profiles differ according to the type of occlusion and the texture of the food.

The transverse movements of the lower jaw (i.e. lateral excursions or side-to-side movements as viewed from above) are illustrated in Fig. 6.7. These movements involve bilaterally asymmetric movements of the mandible. They are produced by protrusion of the mandibular condyle down the articular eminence of the temporal bone on one side with reactive movements of the other condyle (rotation around a laterally shifting axis). The illustration describes the changing positions of the long axes of the mandibular condyles during lateral movements of the mandible to the left. The figure also shows the change in the horizontal band of the temporomandibular ligament passing from the articular eminence to the lateral surface of the condyle during lateral movements. Tension generated in the horizontal band produces a slight lateral shift in the condyle (Bennett shift).

The control of mastication

There has in the past been much controversy concerning the origin and control of the rhythmic activity of the jaws during mastication. One view, the cerebral hemispheres theory, held that mastication was a conscious act, a patterned set of instructions originating in the higher centres of the central nervous system (in particular the motor cortex) and descending to directly drive the motoneurones within the brainstem (trigeminal, facial and hypoglossal motoneurones). Another idea, the reflex chain theory, held that mastication involved a series of interacting chains of reflexes. Accordingly, sensory input from the region of the mouth (e.g. pressure on the teeth) triggered the motoneurones in the brainstem to elicit a jaw opening movement. In turn, this movement produced another sensory input (e.g. from stretch receptors in the jaw muscles), which resulted in a jaw closing reflex. Such a theory could explain the rhythmic jaw movements seen in decerebrate animals. Although there are several well recognised types of jaw reflexes (see Fig 6.8–6.10 for examples), objections to the reflex chain theory have been raised on the basis that masti-

cation involves prolonged bursts of muscle activity and not the brief and abrupt behaviour usually associated with reflex activation of muscle. A third theory, the rhythm (pattern) generator theory, has more recently been proposed to explain rhythmic jaw functioning. This theory is based upon the proposition that there are central pattern generators (CPGs) within the brainstem, which, on being stimulated from either higher centres or sensory inputs in the region of the mouth, are driven into rhythmic activity. This idea could account for rhythmic activity obtained by stimulating either the motor cortex or, in decerebrate animals, the oral cavity. This theory, supported by comparisons with other physiological systems that require pattern generators (e.g. respiration), is now generally accepted.

A CPG is a set of closely interconnected neurones that generates a series of rhythmic outputs passing to the different groups of motor neurones involved in a particular movement (e.g. suckling, chewing). Consequently, each motor neurone group, and therefore each muscle, is activated at the correct time for that rhythmic movement. The activity of this generator depends upon excitation descending in pathways from cerebral cortical areas and upon excitation deriving from peripheral stimulation (i.e. the rhythmic activity can be generated by conscious drive and/or by the presence of food in the mouth). However, the relative importance of the two sources of excitation seems to vary with age. The human adult may be unable to feed at all after damage to the cerebral cortex while, in the anencephalic infant (one born without any cerebral hemispheres), suckling movements can be elicited simply by stimulating the lips.

During mastication, the cycles of jaw movement differ, depending upon the consistency of the food initially ingested and upon the stage of breakdown of that food. This indicates that the cyclic activity generated by the CPG is subject to modification by sensory input from the mouth. However, if equivalent types of sensory input are generated experimentally by controlled stimuli applied to oral sites then reflex responses can be generated quite independently of any pre-existing rhythmic activity (i.e. whether a particular sensory input elicits a reflex, fails to elicit a reflex or modifies ongoing activity simply depends upon what else is going in the central nervous system).

In the last 100 years, at least a dozen oral reflexes have been described, forgotten and redescribed. Only the two least contentious and most commonly known are described here: the jaw jerk and the jaw opening reflex.

The jaw jerk

The jaw jerk is produced when the jaw closing muscles are stretched by tapping the chin downwards so that the jaw opens suddenly. The monosynaptic reflex is due to stimulation of stretch-sensitive receptors (muscle spindles) in the masseter and temporalis muscles. The stretch produces a burst of impulses in the sensory nerves that is conveyed back to the motor neurones of those muscles. The muscles are consequently activated briefly to produce a short-lived contraction (Fig. 6.8).

Jaw opening reflex

The jaw opening reflexes are more complex (polysynaptic) and can be produced by applying mechanical or electrical stimuli to oral mucosa, periodontal ligament or teeth; the stimuli do not have to be painful to elicit the reflex but stronger stimuli do produce correspondingly more vigorous responses. In humans the reflex is characterised by a brief period of inhibition of

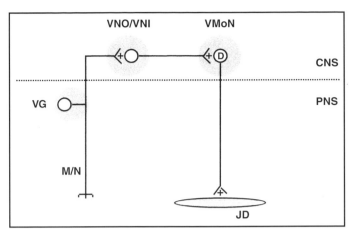

Fig. 6.10 *Schematic representation of pathway of jaw opening reflex involving the digastric muscle. There are disynaptic connections between afferent nerves from orofacial mechano receptors and nociceptors (M/N) through the trigeminal sensory nuclei oralis (VNO) and/or interpolaris (VNI) to jaw depressor motoneurones (D). Shaded areas represent ganglia or brainstem nuclei. VG = Trigeminal ganglion; VMoN = trigeminal motor nucleus; CNS = central nervous system; PNS = peripheral nervous system; + = excitatory synapse; JD = jaw depressor muscle. Courtesy of Doctors S.W. Cadden and R. Orchardson, and Karger, Basel.*

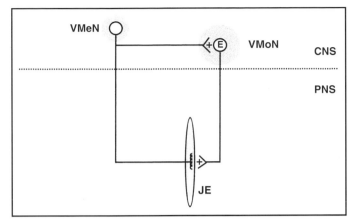

Fig. 6.8 *Schematic representation of pathway of the jaw jerk reflex. There are monosynaptic connections between afferent nerves and from spindles in the jaw elevator muscles (JE) and the motoneurones to these same muscles. Shaded areas represent brainstem nuclei. VMeN = Trigeminal mesencephalic nucleus; VMoN = trigeminal motor nucleus; CNS = central nervous system; PNS = peripheral nervous system; + = excitatory synapse; E = jaw elevator motoneurone. Courtesy of Doctors S.W. Cadden and R. Orchardson and Karger, Basel.*

activity in the motor neurones of the jaw closing muscles (Fig. 6.9). However, in other mammals (and in some neurological disorders in humans) there is in addition a simultaneous activation of the jaw opening muscles (e.g. digastric and infrahyoid muscles) (Fig. 6.10).

SWALLOWING

Swallowing (deglutition) involves an ordered sequence of events that carry food (or saliva) from the mouth into the stomach. Although a continuous activity, swallowing is subdivided into stages for descriptive convenience. Humans swallow approximately 600 times every 24 hours, but only about 150 of these are concerned with food and drink; the rest simply clear saliva from the mouth. It is important to appreciate that, alongside muscle activity required to move the bolus, there must be mechanisms to protect the airway (e.g. closure of the nasopharynx by the soft palate, elevation of the larynx, closure of the laryngeal inlet by the epiglottis).

In preparation for swallowing, a softened or liquid food bolus is moved through the mouth by the action of the tongue. The bolus is first moved to lie in a longitudinal midline furrow formed in the tongue dorsum; the floor of this furrow is then progressively raised from before backwards, squeezing the bolus back against the hard palate. The kinetic energy imparted to the bolus moves it into and through the pharynx, where contractions of the circularly arranged pharyngeal constrictor muscles complete the movement of the bolus down to the oesophagus, where peristalsis (a moving wave of contraction) conveys the bolus onwards to the stomach. This process requires that the upper (cricopharyngeal) and lower oesophageal (cardiac) sphincters relax at the correct time to allow the bolus to pass. The classical division of the above components of the

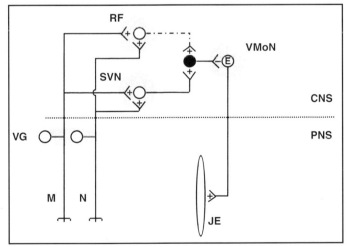

Fig. 6.9 *Inhibitory exteroceptive jaw reflexes: schematic representation of probable pathways. These reflexes can be produced most effectively by stimulation of mechanoreceptors (M) or nociceptors (N) from the mouth and face. Two responses can be identified: a short-latency one mediated by a di- or trisynaptic pathway through the supratrigeminal nucleus and a long-latency one mediated by a polysynaptic pathway through the reticular formation. Shaded areas represent ganglia or nuclei. VG = Trigeminal ganglion; SVN = supratrigeminal nucleus; RF = reticular formation; VMoN = trigeminal motor nucleus; CNS = central nervous system; PNS = peripheral nervous system; + = excitatory synapse; − = inhibitory synapse; E = jaw elevator motoneurone; JE = jaw elevator muscle. Broken line represents uncertainty about the number of synapses involved in that pathway. Courtesy of Doctors S.W. Cadden and R. Orchardson, and Karger, Basel.*

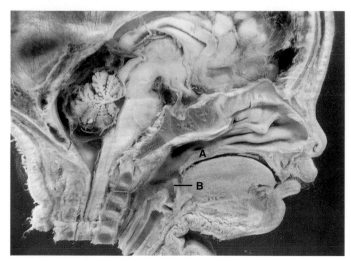

Fig. 6.11 Sagittal section of the head of a neonate. Note the relatively high position of the larynx, the opening being at the level of the soft palate (A). B = Epiglottis.

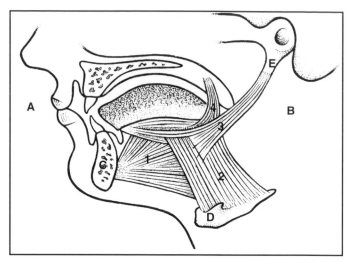

Fig. 6.12 Sagittal section of an adult head. Compared with Fig. 6.11, the opening of the larynx lies well below the level of the soft palate (A). B = Epiglottis.

swallow in the human adult is into three phases: the oral phase, the pharyngeal phase and the oesophageal phase.

In the adult human, the process of swallowing is complicated by the fact that the pharynx also forms part of the airway leading from the nose to the larynx. Consequently, swallowing and breathing cannot safely occur at the same time. In contrast, in the human newborn and generally in other mammals (both infant and adult) the larynx occupies a relatively higher position (Fig. 6.11). In these cases the laryngeal opening is usually above the level of the soft palate, the lateral part of which extends around the larynx. In this situation there is a degree of anatomical separation of the respiratory tract and the alimentary tract (in some animals the high larynx completely divides the pharynx into two passages, which pass laterally either side of the larynx, rejoining behind and below it). The timed separation of swallowing and breathing is consequently less critical in this situation than it is in adult humans.

The anatomical differences between adults and neonates also produce differences in the way that the swallow is executed. In the case of the high larynx in the infant, where the epiglottis contacts the posterior edge of the U-shaped soft palate, a space is formed which is bounded above by the soft palate, behind by the anterior surface of the epiglottis/larynx and in front and below by the tongue dorsum. During feeding this space accumulates food before its onward passage via the pharynx and oesophagus to the stomach. The space (filled by the posterior part of the tongue – Fig. 6.11) includes, but is usually significantly larger than, the valleculae (the pockets formed between the larynx and the surface of the back of the tongue). For convenience this storage area will be referred to as the 'vallecular space'.

Growth in length of the human pharynx (starting a few months after birth) causes the larynx to take up a relatively lower position in the pharynx so that its contact with the soft palate is lost (Fig. 6.12). There is consequently no longer an enclosed space in which food can be stored or accumulated and the airway is no longer anatomically separated from the food passage. A variety of measures operate to protect the airway during swallowing in this situation, including interruption

of breathing, closure of the glottis, tipping the larynx forward so that the back of the tongue bulges over it during swallowing, bending of the epiglottis back and down over the laryngeal opening. At the same time the nasal airway is closed by elevation of the soft palate against an upper pharynx narrowed by the pharyngeal constrictor muscles. Because of the low position of the larynx, the pattern of swallowing in the adult human is the exception to the general pattern in mammals.

In most mammalian (and human infant) feeding, the 'vallecular space' is gradually filled during the course of a number of food transport cycles (which may include mastication where appropriate). Adequate filling of the 'vallecular space' appears to be the trigger for its periodic emptying. The contents then pass down the pharynx and oesophagus. Unless one includes all of the tongue and jaw movements involved in suckling, lapping or chewing that are associated with filling the vallecular space, the true swallow consists only of emptying that space and the subsequent movement of the bolus down the pharynx and oesophagus. The ratio of the number of cycles filling the vallecular space to the number of cycles in which swallowing (vallecular emptying) occurs varies from about 2:1 to 14:1. The situation is different in the human adult, where the descent of the larynx means that the vallecular space no longer exists as a potentially closed cavity and storage area. Surprisingly, in this situation a swallow is initiated immediately the first trace of food material or saliva enters the true valleculae. The question then becomes one of how vallecular emptying is triggered so readily in the adult human when (unlike other mammals where a significant amount of food is transported into the vallecular space over a number of cycles) only a trace of food or liquid may have reached the region. Furthermore, in humans the movement of the bolus backwards from the mouth to the valleculae is followed by vallecular emptying on a 1:1 basis. Consequently, the transport of the bolus into the valleculae is regarded as part of the swallow and is classically described as the first (or oral phase) of the swallow in adult humans.

In mammals generally, the neural mechanisms involved in swallowing depend upon sensory input from branches of the glossopharyngeal and vagal nerves that supply the mucous membrane of the vallecular space. Through its internal laryngeal branch, the superior laryngeal nerve (a branch of the vagus) carries important sensory input from the larynx, epiglottis and valleculae; this is one of the most powerful sensory pathways involved in eliciting a swallow. In the case of the high larynx, swallowing can be elicited reflexly by fluid in the vallecular space even when there are no connections with those parts of the brain above the brainstem (in decerebrate animals and e.g. in infants with anencephaly, where the cerebral hemispheres are congenitally absent). It can therefore firstly be assumed that all the necessary neural components for swallowing are located in the brainstem. Secondly, it can be assumed that sensory input from the surface of the palate, epiglottis and tongue (the walls of the vallecular space) is alone sufficient to elicit a swallow. The generally accepted view is that the peripheral sensory input activates a set of neural circuits within the brainstem that collectively produce the pattern of motor activity constituting a swallow. These circuits constitute a central pattern generator (CPG) for the activity involving the 30 or so muscles that take part in a swallow. The relevant network of brainstem neurones receives not only peripheral sensory input but also excitatory fibres descending from the cerebral cortex, in this way being similar to the CPG for mastication.

However, in the adult human, where there is no longer an enclosed vallecular space and no possibility of significant storage of food, the level of sensory input from the periphery must be less than that arising in other mammals. The initiation of swallowing in adult humans can be explained on the basis of the activity in the excitatory pathway descending from the cerebral cortex exciting the swallowing CPG to a high level, so that it requires only a trace more sensory input from the periphery to trigger the swallow. In other words, the descending drive lowers the threshold for reflex emptying of the valleculae. Because only a weak sensory input is necessary, only a trace of material has to reach the vallecula to elicit its emptying and all the subsequent components of the swallow. The lower threshold does, however, mean that other sensory inputs (e.g. glosso-pharyngeal) play a larger role in eliciting the swallow.

The stages of swallowing

Although the act of swallowing is not discontinuous, classically it has been divided into three stages for descriptive convenience: the oral stage, the pharyngeal stage and the oesophageal stage (Fig. 6.13). At each stage it is necessary to consider not only the movement of the bolus but also how the airway is isolated from the food.

Stage 1 – Oral stage

The jaw is elevated by the action of the masseter and temporalis muscles, and the lips are approximated by the circumoral muscles forming the anterior oral seal. A longitudinal furrow is produced in the upper surface of the tongue by the bilateral action of the styloglossus muscles inserted into the lateral edges of the tongue, by the vertical fibres of the intrinsic musculature

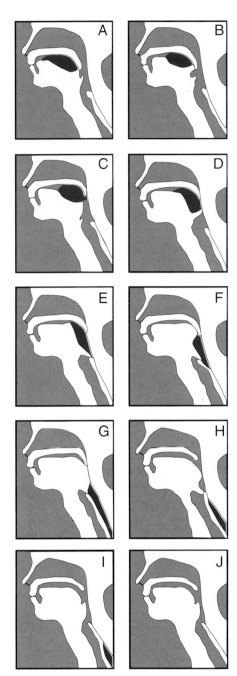

Fig. 6.13 The stages of swallowing. A – C = Oral stage; D – F = pharyngeal stage; G – J = oesophageal stage.

and by the action of the genioglossal muscles inserted close to the midline. The tongue is then elevated against the palate by the action of the mylohyoid muscles and the groove in the tongue is progressively emptied from before backwards, moving the bolus rapidly towards the pharynx. The airway remains open at this stage, with the soft palate lying away from the posterior wall of the pharynx and contacting the posterior surface of the tongue, so forming a posterior oral seal.

Stage 2 – Pharyngeal stage

The bolus passes through the oropharyngeal isthmus into the pharynx because of the kinetic energy imparted by the tongue; as the bolus leaves the oral cavity the palatoglossal folds contract behind the bolus. A wave of contraction within the pharyngeal constrictor muscles then clears the bolus from the pharynx. The tensor veli palatini and levator veli palatini muscles are activated so that the soft palate elevates to contact the posterior wall of the pharynx, closing the nasopharynx. The larynx is elevated and its opening is protected by the bulge of the posterior part of the tongue and by being covered by the epiglottis, which is flexed partly by the drag of the bolus and partly by the action of the aryepiglottic muscles. The laryngeal inlet is also reduced by closure of the glottis.

Stage 3 – Oesophageal stage

Relaxation of the cricopharyngeal part of the inferior constrictor allows the food into the oesophagus, where a peristaltic wave moves the bolus towards the stomach. Once the bolus is in the oesophagus, the cricopharyngeal sphincter closes to prevent reflux. The passage of the bolus into the stomach requires relaxation of the lower oesophageal (or cardiac) sphincter. The airway is re-established during the oesophageal phase: i.e. the soft palate, tongue and epiglottis return to their normal positions.

SPEECH

The acquisition of language is probably the most complex sensorimotor developmental process in a person's life. Sounds are produced initially in the larynx (phonation) by the co-ordinated movements of abdominal, thoracic and laryngeal muscles. Subsequent modification of this laryngeal sound to produce meaningful speech (articulation) occurs principally within the pharyngeal, oral and nasal cavities.

Fig. 6.14 summarises the principal sensory and motor mechanisms in speech. The main speech area of the brain is located within the temporoparietal region of the dominant cerebral hemisphere (i.e. the left cerebral hemisphere for a right-handed person) (see Fig. 6.17). The diagram indicates the many monitoring systems involved in the control of speech (such as hearing, proprioceptive information from the various muscles involved). Note that there has to be co-ordinated activity of respiration, laryngeal behaviour and oral structures to produce effective speech.

The fundamental laryngeal note has a thin and reedy quality. This sound therefore contains a limited amount of speech information and so is modified within resonating chambers and by the activity of organs such as the lips, tongue and soft palate.

By a process of sympathetic vibration, the resonators (Table 6.2) act as acoustic filters, amplifying selected frequencies and attenuating others.

The classification of sounds

Sounds may be voiced (i.e. the vocal folds in the larynx vibrate

Table 6.2 *The vocal resonators*

The following spaces are present in the vocal apparatus, any or all of which might be available as variable resonating chambers.

1. Between the true and false vocal cords
2. Between the larynx and the root of the tongue, possibly involving the epiglottis
3. Between the pharyngeal wall and the soft palate and uvula
4. Between the dorsum of the tongue and the posterior surface of the hard palate
5. Between the dorsum of the tongue and the anterior surface of the hard palate
6. Between the tip of the tongue and the teeth
7. Between the teeth and the lips
8. The nasal passages

Fig. 6.14 The principal sensory and motor mechanisms in speech.

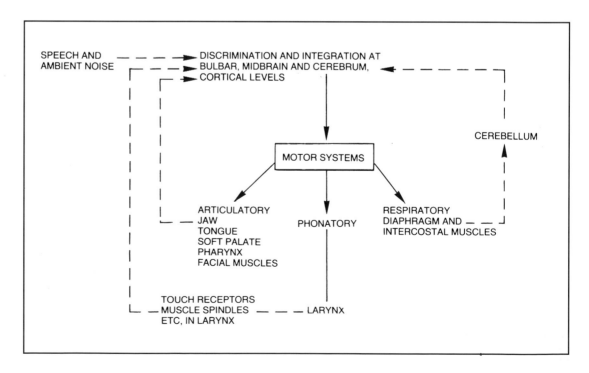

Table 6.3 *Classification of consonant sounds based upon place and manner of articulation*

Manner of articulation	Bilabial	Labiodental	Linguodentals Dental	Linguodentals Alveolar	Linguopalatals Alveolar	Linguopalatals Palatal	Glottal
Voicing	− +	− +	− +	− +	− +	− +	− +
Plosives	p b			t d		k g	
Fricatives		f v	θ ð	s z	ʃ ʒ		h
Affricatives				tʃ			
				tr dr		j	
Nasals	m			n		ng	
Laterals							
Semi-vowels	w			l			

for sound production) or breathed (i.e. the vocal folds do not vibrate). The two main groups of speech sounds are vowels and consonants.

Vowel sounds are modified by resonance and voiced consonants are modified by resonance and air flow obstruction. All vowel sounds are voiced. They are produced without interruption of the air flow, the air being channelled or restricted by the position of the tongue and lips (Fig. 6.15).

A consonant is produced when the air flow is impeded before it is released. Consonants may be voiced (e.g. b, d, z) or breathed (e.g. p, t, s). Consonant sounds are of low amplitude (vowels are created by high amplitude waves) and are classified in two ways: according to the place of articulation or according to the manner of articulation. For the classification based upon the place of articulation (Table 6.3), consonants are categorised into bilabial, labiodental, linguodental, linguopalatal and glottal sounds. In bilabial sounds (e.g. b, p, m) the two lips are used; in labiodental sounds, the lower lip meets the maxillary incisors (e.g. f, v). Linguodental sounds (e.g. d, t)

involve the tip of the tongue contacting the maxillary incisors and the adjacent hard palate; for linguopalatal sounds the tongue meets the palate away from the region of the maxillary incisors (e.g. g, k). For the classification of consonant sounds based upon the manner of articulation (Table 6.4), the degree of stoppage of the air flow is an important criterion. Note that, although one may describe the position of articulators for a particular vowel or consonant, there are no fixed positions during speech, only continuous movement. Both systems for classifying consonant sounds can be linked as in Table 6.3.

The configuration of the oral structures during consonant articulations is illustrated in Fig. 6.16. From this it can be seen that the tongue has a significant role during speech, although all oral structures (including the soft palate) are important. That speech is probably the most complex movement in the body is indicated by the range of muscles involved, by the great number of nerves implicated, and by the large areas of the cerebral hemispheres of the brain associated with speech (Fig. 6.17). The muscles involved include those in the chest, that control breathing, the intrinsic muscles of the larynx that are concerned with phonation (i.e. those required to close the rima glottidis between the cords, to put tension in the cords, and to change the shape of the cords), the muscles in the pharynx and soft palate that help in resonance, and the muscles of the tongue, palate, jaws and facial musculature that produce meaningful speech. The nerves involved may include the

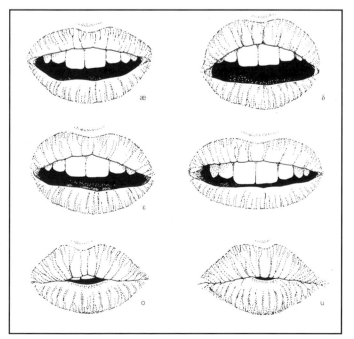

Fig. 6.15 Lip postures during the production of vowel sounds. The short vowel sounds are shown on the left and the long vowel sounds on the right.

Table 6.4 *Classification of consonant sounds based upon manner of articulation*

Plosives	(p, b, t, d, g, k)	Require a complete stoppage of air
Fricatives	(f, v, th)	Require only a partial stoppage
Affricatives	(c, h, j)	Although involving only a partial stoppage of the air, require a rapid release of this air
Nasals	(m, n)	Require obstruction of the mouth with the nasal passages open
Laterals	(l)	Air forced to leave sides of mouth
Rolled	(r)	

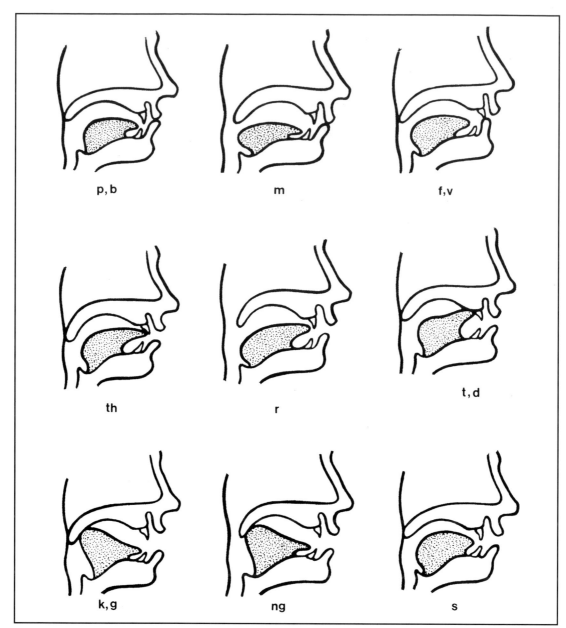

Fig. 6.16 Configuration of the oral structures during consonant articulations.

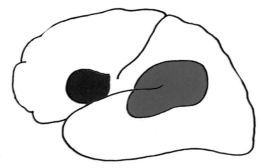

Fig. 6.17 Speech areas of the brain are located in the dominant cerebral hemisphere (i.e. left hemisphere for right-handed persons). The main areas are Broca's area (red), which is concerned with speech production, and Wernicke's area (blue), which is concerned with ensuring that spoken language is comprehensible. A third area (not illustrated), around the angular gyrus and posterior to Wernicke's area, is concerned with 'meaning'. In addition, the insula of the brain co-ordinates the activities of the speech areas. Note the large amount of the cerebral hemisphere given to speech.

intercostals and phrenic nerves, the recurrent laryngeal and superior (external) laryngeal branches of the vagus, nerves associated with the pharyngeal plexus, and the trigeminal, facial and hypoglossal cranial nerves.

The complexity of speech is further indicated by the fact that, although meaningful speech results from the bringing together of very simple sounds so that phonemes become syllables become words become whole sentences and concepts, the brain has to work in the opposite manner so that whole concepts and ideas, if not entirely coherent sentences, have to be established before the physiological process of phonation and articulation. In addition, speech occurs alongside other means of communication – facial expression, hand movements, body posture – and requires feedback from the person(s) to whom one is speaking so that visual and auditory signals must be co-ordinated with speech.

7 Enamel

Before describing enamel, a few introductory remarks are required concerning the dental and supporting tissues. The teeth are composed of three mineralised tissues (enamel, dentine and cementum) surrounding an inner core of loose connective tissue, the dental pulp. Enamel is of ectodermal origin; dentine, cementum and the dental pulp of ecto-mesenchymal origin.

The appearance of the tissues depends upon the method of specimen preparation: in ground sections the hard, mineralised tissues remain intact but the soft connective tissues and epithelia are lost; in decalcified sections the soft connective tissues and the organic matrices of the mineralised tissues remain. Because enamel is almost entirely mineral it is lost completely after most demineralisation procedures and its

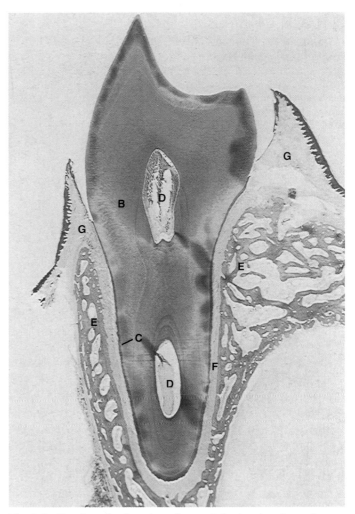

Fig. 7.2 Demineralised section of a tooth *in situ*. A = Enamel; B = dentine; C = cementum; D = dental pulp; E = alveolar bone; F = periodontal ligament; G = gingiva. Compared with Fig. 7.1, the enamel has been lost (× 6). Courtesy of Dr D.A. Lunt.

structural features are mainly described in ground sections (Figs 7.1, 7.2).

Dentine forms the bulk of the tooth and is covered in the crown with enamel and in the root with cementum (Figs 7.1, 7.2). The dental pulp derives from the dental papilla and is responsible for the production of dentine, which goes on throughout life. It also acts as a sensory organ, detecting significant stimuli and toxins that affect the dentine. It has a positive but limited ability to respond to noxious stimuli by laying down additional dentine.

The tissues that support the teeth, known collectively as the periodontium (Figs 7.1, 7.2), include the alveolar bone forming the tooth sockets, the periodontal ligament (a connective tissue that attaches the tooth to the alveolar bone) and the

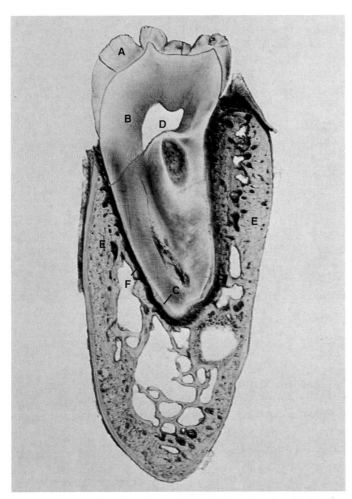

Fig. 7.1 Ground section of a tooth *in situ* showing the distribution of the dental tissues. A = Enamel; B = dentine; C = cementum; D = dental pulp; E = alveolar bone. As the section was embedded in plastic, part of the periodontal ligament (F) has been fortuitously retained (× 4).

gingivae (the component of the oral mucosa that forms a collar around the tooth).

PHYSICAL PROPERTIES

Enamel covers the crown of the tooth (Fig. 7.3). It is thickest over cusps and incisal edges and thinnest at the cervical margin. Over the cusps of unworn permanent teeth it is 2.5 mm thick (over the cusps of deciduous teeth 1.3 mm), and on lateral surfaces up to 1.3 mm. The thickness declines gradually to become a very thin layer at the cervical margin. Enamel is the hardest biological tissue and, while highly mineralised, withstands both shearing and impact forces well. Its abrasion resistance is high, allowing it to wear down only slowly, an important property as enamel can undergo neither repair nor replacement. Although enamel has a low tensile strength and is brittle, it has a high modulus of elasticity and this, together with the flexible support of the underlying dentine, minimises the possibility of fracture. Enamel has a high specific gravity (~ 3).

The properties of enamel vary at different regions within the tissue. Surface enamel is harder, denser and less porous than subsurface enamel. Hardness and density also decrease from the surface towards the interior, and from the cuspal/incisal tip towards the cervical margin.

Enamel is a birefringent crystalline material, the crystals refracting light differently in different directions. Young enamel is white because, although light enters it readily, it is almost entirely internally reflected with no wavelengths differentially absorbed. This results in low translucency and the white colour. The translucency of enamel increases with age and some of the colour of the underlying dentine is then transmitted, resulting in a more yellow appearance. The tissue

Table 7.1 *A comparison of the physical properties of enamel and dentine (typical values)*

	Enamel	Dentine
Specific gravity	2.9	2.14
Hardness (Knoop no.)	296	64
Stiffness (Young's modulus)	131 GN m^{-2}	12 GN m^{-2}
Compressive strength	76 MN m^{-2}	262 MN m^{-2}
Tensile strength	46 MN m^{-2}	33 MN m^{-2}

GN = giganewtons ($N \times 10^9$), MN = meganewtons ($N \times 10^6$)

has an average refractive index of 1.62. These optical properties considerably influence the histological appearance of enamel (for example explaining why there are differences with various mounting media). Some of the physical properties of enamel (and, for comparison, dentine) are listed in Table 7.1.

CHEMICAL PROPERTIES

Hydroxyapatite

Calcium hydroxyapatite $Ca_{10}(PO_4)_6(OH)_2$ is the principal mineral component of enamel, comprising about 88–90% of the tissue by volume, which corresponds to about 95–96% by weight, the remainder being organic material and water. The mineral content increases from the dentine–enamel junction to the surface. Hydroxyapatite is present in the form of crystallites (Figs 7.4, 7.5) about 70 nm in width, 25 nm thick and of

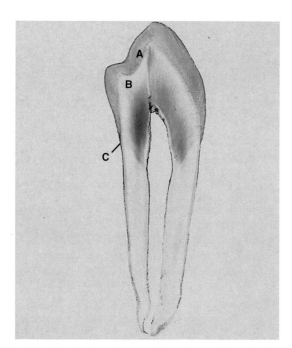

Fig. 7.3 The distribution of enamel. A = Enamel; B = dentine; C = cementum (× 3).

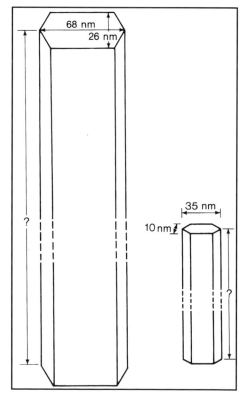

Fig. 7.4 The dimensions of an enamel crystallite (left) and a dentine crystallite (right). Both are impure hydroxyapatite.

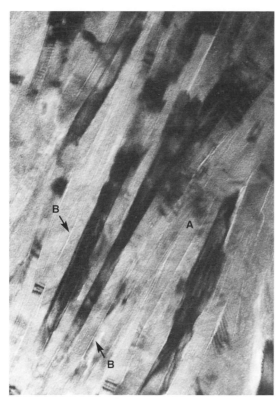

Fig. 7.5 Enamel crystallites in longitudinal section prepared by ion-beam thinning. For this technique a beam of ionised argon is directed obliquely onto the section so that is etched. In such specimens, crystallites (A) up to 100 μm long are seen and it is possible that some crystallites cross the full thickness of the enamel. B = Pores between crystallites (TEM; × 100 000). Courtesy of Doctors H.J. Orams, P.P. Phakey and W. Rachinger and the editor of *Advances in Dental Research*.

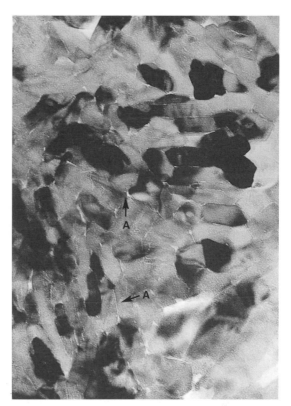

Fig. 7.6 TEM showing enamel crystallites in cross-section prepared by ion-beam thinning, showing the hexagonal pattern of the enamel crystallites (× 120 000). Small gaps or pores (A), which may contain water and organic material, occur between crystallites. Courtesy of Doctors H.J. Orams, P.P. Phakey and W. Rachinger and the editor of *Advances in Dental Research*.

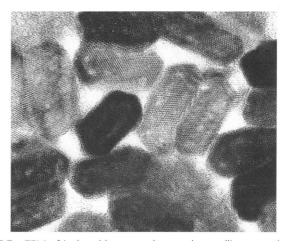

Fig. 7.7 TEM of isolated hexagonal enamel crystallites containing many hydroxyapatite molecules organised in a repeating pattern or lattice (× 800,000). Courtesy of Professor H. Warshawsky.

great length, some possibly extending across the full width of the tissue (the crystallites of dentine, bone and cementum are much smaller). Most crystallites are regularly hexagonal in cross-section (Figs 7.6, 7.7), though some are distorted by crowding during development. The cores of the crystallites differ slightly in composition from the periphery, being richer in magnesium and carbonate. The core of the crystallite is more soluble than the periphery.

The molecular arrangement within each unit cell of the crystallite consists of a hydroxyl group surrounded by three uniformly spaced calcium ions, which in turn are surrounded by three similarly spaced phosphate ions. Six calcium ions in a uniform hexagon enclose the phosphate ions. The crystal consists of this arrangement of planes of ions repeated side by side and in stacked layers.

Although the basic molecular arrangement of the crystal is highly organised, it is subject to variation. 'Normal' ions may be replaced by different ionic species. Carbonate may occur at a phosphate or hydroxyl site (about 90% being found at the phosphate position). Magnesium may occur in the place of a calcium ion or elsewhere in the lattice. Fluoride may substitute for hydroxyl ions, conferring greater stability and resistance to acidic dissolution. Fluoride levels (unlike magnesium and carbonate) decline from the outer surface towards the dentine,

perhaps because the fluoride is acquired during enamel maturation. Chloride, lead, zinc, sodium, strontium and aluminium ions may also substitute into the apatite lattice. Another change in the molecular arrangement occurs if one plane of ions 'slips' from the usual uniform arrangement with its neighbour.

It has been suggested, though not established with certainty, that small quantities of non-apatitic minerals may also be present in mature enamel. These possibly include octacalcium phosphate, which may be a hydroxyapatite precursor.

Water

Water constitutes about 2% by weight of enamel, corresponding to 5–10% by volume. The presence of water is related to the porosity of the tissue. Some of the water may lie between crystals and surround the organic material, some may be trapped within defects of the crystalline structure and the remainder forms a hydration layer coating the crystals. As ions such as fluoride would travel through the water component its distribution is of clinical importance.

Organic matrix

Mature enamel contains only 1–2% of organic matrix. The organic component of regions where the prismatic and crystallite arrangement is straight and regular may be as low as 0.05% w/w; where the prisms and crystallites are more irregular it may be as high as 3%. The protein component has been the most widely studied.

A wide variety of organic molecules occur in enamel, ranging from free amino acids to large unique proteins complexes. These proteins are the amelogenins and non-amelogenins (enamelins) and are considered in detail in Chapter 22. Between 50 and 90% of the matrix is composed of small molecules, peptides and free amino acids (including large amounts of glycine and glutamic acid). Larger molecular weight material (> 30,000 Da) contains components rich in carbohydrate (80–95% sugars, 5–20% amino acids).

The concentration of protein is highest within the enamel tufts at the dentine–enamel junction. This tuft protein extends in lesser amounts beyond the tufts and possibly throughout the enamel, and seems to be localised in the periphery of the prisms.

Although little studied, the lipid content of enamel appears to approximate that of protein (approximately 1% by weight). It may represent the remnants of cell membranes remaining from development

ENAMEL PRISMS

The basic structural unit of enamel is the enamel prism or rod (Fig. 7.8), consisting of several million hydroxyapatite crystallites packed into a long thin rod 5–6 μm in diameter and up to 2.5 mm in length. Although the units are not strictly prismatic in outline, this term for the enamel unit has become accepted by widespread usage. Prisms run from the enamel–dentine junction to the surface. The boundaries of the prisms reflect sudden changes in crystallite orientation that give an optical effect different from that of the prism core or body: at the boundaries, the crystallites deviate by 40–60° from those inside the prism. Owing to the resultant increased microporosity at the prism boundary, slightly more organic material can be accommodated.

In cross section the shape of an enamel prism approximates to one of three main patterns (Fig. 7.9). The distribution of the three pattern types varies between species. All three patterns

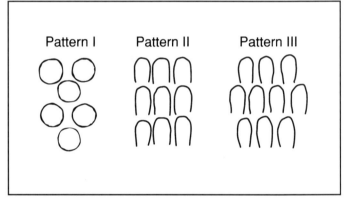

Fig. 7.9 The three prism patterns seen in human enamel. In pattern I enamel the prisms are circular. In pattern II enamel the prisms are aligned in parallel rows. In pattern III enamel the prisms are arranged in staggered rows such that the tail of a prism lies between two heads in the next row, giving a keyhole appearance.

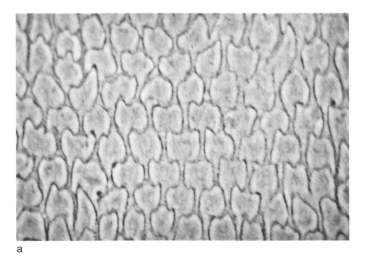

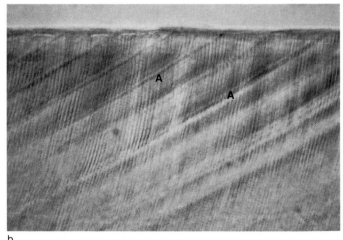

a   b

Fig. 7.8 (a) Enamel prisms in transverse section demonstrating the keyhole pattern seen in most regions of human enamel (phase contrast × 14 500). (b) Enamel prisms cut longitudinally and running towards the surface in the direction of the arrow (× 250). The lines running obliquely (A) are enamel striae. Courtesy of Dr D.F.G. Poole.

are present in humans but pattern III (Figs 7.8a and 7.11), the keyhole pattern, predominates. This is found in the bulk of the enamel with pattern I (Fig. 7.10) near the enamel–dentine junction and near the surface, possibly because the enamel in these regions is formed slowly.

In pattern I enamel the prisms appear circular. The enamel between the prisms has been termed 'interprismatic'. Its composition is similar to that inside the prisms but it has a different optical effect because the crystals deviate by 40–60° from those in the prism.

The keyhole shape of pattern III enamel shows clear 'head' and 'tail' regions, the tail of one prism lying between the heads of the adjacent prisms and pointing cervically. There is an abrupt change in crystal orientation (Figs 7.12–7.14), which is responsible for the refraction of light and the appearance of the prism boundary. As polarised light identifies changes in crystallite orientation it is useful in highlighting features in enamel such as prisms (Fig. 7.15).

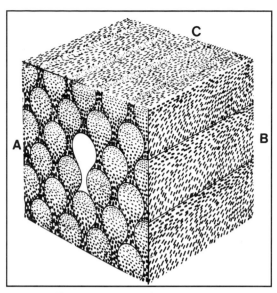

Fig. 7.12 Crystallite orientation and prism structure in a diagrammatic representation of a block of enamel. A = Cross-sectional view; B = lateral surface; C = top surface. The cross-sectional view reveals the characteristic keyhole arrangement of enamel prisms with the tails pointing cervically and the heads occlusally. In the head of the prism the crystallites run parallel to the long axis of the prism. In the tail, the crystallites gradually diverge from this to become angled 65–70° to the long axis. The change within a single prism is gradual such that no clear division between head and tail of the same prism is seen. However, the crystallites in the tail of one prism show a sudden divergence from the crystallites in the head of an adjacent prism. The sudden change in crystallite orientation at the prism boundary can be seen most clearly in the lateral surface of the block (B). On this surface, where the prisms have been cut exactly centrally through the head–tail axis, there are rows of equal but wide prisms. On the top surface (C), where the plane of section has passed through adjacent heads and tails, there is the appearance of broad prisms separated by narrower bands of 'interprismatic' enamel. It must be noted that in preparing histological material the enamel will be sectioned with varying degrees of obliquity, producing a wide variety of prism appearances and crystal orientations. Courtesy of Doctors A.H. Meckel, W.J. Griebstein & R.N. Neal and John Wright, publishers.

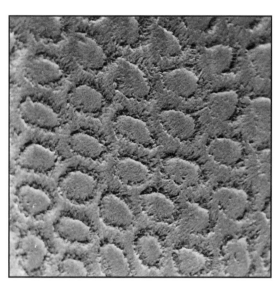

Fig. 7.10 Circular pattern I prisms (SEM × 4300). Courtesy of Professor A. Boyde.

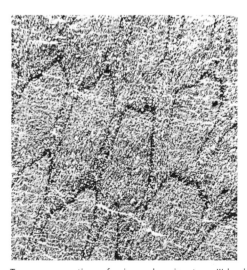

Fig. 7.11 Transverse section of prisms showing type III keyhole pattern (TEM with silver staining × 2000). Courtesy of Dr D.F.G. Poole.

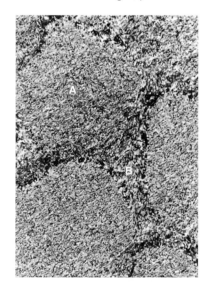

Fig. 7.13 TEM showing enamel prisms cut transversely showing variations in crystal orientation between head (A) and tail (B) regions (× 7000). Courtesy of Dr D.F.G. Poole.

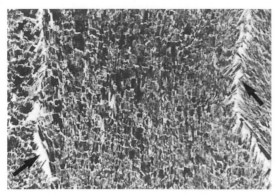

Fig. 7.14 TEM showing enamel prisms cut longitudinally showing sudden change in orientation (arrow) at the prism boundary. The apparent space at the prism boundary represents a preparation artefact (× 13 500). Courtesy of Dr D.F.G. Poole.

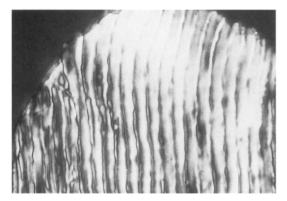

Fig. 7.15 In polarised light, enamel cut longitudinal to the prisms shows a series of light and dark lines which distinguish the prism cores from the prism boundaries. This appearance is due to the abrupt change in orientation of the crystals at the prism boundary (and not to differential degrees of mineralisation). Indeed, the presence of the enamel prism as a subunit of enamel is entirely due to these changes in crystal orientation. (× 600). Courtesy of Dr D.F.G. Poole.

In the head of the prism the crystals run parallel to the long axis of the prism. In the tail the crystals gradually diverge from this to become angled 65–70° to the long axis (Fig. 7.12, face A). The change within a single prism is gradual such that there is no clear division between head and tail of the same prism; however, the crystals in the tail of one prism show a sudden divergence from the crystals in the head of an adjacent prism (Figs 7.12, 7.13). In preparing histological material the enamel will be sectioned with varying degrees of obliquity, producing a wide variety of prism appearances. Although some areas may be termed interprismatic, what appears 'interprismatic' is often the tail of one prism adjacent to another.

When viewed in enamel fractured or sectioned parallel to the long axis of the tooth (Fig. 7.8b), most prisms (3–6 μm in diameter) appear to travel in a straight line from the enamel dentine junction to the surface (however, see Hunter-Shreger bands, below). The prisms meet the surface at varying angles depending on the relative shape of the enamel–dentine junction and the outer surface. Just above the cervical margin prisms meet the surface at right angles whereas more

occlusally they meet the surface at an angle of about 60° (Fig. 7.16). Within fissures prisms make surface angles as acute as 20° (Fig. 7.17).

When viewed in enamel fractured or sectioned longitudinally, prisms follow a parallel sinusoidal path. Between 10 and 13 layers of prisms follow the same direction but blocks above and below follow paths in different directions (Figs. 7.18–7.20). These periodic changes in prism direction give rise to a banding pattern termed the **Hunter-Schreger bands** (Fig. 7.21). These bands are approximately 50 μm wide

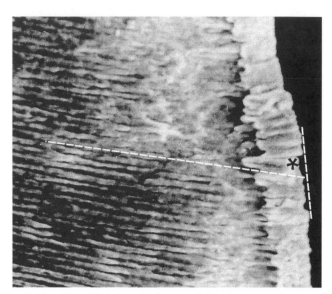

Fig. 7.16 SEM of lightly etched enamel showing enamel prisms reaching the surface at 60° (★) (× 320). Courtesy of Dr R.C. Shore and the CRC Press.

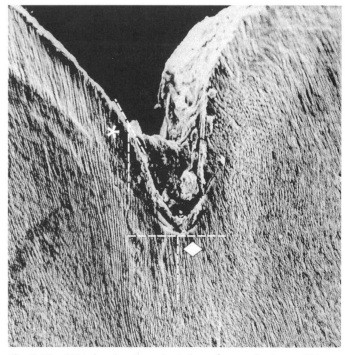

Fig. 7.17 SEM showing the orientation of enamel prisms within an occlusal fissure. Note the acute angle at which the prisms reach the surface in this region (× 100) Courtesy of Dr R.C. Shore and the CRC Press.

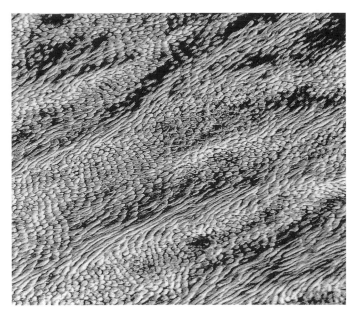

Fig. 7.18 SEM of longitudinally sectioned enamel lightly etched to show alternating bands of transversely sectioned (diazones) and longitudinally sectioned (parazones) prism. (× 160). Courtesy of Dr R.C. Shore and the CRC Press.

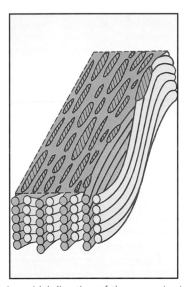

Fig. 7.19 The sinusoidal direction of the enamel prisms in alternating sheets results in alternately reflecting bands on the cut surface. Different sheets exhibit different crystal orientations and thus different degrees of polarisation.

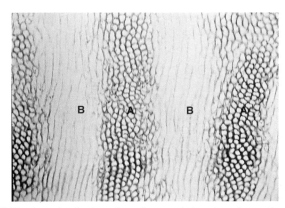

Fig. 7.20 Longitudinal section of enamel showing alternating regions with groups of prism sectioned more transversely (A) or more longitudinally (B) that give rise to the appearance of Hunter-Schreger bands (× 300). Courtesy of Dr B.A.W. Brown.

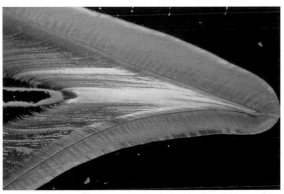

Fig. 7.21 Longitudinal section of enamel showing Hunter-Schreger bands in reflected light (× 12).

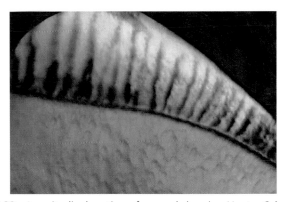

Fig. 7.22 Longitudinal section of enamel showing Hunter-Schreger bands in polarised light. Note that the bands do not completely reach the outermost surface of the enamel (× 25).

and are visible as the different bands of prisms reflect or transmit light in different directions. In sections of enamel cut parallel to the long axis of the tooth, the individual crystals will be oriented differently in the groups of prism cut more transversely or more longitudinally. The bands of prisms that are cut longitudinally are known as parazones and those cut transversely as diazones. The angle between parazones and diazones is 40°. This complex pattern of prisms makes enamel resistant to fracture and, when exposed on the surface, leads to a micro-ridged grinding surface. In approximately the outer quarter of enamel the prisms all run in the same direction and no Hunter-Schreger bands are present (Fig. 7.22).

As prisms are arranged in a spiral pattern, in some areas beneath the cusps and incisal edges the changes in direction of the prisms appear more marked and irregular. Groups of prisms seem to spiral around others, giving the appearance of 'gnarled' enamel (Fig. 7.23).

APRISMATIC ENAMEL

The outer 20–100 μm of enamel of newly erupted deciduous

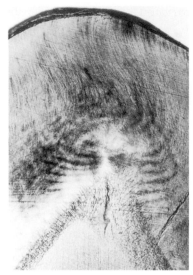

Fig. 7.23 Longitudinal section of a cusp showing gnarled enamel (× 25).

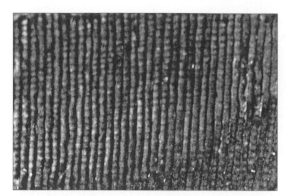

Fig. 7.25 Phase-contrast microscopy of longitudinal section of enamel showing cross-striations (horizontal lines) along the enamel prisms (× 350). Courtesy of Dr D.F.G. Poole.

teeth and the outer 20–70 µm of newly erupted permanent teeth is aprismatic (prismless). Here, the enamel crystallites are aligned at right angles to the surface and parallel to each other. This surface layer is more highly mineralised than the rest of the enamel due to the absence of prism boundaries where most organic material is located. Its thickness is variable (Fig. 7.24). Aprismatic enamel occurs as a result of the absence of Tomes processes on the ameloblasts in the final stages of enamel deposition (see Chapter 22).

INCREMENTAL LINES

Enamel is formed incrementally, periods of activity alternating with periods of quiescence. This results in structural markings known as incremental lines. There are two types: short period (cross-striations) and long period (enamel striae).

Cross-striations

Cross-striations are seen as lines traversing the enamel prisms at right angles to their long axes (Fig. 7.25). The cross-

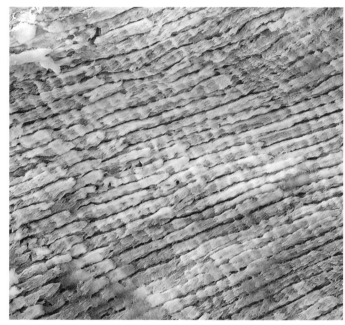

Fig. 7.26 SEM of fractured enamel surface showing cross-striations along the length of prisms seemingly corresponding to sites of narrowing of the prism width (× 600). Courtesy of Professor M.C. Dean.

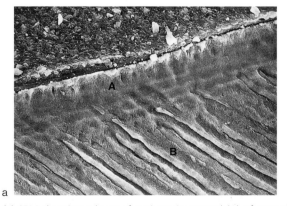

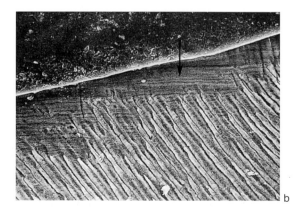

Fig. 7.24 (a) SEM showing a layer of aprismatic enamel (A) of even thickness overlying a layer of prismatic enamel (B) (× 63). (b) SEM showing a layer of aprismatic enamel (arrow) of uneven thickness overlying prismatic enamel. Courtesy of Dr D.K. Whittaker.

striations reflect a diurnal rythm. Their appearance may relate to regular variations in width (Figs 7.26 and 7.27) thought to reflect diurnal variations in the rate of secretion by ameloblasts (daily increments of growth). An alternative, but less likely, explanation is that these lines are a result of the crystals within the prism following a spiral path (Fig. 7.28), although this variation may also be diurnal in nature. At low power cross-striations appear as lines 2.5–6 μm apart, being closer together near the enamel–dentine junction. It has also been suggested that cross-striations are the result of subtle changes in the nature of the organic matrix and/or crystallite orientation and/or composition (especially in the carbonate component). Cross-striations have yet to be observed under the transmission electron microscope.

Enamel striae

When sections of enamel cut along the longitudinal axis of the crown are viewed, structural lines are seen to run obliquely across the prisms from near the enamel–dentine junction to the surface (Fig. 7.29). These represent incremental lines and are known as the enamel striae (of Retzius). In horizontal sections of the crown, the enamel striae run circumferentially, like the rings of a tree (Fig. 7.30).

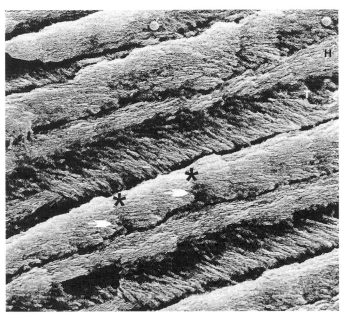

Fig. 7.27 SEM of lightly etched enamel showing individual enamel crystallites (arrows) terminating at constrictions of prisms (∗) (× 1600). Courtesy of Dr R. Shore and the CRC Press.

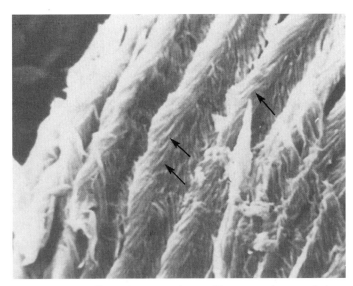

Fig. 7.28 SEM illustrating enamel crystallites appearing to spiral within prisms (arrow) (× 1400). Courtesy of Dr R.C. Shore and the CRC Press.

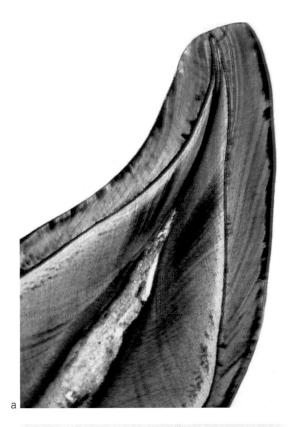

a

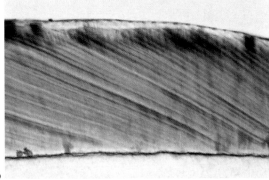

b

Fig. 7.29 (a) Longitudinal section of enamel showing enamel striae running obliquely across the tissue. Wear at the tip of the cusp has exposed some of the striae on the surface at this site. Along the slopes of the tooth the striae naturally reach the surface (× 15). (b) Higher-power view (× 40) of enamel striae in enamel (A) along the side of the tooth running from the enamel–dentine junction (B) to the surface.

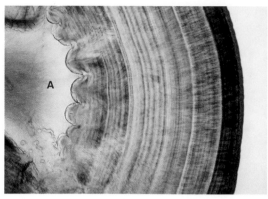

Fig. 7.30 Transverse section of enamel showing enamel striaie running circumferentially. A = Dentine (× 120). Courtesy of Dr M.E. Atkinson.

Although following routine demineralisation all enamel structure is lost due to the low content of the organic matrix, leaving an enamel space (see Fig. 7.2), controlled (and probably incomplete) demineralisation will allow retention of some organic material for subsequent staining. Many of the structural features seen in ground sections will be retained. The keyhole pattern of the prisms can be clearly seen (Fig. 7.31a). Although it is known that the prism lacks an organic sheath, the level of organic material and water is likely to be higher at

the prism boundary because of the larger pores produced by the abutment of hydroxyapatite crystallites at this junction. This, and the apparently lower solubility of the organic matrix at the prism boundary, can explain the deeper staining at these sites. Enamel striae are also observed in demineralised sections (Fig. 7.31b).

· Due to the manner in which enamel is deposited (see pages 316–317), the striae overlying the cusps and incisal edges do not reach the surface (Fig. 7.32) unless there has been enamel loss (Fig. 7.29). In the case of unworn incisors, the first 25–30 striae do not reach the surface.

In human teeth there are 7–10 cross-striations between adjacent striae in any one individual (Fig. 7.33). The striae are therefore formed at about weekly intervals. As the average distance between two cross-striations is about 4 μm, enamel

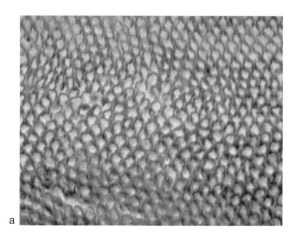

a

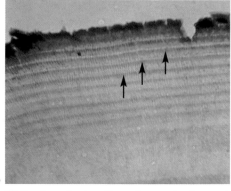

b

Fig. 7.31 (a) Demineralised section of enamel prisms cut transversely showing retained enamel matrix presenting a prismatic appearance (Light blue stain; × 600). (b) Demineralised transverse section of enamel showing enamel striae patterns (arrows) in the retained enamel matrix (Light blue stain; × 150).

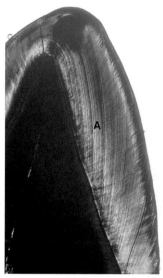

Fig. 7.32 Longitudinal section of unworn enamel (A) showing that striae passing over the cusp do not reach the outer tooth surface, but those more laterally do (× 20). Courtesy of Doctors R.J. Hiller and G.T. Craig.

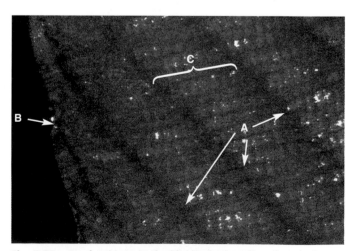

Fig. 7.33 Confocal image of a longitudinal section of enamel showing enamel striae (A) reaching the surface at perikymata grooves (B). Between adjacent striae, about seven cross-striations (C) are evident as vertical lines (× 850). Courtesy of Professor M.C. Dean.

striae in the middle portion of enamel are about 25–35 μm apart. In cervical enamel, where enamel is formed more slowly and cross-striations may be only about 2 μm apart, the striae are closer together and may be separated by only 15–20 μm. Accentuated striae may be due to metabolic disturbances occurring during the time of mineralisation.

Over the whole of the lateral enamel, enamel striae reach the surface in a series of fine grooves running circumferentially around the crown. These features are known as the **perikymata grooves** and are separated by ridges, the **perikymata ridges** (Figs 7.34, 7.35; see also Figs 7.39 and 7.40). The distance between perikymata reflects the data already given for that of enamel striae: they are close together near the cervical margin (about 15–20 μm) but as they reach the surface obliquely may be up to 100 μm apart towards the cusp of the tooth. The process that results in the production of the enamel striae is unknown.

In deciduous teeth, enamel striae and perikymata are only ever clearly seen in the cervical enamel of deciduous second molars.

The exaggeration of striae in different teeth forming at the same time suggests a common systemic influence. One hypothesis is that there may be a rhythm with a 27-hour cycle in addition to a diurnal daily rhythm. The two rhythms would

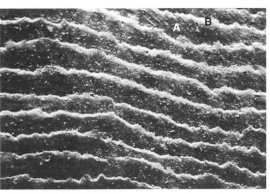

Fig. 7.35　Higher power view of surface enamel with perikymata grooves (A) separated by perikymata ridges (B) (SEM, × 400). Courtesy of Dr D.F.G. Poole.

coincide approximately every seven or eight days, producing a fault in the developing enamel. The underlying reason for the structural feature apparent as a stria in ground section is due to differential light-scattering effects at this fault line, possibly due to a slight change in prism direction/thickness or slight differences in crystallite composition/ orientation and/or differences in organic content. That the striae are seen in partially demineralised sections has been interpreted by some as being due to the site of striae having a higher carbonate content which causes greater solubility of the crystals and greater porosity.

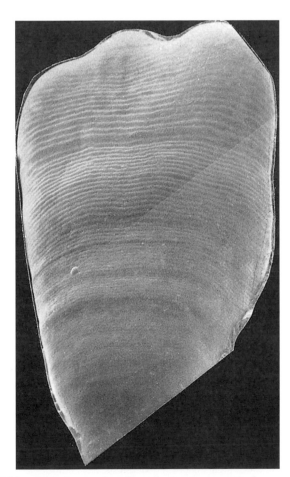

Fig. 7.34　SEM of enamel surface of a human lower incisor showing numerous transversely running perikymata grooves and ridges. (× 10). Courtesy of Professor M.C. Dean and the *Journal of Human Evolution*.

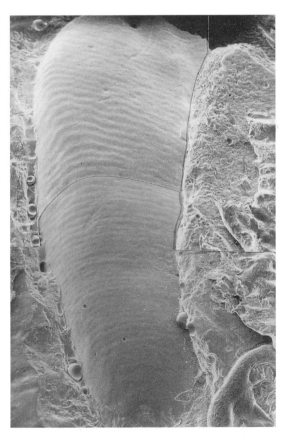

Fig. 7.36　SEM showing perikymata on the surface of a lower incisor from *Paranthropus robustus* (× 10). Courtesy of Professor M.C. Dean.

It is possible to use the incremental markings in enamel (cross-striations, enamel striae and perikymata) to assess the time taken to form the crown of the tooth, and to help age material. As impressions of the surface enamel can record the perikymata, rare teeth of fossil hominids have also been studied (Fig. 7.36). Assuming adjacent perikymata are separated by 7–10 day intervals, the total number of perikymata on a crown indicates the time taken for the crown to form, if about 6–9 months are added to this total to account for the 25–30 striae over the top of the crown that do not reach the surface (Fig. 7.31). From such studies it has been found, for example, that the teeth of apes and many extinct hominids develop and erupt more quickly than those of modern humans. There is some evidence in primates that the number of cross-striations between two adjacent striae reflects body size; in monkeys, there are only 4–5 cross-striations between striae.

Enamel striae are less pronounced or absent from enamel formed before birth. A particularly marked stria is formed at birth – this is the neonatal line (Fig. 7.37), and reflects the metabolic changes at birth. Prisms appear to change both direction and thickness at the time of this event (Fig. 7.38).

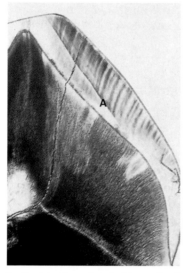

Fig. 7.37 Longitudinal section of a deciduous tooth showing a neonatal line (A) (× 6). Courtesy of Doctors R.J. Hillier and G.T.

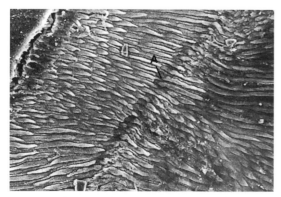

Fig. 7.38 SEM of an etched longitudinal section of deciduous enamel showing enamel prisms changing in both thickness and direction at the neonatal line (A) (× 400). Courtesy of Dr D.K. Whittaker.

SURFACE ENAMEL

The surface of the enamel is, perhaps, its most clinically significant region. It is here that the tooth comes into contact with food, that caries is initiated, restorations are attached or abutted, orthodontic brackets cemented and toothpaste, bleaches and fluoride/remineralization preparations applied.

Both physically and chemically surface enamel differs markedly from subsurface enamel. Surface enamel is harder, less porous, less soluble and more radio-opaque than subsurface enamel. It is richer in some trace elements (especially fluoride) but contains less carbonate. The enamel surface presents a variable appearance, exhibiting features such as aprismatic enamel, perikymata, prism-end markings, cracks, pits and elevations.

The outer enamel, if unabraded, is in most areas aprismatic and thus more highly mineralised and resistant to caries (see Fig. 7.24). This may help explain why acid etching, unless sufficient to penetrate to the prismatic enamel, may not always enhance adhesion. Although the enamel is aprismatic, the incremental striae of Retzius reach the surface and appear as perikymata grooves, wave-like concentric surface rings parallel to the cementum–enamel junction. The perikymata grooves are separated from each other by the wavelike perikymata ridges (Fig. 7.39, see also page 111). Attrition and abrasion remove these features after eruption but they may persist in protected cervical areas. In some areas, particularly cervically where the reduced enamel epithelium persists for some time after eruption, small pits are seen within the perikymata. These are the impressions of the ends of the ameloblasts and are 1–1.5 μm in depth (Fig. 7.40).

Small cracks are frequently found in surface enamel, although it is difficult to know whether many of these were present *in vivo* or were induced by the procedures necessary to examine the tissue. They represent potential areas of weakness. Small elevations 10–15 μm across (enamel caps, Fig. 7.41)

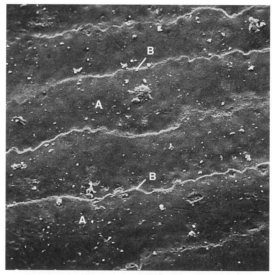

Fig. 7.39 SEM of enamel surface showing perikymata grooves (A) separated from each other by perikymata ridges (B) (× 500). Courtesy of Professor H.N. Newman.

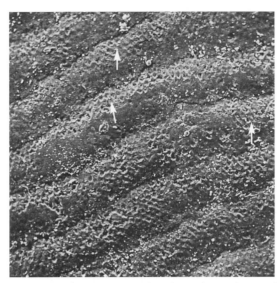

Fig. 7.40   SEM showing prism-end markings (arrows) on surface of enamel. Compare with Fig. 7.39, which lacks this feature. (× 300). Courtesy of Professor H.N. Newman.

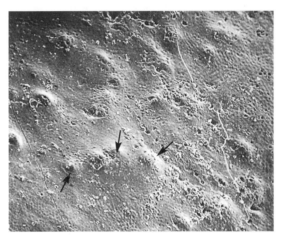

Fig. 7.41   SEM of enamel surface showing enamel caps (arrow) (× 150) Courtesy of Professor H.N. Newman.

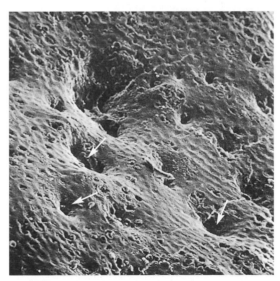

Fig. 7.42   SEM of enamel surface showing focal holes (arrow) (× 400). Courtesy of Professor H.N. Newman.

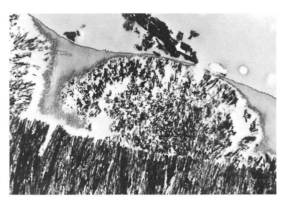

Fig. 7.43   TEM showing an enamel broch (× 10 000). Courtesy of Professor H.N. Newman.

or depressions (focal holes, Fig. 7.42) are also found, particularly on lateral surfaces. The caps are thought to result from enamel deposition on top of small deposits of non-mineralisable debris late in development. The focal holes result from loss of the cap and underlying material by abrasion or attrition.

Larger surface elevations, enamel brochs 30–50 μm in diameter, also occur occasionally and consist of radiating groups of crystals (Fig. 7.43). They seem to be more common in premolars but are of unknown origin.

ENAMEL–DENTINE JUNCTION

The boundary between enamel and dentine has a scalloped pattern (Fig. 7.44) in areas where shearing forces would be high (such as beneath cusps and incisal edges) but is smooth on the lateral surfaces. The convexities are on the enamel surface (Fig. 7.45) and the concavities on the dentinal surface (Fig. 7.46). Dentine crystals are much smaller than those of enamel and the transition from one to the other at the junction of the tissues is generally clear (Fig. 7.47); however, there may be areas in which crystals of intermediate size exist and there is a more gradual blending of the tissues.

A number of features can be seen at the enamel–dentine junction (amelodentinal junction), extending from the dentine surface into the enamel. These include enamel spindles, tufts and lamellae (Fig. 7.48).

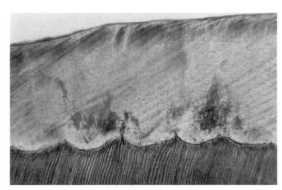

Fig. 7.44   Scalloped appearance of the enamel–dentine junction beneath the cusp of a tooth (× 60).

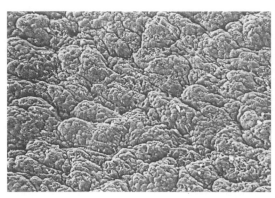

Fig. 7.45 SEM of the enamel surface which lies in contact with the dentine, separation having been achieved following dehydration and fracture. The enamel surface is convex at this site. (× 250). Courtesy of Dr D.K. Whittaker.

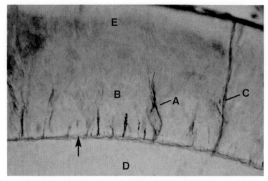

Fig. 7.48 Transverse section showing the enamel dentine junction. A = Enamel tuft; B = enamel spindle; C = enamel lamella; D = dentine; E = enamel (× 60). Courtesy of Dr R. Sprinz.

Enamel spindles

Narrow (up to 8 μm in diameter), round, sometimes club-shaped tubules – the enamel spindles – extend up to 25 μm into the enamel (Fig. 7.49). They are not aligned with the prisms and are thought to be the result of some odontoblast processes that, during the early stages of enamel development, insinuated themselves between the ameloblasts. The size of some would exceed the usual dimension of dentinal tubules. It has also been suggested that they may be dentinal collagen or the remnants of dead odontoblasts (Fig. 7.50). Enamel spindles are most common beneath cusps where most crowding of odontoblasts would have occurred. In the erupted tooth these tubules do not contain cell processes. Due to their alignment, they are best seen in longitudinal sections of enamel.

Enamel tufts

Enamel tuft is the term given to junctional structures in the inner third of the enamel that, in ground sections, resemble tufts of grass (Fig. 7.51). They appear to travel in the same

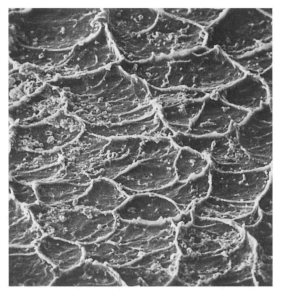

Fig. 7.46 SEM of dentine surface at the enamel dentine junction, following removal of enamel by demineralisation. The dentine at this site shows a series of concavities (× 400). Courtesy of Dr. B.G.H. Levers.

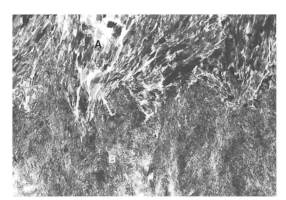

Fig. 7.47 TEM showing enamel (A) and dentine (B) crystallites at the enamel–dentine junction (arrow). Note the larger size of the enamel crystallites (× 18000). Courtesy of Professor H.N. Newman.

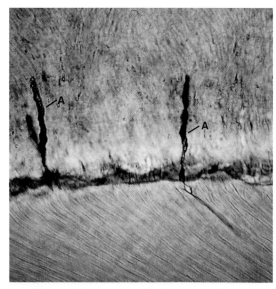

Fig. 7.49 Longitudinal section of enamel showing enamel spindles (A) (× 250). Courtesy of Dr R. Sprinz.

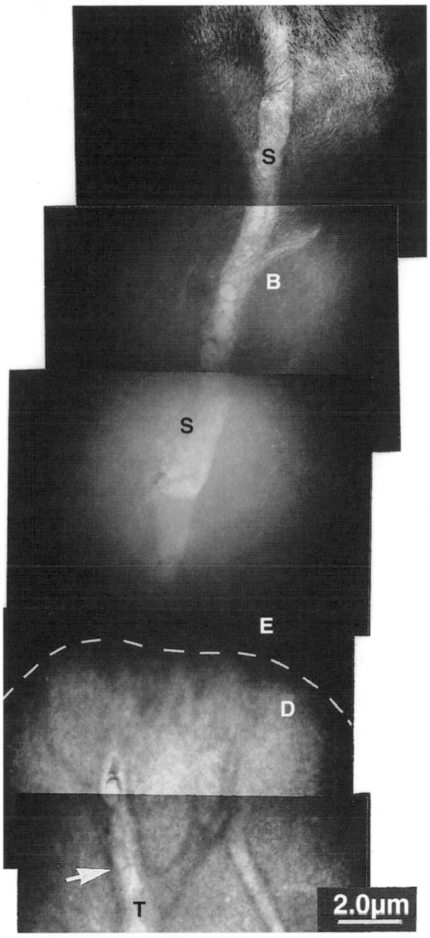

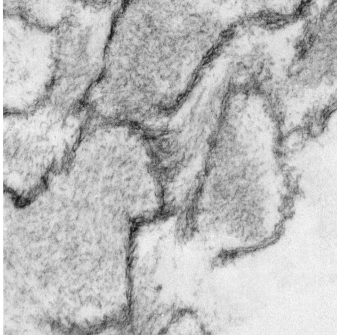

Fig. 7.52 TEM of an enamel tuft separated from the dentine surface after demineralisation of the enamel. The dense staining areas are presumptive prism boundaries representing organic matrix (× 11000). Courtesy of Dr R.C. Shore and the CRC Press.

is not amelogenin, the major developmental enamel protein, but the minor non-amelogenin fraction.

Enamel lamellae

Enamel lamellae are sheet-like apparent structural faults that run through the entire thickness of the enamel (Fig. 7.53). They are hypomineralised and narrower, longer and less common than enamel tufts but, like tufts, are best visualised in transverse sections of enamel. In routine ground sections, many

Fig. 7.50 TEM showing an enamel spindle (S) appearing as the continuation of a dentinal tubule (T) from dentine (D) into enamel (E) (× 6500). Courtesy of J. Palamara, P.P. Phakey, W.A. Rachinger and H.J. Orams and the editor of *Advances in Dental Science*.

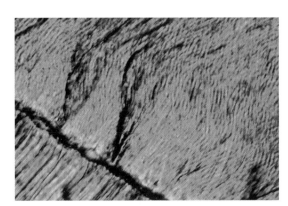

Fig. 7.51 Transverse section of enamel showing enamel tufts (arrow) (× 200).

direction as the prisms and, in thick sections, undulate with sheets of prisms. They are hypomineralised and recur at approximately 100 μm intervals along the junction. Each tuft is several prisms wide. Owing to their alignment, tufts are best visualised in transverse sections of enamel.

It has been suggested that this appearance results from protein, presumed to be residual matrix, at the prism boundaries of hypomineralised prisms (Fig. 7.52). Tuft protein, however,

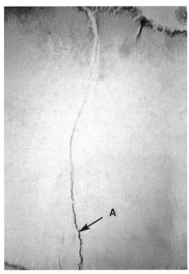

Fig. 7.53 Demineralised section of enamel sectioned transversely to show an enamel lamella (A) (Light blue stain; × 150).

lamella-like structures are simply cracks produced during section preparation. This can be confirmed by demineralising the section, when cracks (but not true lamellae) will disappear.

Lamellae may arise developmentally due to incomplete maturation of groups of prisms (in which case they would contain enamel proteins) or after eruption as cracks during function (containing saliva and oral debris).

MICROPOROSITY OF ENAMEL

In vivo, the pores in enamel are water-filled spaces between the crystallites. Figures as high as 10–12% have been quoted for pore volume based on thermogravimetric analysis. These values, however, may be inflated because of the release of water that is normally a structural part of the enamel crystallites. From studies based upon water absorption techniques, enamel appears to have a porosity of about 3–5% by volume, but even this figure may not be a true reflection of the porosity as it may incorporate a factor related to water that is bound to the organic material. Within the prisms most pores exist as very narrow gaps between closely packed crystallites but some, though they are still small, appear elongated and tube-like. Most of the pores are accessible only to small molecules such as water. Polarised light studies, internal surface area measurements and etching studies suggest that most, if not all, of the pores that are accessible to molecules larger than water are distributed in the prism boundaries, while the pores that are accessible only to small molecules are found throughout the rest of the enamel. The prism boundaries may thus be thought of as main highways through the enamel, while the rest of the porosity may be thought of as a fine network of footpaths connecting occasionally with the main highways so that access through them is slow and restricted. The pathways for diffusion and, to a lesser extent, electrochemical effects arising from the charge on the pore walls have an important influence on the formation of a carious lesion. Putative micropores are shown in Figs 7.5 and 7.6.

AGE CHANGES IN ENAMEL

Enamel wears away slowly with age, dependent on diet and masticatory habits. It seems to darken in colour, which may be in part due to the reduced translucency of the tooth as secondary dentine forms and enamel thins and in part due to the accumulation of surface coatings and stains. The composition of the surface enamel alters as a result of additions and exchanges with the oral fluids. Fluoride can beneficially be incorporated into surface enamel. This reduces its porosity and susceptibility to caries.

CEMENT–ENAMEL JUNCTION

This feature is discussed with cementum on pages 168–169.

CLINICAL CONSIDERATIONS

Defects in enamel

Surveys report the presence of developmental enamel defects in 68–95% of the population. Defects may be of environmental or genetic origin. Disturbances of initial enamel formation result in hypoplasia and those of maturation in hypomineralisation. Hypoplasia usually manifests as pits and grooves on the enamel surface. In hypomineralisation the surface is generally intact but opaque rather than translucent. Hypoplasia is often induced by the infectious diseases of childhood such as measles, which leave a defect in those parts of the teeth actively developing at the time of the infection. The hypomineralisation of the enamel is related to a delay in the removal of amelogenins during maturation. Birthing difficulties and dietary deficiencies also commonly disturb development. Mottled enamel occurs as a result of a diet containing relatively high levels of fluoride. This fluorisis appears as a diffuse bilateral opacity of the enamel, and surface pitting occurs in severe cases.

Enamel structure and dental caries

In tooth decay (dental caries), acids produced by plaque dissolve enamel mineral. Because there is very little matrix the histologically observable changes are due to demineralisation. The basic description of the structure of the carious lesion is based on the observation of ground sections in polarised light (Fig. 7.54), as this approach gives an appearance related to crystallite content. In early lesions before cavitation occurs the surface enamel shows relatively little change but beneath it, in the 'body' of the lesion, 20–50% of the mineral is lost. When mineral is dissolved the loss begins at the periphery of the prism. The mineral is not necessarily lost permanently as remineralisation does occur (saliva is saturated with mineral). During carious attack a repeating cycle of demineralisation and remineralisation occurs: clearly, if demineralisation dominates the caries progresses. That the possession of a relatively intact surface layer (despite considerable subsurface demineralisation) in the carious lesion does not reflect unique features of the surface enamel (but more a process of reprecipitation of mineral) is evident from *in vitro* studies, in which the surface layer of enamel was ground away to a considerable depth and carious-like lesions induced artificially. In such lesions an intact surface lesion still appeared as a characteristic feature of the carious lesion.

The basis of the treatment of early caries and the prevention of caries is to tip the balance in favour of remineralisation and away from demineralisation. Thus, caries is prevented by procedures that minimise plaque formation (diet and oral hygiene), starve such plaque biofilm as is present of acid-producing substrates (diet), render the enamel mineral less soluble (fluoride) and encourage remineralisation (diet, fluoride mouthwash and toothpaste).

Enamel structure and restorative dentistry

Many of the structural features of enamel are acutely relevant

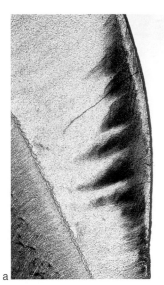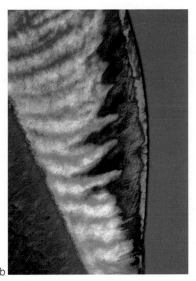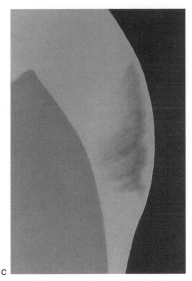

Fig. 7.54 An early carious lesion, which clinically would appear as a 'white spot' without cavitation. (a) A ground section showing an apparently intact surface zone but darker regions beneath it where mineral has been lost. (b) the same section seen in polarising light. (c) The same section as a microradiograph with a darker (less radiodense) subsurface zone (× 24). Courtesy of Dr B. H. Clarkson.

to restorative dentistry. The understanding of the initiation and progress of dental caries has been based on a knowledge of enamel composition and morphology and has led to a much more conservative approach by utilising the phenomenon of remineralisation and reducing the need for the removal of sound tissue. This reduced sacrifice of sound tooth structure has also been brought about by the development of adhesives that will bond to enamel, a development that is based on an understanding of the prismatic structure of enamel and the controllable effects of acids on it. Different acids at different concentrations can produce a variety of patterns of partial prism dissolution to provide a roughened surface suitable for adherence of restorative materials (acid conditioning). This reduces or eliminates the need for mechanical retention cut into sound tissue. For agents mechanically binding to enamel, it is necessary to produce microporosities in the surface by acid-etch techniques (Fig. 7.55). Thus when bonding agents are applied to such as surface, microscopic tags can be seen invaginating into the roughened surface (Fig. 7.56).

When cavities are prepared a knowledge of the microanatomy of enamel, particularly in terms of prism orientation, is essential to conserve as much as possible of the original strength of the tissue. Cutting cavities into enamel with rotary instruments will inevitably lead to subsurface cracking. Fortunately, some of the adhesive materials are capable of reinforcing this weakened substrate (Fig. 7.57).

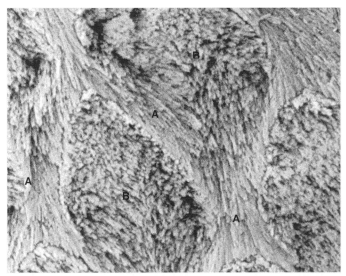

Fig. 7.55 SEM of enamel prisms etched end-on with an acid (maleic acid), showing a differential etch pattern between the prism boundary region (A) and the prism core region (B). This produces a microscopically rough surface suitable for the retention of a resin-based adhesive (× 6000). Courtesy of Professor B. Van Meerbeek.

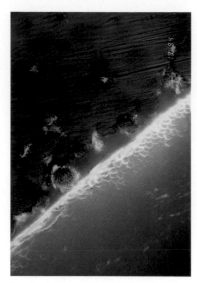

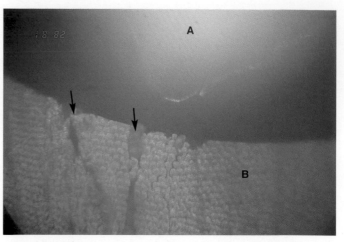

Fig. 7.56 Confocal microscope image showing the penetration of a (yellow) dye-labelled bonding agent into acid-etched enamel. Note tags of resin around the prism boundaries made porous by acid etching (× 450). Courtesy of Professor T. Watson.

Fig. 7.57 Confocal microscope image of the interface between a dental bur (A) and the enamel wall (B) taken during the actual cutting of a cavity. Note the fracture lines (arrows), the prism boundaries, the enamel prisms being viewed in cross-section (× 450). Courtesy of Professor T. Watson.

Enamel pearls

These are small isolated spheres of enamel that are occasionally found on the root towards the cervical margin (see page 348). They are particularly common in the root bifurcation region. They may predispose to plaque accretion following gingival recession.

8 Investing organic layers on enamel surfaces

Throughout its life, the crown of a tooth is covered by an organic layer or integument. Before the tooth erupts into the oral cavity the crown is covered by the overlying oral mucosa, the coronal part of the dental follicle, and the vestiges of the enamel organ (plus its associated primary enamel cuticle). For information concerning the origins of the enamel organ and the dental follicle during early tooth development, see Chapter 21. After emerging into the mouth, parts of the integument of enamel organ origin are lost by degeneration of its epithelial component and by attrition or abrasion of the underlying cuticular component. In the region of the gingival crevice or sulcus the primary (or pre-eruptive) enamel cuticle acquires additional matter from the lining epithelium and, coronal to the gingival margin, from saliva. The salivary layer is known as the acquired pellicle. Oral bacteria adhere initially to the enamel cuticle and later to the acquired pellicle, to form the dental plaque.

INVESTING LAYERS ASSOCIATED WITH THE CROWNS OF UNERUPTED TEETH

The soft tissues covering an erupting tooth comprise oral mucosa and the subjacent connective tissue of the dental follicle. Between the dental follicle and the enamel is an epithelial layer that is the remains of the enamel organ – the reduced enamel epithelium (Fig. 8.1). The appearance of this epithelium varies from a thin, flattened layer of cells to a more organised layer of recognisable cuboidal or columnar reduced ameloblasts, deep to which may be additional cell layers (Fig. 8.2). Although it is

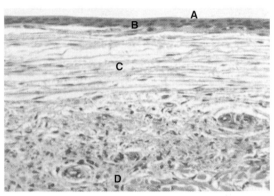

Fig. 8.2 Immediately adjacent to the enamel space (A) is the reduced enamel epithelium (B). In this section, the reduced enamel epithelium appears flattened. Superficial to the reduced enamel epithelium is the fibrous connective tissue of the dental follicle (C), and superficial to this is the oral submucosa (D) (Demineralised section, H & E; × 160).

not evident at the light microscope level, a basal lamina (primary enamel cuticle) is interposed between the enamel surface and the reduced enamel epithelium. The reduced enamel epithelium and the basal lamina comprise **Nasmyth's membrane**. The enamel organ associated with an occlusal fissure appears to be the last to change to a reduced enamel epithelium and the cells adjacent to the enamel in this region may retain a columnar appearance for some considerable time (Fig. 8.3). The reduced enamel epithelium covering the crown of unerupted teeth can be demonstrated with special staining (Fig. 8.4)

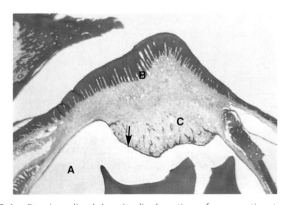

Fig. 8.1 Demineralised, longitudinal section of an erupting tooth *in situ*. A = Enamel space; B = oral epithelium, immediately beneath which is its associated lamina propria and submucosa; C = dental follicle associated with the underlying erupting tooth. Reduced enamel epithelium (arrow). (H & E; × 10).

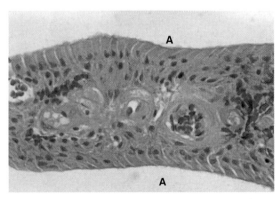

Fig. 8.3 The reduced enamel epithelium in an occlusal fissure. Although the reduced enamel epithelium covering the rest of the crown comprises cells with a flattened morphology, the cells immediately adjacent to the enamel space (A) still retain a columnar appearance. Note the vascularity of the tissue in this region (Demineralised section, Mallory's trichrome; × 80). Courtesy of Professor H.N. Newman.

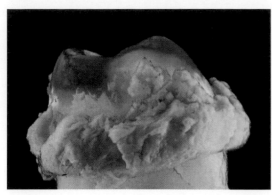

Fig. 8.4 This unerupted permanent third molar has been stained to show the remains of the dental follicle (yellow) and the vestigial enamel organ (blue). Note that part of the follicle has been lost during the surgical removal of the tooth and that the underlying vestigial enamel organ covers the entire crown (Alcian blue after fixation in Bouin's solution; × 4). Courtesy of Professor H.N. Newman.

INVESTING LAYERS ASSOCIATED WITH THE CROWNS OF ERUPTED TEETH

The organic layers covering the erupted healthy tooth can be revealed by special stains (Fig. 8.5). That part of the crown well exposed in the mouth is covered by loosely adherent reduced enamel epithelium, which is soon lost, leaving the

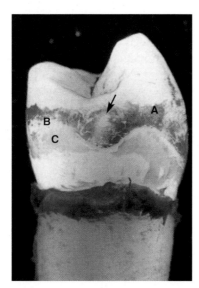

Fig. 8.5 Approximal view of a partially erupted premolar, showing the zones of its organic integument. Two zones are stained. The dark blue layer (A) is the plaque. The light blue layer (C) is the attachment or junctional epithelium, which in life links the tooth to the gingiva coronal to the periodontal ligament. The unstained zone between them (B) comprises the primary (or pre-eruptive) enamel cuticle. Note that the plaque corresponds to a position above the crest of the gingival margin and around the contact point (arrowed) where adjacent teeth meet, and that the cuticle lies in the region of the gingival crevice. Apical to the junctional epithelium, the enamel was covered *in vivo* by loosely adherent reduced enamel epithelial cells, which were lost during extraction. Coronal to the plaque the crown is covered by the primary enamel cuticle together with an organic element of salivary origin (the acquired pellicle) (Alcian blue–Aldehyde fuchsin; × 4). Courtesy of Professor H.N. Newman.

primary enamel cuticle, which immediately acquires an organic element of salivary origin, the acquired pellicle. Passing towards the gingiva but above the gingival margin, the tooth is likely to be covered by plaque. In the region of the gingival crevice the tooth will be covered only by the primary enamel cuticle. Below this layer the tooth will be covered by the junctional epithelium, its extent being related to the stage of tooth development. Using careful demineralising techniques it is possible to lift off the organic integument; consequently the plaque, primary enamel cuticle and junctional epithelium appear as a single continuous entity (Figs 8.6, 8.7). The surface of this organic film adjacent to the enamel may even show prism-end markings in the region of the gingival crevice where it is formed only by the primary enamel cuticle, indicating its intimate association with the enamel surface (Fig. 8.8).

The three distinct zones forming the enamel integument as seen in Figures 8.5 and 8.6 are clearly distinguishable at the ultrastructural level. Beneath the gingival crevice in the region of the junctional epithelium the enamel integument covering the enamel surface consists of the junctional epithelial cells and the primary enamel cuticle (Fig. 8.9). The junctional epithelium is described further on pages 235–239. Immediately coronal to this, in the region of the gingival crevice, the enamel

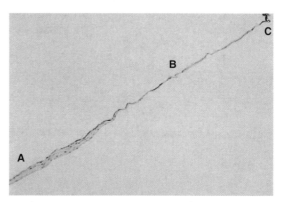

Fig. 8.6 The organic integument removed from the enamel surface of an erupted tooth following careful demineralisation. A = Epithelium; B = primary enamel cuticle; C = plaque (Ollett's modification of Twort; × 100). Courtesy of Professor H.N. Newman.

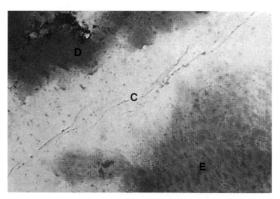

Fig. 8.7 High-power view of the external surface of part of organic integument removed from enamel by careful demineralisation. D = Plaque; C = primary (pre-eruptive) enamel cuticle; E = junctional epithelium (Toluidine blue and erythrosin; × 20). Courtesy of Professor H.N. Newman.

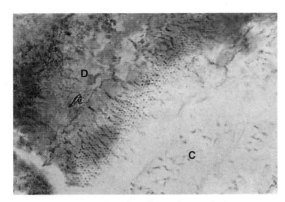

Fig. 8.8   Deep enamel-related surface of organic integument removed from enamel by careful demineralisation, revealing a zone of prism end markings (arrowed) in the primary enamel cuticle (C) just beneath the plaque (D) (Alcian blue and erythrosin; × 20). Courtesy of Professor H.N. Newman.

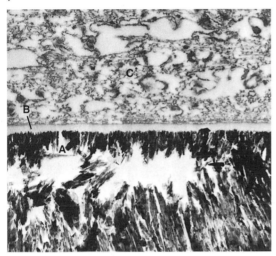

Fig. 8.9   The enamel integument at the level of the junctional epithelium. This micrograph is taken from a region at the coronal limit of the gingival crevice. The enamel surface (A) is covered by the primary enamel cuticle (B) and the remaining vestige of an attachment or junctional epithelial cell (C) (TEM; × 13 000). Courtesy of Professor H.N. Newman.

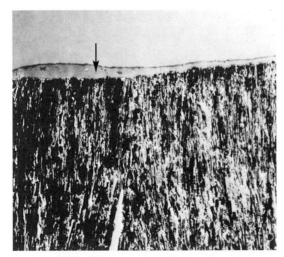

Fig. 8.10   The enamel integument immediately coronal to the junctional epithelium showing the primary enamel cuticle (arrowed) on the enamel surface. This section is in the region of the gingival crevice coronal to that illustrated in Fig. 8.9 and therefore lacks a junctional epithelial cell. Note that the cuticle usually has an electron-dense outer border (TEM; × 10 000). Courtesy of Professor H.N. Newman.

surface is covered only by the primary enamel cuticle, the junctional epithelium having been lost (Fig. 8.10). Above the gingival crest, the primary enamel cuticle exposed in the mouth will become coated with an acquired pellicle derived from saliva and this will become colonised by bacteria to form dental plaque (Fig. 8.11). In health, the firm apposition of the gingiva to the tooth limits the plaque to the gingival margin (Fig. 8.12). Excessive plaque accumulation is associated with both dental caries and chronic inflammatory periodontal disease.

The primary enamel cuticle is in intimate contact with the underlying organic enamel matrix. Generally approximately 30 nm thick, the cuticle acquires accretions in the region of the gingival crevice, which derive from crevicular epithelium

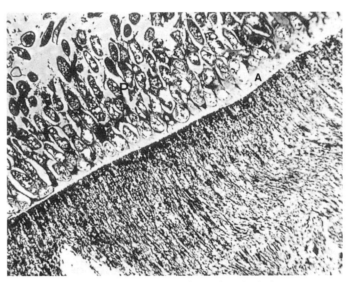

Fig. 8.11   The enamel integument above the gingival crest showing bacterial colonisation forming dental plaque. This micrograph shows early approximal surface plaque on a clear layer (A), which is probably combined primary enamel cuticle and pellicle, above which is a layer of plaque (P) (TEM; × 1250). Courtesy of Professor H.N. Newman.

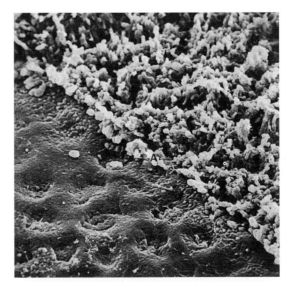

Fig. 8.12   In health, the firm apposition of the gingiva to the tooth limits the plaque to the gingival margin. There is a sharp boundary to the dental plaque (A), below which lies the plaque-free surface of enamel in the region of the gingival sulcus (SEM; × 1500). Courtesy of Professor H.N. Newman.

and from plasma and may increase the cuticle to about 5 μm thick (Fig. 8.13). Localised thickening of the primary enamel cuticle may also occur on its deep aspect, where enamel maturation is incomplete because of the presence at this site of a stria of Retzius reaching the surface (Fig. 8.14). The primary enamel cuticle is thought to be composed of protein. Its accretions are mainly proteoglycan or glycoprotein elements from the contiguous soft tissues. Plasma contributions include immunoglobulins (Fig. 8.15), which form part of the host defence system against plaque.

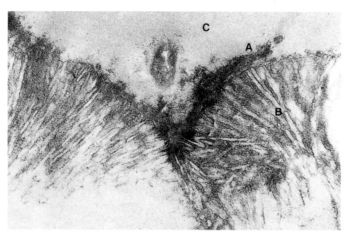

Fig. 8.13 The thin primary enamel cuticle (A) is in intimate contact with the underlying organic enamel matrix (B). Note the lathe-like spaces occupied *in vivo* by enamel crystals. In the region of the gingival crevice, the cuticle aquires accretions (C) and appears thicker (Demineralised section, TEM × 30 000). Courtesy of Professor H.N. Newman.

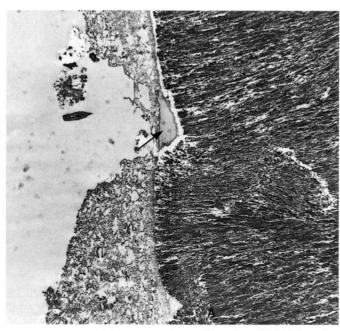

Fig. 8.14 Localised thickening of the primary enamel cuticle at the enamel surface in relation to an enamel stria reaching the surface (arrow) (TEM micrograph; × 5100). Courtesy of Professor H.N. Newman.

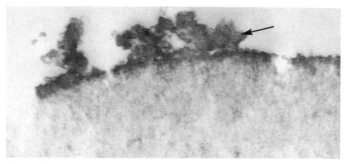

Fig. 8.15 The primary enamel cuticle at the enamel surface showing positive staining for the immunoglobulin IgG (arrow). This forms part of the host defence system against plaque (TEM with antibody to human IgG; peroxidase method for localisation of IgG; × 34 500). Courtesy of Professors H.N. Newman and S.J. Challacombe.

Where the enamel surface is exposed to wear, either by attrition or abrasion, the vestigial enamel organ is worn away, but the enamel rapidly acquires a layer of acquired pellicle. Indeed, this pellicle always forms a protective coat following any wear. This acellular layer is derived mainly from salivary proteins, but includes elements from crevicular fluid and bacteria.

Dental plaque is the combination of bacteria embedded in a matrix of salivary proteins and bacterial products superimposed on the acquired pellicle (see Fig. 8.11). Dental plaque is an example of a biofilm, a term used to describe communities of microbes attached to surfaces. Early plaque is composed of mainly Gram-positive, facultative, anaerobic cocci and filaments (Fig. 8.16). With time, the deposit will thicken, although in non-pathological, supragingival situations its microfloral composition is unlikely to vary greatly (see Fig. 8.12).

Where the plaque is associated with chronic inflammatory periodontal disease and becomes subgingival, a more complex flora develops with anaerobic Gram-negative organisms predominating, to include cocci, rods, filaments and many motile forms (particularly spirochaetes) (Figs 8.17, 8.18). The microbial

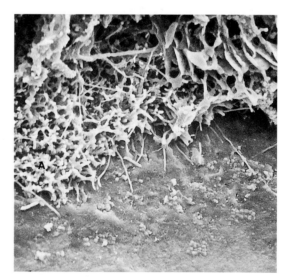

Fig. 8.16 SEM showing apical border of early plaque composed mainly of cocci (A) and filaments (× 1300). Courtesy of Professor H.N. Newman and the editors of the *British Dental Journal*.

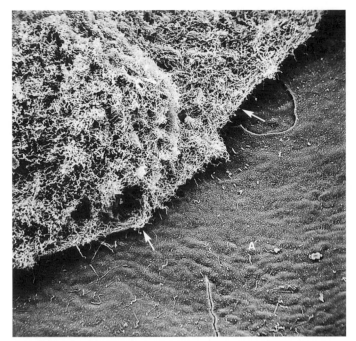

Fig. 8.17 SEM showing apical border of subgingival plaque (arrow) associated with advanced chronic inflammatory periodontal disease. The predominant organisms are spirochaetes. The details of cementum (A) are obscured by a dental cuticle on which isolated spirochaetes are seen (× 430). Courtesy of Professor H.N. Newman and Academic Press, London.

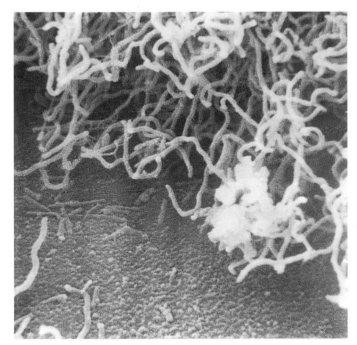

Fig. 8.18 SEM showing high power of the apical border seen in Fig. 8.17. The subgingival plaque is composed mainly of spirochaetes (× 4000). Courtesy of Professor H.N. Newman and Academic Press, London.

composition of dental plaque will vary, not only with the stages of maturity of the deposit but also from individual to individual, from tooth to tooth, from site to site and from surface to surface. Plaque can be seen on all tooth surfaces that are not subject to constant abrasion, especially in areas

that are difficult to clean (such as occlusal pits and fissures, interproximal regions and at the gingival margin). Its presence may be more readily visualised clinically by the use of disclosing solutions (Fig. 8.19). Many plaque bacteria metabolise dietary carbohydrates, often producing polysaccharides, which may be stored intracellularly, on the cell surface, and extracellularly in the matrix.

Dental calculus is mineralised plaque (Fig. 8.20). Saliva is supersaturated with minerals (such as calcium and phosphate) that have the potential to mature newly erupted enamel, protect exposed tooth surfaces from acid action and remineralise areas in the early stages of demineralisation. Salivary inhibitors prevent precipitation and crystallisation of minerals in saliva, but bacterial enzymes can degrade these inhibitors. Thus, under suitable conditions (e.g. with high concentrations of minerals derived from saliva), precipitation and crystallisation may occur within dental plaque. Early calculus formation includes deposition in the matrix of poorly crystalline calcium phosphate types, including octacalcium phosphate and dicalcium phosphate dihydrate, and dying bacterial cells. With

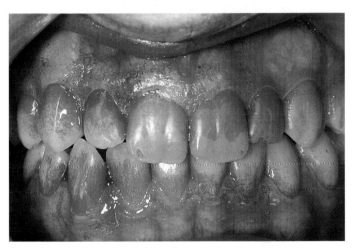

Fig. 8.19 Plaque stained red and exposed by the use of a disclosing solution. Courtesy of Professor R. Palmer.

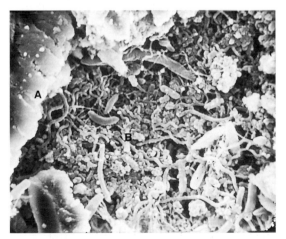

Fig. 8.20 SEM of calculus showing mineralised (A) and unmineralised areas of plaque composed of a mixed flora (B) (× 3000). Courtesy of Professor H.N. Newman and Academic Press, London.

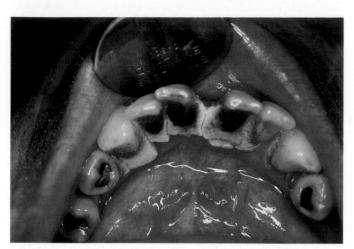

Fig. 8.21 View of mouth showing presence of supragingival calculus associated with the lingual surfaces of heavily stained anterior mandibular teeth. Courtesy of Dr M. Ide.

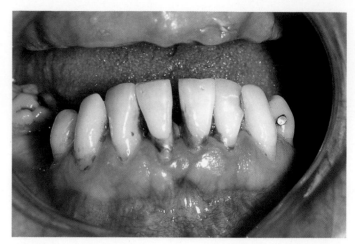

Fig. 8.23 Subgingival calculus exposed following gingival recession associated with chronic inflammatory periodontal disease. Courtesy of Professor R. Palmer.

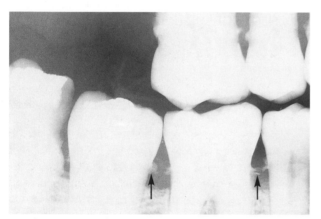

Fig. 8.22 Subgingival calculus (arrowed) evident in a bitewing radiograph. Courtesy of Dr M. Ide.

time more structured crystalline elements, including hydroxyapatite and whitlockite, are formed.

Supragingival dental calculus is seen predominantly on the lingual surfaces of the anterior mandibular teeth (near the opening of the submandibular and sublingual glands (Fig. 8.21) and on the buccal surfaces of the maxillary molars (near the openings of the parotid glands). Subgingival calculus can occur throughout the dentition from minerals in the inflammatory exudate associated with periodontal disease. Large deposits of subgingival calculus are sometimes identified on interproximal surfaces in dental radiographs (Fig. 8.22). It may also be exposed when the gingiva recedes from the teeth following chronic inflammatory periodontal disease (Fig. 8.23).

Dental calculus is always covered with a biofilm of living organisms (see Fig. 8.21).

CLINICAL CONSIDERATIONS

The presence of dental plaque predisposes to the onset of the two main dental pathologies: dental caries and periodontal disease. However, different microorganisms are thought to be involved in the two diseases. Dental caries is associated with the metabolism of dietary sugar to acid by predominantly Gram-positive organisms (e.g. *Streptococcus mutans*) in supragingival plaque. Frequent intake of sugar induces a cariogenic plaque in which organisms capable of surviving at low pH are favoured. Periodontal disease is associated with the persistent presence of mature plaque at the gingival margin, and exacerbated by an increase in Gram-negative organisms and obligate anaerobes, which are favoured by the environment of periodontal pockets. Gingival inflammation and periodontal destruction are the result of direct action of bacterial products (such as proteases) and indirect promotion of potentially damaging immune responses. The challenge of dental plaque can be limited by reducing dietary sugar intake, mechanical removal of the plaque and modifying the pathogenic potential. Toothbrushing, flossing or professional scaling and root planing may achieve mechanical removal. Pathogenic potential may be modified by the use of personal oral hygiene products such as toothpastes, mouth rinses and gels containing antimicrobials, or delivery of antibiotics as local or systemic treatments by the general practitioner.

9 Dentine

Dentine is the mineralised tissue that forms the bulk of the tooth. In the crown it is covered by enamel, in the root by cementum (Fig. 9.1). It is a rigid but elastic tissue consisting of large numbers of small parallel tubules in a mineralised collagen matrix. The tubules contain the long processes of the cells responsible for forming the tissue, the odontoblasts, as well as a small volume of extracellular (dentinal) fluid. The cell bodies of the odontoblasts line the deep surface of the dentine defining the outer border of the dental pulp. The combination of enamel and dentine provides a rigid hard structure suitable for tearing and chewing that resists both abrasion and fracture. The cementum covering the dentine of the root anchors the tooth to the bone of the socket via the periodontal ligament. The junctions of the dentine with these two other hard tissues are biologically unique as is the tissue itself. Two major properties distinguish dentine from enamel. Firstly, dentine is sensitive. Secondly, dentine is formed throughout life, increasing in thickness at the expense of the dental pulp. This is reflected in the presence of an unmineralised layer of dentine matrix at the pulpal surface known as predentine. The physical properties of enamel and dentine are complementary. Thus, although enamel is extremely hard, it is unyielding and may fracture during mastication if the underlying dentine did not provide a degree of deformability.

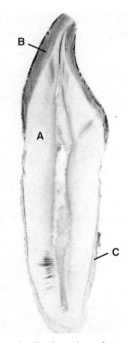

Fig. 9.1 Ground longitudinal section of a tooth showing dentine (A) forming the bulk of the tooth, covered in the crown by enamel (B) and in the root by cementum (C). The dental pulp has been lost during preparation and the pulp chamber and root canal are empty (× 4).

PHYSICAL PROPERTIES

Fresh dentine is pale yellow in colour and contributes to the appearance of the tooth through the translucent enamel. Dentine is harder than bone and cementum but softer than enamel. Its organic matrix and tubular architecture provide it with greater compressive, tensile and flexural strength than enamel. Dentine is permeable, the permeability depending on the size and patency of the tubules which will decline with age. Some of the physical properties of dentine (compared with those of enamel) are listed in Table 7.1, page 102.

CHEMICAL PROPERTIES OF DENTINE

The gross composition of dentine approximates to 70% inorganic, 20% organic and 10% water by weight; 50% inorganic, 30% organic and 20% water by volume.

The inorganic, mineral component is in the form of calcium hydroxyapatite crystals. The percentage dry weight of some of the important elements is shown in Table 9.1. The crystallites are calcium poor and carbonate rich in comparison to pure hydroxyapatite and, although similar in shape, are very much smaller (approx. $35 \times 10 \times 100$ nm) than those in enamel (see Fig. 7.4). The crystallites contain other trace elements including fluoride. The hydroxyapatite crystallites in the mineralised dentine are found on and between the collagen fibrils.

Organic matrix

The organic matrix of dentine in which the crystallites are embedded has a composition similar to that of bone. The organic matrix consists of fibrils embedded in an amorphous ground substance. The fibrils are collagen and comprise over 90% of the organic matrix.

The principal collagen fibril is the ubiquitous type I collagen. Traces of type III and type V collagen, which are present in sizeable amounts in the pulp, have also been detected. Most of the collagen fibrils in dentine run parallel to the pulpal surface

Table 9.1 *The major inorganic elements of dentine*

Constituent	% of dry weight
Calcium	26.9
Phosphorus	13.2
Carbonate	4.6
Sodium	0.6
Magnesium	0.8

(Fig. 9.2). In mineralised dentine the collagen fibrils are of larger diameter (100 nm) and are more closely packed than in predentine. Collagen fibrils in dentine are not assembled into bundles as they are in many non-mineralised connective tissues such as tendon or periodontal ligament.

Proteins

Though comprising only a relatively small percentage of the organic matrix compared with collagen, the non-collagenous proteins of dentine have important, but as yet poorly understood, biological functions. They include dentine phosphoproteins, proteoglycans, Gla-proteins, other acid proteins and growth factors.

Dentine phosphoproteins

These represent the main non-collagenous protein. There are several types, but the term dentine phosphoprotein (phosphophoryn or PP-H) relates to the highly phosphorylated protein species. Owing to its very high phosphate content it represents the most acidic protein known. Indeed, about 80% of the amino acid residues carry negatively charged phosphate or carboxyl groups. Its high calcium ion binding properties have implicated PP-H in the process of mineralisation.

Proteoglycans

These also form a significant component of the non-collagenous proteins. In dentine, they are represented by the smaller-molecular-weight types known as biglycan and decorin. The glycosaminoglycans are primarily chondroitin-4-sulphate and chondroitin-6-sulphate. Among the important functions of proteoglycans in general are their role in collagen fibril assembly and their cell-mediated effects such as cell adhesion, migration, proliferation and differentiation. As significant biochemical changes occur at the mineralising front, it can be assumed that proteoglycans have an important but as yet incompletely understood role in mineralisation. They appear to bind calcium non-specifically. They may be inhibitors of calcifications that need to undergo some degree of degradation before mineralisation will occur.

γ-Carboxyglutamate-containing proteins (Gla-proteins)

Little is known about the function of these small proteins, present in low amounts in dentine. They bind strongly, but reversibly, to hydroxyapatite crystallites and may play some role in mineralisation.

Other acidic proteins

Osteonectin, a protein containing high levels of glutamic and aspartic acid, is found in dentine at levels of about 5% of total protein. Osteopontin, a phosphorylated glycoprotein has been identified in predentine and contains the receptor binding sequence Arg-Gly-Asp (RGD). The precise role of osteonectin and osteopontin in dentine (as in bone) is not known.

Growth factors

Like bone, numerous growth factors can be isolated from dentine matrix and are presumably absorbed from circulating tissue fluid. Unlike bone, which is continually turning over and releasing the bound-up growth factors that might play a role in subsequent bone activity, it is difficult to envisage a similar active role for such growth factors in dentine. These factors include insulin-like growth factor and transforming growth factor.

Lipids

These comprise about 2% of the organic content of dentine and, as they are conspicuous at the mineralising front, are thought to play a role in mineralisation. Phospholipids have been detected in both predentine and mineralised dentine. They occupy the same areas of the tissue as proteoglycans. In the predentine, they are most heavily concentrated near the mineralising front. In dentine, phospholipids are needle-like 'crystal ghosts' and may be involved in the formation and growth of crystals. They seem to be absent from the centres of calcospherites but present in interglobular dentine.

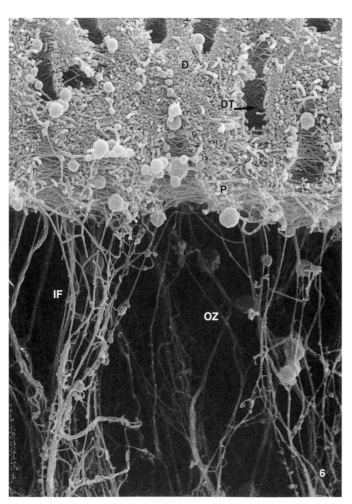

Fig. 9.2 SEM of predentine (P) with mineral and odontoblast cells removed revealing the pattern of collagen fibres. In predentine most of the dentinal collagen fibres run parallel to the pulpal surface. Collagen fibres in the odontoblast layer parallel the long axis of the cell bodies; OZ = odontoblast zone; IF = intercellular fibres (× 3500). Courtesy of B. Sogaard-Pedersen, H. Boye and M. Matthiessen and the editor of *Scandinavian Journal of Dental Research.*

DENTINE TUBULES

Dentine is permeated by tubules, the dentine tubules, that run from the pulpal surface to the enamel–dentine and cementum–dentine junctions (Fig. 9.3). The dentine tubules follow a curved, sigmoid course – the **primary curvatures**. The convexity of the primary curvatures nearest the pulp chamber faces rootward. In the root and beneath the cusps, the primary curvatures are less pronounced, the tubules running a straighter course. In transverse section the tubules are approximately circular although their appearance is obviously dependent on the plane in which the tissue is sectioned (Figs 9.4, 9.5). The dentine between the tubules is termed intertubular dentine.

The tubules taper from approximately 2.5 μm in diameter at their pulpal ends to 1 μm or less peripherally. During the formation of dentine tubules by the odontoblasts the cells migrate inwards and occupy a smaller surface area. Hence, the tubules are more widely separated at their peripheries. Approximately 22% of the cross-sectional area of the dentine near the pulp is composed of tubules, while near the enamel–dentine junction the tubules comprise only about 2.5%. Estimates of the number

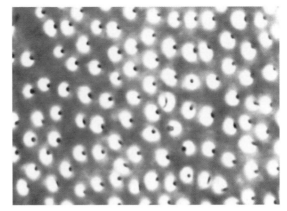

Fig. 9.5 A demineralised section of dentinal tubules cut transversely. This treatment results in the loss of the peritubular/intratubular dentine, which has little organic matrix. The dark-staining odontoblast processes occupy only a small proportion of the resulting lumen (Haemotoxylin; × 1000). Courtesy of Professor E.W. Bradford.

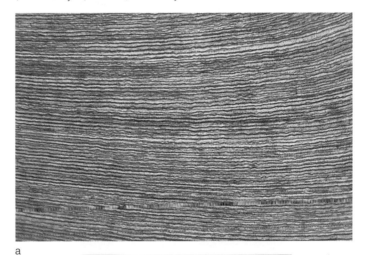

a

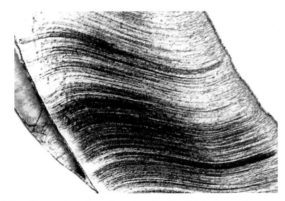

Fig. 9.3 Ground section showing dentinal tubules cut longitudinally and demonstrating the sinusoidal primary curvatures (× 25).

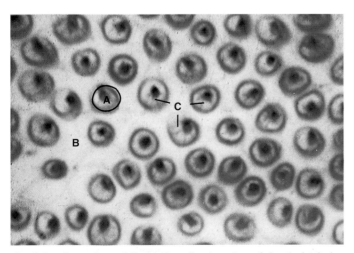

Fig. 9.4 Ground, partially demineralised section of dentinal tubules cut transversely. A indicates the perimeter of a tubule as initially laid down; B = intertubular dentine; C = peritubular/intratubular dentine. (Eosin stain; × 1500). Courtesy of Dr. R. Sprinz.

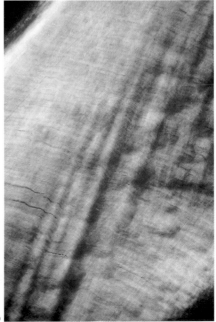

b

Fig. 9.6 (a) Decalcified section showing dentinal tubules cut longitudinally. The lumens of the tubules have been stained with picrothionin and demonstrate secondary curvatures (× 200). Courtesy of Professor M.M. Smith. (b) Ground section showing dentinal tubules cut longitudinally and exhibiting contour lines (arrows) due to coincidence of secondary curvatures (× 150). Courtesy of Dr R.P. Shellis.

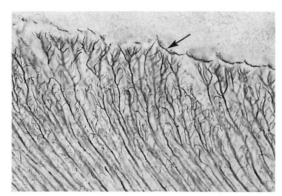

Fig. 9.7 Ground section of dentine near the enamel–dentine junction (arrow) showing branching of dentinal tubules (× 320).

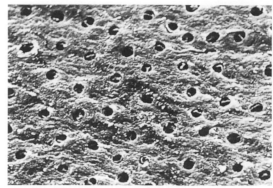

Fig. 9.8 SEM of transversely sectioned dentinal tubules close to the pulp and lacking peritubular dentine (× 540). Courtesy of Professor B.R.R.N. Mendis.

of tubules vary somewhat between reports due to differences in tooth age and type and the thickness of the dentine. A reasonable rounding of the numbers suggests 20 000/mm^2 in outer dentine, 50 000/mm^2 in inner dentine and 40 000/mm^2 in the middle.

The tubules also show changes in direction of much smaller (a few μm) amplitude. These are known as the **secondary curvatures** (Fig. 9.6). In some region the secondary curvatures may coincide in adjacent tubules. At low magnification, this gives the appearance of a line crossing the dentine, a **contour line** (of Owen) (Fig. 9.6). These are not commonly seen in most of the dentine, but one such line is usually evident at the junction of primary and secondary dentine where, during deposition, all the odontoblasts seem to take a simultaneous and similar change in direction (see Fig. 9.48).

Dentinal tubules branch. The most profuse branching is in the periphery near the enamel–dentine junction (Fig. 9.7), presumably a reflection of the numerous processes the early odontoblast has. Many small side branches appear to end blindly but some may unite with branches of other tubules. In the root, the terminal tubule branches and the branches loop. This looping is thought by some to be responsible for the appearance of the granular layer of Tomes seen in this region in ground section (see page 136). Branching is not obvious in much of the dentine beneath the periphery but becomes notable in the uncalcified predentine near the pulp. Presumably during mineralisation many of the odontoblastic branches retract or atrophy and the small canals they occupied fill in.

PERITUBULAR DENTINE

The walls of the dentinal tubules in recently formed intertubular dentine at the pulp surface are comprised of mineralised type I collagen (Figs 9.8, 9.9). With maturation, another type of dentine is deposited on the walls of the dentinal tubule, narrowing the size of the lumen (Figs 9.10, 9.11). This type of dentine is known as peritubular dentine (more properly, but not more popularly, known as **intratubular dentine**), and deposition often eventually leads to obliteration of the tubule (Fig. 9.12). Peritubular dentine differs from intertubular dentine in lacking collagenous fibrous matrix.

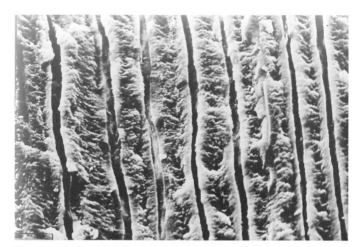

Fig. 9.9 SEM of longitudinally sectioned dentinal tubules close to the pulp showing little evidence of peritubular dentine (× 540). Courtesy of Professor B.R.R.N. Mendis.

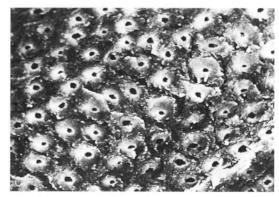

Fig. 9.10 SEM of dentine tubules cut in cross section in the middle of the dentine. They reveal a distinctive zone of peritubular dentine, narrowing the original tubule (× 1200). Courtesy of Professor B.R.R.N. Mendis.

Peritubular dentine can also be distinguished from intertubular dentine as a zone of increased radiographic (Fig. 9.13) and electron density (Fig. 9.14) lining the internal surface of the dentinal tubule. Peritubular dentine is about 15% more mineralised than intertubular dentine. When dentine is routinely demineralised, the peritubular dentine will be lost as it lacks the stabilising feature of collagen. The dimensions of

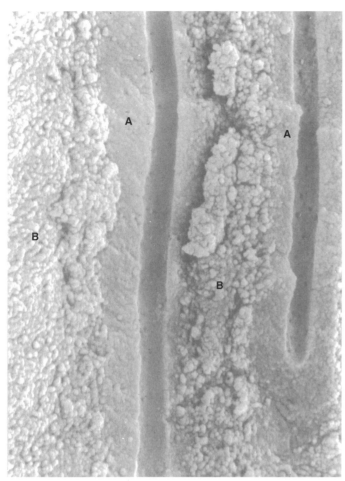

Fig. 9.11 SEM of dentine tubules cut longitudinally and showing peritubular dentine (A) deposited on the tubule wall. B = Intertubular dentine (× 7000). Courtesy of Professor M.M. Smith.

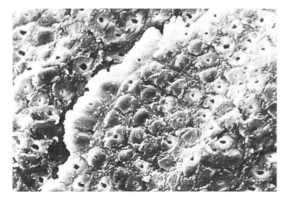

Fig. 9.12 Dentine tubules sectioned transversely close to the enamel–dentine junction showing peritubular dentine formation obliterating the lumen (× 1200). Courtesy of Professor B.R.R.N. Mendis.

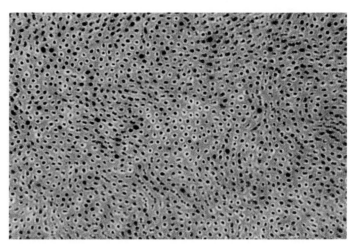

Fig. 9.13 Microradiograph of transversely sectioned dentinal tubules surrounded by a more radio-opaque (and therefore denser) zone of peritubular dentine (× 650). Courtesy of Dr G. McKay.

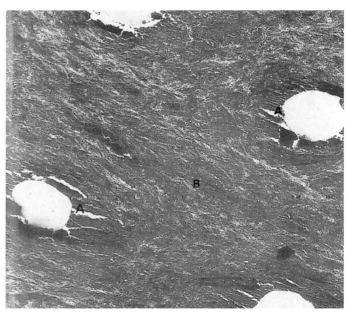

Fig. 9.14 TEM of peritubular dentine (A) seen in an ultrathin undecalcified section. The peritubular dentine appears non-fibrillar and more electron opaque. It is more fragile than intertubular dentine (B) and shatters during sectioning (× 6000). Courtesy of Professor N.W. Johnson.

the dentine tubules will thus be increased to their initial dimensions (compare Figs 9.4 and 9.5). Peritubular dentine is found in unerupted teeth.

The main protein of peritubular dentine has a higher molecular weight and an amino acid composition quite different from the phosphophoryn found in intertubular dentine. In demineralised sections at the electron microscope level the matrix appears as an amorphous material. The mineral component of peritubular dentine is mainly carbonated apatite but its crystalline form is distinct from that of intertubular dentine. Some crystallites have a hexagonal shape and appear as compact platelets slightly smaller than (but similar to) those of intertubular dentine. Other crystalline species may also be present. In tubules exposed by attrition, some occluding components may be derived from saliva. Although the bulk of peritubular dentine is hypercalcified relative to the intertubular dentine, hypocalcified areas bound its inner and outer surfaces. Peritubular dentine is formed at about the same time as (or soon after) intertubular dentine. By the time primary dentine formation is complete, all peripheral tubules have a lining of peritubular dentine that extends from the enamel dentine junction to within 100–50 μm of the predentine. In outer dentine, peritubular dentine occupies two-thirds of the cross-sectional area of the tissue; near to the predentine it occupies only approximately 3% (Fig. 9.8).

Associated with physiological ageing, especially in root dentine, the dentinal tubules become completely occluded by peritubular dentine formation. The contents of the tubule acquire the same refractive index as the intertubular dentine. When a ground section of a root is placed in water (which has a refractive index different from that of dentine), regions blocked by peritubular dentine will appear translucent ('translucent dentine'), while regions with patent tubules will fill with water and appear opaque (Fig. 9.15). Dentine tubules become infilled at the root apex adjacent to the cementum and extend cervically and towards the root canal with age. In cross section, translucent zones have a butterfly shape owing to the convergence of the tubules pulpally, being wider at the mesial and distal margins (Fig. 9.16). The amount of translucent

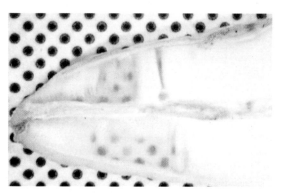

Fig. 9.15   Old tooth root sectioned longitudinally and placed in water. The presence of peritubular dentine completely occluding the tubules in much of the apical tissue results in this part appearing translucent as water is excluded. Towards the cervical margin (right side), patent tubules become filled with water, which has a refractive index that differs from that of the intertubular dentine. This results in the tissue appearing opaque (× 5). Courtesy of Professor A.G.S. Lumsden.

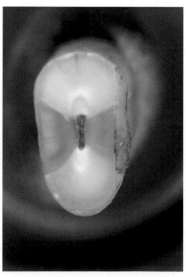

Fig. 9.16   Transverse section of mandibular premolar showing butterfly-shaped outline of translucent dentine (× 5). Courtesy of Dr R. O'Sullivan.

dentine increases linearly with age and is not affected by function or external irritation. This feature is used in forensic dentistry to age teeth. Translucent dentine is is also referred to on page 140; sclerotic dentine, which has features similar to translucent dentine, is discussed on page 143.

CONTENTS OF THE DENTINAL TUBULES

The dentinal tubules contain the processes of the odontoblasts that are responsible for their formation. In some parts of the tissue they also contain afferent nerve terminals. It is also possible that processes from antigen-presenting cells in the peripheral pulp may extend for a short distance into the tubules. Technical limitations prevent a definitive figure being given for what proportion of the tubule is occupied by cell processes and how far along the tubule the processes extend. It seems likely, however, that there is a periodontoblastic space, and possibly a postodontoblastic space, from which the process has receded. These spaces are thought to be filled with extracellular 'dentinal' fluid, the precise composition of which is unknown. Some studies have suggested a composition that differs from extracellular fluids elsewhere in having a relatively higher concentration of potassium ions and a relatively lower concentration of sodium ions. Such a balance could affect the membrane properties of the nerve endings and odontoblast processes in the tubules. If dentine is fractured, fluid exudes from the tubules and forms droplets on the surface of the dentine. This suggests that there is a positive force, presumably pulpal tissue pressure, that is exerted outwards (p. 159). This could help limit the progress of chemicals or toxins on, or in, dentine towards the dental pulp.

The cell body of the odontoblast is described in detail in the section on the dental pulp (pages 152–154). The process of the odontoblast that extends into the dentine varies in structure at different levels in the tissue, organelles being most numerous in the predentine whereas, in mineralised dentine, few are present (Fig. 9.17).

There are two technical problems that limit our interpretation of available histological data on the contents of the dentinal tubules. One is the difficulty of fixing small amounts of tissue deep in mineralised tissue. Fixation tends to shrink tissue, and even when this can be minimised the slowness with which most fixatives penetrate means that post-mortem changes will often occur. The second problem is that, in extracting a tooth, it is often compressed by forceps. Releasing the compression often draws tissue up into the tubules (e.g. 'aspiration' of odontoblast nuclei) that is not normally there. Thus, the interpretation of images of tubule contents should be approached with caution. More indirect approaches, such as labelling the tissue *in vivo* with, for example, a radioactive tag or using immunohistochemical techniques which mark the presence of cell components, can add considerably to our understanding.

Microtubules and intermediate filaments run longitudinally throughout the odontoblast process. Mitochondria are sometimes present in the process in the predentine; strands of rough endoplasmic reticulum are also occasionally seen. Vesicles of a

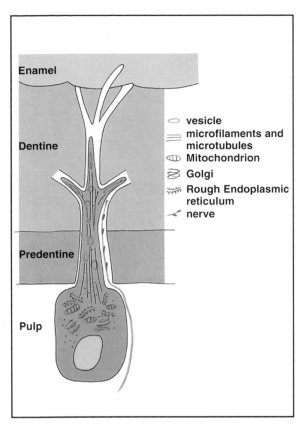

Enamel

Dentine

Predentine

Pulp

◯ vesicle
≡ microfilaments and microtubules
⬭ Mitochondrion
〰 Golgi
〰 Rough Endoplasmic reticulum
↙ nerve

Fig. 9.17   Diagram of an odontoblast and its main process extending into the dentine. The true extent of the process is controversial, as is the existence of the periodontoblastic space.

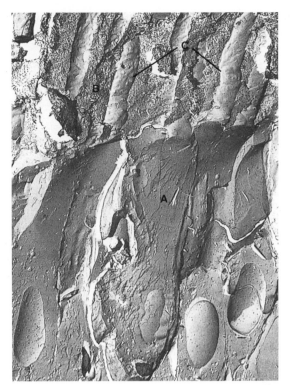

Fig. 9.18   TEM of a surface replica of the pulp–predentine junction. The odontoblasts (A) form a continuous layer on the surface of the predentine (B) and their processes (C) completely fill the dentinal tubules with no evidence of a periodontoblastic space. The technique involves fracturing the frozen tissue, coating the surface with vaporised metal and then separating the ultrathin coating for examination in the microscope. This complex technique is thought to cause minimal, if any, shrinkage (× 2 000). Courtesy of Doctors A. Riske-Anderson and A. Koling and the editors of *Acta Scandinavica Odontologica*.

variety of sizes are present, being more dense near the cell membrane. Their incidence declines in the more distal parts of the process.

In the predentine and very innermost mineralised circumpulpal dentine the odontoblast process seems to occupy the full width of the dentinal tubule with no discernable periodontoblast space (Figs 9.18–9.20). At these levels afferent nerve axons are also seen within the tubule and in close apposition to the odontoblast process. The axons contain several mitochondria and an occasional vesicle. They do not contain large accumulations of vesicles as are found in synapses although proteins associated elsewhere with synaptic vesicle exocytosis have been demonstrated in dentinal tubules. It is not possible by electron microscopy to recognise cell processes in the dentine tubules of peripheral dentine (Figs 9.21, 9.22).

Although the structural characteristics of cells may be lost due to poor fixation, remnants characteristic of cells may still be found (eg. tubulin–Fig. 9.23). The microtubule and intermediate filament systems are characteristic of cell processes and made up of proteins such as actin, tubulin and vimentin. Some of these proteins can be demonstrated in peripheral dentinal tubules even though no structurally recognisable process can be seen. One possible interpretation for this finding might be that the odontoblast process has degenerated, leaving remnants containing tubulin or microfilamentous material behind.

Clearly, the odontoblast process must occupy the entire dentinal tubule it forms in the early stages of development

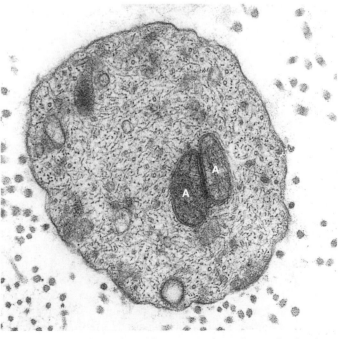

Fig. 9.19   TEM of an odontoblast process from the predentine in cross section, A = Mitochondrion (× 80 000).

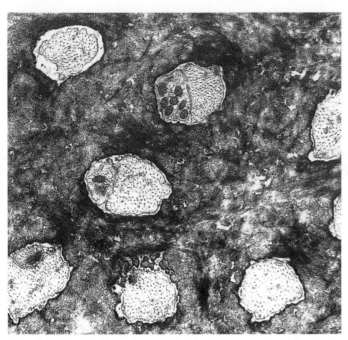

Fig. 9.20 TEM of dentinal tubules in inner calcified dentine in cross section. Three of the tubules contain naked nerve endings as well as odontoblast processes. The periodontoblastic space is either small or absent (× 10 000).

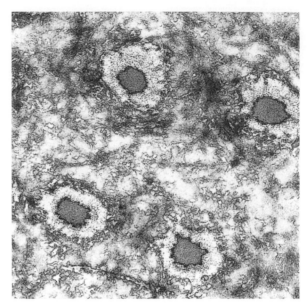

Fig. 9.22 TEM of dentinal tubules in peripheral dentine. The tubules contain amorphous, non-cellular material (× 8000).

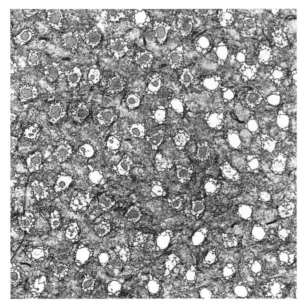

Fig. 9.21 TEM of dentinal tubules from the middle region of coronal circumpulpal dentine. Some tubules appear to contain cell processes, some contain non-cellular material and some are empty. (× 3000).

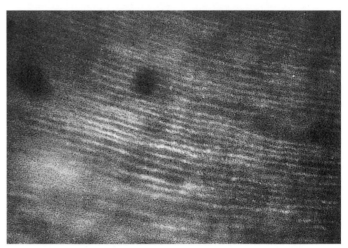

Fig. 9.23 Components of the cytoskeleton in peripheral dentine. A fluorescent label marks the presence of tubulin, a component of intracellular microtubules (× 4200). Courtesy of Doctors M. Sigal, S. Pitaru, J. Aubin and A.R. Ten Cate and the editor of *Anatomical Record*.

when the dentine is thin. There are three hypotheses for what might happen later and these are illustrated in Fig. 9.24. In A, the process grows in length as dentine is deposited and its peripheral termination remains at the outer end of the tubule. This would result in a metabolically unsupported cell process several millimeters long, an arrangement unknown elsewhere in the body where axons (except at their terminations) are supported by Schwann cells. In B, the process reaches a pre-

determined length and then moves pulpally as dentine is formed, leaving behind an empty tubule in which peritubular dentine forms. Perhaps peritubular dentine differs from inter-tubular dentine in being formed by a process that does not directly involve the odontoblast. In C, the peripheral end of the processes degrades sequentially and its remains form part of the matrix for the peritubular dentine.

The possible existence of an odontoblast process in outer dentine is also complicated by the presence of a very thin, apparently proteinaceous membrane termed the **lamina limitans** lining the wall of the dentinal tubule. Its composition is unknown but, in certain preparations, it may give rise to the erroneous impression of an odontoblast process (Figs 9.25, 9.26).

In some parts of the dentine, most commonly beneath cusps, the tubules in inner dentine can contain additional small

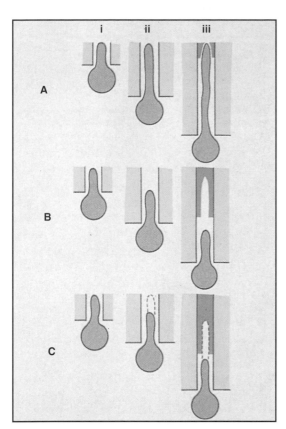

Fig. 9.24   Three hypotheses describing the pulpward migration of the odontoblast as dentine is deposited (see text for details).

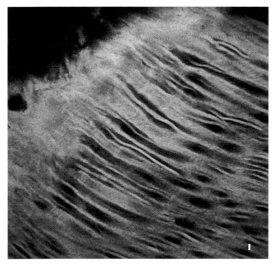

Fig. 9.25   Dentinal tubules from peripheral to tertiary dentine showing the presence of tubular structures in an area from which the odontoblasts have been lost and which probably represent the lamina limitans (Confocal microscopy of a demineralised section × 1700). Courtesy of Doctors G. Goracci, G. Mori, F. Marci and M. Baldi and the editor of *Minerva Stomatologica*.

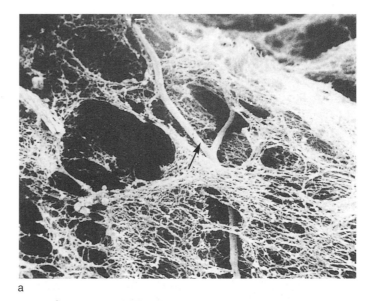

a

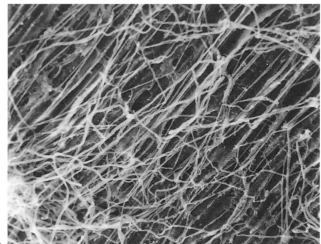

b

Fig. 9.26   (a) SEM of a tubular branching structure in peripheral dentine (arrowed) following collagenase treatment. It is difficult to establish whether this is a true odontoblast process or the lamina limitans. (× 3000) Courtesy of Doctors M. Sigal, S. Pitaru, J. Aubin and A.R. Ten Cate and the editor of *Anatomical Record*. (b) SEM of demineralised dentine also treated with collagenase to remove the bulk of the organic matrix. The remaining tubular structures seen in this micrograph are thought to represent the lamina limitans as complimentary TEM studies show them to possess no cellular characteristics (× 1000). Courtesy of Dr H.F. Thomas.

processes (Fig. 9.27). Some of these could be smaller odontoblastic processes that are lost during later deposition, others will be the processes of the immunocompetent antigen-presenting cells that are found in several areas of the pulp particularly in the periphery within and beneath the odontoblast layer (see pages 156–157). These, and their extensions into the dentinal tubules, are found even in unerupted teeth in small numbers, with intratubular processes limited to the predentine in the coronal pulp. In intact erupted teeth, these processes are present over a much wider area although still limited to predentine. In dentine beneath dental caries, the processes of the immunocompetent cells extend much deeper into the tubules of the circumpulpal dentine. However, in all tubules there is one large odontoblast process.

Sensory terminals have been firmly identified within the dentinal tubule, but special techniques are needed to distinguish them from smaller branches of the odontoblast process. Like the odontoblast process, their extent into dentine is not known for certain. Nerve terminals are limited mainly to the dentine of the crown beneath the cusps (where they may be found in up to 80% of the tubules) and are sparse in cervical and root dentine. The axon in an innervated tubule is narrower than the odontoblast process and contains microtubules, a few microfilaments and often mitochondria. Vesicles are rare in nerve terminals (or in the odontoblast process adjacent to them) and structurally specialised contacts between the nerve terminal and the odontoblast process seem to be absent (Fig. 9.27).

The sensory nature of intratubular axons can be demonstrated by tracer techniques. Radioactive amino acids (eg. tritium-labelled proline) injected into the trigeminal ganglion are converted into proteins and transported down the axons to the peripheral terminations (Fig. 9.28).

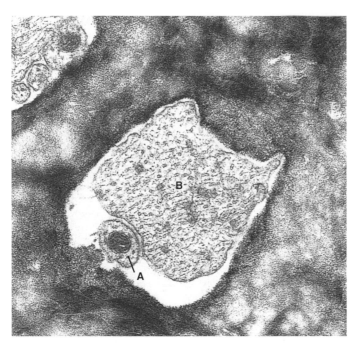

Fig 9.27 TEM showing multiple processes within a single dentinal tubule. The larger process is the odontoblast process, the smaller ones presumptive nerve terminals (× 65 000).

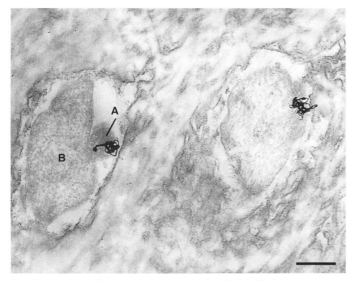

Fig. 9.28 TEM showing autoradiographically labelled nerve (A) adjacent to an odontoblast process (B). The labelled amino acid was originally injected into the trigeminal ganglion (× 20 000). Courtesy of Dr M.R. Byers.

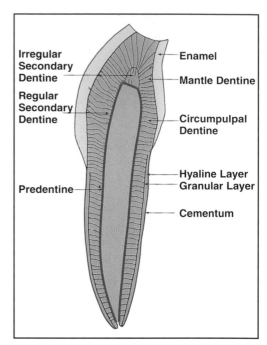

Fig. 9.29 The regions of varying dentine structure.

REGIONAL VARIATIONS IN DENTINE STRUCTURE AND COMPOSITION

Several different regions can be recognised in dentine (Fig. 9.29). The most peripheral region beneath the enamel and dentine has a number of special characteristics bestowed on it by being the earliest formed part of the tissue. In the crown this first-formed layer is known as mantle dentine. In the root there are two morphologically recognisable outer zones: the hyaline layer and the granular layer (of Tomes). There is some controversy (discussed below) as to whether the hyaline layer is properly a component of dentine or cementum or is a mingling of components of both tissues. Predentine is the innermost unmineralised layer, where new dentine is being deposited throughout life. Just peripheral to the predentine is a zone of mineralisation, which is recognisable even in decalcified tissue samples as, simultaneously with mineral deposition, the matrix undergoes considerable modification that results in different staining properties. This region has sometimes been called intermediate dentine. The bulk of the dentine between the mantle layer and the zone of mineralisation is the circumpulpal dentine. The outer part of the circumpulpal dentine beneath the mantle layer is often incompletely mineralised and has a characteristic appearance when seen in ground sections, referred to as 'interglobular dentine'. In older teeth the inner, pulpal part of the circumpulpal dentine differs somewhat in structure from the bulk of the tissue. This secondary dentine is laid down as an age-related change in the rate of dentine formation once a (presumably) genetically predetermined thickness of primary circumpulpal dentine has been deposited and root development (at least in terms of length) is complete. In teeth that have been subject to external stimuli (such as attrition, dental caries and cavity preparation), another layer of dentine is found pulpal to the circumpulpal (and in older teeth secondary) dentine and restricted to the region beneath the irritation. This tertiary dentine is not formed by the original odontoblasts but by odontoblast-like cells that have differentiated from the dental pulp. It is much more irregular than circumpulpal dentine and has been given a variety of names such as reactionary dentine, reparative dentine, response dentine and irregular secondary dentine. There has been broad, although not complete, acceptance of the term tertiary dentine in preference to other terms (see page 141).

Mantle dentine

The outer layer of dentine in the crown differs from the bulk of the circumpulpal dentine in four features:

- It is slightly (approx. 5%) less mineralized.
- The collagen fibres are largely oriented perpendicular to the enamel–dentine junction (see also pages 322–323). For this reason, it can be distinguished from the circumpulpal dentine beneath using polarised light (Fig. 9.30).
- The dentinal tubules branch profusely in this region (Fig. 9.31).
- It undergoes mineralisation in the presence of matrix vesicles (see page 326).

These features give the mantle region an appearance distinct from that of the circumpulpal dentine when seen in polarising light microscopy of ground, undermineralised sections.

The mantle layer varies in width from 20 to 150 μm. The three-dimensional scalloped architecture of the enamel–dentine junction and the extension of some dentinal tubules into the enamel as enamel spindles have been described in Chapter 7.

Interglobular dentine

Much of the mineral in dentine is deposited as globules or calcospherites. These, in most areas, fuse to form a uniformly calcified tissue. However, in some areas, usually beneath the mantle layer in the crown and beneath the granular layer in the root, the fusion may be incomplete. When ground sections are viewed in transmitted light, internal reflection of the light

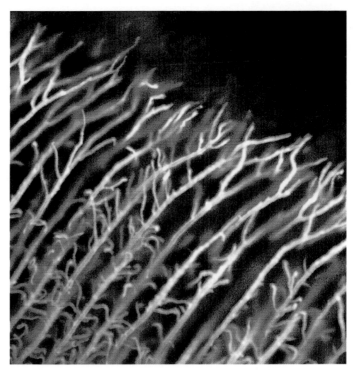

Fig. 9.31 Confocal image of dentinal tubules branching in the region of the mantle dentine (Alizerin red; × 1200). Courtesy of Doctors M. Kagayama, Y. Sasao, S. Kamakura, K. Motegi and I. Mizoguchi and the editor of *Anatomy and Embryology*.

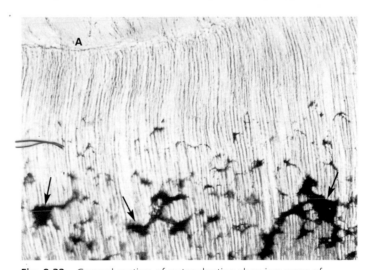

Fig. 9.32 · Ground section of outer dentine showing areas of interglobular dentine (arrowed). A = Enamel (× 300). Courtesy of R.V. Hawkins.

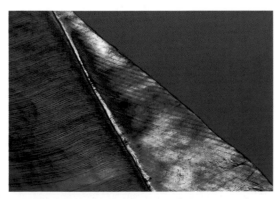

Fig. 9.30 Ground longitudinal section of the crown of a tooth viewed in polarised light (with a quartz filter). Due to the different orientation of the collagen fibres, the mantle layer immediately beneath the enamel–dentine junction appears red, in contrast to the blue appearance of the rest of the circumpulpal dentine (× 50).

makes the uncalcified, interglobular areas appear dark (Fig. 9.32). Dentinal tubules pass without deviation through interglobular areas (Fig. 9.33). As interglobular areas remain uncalcified, peritubular dentine is also absent from the tubules as they pass through interglobular dentine.

Granular layer

In ground sections the periphery of the dentine in the root is marked by the presence of a dark granular zone, the granular layer (Figs 9.34, 9.35). Various explanations for this appear-

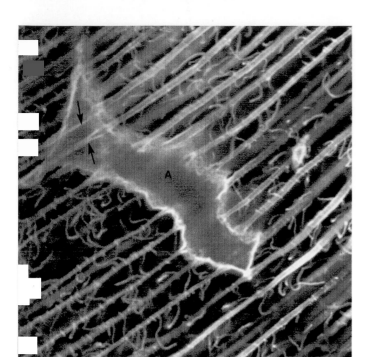

Fig. 9.33 Confocal image of dentinal tubules (arrow) passing through an area of interglobular dentine (A). (Alizerin red, × 1200). Courtesy of Doctors S. M. Kagayama, Y. Sasao, S. Kamakura, K. Motegi and I. Mizoguchi and the editor of *Anatomy and Embryology*.

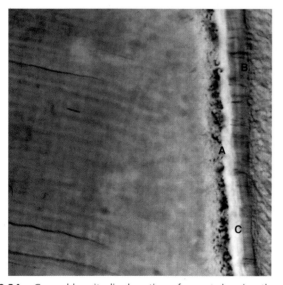

Fig. 9.34 Ground longitudinal section of a root showing the granular (A) and hyaline (C) layers beneath a layer of acellular cementum (B) (× 160).

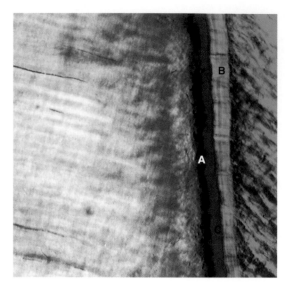

Fig. 9.35 The same section as in Fig. 9.34 viewed in polarised light with a quartz tint. The hyaline layer can be distinguished from the rest of the underlying dentine and the cementum by the difference in the orientation of its collagen fibres. A = Granular layer, B = cementum, C = hyaline layer (× 160).

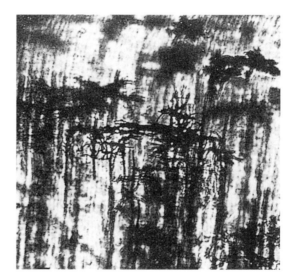

Fig. 9.36 Ground thick section of root impregnated with silver stain in region of granular layer showing peripheral terminations of tubules exhibiting profuse branching in three dimensions (× 490).

ance have been suggested. That currently most accepted is that the dentinal tubules in this area branch more profusely and loop back on themselves, creating air spaces in ground sections that result in internal reflection of transmitted light. Differences in the rate of formation of coronal and radicular dentine could explain why this appearance is seen in the root but not the crown. Stain-filled tubules viewed in thick sections have a 'tree-top' appearance somewhat supporting this idea (Fig. 9.36). The granular layer is hypomineralised in comparison to circumpulpal dentine, but this may be the result of the presence of more tubular branches. An alternative explanation for the granular appearance is that it is due to the incomplete fusion of calcospherites.

Hyaline layer

Outside the granular layer is a clear hyaline layer usually included as a component of the dentine but whose origin is obscure. This narrow band (up to 20 μm wide) appears to be non-tubular and relatively structureless (Figs 9.34, 9.35). The hyaline layer may serve to bond cementum to dentine and may be of considerable clinical significance when considering periodontal regeneration. It is discussed further on page 327.

Circumpulpal dentine

The basic structure of dentine as described throughout this chapter is that of circumpulpal dentine. It forms the bulk of the dentine and is uniform in structure except at its edges where, peripherally, interglobular dentine marks incomplete initial mineralisation and, centrally, the mineralising front represents ongoing mineralisation. In older teeth its tubular pattern is modified on the pulpal surface due to the age-related deposition of secondary dentine.

Predentine

In demineralised sections stained with hematoxylin and eosin, the innermost layer of dentine, the predentine, has a distinct pale-staining appearance (Fig. 9.37). This reflects a difference in the composition of its matrix from that of the matrix of the mineralised circumpulpal dentine. The mineralising front may show a globular (Fig. 9.37) or a linear outline, reflecting the mineralisation process (see pages 324–327). The predentine is the initially laid down dentine matrix before its mineralisation. During mineralisation, the matrix undergoes considerable modification. The principal role of the odontoblast process in predentine is the secretion of matrix components. In mineralising dentine the role of the odontoblast process is to participate in the modification of that matrix and, perhaps, also in its mineralisation (see pages 324–327). The width of the predentine can vary from 10 to 40 μm, depending on the rate at which dentine is being deposited: it is, for example, thicker in young teeth.

Structural lines in dentine

In sections of dentine viewed by different techniques, a variety of lines approximately perpendicular to the dentinal tubules can be seen. The descriptions and explanations of these lines vary considerably. Some have had the name of the individual who first described them attached to them, causing confusion when later investigators use those names to include somewhat different structures. The description given here will rely on the functional origin of the lines as best understood but will include the eponym to retain the historical flavour these lines have acquired.

There are two related groups of lines: those originating from curvatures in the dentinal tubules and those arising from the incremental deposition of dentine and its subsequent mineralisation.

Lines associated with the primary curvatures of the dentinal tubules

In some longitudinal sections the peaks of the sigmoid primary curvatures coincide to form broad bands in the dentine. These are not apparent in many sections, and rarely can two be seen. They are more difficult to see in horizontal sections where they would be seen as broad concentric bands in the circumpulpal dentine. These lines are known as Schreger lines (Fig. 9.38).

Lines associated with the secondary curvatures of the dentinal tubules

When the secondary curvatures coincide they also give rise to an optical effect, resulting in the appearance of lines, the contour lines of Owen (Fig. 9.39). They are unusual in primary dentine but are sometimes seen. An exaggerated line is found at the border of primary and secondary dentine (see pages 138–139) and between dentine formed before and that formed after birth. This latter **neonatal line** may include compositional variations in matrix and mineralisation.

Incremental lines associated with matrix deposition and mineralisation

Dentine has regular, incremental, short-period and long-period markings. The lines may be seen in normal ground sections (Fig. 9.40), demineralised sections, under polarised light (Fig. 9.41) and in microradiographs. They can be

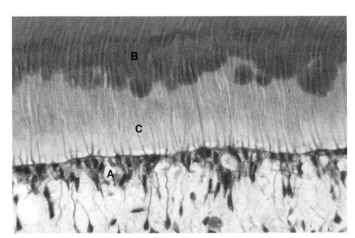

Fig. 9.37   Decalcified section of the pulpodential region showing the odontoblast layer (A) and predentine (C). Note the different staining reaction of the predentine to that of the mineralised dentine matrix (B). The mineralising front at B is globular (H & E; × 500).

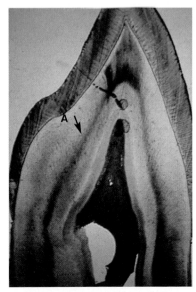

Fig. 9.38   Ground longitudinal section of a crown showing a broad Schreger line (A), coincident with the apex of one of the primary curvatures of the dentinal tubules. Only one is visible although, hypothetically, two are possible (× 5).

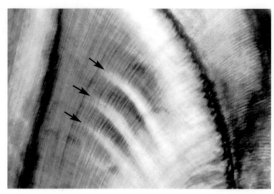

Fig. 9.39 Ground longitudinal section viewed in polarised light of a crown showing contour lines associated with the coincidence of secondary curvatures (arrows) of the dentinal tubules (× 120).

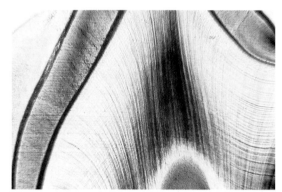

Fig. 9.40 Ground longitudinal section of a crown showing, on the right side, horizontally running long-period incremental lines (× 12). Courtesy of Dr B.A.W. Brown.

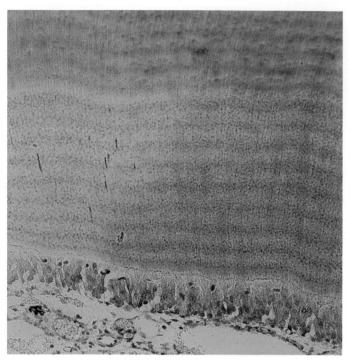

Fig. 9.42 This decalcified section is taken from a rat injected with tritiated proline. The amino acid is incorporated rythmically into the collagen of the dentine matrix, as shown by the periodic presence of silver grains developed by the radioactivity from the photographic emulsion layered onto the section. The section is also lightly stained to show incremental lines and how these coincide with the incorporation of proline (H & E; × 350). Courtesy of Doctors M. Ohtsuka, S. Saeki, K. Igarashi, H. Shinoda and the editor of the *Journal of Dental Research*.

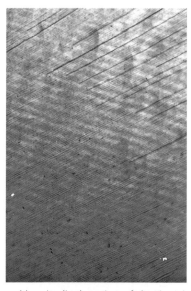

Fig. 9.41 Ground longitudinal section of dentine viewed in polarised light showing alternate light and dark bands representing long-period incremental lines. The bands are approximately orientated at right angles to the direction of the dentinal tubules (× 250).

attributed to circadian fluctuations in acid–base balance that affect both the mineral content and the refractive index of forming hard tissues. The long-period lines, at least, are greatly enhanced when viewed in polarised light (Fig. 9.41), suggesting that they are associated with changes in collagen fibril orientation.

Short-period markings may be seen as alternating dark and light bands, each pair reflecting the diurnal rhythm of dentine formation (Fig. 9.42). These fine lines are sometimes referred to as **von Ebner's lines**. In cuspal dentine, where deposition is most rapid, the amount of dentine formed each day and the distance between adjacent dark bands is approximately 4 μm (Fig. 9.43). In the root peripherally near the granular layer, where the dentine has a calcospheritic pattern, the distance between lines is nearer 2 μm (Fig. 9.44). In demineralised sections the values are smaller, presumably due to shrinkage caused by processing of the tissue.

The coarser, long-period lines **(Andresen lines)** are approximately 16–20 μm apart (Figs 9.40, 9.41, 9.45). Between each long-period line there are 6–10 pairs of short-period lines (Fig. 9.45). The cause for the 6–10 day periodicity is unknown. The same periodicity exists between the long-period striae of Retzius in enamel and the long-period Andresen lines in dentine, making it likely that a common mechanism exists.

As with enamel, an exaggerated line, the **neonatal line** (Fig. 9.46), can be seen in teeth mineralising at birth.

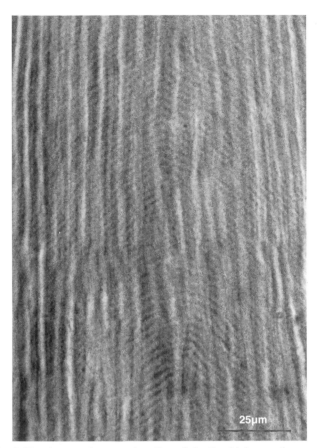

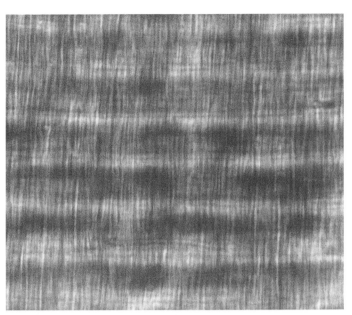

Fig. 9.45 Ground section of dentine viewed in polarised light. The long period lines are about 20 μm apart and between them are seven or eight short-period incremental lines (× 900). Courtesy of Professor M.C. Dean and the editor of *Archives of Oral Biology*.

Fig. 9.43 Anorganic ground section of dentine high over the cuspal region of a premolar showing short-period incremental lines running across the field approximately 4 μm apart (× 720). Courtesy of Professor M.C. Dean and the editor of *Archives of Oral Biology*.

Age-related and posteruptive changes

Once the tooth is erupted and fully formed, dentine can undergo a number of changes that are either related to age or occur as a response to a stimulus applied to the tooth, such as caries or attrition. With regard to physiological age changes, secondary dentine and translucent dentine will be considered.

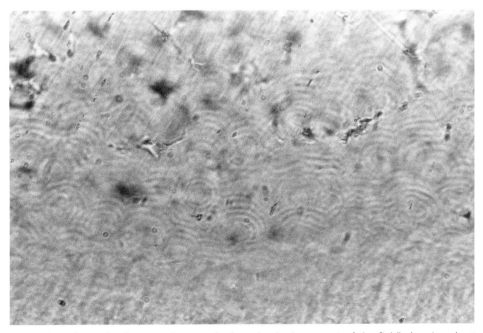

Fig. 9.44 Anorganic preparation of root dentine near the granular layer (at the lower part of the field) showing short-period incremental lines about 2 μm apart and having a calcospheritic outline (× 800). Courtesy of Professor M.C. Dean and the editor of *Archives of Oral Biology*.

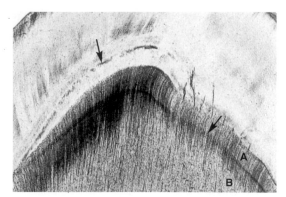

Fig. 9.46 Ground longitudinal section of a deciduous tooth showing neonatal lines (arrows) in enamel and dentine. These are exaggerated in this example as the tooth came from a patient who suffered from icterus neonaturium (newborn jaundice) (× 25). A = Dentine formed prenatally, B = dentine formed postnatally.

Concerning the response of dentine to stimuli, tertiary dentine, sclerotic dentine and dead tracts will be discussed.

Secondary dentine

The most conspicuous age-associated change in dentine is the formation of secondary dentine. Its structure is very similar to that of primary dentine and it may be difficult to distinguish between the two. However, primary and secondary dentine are often delineated as a result of a change in direction of the

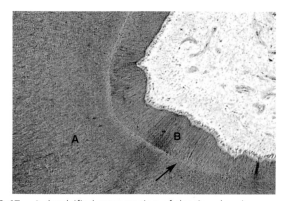

Fig. 9.47 A decalcified cross section of dentine showing a pronounced contour line separating primary dentine (A) from secondary dentine (B) (Silver staining, × 32).

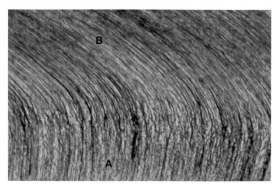

Fig. 9.48 Ground longitudinal section of dentine illustrating the change in direction of dentinal tubules as they pass from primary (B) to secondary (A) dentine (× 125).

dentinal tubules with coincidence of secondary curvatures. This produces a particularly pronounced contour line (of Owen) (Figs 9.47–9.50). The same odontoblasts continue to lay down similar dentine and the tubules of primary and secondary dentine are continuous. The increased crowding of

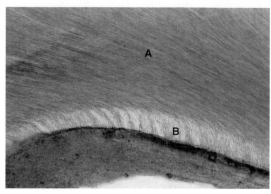

Fig. 9.49 Ground longitudinal section showing primary (A) and secondary (B) dentine (× 80).

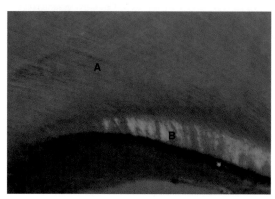

Fig. 9.50 Same section as Fig. 9.49, but viewed in polarised light with a quartz tint. The difference in colour between primary (A) and secondary (B) dentine is presumably due to the difference in orientation of collagen fibres and/or crystals (× 80).

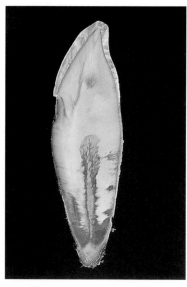

Fig. 9.51 A section of a whole tooth showing the translucent dentine predominantly in the apical part of the root (Ground section; × 2). Courtesy of Doctors A.M. Sengupta, D. K. Whittaker and P. R. Shellis and the editor of *Archives of Oral Biology*.

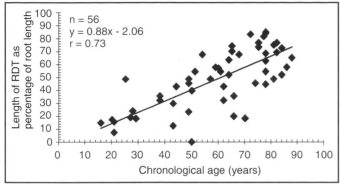

Fig. 9.52 The relationship between age and the area of translucent dentine (RDT). Courtesy of Doctors A.M. Sengupta, D. K. Whittaker and P. R. Shellis and the editor of *Archives of Oral Biology*.

odontoblasts as secondary dentine formation continues throughout life, and the slower rate of deposition make the tubular pattern of secondary dentine a little less regular than that of primary dentine and the incremental markings somewhat closer together. Secondary dentine formation begins at the completion of root formation as the tooth comes into occlusion. The main coincidence would seem to be the apparent completion of root formation as secondary dentine still forms in unerupted, impacted teeth. Secondary dentine forms most rapidly on the pulpal floor. Its continuing deposition leads to smaller pulp chambers and narrower root canals in older patients.

In physiological ageing, especially in root dentine, the tubules can become completely occluded with peritubular dentine to form **translucent dentine**. With age, translucent dentine is particularly pronounced at the root apex and increases linearly with age (Figs 9.51, 9.52). For this reason it is used in forensic dentistry to help determine the age of a person from the teeth. Translucent dentine is discussed further on page 143.

Tertiary dentine

The dental pulp may be induced to produce calcified material in addition to its 'usual' primary and secondary dentine by a variety of outside stimuli including caries, attrition, cavity preparation, microleakage around restorations and trauma. Stimuli of different types and extent may be applied to teeth at different stages of development or ageing, resulting in a response tissue that may vary considerably in appearance and composition: it may resemble secondary dentine in having a regular tubular structure; it may have few and/or irregularly arranged tubules; or it may be relatively atubular (Figs 9.53–9.55). Continuity of dentinal tubules between normal dentine and tertiary dentine will therefore be lost in many instances (Fig. 9.56).

Because of this wide range of presentations, this response tissue has been given a variety of names, including irregular secondary dentine, reparative dentine, reactionary dentine, response dentine and osteodentine. It seems sensible to rationalise this nomenclature and use the term 'tertiary dentine' for all hard tissue deposited on the pulpal surface in response to an external stimulus.

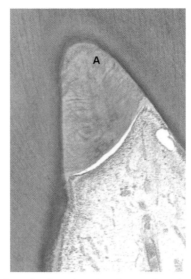

Fig. 9.53 Demineralised section showing tertiary dentine (A) having an irregular appearance in a pulp horn (H & E; × 50).

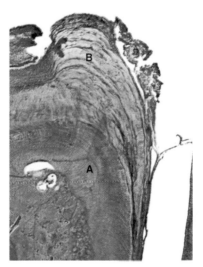

Fig. 9.54 Tertiary dentine (B) overlying primary dentine (A) on the floor of a pulp chamber extending around the orifice of a root canal (demineralised section stained with Weigerts and van Gieson) (× 20).

The pulp does not seem to respond to stimuli by increasing the rate of deposition of secondary dentine but by inducing previously quiescent odontoblast-like cells to produce mineralised tissue. The different appearances of tertiary dentine are thus probably due to its production by newly differentiated mesenchymal cells rather than by the odontoblasts that have produced primary and secondary dentine (although recent studies suggest that, at least on some occasions, primary odontoblasts may be involved in the initial stages of tertiary dentine formation). The newly differentiated cells responsible for tertiary dentine formation are very similar to odontoblasts in that they produce type I collagen and dentine sialoprotein, a dentine-specific protein.

The term **reactionary dentine** refers to the dentine forming in response to an insult in which, although some damage has been sustained and some odontoblasts die, the

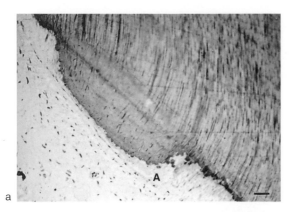

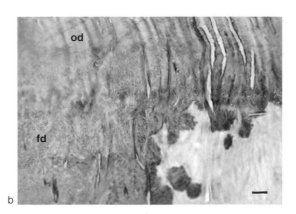

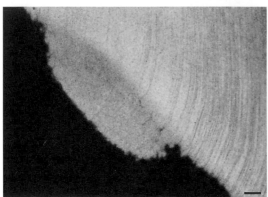

Fig. 9.55   Tertiary dentine formation in response to deep caries. (a) Zone of tertiary dentine (adjacent to A) at dentine–pulp interface projecting from normal dentine (B) (H & E; × 300). (b) Higher power view, showing calcospherites in tertiary dentine (H & E; × 1500). (c) Microradiograph of undemineralised lesion similar to that seen in (a), revealing a difference in mineralisation levels between normal and tertiary dentine, there being less mineral in tertiary dentine (× 300). Courtesy of Doctors L. Bjorndal and T. Darvann and the editor of *Caries Research*.

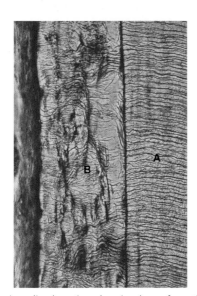

Fig. 9.56   Demineralised section showing loss of continuity of many dentinal tubules between normal dentine (A) and tertiary dentine (B) Picrothionine stain; × 100). Courtesy of Professor M.M. Smith.

the origin of odontoblasts during normal tooth formation (see page 320), reciprocal epithelial/mesenchymal interactions are an essential feature. However, it is clear that odontoblast-like cells arising from the adult pulp after a suitable stimulus do so in the absence of epithelial cells. There are two possible explanations for this. It might be that during initial dentine formation epithelial/mesenchymal interactions guide some cells on the path to becoming odontoblasts, but that these cells remain dormant in the pulp awaiting a later stimulus for them to complete their lifecycle and form reparative dentine. A more likely explanation, however, is that odontoblast-like cells are

existing odontoblasts recover and continue to form dentine. There will be some irregularity in dentine structure depending on the strength of the stimulus and the dentine will have an irregular appearance with fewer tubules.

The term **reparative dentine** relates to dentine forming after a stimulus in which the original odontoblasts in the associated region have been destroyed and new calcified tissue (reparative dentine) has been formed by newly differentiated cells referred to here as 'odontoblast-like' cells. In considering

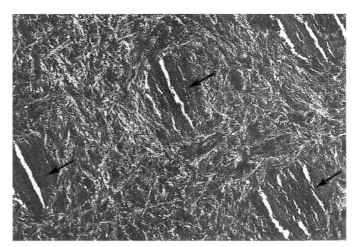

Fig. 9.57   TEM of a zone of sclerotic dentine adjacent to a carious cavity showing transversely sectioned tubules completely occluded, (arrows) forming a zone of sclerotic dentine (× 7000). Courtesy of Professor N.W. Johnson.

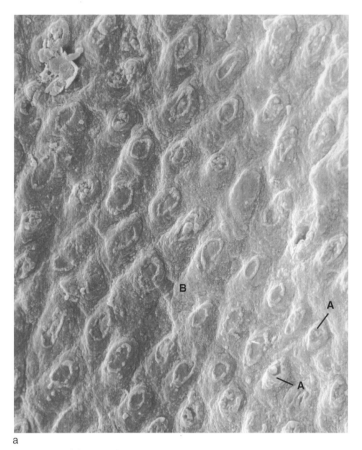

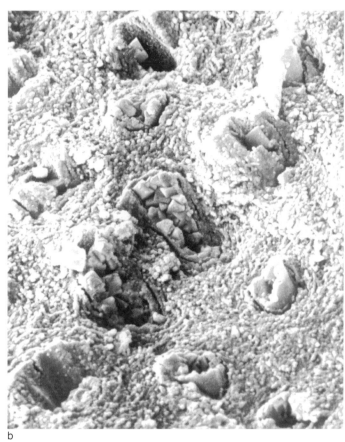

a   b

Fig. 9.58 (a) SEM of fractured surface through a region of sclerotic dentine. In the lower part of the micrograph, within an initial layer of peritubular dentine (A), an additional central plug of mineral has been deposited to occlude the tubule. B = intertubular dentine. In the upper part of the micrograph, the dentinal tubules remain patent (× 1500). (b) High-power view of sclerotic dentine from (a), showing central plug of dentinal tubules containing large rhombohedral crystals (probably whitlockite) (× 5000). Courtesy of Professor M.M. Smith.

differentiated from a stem cell population in the absence of any epithelial contribution. It is envisaged that the appropriate bioactive molecules necessary for such differentiation (eg. cytokines, growth factors) are locally synthesised and released during the inflammatory process accompanying the stimulus (such as dental caries). To this effect, a number of factors have been shown to induce the formation of repair dentine in the pulp of experimental animals, such as pieces of native dentine, pieces of demineralised dentine, crude extracts of dentine matrix, fibronectin products and bone morphogenetic protein. It might be envisaged that the addition of suitable activating substances to the region of pulp exposures might aid and speed up clinically the formation of repair dentine over pulp exposures. Recent work, however, also suggests that healing can occur naturally providing that the cavity is completely sealed at its margins.

Sclerotic dentine

In addition to infilling with peritubular dentine as a physiological response to ageing (eventually forming translucent dentine – see page 140), dentinal tubules commonly fill in as a response to an external stimulus such as under slowly advancing caries or beneath areas of severe attrition (Figs 9.57 and 9.58). This type of dentine is termed sclerotic dentine and, like translucent dentine, will present as areas of dentine that

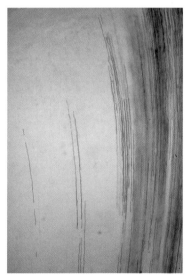

Fig. 9.59 A longitudinal ground section (mounted in water) of sclerotic dentine on the left of the micrograph showing a loss of tubular structure and appearing transparent as the dentinal tubules have been completely occluded by mineral. The unaffected right edge of the micrograph shows a more normal tubular morphology (× 20).

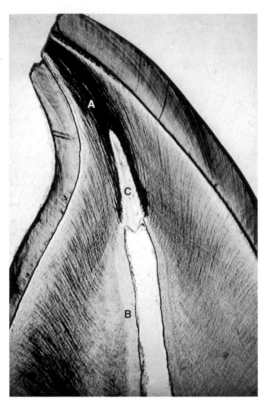

Fig. 9.60 Ground longitudinal section of a crown showing a dead tract (A) beneath a region of attrition that is sealed pulpally by tertiary dentine (C). Secondary dentine (B) lines the rest of the pulp chamber (× 15).

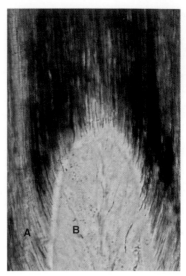

Fig. 9.61 Ground longitudinal section of coronal dentine showing secondary dentine (A) and tertiary dentine (B) beneath a dead tract (× 50).

lack structure and appear transparent (Fig. 9.59). Little is known about the precipitated material but it appears to differ from peritubular dentine and is thus thought not to be formed by the odontoblast. The mineral is crystalline and possibly an apatite, although plate-like crystals of octocalcium phosphate have also been reported. In tubules exposed by attrition or caries some occluding components may be derived from saliva.

Dead tracts

If the primary odontoblasts are killed by an external stimulus, or retract before peritubular dentine occludes the tubules, empty tubules will be left. They may be sealed at their pulpal end by tertiary dentine. When ground sections are prepared and mounted, the mounting medium will not enter these sealed off tubules and they will remain air filled. Under the microscope transmitted light will be totally internally reflected and these tubules will appear dark (Figs 9.60, 9.61). This appearance, which is due partly to the pulpal response and partly to the preparatory procedure, has been termed a 'dead tract'.

CLINICAL CONSIDERATIONS

Permeability of dentine

The tubular structure of dentine allows for the possibility of substances applied to its outer surface being able to reach and affect the dental pulp. This depends on a number of factors:

- That the dentine surface be exposed by caries, attrition, abrasion or trauma.
- That the tubules be patent. Tubules may be occluded physiologically by peritubular (intratubular) dentine or by exogenous material precipitated in them peripherally. They may also be sealed off from the pulp by tertiary dentine.
- That the outward movement of interstitial 'dentinal ' fluid does not wash them out of the tubule.
- That they are able to pass through the odontoblast layer, which presents a barrier to molecules of higher molecular weight.

Given that these factors are overcome, the most significant materials to travel down the tubules are the bacteria of dental caries and, more importantly, the toxins they produce. It is possible, but unproven, that molecules capable of exciting sensory nerves in the pulp may follow this route and induce pain. Components of dental materials, or etchants used to prepare for their placement, may pass through the dentine and kill or damage the dental pulp. This does not seem to be as large a concern as it may seem. The poor pulpal response to some restorative materials is more likely to be due to the poor marginal seal the material provides, allowing microleakage and the presence of bacteria on the surface of the dentine, whose toxins affect the pulp. Although *in vitro* some components of dental materials pass through dentine, *in vivo* the outward flow of dentinal fluid opposes this.

Response to external stimuli (e.g. caries, attrition)

The response to outside stimuli comes from the dental pulp, but is manifest in the structure of the dentine it produces. The deposition of tertiary dentine provides a barrier to the progress of caries and toxins. The presence of secondary dentine and its continuing deposition throughout life, although not a response to external stimuli, contributes to the barrier function of the dentine.

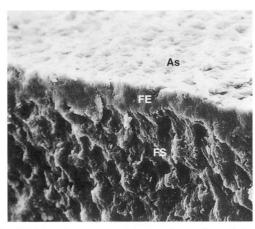

Fig. 9.62 SEM showing a smear layer on the surface of dentine cut with a high- speed bur; As = abraded surface; FE = smear layer on fractured edge; FS = fractured surface (× 35). Courtesy of Dr J. Dennison.

Adhesion of dental materials to dentine

Many of the advances in restorative dentistry are a result of the development of materials that will adhere to enamel and dentine. This allows more conservative cavity preparations, less pulpal injury and improved aesthetic results. Adhesion to dentine is more complex than that to enamel because of the high organic content of the tissue and its tubular architecture. In addition, when dentine is cut with a dental bur a smear layer (Fig. 9.62) forms on its surface, consisting of dentine that has been melted and reset; it may also contain embedded in it bacteria from caries that was being removed. Smearing

has an advantage in that it occludes the dentinal tubules but a disadvantage in that it may harbour bacteria and provides a difficult surface to adhere to. Removing the smear layer is therefore a prerequisite before applying bonding agents. Like enamel, dentine is first etched with strong acids to remove the smear layer and to provide a porous surface that can be infiltrated by the bonding agent (Fig. 9.63) The bonding agent will then penetrate the dentinal tubules and the exposed collagen in the intertubular dentine (Figs 9.64, 9.65).

Endodontics

The continuing deposition of secondary dentine throughout life and the development of tertiary dentine in response to caries and restorative procedures can lead to a reduction in size – even, effectively, obliteration of the pulp chamber and root canals (Fig. 9.66). Root canal therapy (endodontics) consists of cleaning, shaping and filling the root canal system. When the root canals are small and hard to locate, effective treatment becomes difficult and the prognosis is poorer.

Sensitivity

Exposed dentine is often (but not always) sensitive. Three main hypotheses have been put forward to account for its sensitivity, implicating:

- nerves in dentine
- the odontoblast processes;
- fluid movements in the dentinal tubules.

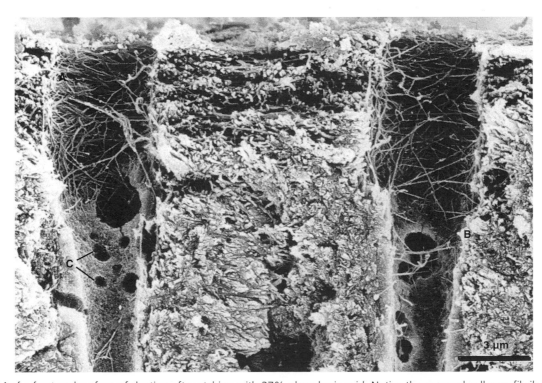

Fig. 9.63 SEM of a fractured surface of dentine after etching with 37% phosphoric acid. Notice the exposed collagen fibrils in the superficial layers (A) and loss of peritubular dentine (seen in deeper layers, B). Open lateral tubules (C) are visible. Mineralised collagen fibrils (arrow) are evident in the intertubular dentine (× 6500). Courtesy of Professor B. Van Meerbeek.

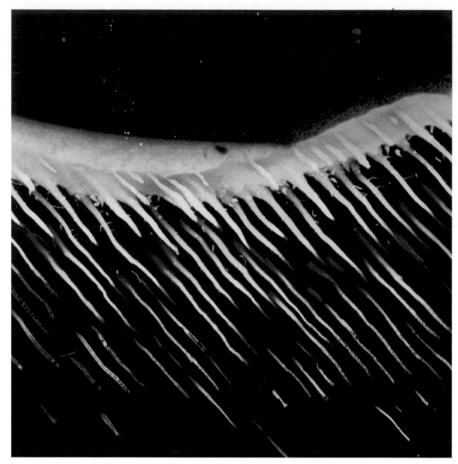

Fig. 9.64   Confocal image of acid-etched dentine infiltrated with a multiple dye-labelled bonding agent. Notice the penetration of the bonding agent into the tubules and the intertubular region at the surface forming a 'hybrid zone' (× 1000). Courtesy of Professor T. Watson.

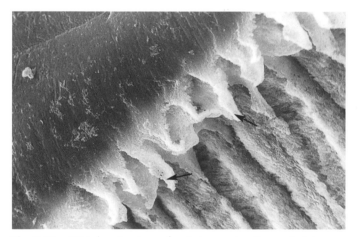

Fig. 9.65   SEM showing tags of resin in a restorative material (arrow) conforming to the dentinal tubules in etched dentine and enhancing retention of the restoration (× 35). Courtesy of Dr J. Dennison.

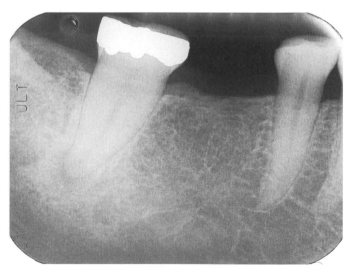

Fig. 9.66   Clinical radiograph of a molar tooth in which the root canals have been obliterated by mineralisation.

Arguments against the view that pain is due to direct stimulation of nerves in the dentine relate to their relative scarcity and to the fact that they appear to be absent in the outer parts of dentine. In addition, the application of local anaesthetics to the surface of dentine does not abolish the sensitivity.

Referring to the second hypothesis, there is no physiological evidence to date that indicates that the odontoblast process is analogous to a nerve fibre and can similarly conduct impulses pulpwards. Furthermore, the process may not extend to the enamel–dental junction, nor is the application of substances designed to prevent transmission of such impulses effective. Odontoblasts have not been shown to be synaptically connected to nerve fibres.

The most plausible hypothesis to explain the transmission of sensory stimuli suggests that all effective stimuli applied to dentine cause fluid movement through the dentinal tubules, and that this movement is sufficient to depolarise nerve endings in the inner parts of tubules, at the pulp–predentine junction and in the subodontoblastic neural plexus. Some stimuli, such as heat, osmotic pressure and drying, would tend to cause fluid movement outwards while others, such as cold, would cause movement inwards (Fig. 9.67). Movement in either direction would mechanically distort the terminals. These stimuli have been shown to cause such fluid movement *in vitro*. Chemicals (in strong solution) and thermal stimuli induce a response much more quickly than can be explained by conduction or diffusion. This, too, is consistent with the hydrodynamic hypothesis. In animal experiments, however, the response of intradental nerves to chemical stimuli is often slow and may be more readily explained by diffusion. It may be that both 'direct' and 'hydrodynamic' mechanisms operate, but that the hydrodynamic force predominates whenever there is pulpal inflammation and a lowering in threshold of intrapulpal nerves to the small mechanical forces generated by fluid flow.

Exposed dentine that is sensitive is sometimes described as 'hypersensitive'. Such dentine has tubules that are patent (Fig. 9.68). Exposed dentine in which the tubules are not patent is not sensitive (Fig. 9.69).

Eliminating or reducing the sensitivity of exposed dentine is not always easy. The most effective approach is to occlude the dentinal tubules either by smearing or by the precipitation of crystalline fluorides or oxalates.

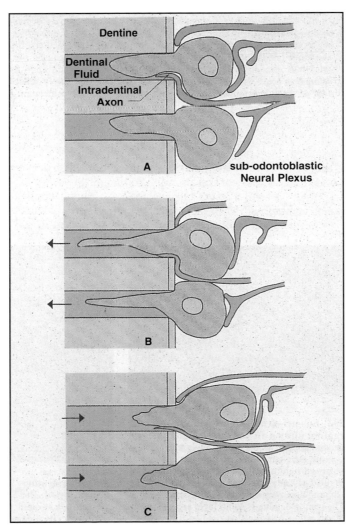

Fig. 9.67 The effects of outward (B) and inward (C) fluid movement in the dentinal tubules.

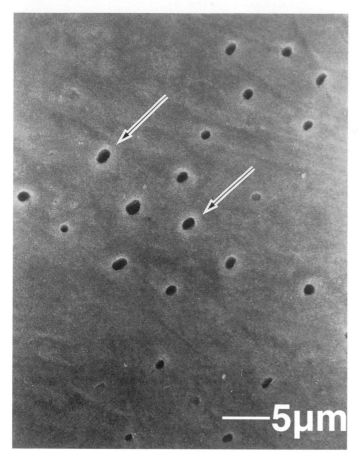

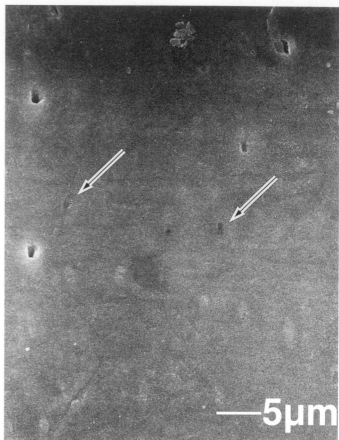

Fig. 9.68 SEM of an exposed dentine surface of a hypersensitive area. A large proportion of dentinal tubules (arrows) are seen to be open (× 2400). Courtesy of Dr M. Yoshiyama and the editor of the *Journal of Dental Research*.

Fig. 9.69 SEM image of the exposed dentine surface of a naturally desensitised area. The lumens of dentinal tubules (arrows) are mostly occluded (× 2400). Courtesy of Dr M. Yoshiyama and the editor of the *Journal of Dental Research*.

10 Dental pulp

The dental pulp is the tissue responsible for the formation of dentine. It is contained within the pulp chamber and root canals of the tooth (see page 28). At the apical constriction of the root canal it becomes continuous with the periodontal ligament (Fig. 26.6). Although the pulp contributes most significantly during development and eruption of the tooth, it remains active throughout life as secondary dentine is formed and it is able to respond (within certain important limits) to applied stimuli such as caries, trauma and restorative procedures by producting tertiary dentine (see page 141).

ORGANISATION

The dental pulp is a specialised connective tissue with a specific anatomical arrangement dictated by its position inside a rigid chamber and by its role of forming hard tissue on the walls of that chamber (Fig. 10.1). The cells directly responsible for dentine deposition (the odontoblasts) lie at the periphery of the tissue. Also in this region are two elements capable not only of detecting external stimuli but also of initiating and participating (at least in part) in the response to them. These are the nerve terminals of trigeminal afferents and specialised antigen-presenting cells. The rest of the dental pulp acts as a support system for these anatomically peripheral, but functionally pivotal, components. Blood vessels and nerves enter

and leave the root canals through an apical foramen at the root end. Each root has at least one canal; many have two. Smaller accessory canals with their own foramina also occur most commonly on the apical third of the root (Fig. 10.2). These canals join the larger canal. In multirooted teeth there are commonly small vascular canals entering the pulp chamber from the bone between the roots. Lateral root canals lead from the main canal to the lateral aspect of the root and are most common in the apical third of the root, connecting with the periodontal ligament.

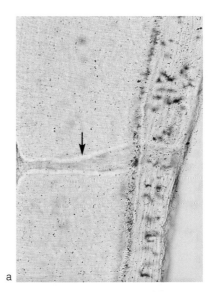

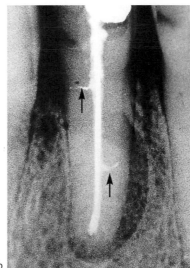

Fig. 10.2 (a) Ground section of root showing a lateral branch from the main root canal (arrow) (× 12). Courtesy of Dr M.E. Atkinson. (b). Radiograph of a root-filled tooth showing accessory canals (arrows). Courtesy of Dr J. Souyave.

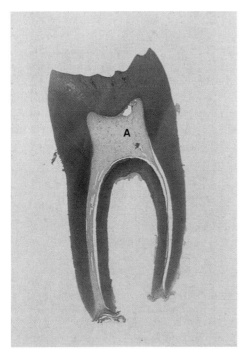

Fig. 10.1 Decalcified section of a whole tooth showing the general disposition of the dental pulp (A), (H & E; × 3).

COMPOSITION

The dental pulp is a loose connective tissue and made up of a combination of cells embedded in an extracellular matrix of fibres in a semi-fluid gel. It contains 75% by weight of water and 25% organic material. As with most connective tissues the matrix is more plentiful than the cells. The extracellular matrix is made up of a versatile group of polysaccharides and proteins secreted by the cells of the tissue and assembled into a complex framework closely associated with the cells. The matrix forms a scaffold that stabilises the structure of the tissue, but it is far from inert: indeed, in the dental pulp, where there is a rigid supporting and protecting hard shell, the skeletal function is minimal. The matrix plays a very active role in controlling the activity of the cells within it. It affects their development, migration, division, shape and function. Collagen is the predominant extracellular matrix component comprising 25–32% of the dry weight. The composition of the dental papilla and dental pulp change during development and can vary between tooth type. Much of the data that is available is from animal tissues, which may differ somewhat from human.

Fibres

The principal fibrous component of the dental pulp is type I **collagen** (Fig. 10.3), the characteristic collagen of bone, cementum, skin, tendon and dentine. The collagen is present

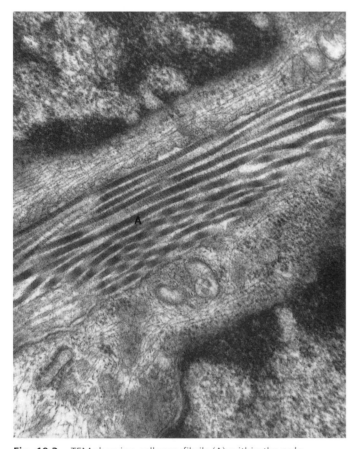

Fig. 10.3 TEM showing collagen fibrils (A) within the pulp (× 134 000).

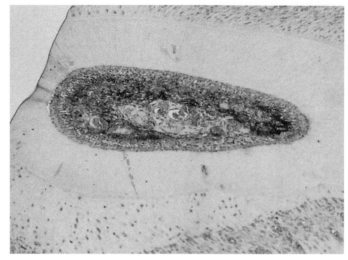

Fig. 10.4 Section of developing mouse molar root showing type III collagen stained brown by immunohistochemical methods (× 30). Courtesy of Dr. Y.Ohsaki and the editor of *Anatomical Record*.

as fibrils thinly scattered through the pulp in the young tooth (see Fig. 10.13). It is present as fibrils 50 nm in diameter and several micrometres long that combine into bundles as fibres of varying size. Their arrangement in the pulp is irregular, except in the periphery, where they become aligned approximately parallel to the forming predentine surface. During early development some of the bundles are arranged at right angles to the developing dentine, contributing to the appearance of 'von Korff' fibres in outer dentine. There are also large amounts of type III collagen (Fig. 10.4), which, while having a similar 67 nm banding pattern to type I collagen, differs from type I collagen. Although type I collagen contains α1 and α2 molecular chains, type III collagen contains only α1 chains. About 56% of pulpal collagen is type I and 41% type III. The functional significance of the high levels of type III collagen is not known: in other sites it has been associated with rapid remodelling and with controlling collagen fibril diameters. Small amounts of type V and type VI collagen are also present. Overall, collagen forms 3–5% of the wet weight of the pulp, a low proportion in comparison with other loose connective tissues. Microfibrils of smaller diameter than collagen have also been detected. These are **fibrillin**, a large glycoprotein that forms beaded fibrils 10–14 nm in diameter. In other tissues, this is associated with elastic fibres but these are absent from the dental pulp.

Non-fibrous matrix

The macromolecules that make up the non-fibrous component of the extracellular matrix fall into two main groups: glycosaminoglycans and other adhesion molecules.

Glycosaminoglycans (GAGs)

GAGs are polysaccharide chains composed of repeating disaccharide units, which, when covalently linked to proteins, form glycoproteins. All four GAGs found in connective tissues (chondroitin sulphate, dermatan sulphate, heparan sulphate and hyaluronan are present in the dental pulp. Chondroitin sulphate (Fig. 10.5) predominates quantitatively and dermatan sulphate is present only in small amounts. Because GAGs are bulky molecules and hydrophilic, they readily form gels that fill most of the extracellular space. These molecules swell when hydrated, which may contribute to the high tissue fluid pressure of the pulp. This provides mechanical support but also allows easy movement of water-soluble molecules and cells.

Hyaluronan is the only GAG found in quantity unbound to protein. As well as having a mechanical function it is thought to facilitate cell migration. It is thus particularly prevalent during development.

In mature pulp 60% of the GAG content is hyaluron, 20% dermatan sulphate and 12% chondroitin sulphate. In the developing pulp chondroitin sulphate is the major GAG, with hyaluron only a minor component.

Proteoglycans

Proteoglycans consist of a core protein (of variable size) surrounded by GAGs and perhaps other sugars. Proteoglycans are members of a larger class of molecules, the glycoproteins, which by definition have GAGs as at least part of their side chains.

Proteoglycans are very diverse molecules with a wide range of potential and actual roles. Many, such as versican (Fig. 10.6), contribute to the bulk of the matrix; some, such as syndecan, are integrated into or attached to cell membranes and act as adhesion molecules or bind signalling molecules such as growth factors. Table 10.1 summarises the proteoglycans present in the pulp and their possible functions.

Other adhesion molecules

Fibronectin (Fig. 10.7) is a glycoprotein (although not a proteoglycan as it does not contain GAGs) that has a major role not only in attaching cells to extracellular matrices but also (by attachment to the cytoskeleton) in regulating cell

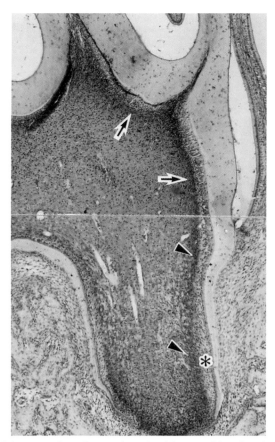

Fig. 10.6 A section of rat pulp stained immunohistochemically for the proteoglycan versican (black stain). Distribution is more concentrated peripherally and it is apparently absent around the central neurovascular bundle (× 1000). Courtesy of Dr S. Shibata and the editor of *Archives of Oral Biology*.

Table 10.1 *Proteoglycans of the dental pulp*

Proteoglycan identified in the dental pulp	Possible role
Decorin	Binds to type I collagen and transforming growth factor β
Biglycan	Regulatory effect on collagen fibrinogenesis
Versican	Participation in large hydrated proteoglycan aggregates
Syndecan	Attaches cell surface to fibrous collagens and other matrix proteins; binds fibroblast growth factor
Tenascin	Can promote or inhibit cell adhesion, guides cell movements
Fibronectin	Cell adhesion (via integrins in the cell membrane) to matrix

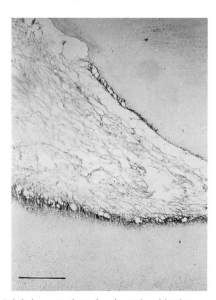

Fig. 10.5 Adult human dental pulp stained by immunohistochemical methods for chondroitin sulphate (staining black at the pulp–dentine junction), showing widespread presence but a greater concentration peripherally in the odontoblast layer, suggesting (circumstantially) a role for this molecule in the development of dentine (× 40). Courtesy of Doctors P.M. Bartold and U. Schlagenhauf, and the editor of *International Endodontic Journal*.

shape, migration and differentiation. It is widely distributed in the pulp. Fibronectin is a member of a family of cell adhesion molecules, the integrins. Another integrin, laminin, is present (with several other components) in basement membranes binding epithelial cells to the extracellular matrix as well as

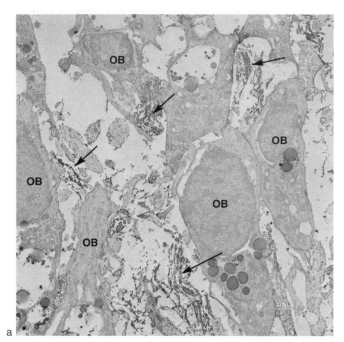

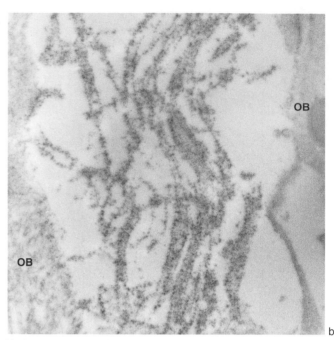

Fig. 10.7 (a) Light micrograph showing immunolabelling for fibronectin (dark staining, arrows) on surface of collagen fibres of the odontoblast layer (OB). There is little staining in the predentine (× 170). (b) Immunoelectron micrograph showing presence of fibronectin as dark-staining fibrillar fascicles between odontoblasts (OB) (× 3600). Courtesy of Dr N. Yoshiba et al. and the editor of *Archives of Oral Biology*.

binding some signalling molecules. Laminin is present in the dental pulp but only around the endothelial cells of blood vessels and the Schwann cells of nerve fibres. Although odontoblasts do not have a basement membrane both their cell bodies and processes are coated with laminin.

Cells

Odontoblasts

The odontoblast (Figs 10.8–10.11) is responsible for the

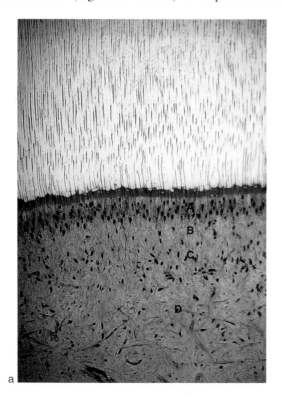

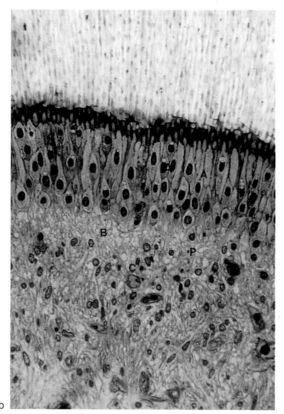

Fig. 10.8 (a) Low-power micrograph showing some cell types and their distribution in the pulp. A = Odontoblast layer adjacent to dentine; B = cell-free zone; C = cell-rich zone; D = central pulp showing principally fibroblasts (Toluidine blue; × 200). (b) Higher power view showing pseudostratified odontoblast layer (A). B = Cell-free zone; C = cell-rich zone; D = dentine (Toluidine blue; × 650).

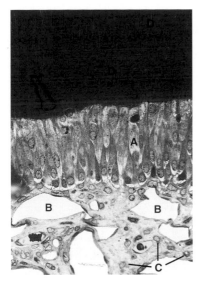

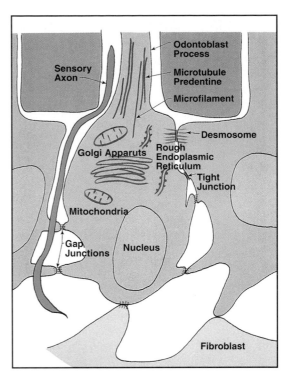

Fig. 10.9 Semithin section showing pseudostratified odontoblast layer (A). B = Subodontoblastic capillary plexus; C = pulp fibroblasts; D = dentine (Toluidine blue; × 450).

Fig. 10.10 The ultrastructure of the odontoblast in a mature tooth is typical of a polarised protein-synthesizing cell of low activity containing all the organelles associated with this process (mitochondria, rough endoplasmic reticulum, Golgi apparatus) in the supranuclear region. One large process enters a dentinal tubule but many smaller ones link the odontoblasts to its neighbouring odontoblasts and fibroblasts.

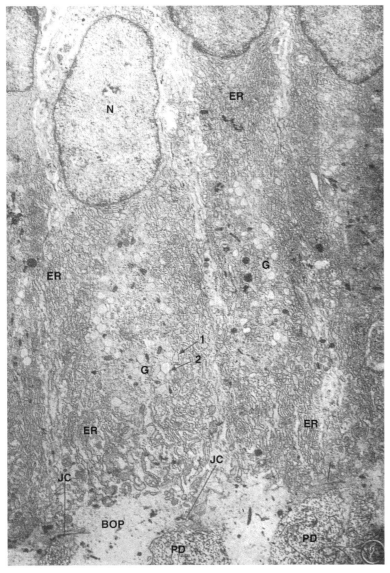

Fig. 10.11 TEM of an odontoblast. N = Nucleus; ER = rough endoplasmic reticulum; G = Golgi complex; JC = junctional complex; PD = predentine; BOP = base of odontoblast process (× 12 000). Courtesy of Professor M.M. Smith.

formation of dentine. The origin and differentiation of these cells are described on pages 320–322. In the fully developed tooth the odontoblasts continue to lay down secondary dentine throughout life and survive for as long as the tooth remains vital. If the tooth is subjected to a severe insult, such as dental caries, the ability of the odontoblast to respond by laying down secondary dentine more rapidly is extremely limited. The odontoblast is a postmitotic cell and cannot divide: insult or injury will result in the death of odontoblasts. However, sub-odontoblastic cells can, in these circumstances, divide and differentiate and lay down a protective barrier of tertiary dentine. Growth factors, especially members of the transforming growth factor-beta (TGF-β) family, play an important role in controlling the synthetic activity of odontoblasts during development. They may also be significant in initiating the production of tertiary dentine in response to dental caries as they seem to be sequestered within mature dentine and may be released during carious breakdown. Odontoblasts in both healthy and diseased teeth express membrane receptors for the TGF-β family well above the level seen for other cells in the pulp.

The fully differentiated odontoblast (Figs 10.8–10.11) is a polarised columnar cell with a single long cell process that extends into the predentine and dentine within a dentinal tubule. The cell body is approximately 50 μm long and 5–10 μm in width. The nucleus is usually in the basal (pulpal) half of the cell with the other organelles involved in dentine synthesis – the rough endoplasmic reticulum, Golgi complex and mitochondria – above it. These organelles are much more pronounced in an actively secreting cell (Fig. 10.11). As well as one large main process the odontoblast has numerous smaller processes, which link it to adjacent odontoblasts and other pulp cells.

In the mature tooth the odontoblasts form a layer of single cells attached to the predentine surface with single cell processes extending into the dentinal tubules. The odontoblasts in the crown are distinctly columnar in outline; in the root they are commonly more cuboidal. The nuclei of adjacent cells in the layer lie at different levels and when the layer is sectioned obliquely this gives the false appearance of multiple layers ('pseudostratification'– Figs 10.8 and 10.9).

The odontoblast layer provides a controlled barrier between the pulp and the dentine. The dentine is formed almost exclusively by the odontoblasts with very little material from the pulp being incorporated into it, except possibly during the initial dentine formation that results in the mantle layer (see page 134). The layer also contributes to the protection of the dental pulp from outside irritants. Stimuli that affect the pulp sufficiently to initiate pain do so largely by causing fluid to move along the dentinal tubules and inducing pressure changes in the pulp. The diffusion of molecules pulpwards is opposed by the outward flow of dentinal fluid and by the almost membrane-like properties of the odontoblast layer.

Cell junctions

The integrity of the odontoblast layer and its limited per-meability are maintained by numerous cell to cell junctions (Fig. 10.12). These are of three types.

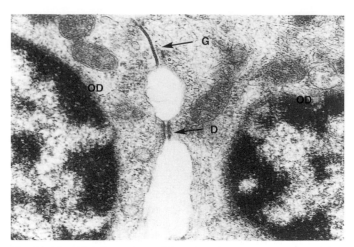

Fig. 10.12   TEM illustrating cell junctions between two odontoblast cell bodies (OD). G = Gap junction; D = desmosome (× 45 000).

- The macula adherens junctions (desmosomes) have a clear intercellular component as well as an intracellular system of anchoring fibrils and are largely responsible for mechanical union. Junctions that would completely encircle the cells (zonula type) are not present.
- Tight junctions, which appear almost as a fusion of apposing cell membranes, limit permeability; the more tight junctions and the closer they are together, the lower the permeability will be. In the odontoblast layer, these junctions do not seem to completely encircle the cells and so limit rather than eliminate permeability. The tight junctions also add to the mechanical integrity of the layer. An arrangement like the 'terminal bar' apparatus found in epithelia (in which a regular pattern of both tight and adherens type junctions is arranged uniformly at the outer margin of the cell layer – Figs 22.12 and 22.15) is not seen in the odontoblast layer. The odontoblast layer is not an epithelium.
- The third type of junction seen between odontoblasts is the gap junction. This allows the movement of small molecules directly between adjacent cells. It is important in cell com-munication and would, presumably, have a key role in synchronising the activity of all the odontoblasts in the layer.

As well as forming junctions with themselves, odontoblasts also unite with other pulpal cells. In histological sections, it is difficult to recognise the origin of most of the cell processes: small processes from an odontoblast, fibroblast, mesenchymal cell, possibly even defence cells or an unsheathed axon have a similar appearance. Odontoblasts have a close relationship with dendritic antigen-presenting cells (see page 157), although the functional nature of the relationship is unknown. Recent *in vitro* studies have suggested that odontoblasts themselves are capable of producing proinflammatory mediators in response to bacterial toxins. Nerve endings are very closely apposed to odontoblast processes in the dentinal tubules and many nerve endings occur in and around the odontoblast layer. It has frequently been suggested that odontoblasts may act as sensory receptors, passing on signals from the surface of the dentine to nerve endings via synapses, either chemical or electrical. There is no direct evidence of chemical synapses involving odontoblasts though proteins specific to exocytosis, the process whereby synaptic vesicles are released, have been demonstrated in dentinal tubules. Gap junctions can act as electrical synapses and are, in fact, morphologically identical to such junctions in the central nervous system. Although there are innumerable gap junctions in the odontoblast layer there is currently little convincing evidence that they link nerves and odontoblasts synaptically. Most of the cell processes making junctions with the odontoblasts originate from other odontoblasts or fibroblasts. It is possible that some of the cells involved in these junctions are mesenchymal cells that can differentiate into hard tissue-forming cells.

Odontoblasts may participate in the pulp's initial response to injury as well as in the later stages of repair. They are the first cells to encounter dental pathogens. They are, *in vitro*, able to express interleukin-8 (IL-8) when challenged with bacterial toxin. IL-8 is a proinflammatory chemokine which can participate in the recruitment of neutrophils.

Fibroblasts

The fibroblast is the ubiquitous cell of unmineralised connective tissues. In the dental pulp, they form a loose network throughout the tissue (Figs 10.8, 10.9), linked by adherens type junctions and gap junctions. Their morphology is highly variable but is most aptly described as stellate, with the arms of the stars linking fibroblast to fibroblast or fibroblast to odontoblast (Fig. 10.13). Their most obvious role in the development of the tissue is the production of extracellular fibres and ground substance for the dental pulp. As this production (and presumably turnover) is relatively slow, pulpal fibroblasts show only moderate amounts of associated intracellular organelles such as endoplasmic reticulum, Golgi complex or mitochondria (Fig. 10.13). They make little or no contribution to the production of dentine.

Much of what is known about pulpal fibroblasts has been obtained from experiments in which they have been maintained in cell culture. These studies show that the pulpal fibroblast, as well as being able to secrete the components that form the extracellular matrix, can participate in their degradation. It thus seems likely that, in the mature tooth, the fibroblasts slowly turn over the matrix. In cell culture these cells have been shown to be capable of forming hard tissue after appropriate stimulation. This is an important component of the dental pulp's response to injury. The mineralised tissue that fibroblasts produce more closely resembles bone than dentine. Cultured dental pulp cells have been shown to respond to a number of stimuli. They respond to the application of calcitonin gene-related peptide by producing bone morphogenetic protein, a factor in formation of hard tissue. In common with fibroblasts elsewhere, pulpal fibroblasts are able to produce a variety of growth factors and cytokines with roles in controlling development, growth and the response to injury. Cultured pulpal fibroblasts do undergo cell division, although mitotic figures are rarely encountered in the normal, uninjured dental pulp. Apoptosis (programmed cell death) has been demonstrated in the continuously growing incisor of the rat. It seems

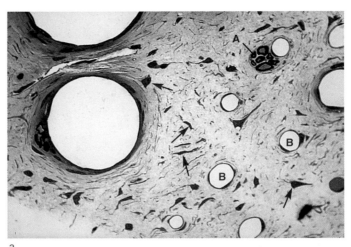

a

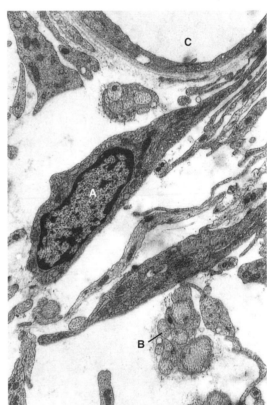

b

Fig. 10.13 (a) Semithin section of the central portion of the pulp showing the appearance of pulpal fibroblasts, which may vary from spindle-shaped (small arrows) to a more rounded and stellate shape (large arrow). A = Myelinated fibres; B = capillary (Toluidine blue; × 450). (b) TEM illustrating spindle-shaped pulpal fibroblasts (A). B = Unmyelinated nerve axons; C = capillary. Note the absence of collagen fibrils in the extracellular matrix (× 20 000).

reasonable to expect cell turnover in the pulps of mature teeth of limited eruption.

Defence cells

T lymphocytes are present in small numbers in the normal dental pulp (Fig. 10.14). Their numbers increase enormously when the pulp is injured or subjected to a noxious stimulus. Macrophages (Figs 10.15, 10.16) are also present. In their resting form (sometimes termed histiocytes) they can appear

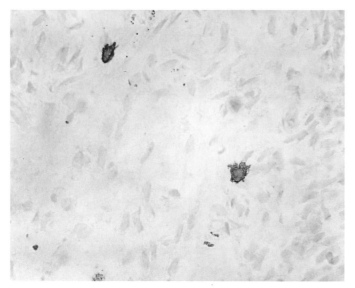

Fig. 10.14 Antibody staining (black) to identify T lymphocytes in the dental pulp (× 500). Courtesy of Dr T. Okiji and the editor of the *Journal of Dental Research*.

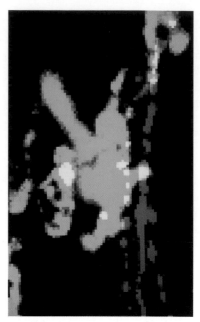

Fig. 10.16 Confocal laser scanning micrograph of a section of dental pulp from the pulp horn of a rat. It is double stained with two fluorescent dyes staining macrophages (green) and substance P- containing nerve fibres (red). This technique allows great depth of focus and, in this case, shows areas (in yellow) where the nerve and macrophage are in close contact (× 1000). Courtesy of Dr T. Okiji and the editor of the *Journal of Dental Research*.

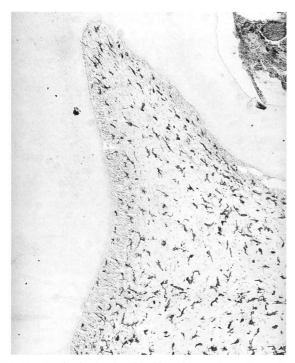

Fig. 10.15 Antibody staining (black) to demonstrate the wide distribution of macrophages in healthy rat dental pulp (× 50). Courtesy of Dr T. Okiji and the editor of the Journal of *Dental Research*.

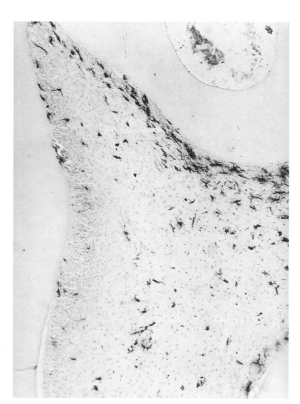

Fig. 10.17 Immunohistochemical stain (black) identifying antigen-presenting cells particularly prominent at the periphery of rat molar pulp (× 70). Courtesy of Dr T. Okiji and the editor of the *Journal of Dental Research*.

in a variety of morphological forms and are difficult to distinguish from fibroblasts in routine histological preparations. Immunohistochemical techniques, however, show that they are widely distributed and in considerable numbers. They are present in the normal dental pulp and are most dense in two areas, around the blood vessels of the inner pulp and around the odontoblast layer.

Dendritic antigen-presenting cells (Figs 10.17, 10.18) are an important component of the normal dental pulp. They are at least 50 μm long and have three or more main dendritic

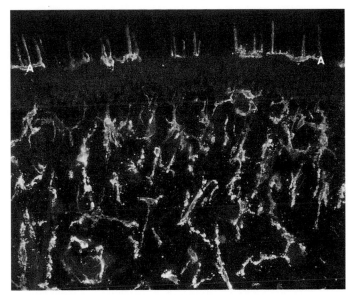

Fig. 10.18 Immunohistochemical stain (white) viewed under fluorescent light showing the distribution of antigen-presenting cells. Note the cells (A) in the periphery of the odontoblast layer have processes extending into the dentine (× 200). Courtesy of Dr N. Yoshiba and the editor of the *Journal of Dental Research*.

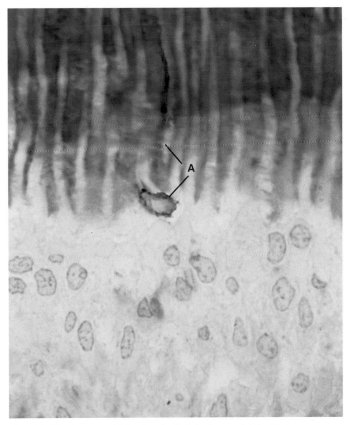

Fig. 10.19 Immunohistochemical stain (brown) identifying an antigen-presenting cell (A) in the outer odontoblast layer and extending a process into the inner dentine (Methylene blue; × 500). Courtesy of Dr N. Yoshiba and the editor of the *Journal of Dental Research*.

processes which branch. Like the macrophages, they are distributed largely around the odontoblasts and the central blood vessels. (Figs 10.18, 10.19).

The dendritic cells act, at least primarily, as antigen-presenting cells stimulating the division and activity of naive T lymphocytes. They initiate the primary immune response and may migrate, with trapped antigen, to regional lymph nodes and induce T-lymphocyte division and differentiation there. The pulp's response to injury includes inflammatory and immune components that are closely integrated. Some features of the inflammatory response are mediated by nerves (see pages 163–164). There is a close structural relationship between nerve fibres and immunocompetent cells (see Fig. 10.15). Mast cells are absent from the dental pulp but there is an intimate relationship between the immune and neural systems such that a combined response to an irritant would result in the release of a cascade of vasoactive molecules.

Undifferentiated cells

Many of the cell types in the dental pulp, including the odontoblasts, defence cells and possibly many fibroblasts, are terminally differentiated and, although able to respond to stimuli in a predetermined manner, are unable to differentiate into another cell type. It has long been known that there is a population of cells in the dental pulp beneath the odontoblast layer, which can, in response to a severe challenge, produce tertiary dentine. This led to the suggestion that the mature pulp holds a population of pluripotential, primitive mesenchymal cells capable of differentiating into a variety of cell types. Real evidence for this is sparse and a modern understanding of molecular events within the cell makes it more likely that some cells can be induced into modifying their activity by changes in gene expression rather than by evolution of a new cell line. Evidence from *in vitro* work suggests that pulpal fibroblasts can produce hard tissue. In responding to dentinal injury it may be pulpal fibroblasts beneath the cavity that are affected rather than a newly differentiated cell line.

BLOOD VESSELS OF THE DENTAL PULP

The architectural arrangement of the blood vessels of the dental pulp closely parallels that of the nerves. It is more easily demonstrated in animal preparations as plastic resins can be perfused through the vascular system and casts prepared (Fig. 10.20).

Arterioles and venules enter the dental pulp via the apical foramina (Fig. 10.20) and lateral canals as components of neurovascular bundles. The larger of these are approximately 150 μm in diameter. They run longitudinally through the root canals. Within the root canals, they send off side branches to the periphery (Fig. 10.21). The vessels divide and narrow to some degree in the root canal but branch profusely once they are within the coronal pulp. Capillary loops extend towards the dentine. A network of vessels beneath the odontoblasts (the subodontoblastic capillary plexus) is more evident in sectioned histological material than it is in three dimensional casts. These capillaries are 6–8 μm in diameter.

Capillaries are present both within (Fig. 10.22) and below the odontoblast layer (Fig. 10.23) and between the odontoblasts and the predentine. Capillaries do not enter the dentinal tubules. The fluid that is present in the dentine is probably an ultrafiltrate of the pulpal interstitial fluid. The arrangement of the blood vessels supplies oxygen and nutrients where they are

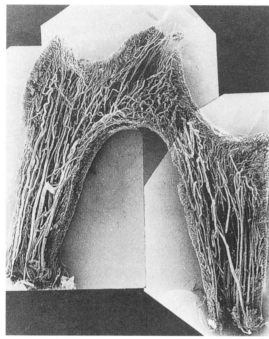

Fig. 10.20 SEM of a vascular cast of a dog mandibular molar. Arterioles run coronally along the sides of the root canal; venules drain in the centre. Larger vessels follow relatively straight pathways. Side branches subdivide to form a capillary network beneath the dentine (× 8). Courtesy of Doctors Y. Kishi, K. Takahashi and K. Kanagawa and the editor of the *Journal of Dental Research*.

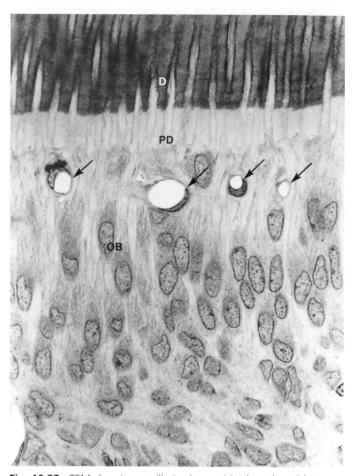

Fig. 10.22 TEM showing capillaries (arrows) in the odontoblast layer (OB), D = Dentine; PD = predentine (× 1200). Courtesy of Doctors S. Yoshida and H. Oshima and the editor of *Anatomical Record*.

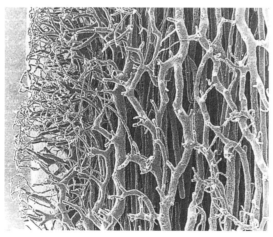

Fig. 10.21 SEM of a vascular cast of terminal capillary network in pulp. There are three layers of the terminal supply to the odontoblast layers: most superficially the flat-ended capillary loops, beneath these the capillary network and under these the venular network. Deep to all these layers are straight arterioles (× 11). Courtesy of Doctors K. Takahashi, Y. Kishi and S. Kim and the editor of the *Journal of Endodontics*.

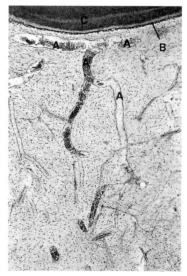

Fig. 10.23 Section of the dental pulp showing rich branching capillaries (A) below the odontoblast layer (B). C = Dentine (H & E; × 100). Courtesy of Professor L. Fonzi.

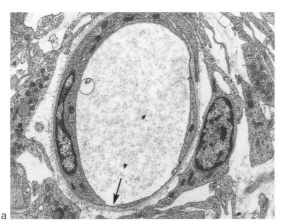

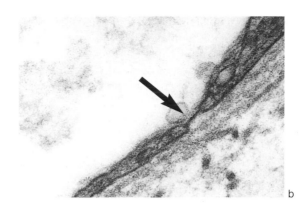

Fig. 10.24 (a). TEM of a subodontoblastic capillary with fenestration (arrowed) (× 12 600). (b) TEM showing a fenestration (arrow) in a capillary wall (× 31 500).

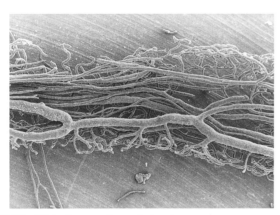

Fig. 10.25 SEM of a vascular cast showing a venous–venous anastamosis (× 160). Courtesy of Doctors Y. Kishi and K. Takahashi.

most needed during dentinogenesis. Approximately 4–5% of the capillaries in the subodontoblastic zone are fenestrated (Fig. 10.24). Fenestrations are 60–80 nm in diameter. Only basement membrane is present at the fenestrations, presumably allowing rapid movement of materials out of the capillary (see also pages 198–199).

Numerous arteriovenous and venous–venous anastomoses (Fig. 10.25) are found between peripheral pulpal vessels presumably to allow rapid changes in blood perfusion.

It is difficult to differentiate lymphatic vessels in the dental pulp. Structures consistent with their known structure elsewhere (like capillaries but with less completely linked endothelial cells and a less well developed basement membrane) have been found (Fig. 10.26). Vessels whose basement membranes have immunohistochemical characteristics in common with lymphatic vessels elsewhere have also been reported (Fig. 10.27). The presence of lymphatics in the pulp has been established by tracing particulate material kept within the pulp from the pulp to regional lymph nodes. Retrograde lymphography deposits material into pulpal vessels.

Nerve endings are associated with the smooth muscle of the arteriole walls. These are probably largely, if not exclusively, vasoconstrictor. The extensive innervation of the peripheral pulp is also very significantly involved in control of blood flow. The most prevalent neuropeptide in these nerves is calcitonin gene-related peptide (Fig. 10.28), the principal action of which is vasodilatation. Substance P (Fig. 10.29), neuropeptide Y (Fig. 10.30) and nitric oxide synthetase (Fig. 10.31) are also present and potent in this respect. Many of the capillaries have class II molecule-expressing dendritic cells around them with processes that are in close contact with the endothelial cells. They can act as antigen-presenting cells and also, possibly, as phagocytes.

Pulpal blood flow has been estimated to be 20–60 ml/min per 100 g of tissue. The pulp has a high, pulsatile interstitial tissue fluid pressure. This pressure would allow dentinal fluid to move outwards whenever the dentinal tubules were patent peripherally. This may slow the inward movement of irritants during the progression of dental caries.

NERVES OF THE DENTAL PULP

The dental pulp is heavily innervated. For example, approximately 2500 axons enter the apical foramen of a mature premolar; 25% of these are myelinated afferents whose cell bodies lie in the trigeminal ganglion. Of these 90% are narrow Aδ fibres (1–6 μm in diameter), with the rest belonging to the wider Aβ group (6–12 μm in diameter). The unmyelinated C fibres are either afferent or autonomic. Although the nerve fibres enter the dental pulp in bundles, there is only a scant perineurium or epineurium.

The nerve bundles run centrally in the pulp of the root in close association with the blood vessels. A few fibres leave the central bundles in the root and travel to the periphery. Most continue to the coronal pulp where they spread apart and branch profusely (Fig. 10.32). Most of the branches end in the odontoblastic or subodontoblastic regions (Fig. 10.33). In the crown there is a pronounced plexus of nerves beneath the odontoblasts, known as the plexus of Raschkow. This plexus is not evident until after the tooth has erupted. Branches from the plexus pass into the odontoblast layer and form the marginal plexus between the odontoblast layer and the predentine, others continue into the dentine to accompany odontoblast processes in the dentinal tubules. This subodontoblastic plexus may be one of the sites of sensory activation in the pulp. Many of the

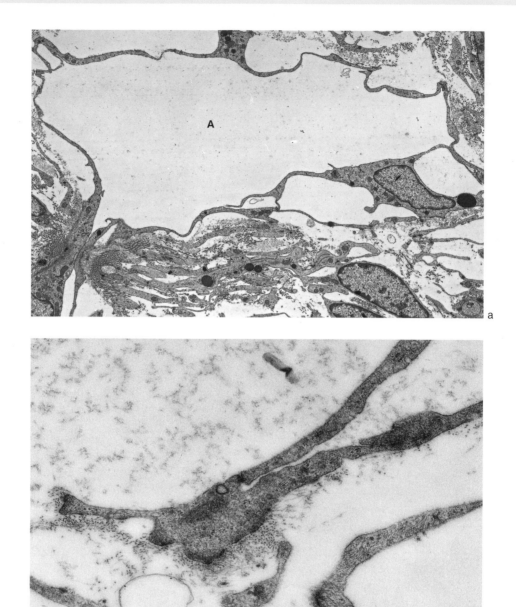

Fig. 10.26 (a) TEM of a lymphatic vessel (A) in the central dental pulp (× 400). (b) Higher power TEM of part of the wall of the lymphatic vessel, showing incomplete junctions between the cells and absence of a basement membrane (× 3000). Courtesy of Dr M. Bishop.

axons are devoid of a Schwann cell covering, either completely or partially, rendering them susceptible to changes in the extracellular environment (Fig. 10.34). The axons branch profusely, providing a broad surface area for activation. Within the Schwann cell, there are often many axons in a single pocket and the spread of signals from axon to axon is possible.

Nerve fibre types

The myelinated nerves (see Fig. 10.13) are trigeminal afferents. They carry sensations of sharp pain centrally. The larger diameter Aβ afferents in some regions carry other non-noxious

sensations but there is no clear evidence that any sensation other than pain can be experienced from the pulp with physiological stimuli. Most of the non-myelinated C fibres are also afferent and involved in the conduction of noxious information centrally. At least as important as the sensory functions of both these afferent nerve groups is their role in axon reflexes. In these reflexes, action potentials generated in one terminal branch travel centrally and then pass anterogradely (central to peripheral) down other branches, resulting in the release of neuropeptides important in the local control of blood flow (but perhaps with other functions as well). It has been suggested that some pulpal nerves may have direct trophic

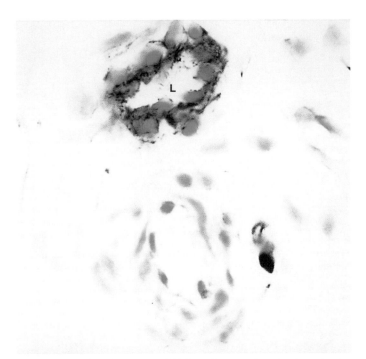

Fig. 10.27 A lymphatic vessel (L) from human dental pulp stained with an antibody against human thoracic duct. The dark-blue stain attaches to the endothelium. Another vessel, presumably a blood capillary (C), nearby remains unstained (× 1000). Courtesy of Doctors Y. Sawa, S. Yoshida, Y. Ashikaga, T. Kim, Y. Yanaoka and M. Suzuki and the editor of *Tissue and Cell*.

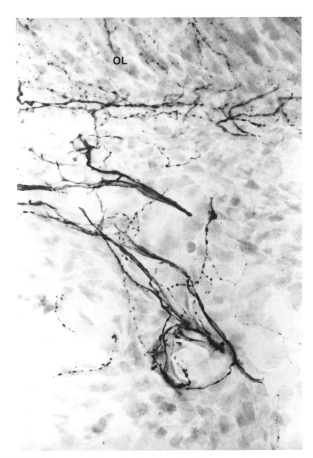

Fig. 10.28 Immunohistochemical method demonstrating varicose CGRP immunoreactive nerve fibres (black) around a blood vessel (V) and in the odontoblast layer (OL) (× 1600). Courtesy of Doctors J-Q. Zhang, K. Nagata and T. Iijima and the editor of *Anatomical Record*.

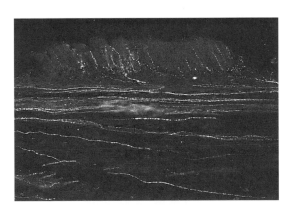

Fig. 10.29 Immunohistochemical staining demonstrating substance P-containing nerve fibres (white) in the odontoblast layer (top) and in the subodontoblastic plexus. (Dark field illumination; × 300).

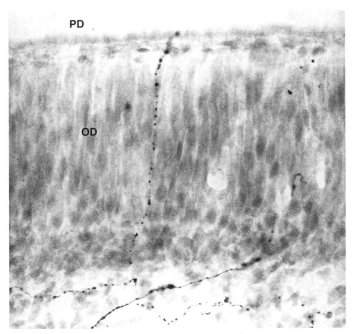

Fig. 10.30 Immunohistochemical stain showing neuropeptide Y-containing nerve fibres in and below the odontoblast layer (OD). PD = Predentine (× 1600). Courtesy of Doctors J-Q. Zhang, K. Nagata and T. Iijima and the editor of *Anatomical Record*.

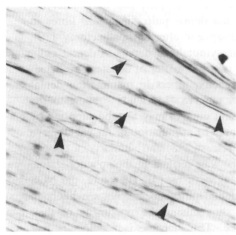

Fig. 10.31 Immunohistochemical staining to show nerve fibres (arrrowed) staining for nitric oxide synthetase in dog coronal pulp (× 16 000). Courtesy of Doctors Z. Lohinai et al. and the editor of *Neuroscience Letters*.

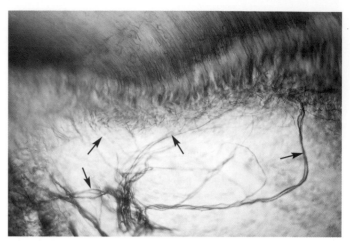

Fig. 10.33 Terminal branching of sensory fibres (arrows) in the dental pulp. This very thick section allows the axons at several levels to be seen, including the subodontoblastic nerve plexus of Raschkow (Silver stain; × 140). Courtesy of Dr R. O'Sullivan.

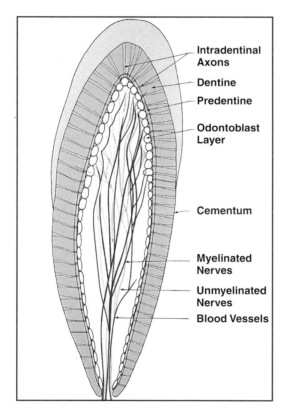

Intradentinal Axons
Dentine
Predentine
Odontoblast Layer
Cementum
Myelinated Nerves
Unmyelinated Nerves
Blood Vessels

Fig. 10.32 General distribution of myelinated nerves (dark green), non-myelinated nerves (light green) and blood vessels (red) in the pulp.

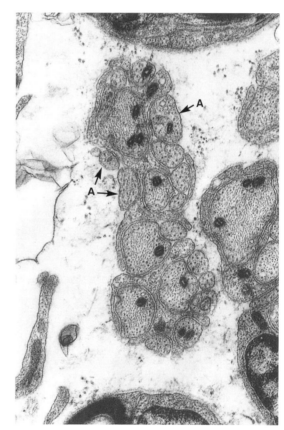

Fig. 10.34 TEM showing nerve fibres in the sub-odontoblastic plexus. Many of the axons are incompletely sheathed by Schwann cells (A), perhaps making them more susceptible to changes in the local environment (× 40 000).

effects, perhaps controlling, in part, the activity of odontoblasts. There is, however, no convincing evidence of an effect other than one that might be mediated by blood flow changes.

Some of the C fibres are sympathetic efferents and supply arteriolar smooth muscle. As there are only a few arterioles within the dental pulp sympathetic fibres are scarce

(Fig. 10.35). They seem to mediate their vasoconstrictive effect by the release of noradrenaline and neuropeptide Y. Evidence for a parasympathetic innervation of the dental pulp is weak. Acetylcholine, the principal mediator for the parasympathetic system, is rarely detected in the dental pulp. Vasodilatation seems to be effected by axon reflexes involving

Fig. 10.35 TEM demonstrating sympathetic axons from an animal injected with a false neurotransmitter, 6-hydroxydopamine, which is taken up but not released by noradrenergic axons. The false neurotransmitter accumulates as dense-cored vesicles (arrowed) identifying the sympathetic axons. In this nerve fibre the sympathetic axons are contained in the same Schwann cell pocket as unlabelled, presumably sensory, axons. Simultaneous activation of sympathetic axons amplifies the activity in sensory nerves. The close approximation of sensory and sympathetic axons may explain this interaction (× 31 000).

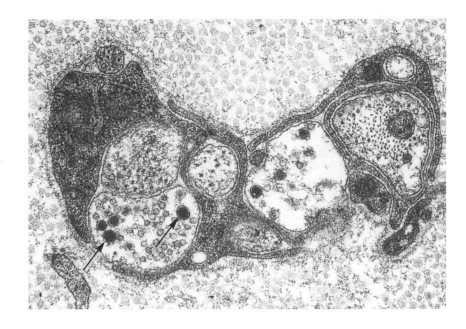

afferent nerves as well as (presumably as in other tissues) by the build-up of metabolites locally. Nitric oxide produced following hypoxia and tissue injury in the dental pulp is the signalling molecule most likely to induce vasodilatation under these conditions.

Nerve endings

It is difficult to determine where all nerve fibres end. Autonomic nerves end on the smooth muscle of the arterioles and special neuromuscular junctions are present. Some of the afferent fibres (probably a proportion of the Aδ fibres) enter the tubules largely in the coronal dentine and predentine. Others may end at the pulp–predentine junction in what is sometimes known as the marginal plexus (Fig. 10.36). Both of these groups would be in an ideal position to detect stimuli applied to the outside of the dentine.

Many axons end in close proximity to odontoblasts. It has been suggested that there are specialised junctions between odontoblasts and nerves but confirmatory evidence is lacking, although recent studies describe the proteins synapsin and synaptotagmin, characteristic of neural junctions, in the dentinal tubules. Whilst odontoblasts participate in many gap junctions (which elsewhere can act as electrical synapses), the cell processes involved in these junctions seem to come from other odontoblasts or from fibroblasts. The nerve–odontoblast relationship may be functionally if not structurally significant as the odontoblast or its process would dominate the local environment in which naked axons were present, especially in the dentinal tubules.

The nerves in the dentinal tubules, at the pulp–predentine border and among the odontoblast cell body have all lost their ensheathing Schwann cells and their axolemmas are exposed directly to the extracellular environment (Fig. 10.36). Changes in the composition of, or movement within, the extracellular fluid could readily affect the membrane properties of these terminals. Most activity in these terminals probably does not reach the level of sensation but presumably results locally in the release of neuropeptides by axon reflexes. The variety of neuropeptides found in the dental pulp is considerable. The most widely distributed and possibly the most significant functionally is calcitonin gene-related peptide (CGRP) (Fig. 10.37a), whose name derives from its first discovery and does not represent the widespread role it is now known to have.

CGRP is a potent vasodilator and quite possibly the principal agent controlling blood flow locally in the periphery of the dental pulp. CGRP is synthesised in the cell bodies of the nerves in the

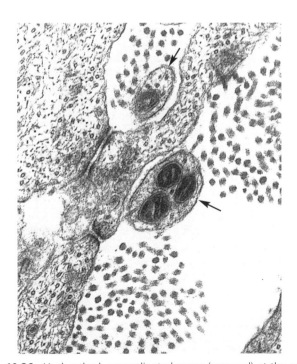

Fig. 10.36 Unsheathed, unmyelinated axons (arrowed) at the pulp (left) predentine border. Such axons may be activated by stimuli applied to dentine that cause fluid movement through the dentinal tubules (TEM; × 85 000).

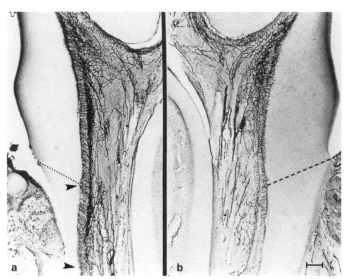

Fig. 10.37 Pulpal nerves stained immunohistochemically (black) for calcitonin gene-related peptide. (a) A tooth in which a cervical cavity was cut 12 days earlier; (b) a normal control tooth. The broken line approximates the boundary bewteen coronal and radicular dentine. There are many more CGRP-staining nerves after cavity preparation (× 650). Courtesy of Doctors R. Taylor and M. Byers and the editor of *Brain Research*.

Table 10.2 *Neuropeptides and neurotransmitters identified in the dental pulp with possible roles (largely interpolated from actions in other tissues)*

Neuropeptide/small molecule transmitter	Possible role
CGRP	Vasodilatation, stimulates cell division in pulpal fibroblasts
Substance P	Vasodilatation, ? nociceptive transmitter, stimulates cell division in pulpal fibroblasts
Neuropeptide Y	Sympathetic vasoconstrictor
Norepinephrine	Sympathetic vasoconstrictor
Enkephalin	Silencer of nociceptors
Somatostatin	Silencer of nociceptors
Endorphin	Silencer of nociceptors
Dopamine	Vasoactive or a precursor of epinephrine
Epinephrine	Vasoconstrictive via smooth muscle in arterioles
Cholecystokinin	Unknown
Vasoactive intestinal polypeptide	? Parasympathetic
Secretoneurin	Axon reflexes
Neurokinin A	Vasodilatation, ? nociceptive transmitter, stimulates cell division in pulpal fibroblasts
Peptide histidine isoleucine amide	? Parasympathetic
? Acetylcholine	? Parasympathetic

trigeminal ganglion and moved peripherally by axonal transport. Clearly a message, presumably a signalling molecule such as nerve growth factor, is carried from the periphery of the dental pulp to the ganglion cell body to modulate the production of CGRP. As well as having a role in pulpal blood flow CGRP may participate in initiating or controlling hard-tissue production. Dental pulp cells, when maintained *in vitro*, respond to the application of CGRP with increased production of bone morphogenetic protein-2, a signalling molecule known to be involved in dentine formation. Nerve growth factor (NGF) and NGF receptors have been detected in the peripheral dental pulp. Both NGF and receptors for it are found on odontoblasts as well as pulpal nerves. NGF appears not to be produced by odontoblasts but donated by neigbouring fibroblasts. The expression of both NGF and its receptors increases in the injured pulp. Apart from a direct neural role NGF may be a chemoattractant for leukocytes in the damaged pulp.

Though something of a paradigm shift from the original division of sensory and motor functions between different components of the nervous system, it seems reasonable to suggest that the major role of the trigeminal afferents in the dental pulp is in controlling the local environment rather than in carrying sensory information centrally. Some neuropeptides may function to control the flow of sensory activity centrally. The experience of toothache makes one realise that the balance of activities is flexible.

Several other neuropeptides and transmitters have been found in the normal dental pulp and it is possible, based on their known activities in other sites, to speculate on their role in the pulp (see Table 10.2). We are a long way from understanding what such a large number of agents contributes in the intact pulp and how they interact. In the injured pulp the number of biologically active molecules present increases

substantially and many of those detectable in normal pulps increase in quantity and distribution. It is likely that the continuous release of such peptides plays a role in the homeostasis of the dental pulp (Fig. 10.37b).

REGIONS

The structure of the dental pulp can be described on a regional basis (see Fig. 10.8).

Beginning from the outside the potential space between the odontoblast layer and the predentine could be described as the supraodontoblast region. In most histological preparations there is shrinkage of the soft pulp away from the dentine, creating a space in this region that is not present in the vital tissue. However, such preparations are useful in demonstrating the presence of odontoblast processes (Fig. 10.38). Two important structures are located in this region.

■ Unsheathed axons, found almost exclusively in the crown. These have been described as the predentinal plexus (of Bradlaw). They are not a true plexus (network) but an area where a number of axons congregate. It is not clear whether many axons end in this plexus. Most, presumably, continue

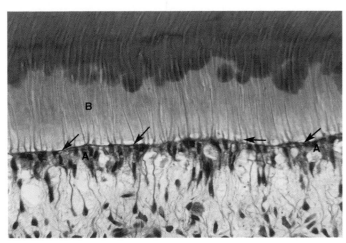

Fig. 10.38 Micrograph of the pulp–dentine boundary exhibiting slight shrinkage and showing continuity of odntoblast processes (arrow) with odontoblast cell bodies (A). B = Predentine (H & E; × 400).

to enter and end within dentinal tubules. These axons are in an ideal position to sense changes in fluid movement through the dentinal tubules as well as changes in the extracellular fluid composition, which, because of the barrier properties of the odontoblast layer, will be delayed in reaching the core of the pulp.

■ Dendritic antigen-presenting cells (described above).

This region thus deserves some special recognition as (after the odontoblast process) the first level at which external stimuli can be detected in the pulp.

The odontoblast layer (see Figs 10.8 and 10.9) is, self-evidently, the effector system of the pulp. All other elements of the pulp are supportive or protective of the cells forming dentine or programmed to replace them should they be killed.

The **subodontoblastic zone** (Fig. 10.8) has several terms associated with it. Immediately beneath the odontoblast layer a **cell-free zone** (of Weil) is commonly described in which, in standard paraffin-embedded sections, no cells are apparent. Many routine stains such as haemotoxylin and eosin stain principally nuclei and areas that lack nuclei appear empty: this is the case with the area immediately beneath the odontoblasts. Electron microscopy reveals that many cell processes of fibroblasts, odontoblasts, axons and capillaries cross this region. More correctly this area could be described as anuclear. The cell-free zone is usually absent from the radicular pulp and usually appears in the pulp once the tooth has erupted. There is no apparent reason for this feature and it has been suggested that it is an artefact of histological processing produced by differential shrinkage of the odontoblast and the deeper pulp.

Immediately deep to the 'cell-free' zone is another region in which there are, apparently, many cells – the so-called **cell-rich zone** (Fig. 10.8). This too may be an artefact induced by contrast to the cell-free zone. In this region there is a high concentration of both capillaries (the **subodontoblastic capillary plexus**) and axons (the **subodontoblastic neural plexus**). The Schwann cells, endothelial cells, etc. associated with these 'plexi' could result in the 'cell-rich' appearance.

Central to the subodontoblastic region is the bulk of the dental pulp which, devoid of its peripheral structures and its central neurovascular core, would be similar to loose connective tissue in many other sites although having a richer nerve and blood supply. The central core itself is most evident in the root canal. Once it enters the crown repeated branching of both nerves and blood vessels renders the neurovascular bundle less obvious.

ROLE OF THE DENTAL PULP

Once differentiated from the dental papilla the dental pulp is a single industry organ dedicated to the production of dentine rapidly during development, slowly during adult life, or suddenly in response to insult. The presence of a soft-tissue core in a tooth affects its physical properties. A young tooth with a large vital pulp is more elastic than a tooth in which most of the pulp has been replaced with secondary dentine or all of the pulp with a filling material as occurs during root canal therapy.

AGE-RELATED CHANGES IN THE DENTAL PULP

The dental pulp gets smaller with age because secondary dentine deposition continues, albeit at a slow rate, throughout life.

The older pulp is less vascular and, apparently, more fibrous than the young pulp. The innervation is reduced. The pulp often mineralises in the form of pulp stones. Many older human teeth show some degree of mineralisation, which can occur as many tiny spicules of mineralised tissue throughout the pulp ('snow storm' calcification, Fig. 10.39) or as discrete pulp stones either singly or in small groups. Pulp stones may resemble dentine in being, at least partially, tubular ('true' denticles) or resemble bone by having cells embedded within them ('false' denticles: Figs 10.39, 10.40). In some (lamellated pulp stones), accretion by layers is evident. Some larger pulp stones may be attached to the dentine. The incidence of pulpal calcifications increases with age and they are generally regarded as an age-related change rather than pathological. If detected in the absence of symptoms or pathological change pulp stones are not an indication for root canal therapy. The presence of pulp stones can complicate root canal therapy when it is indicated for other reasons. The factors determining why some individuals and not others produce pulp stones are not known – nor why, when present, one form or another occurs. If an individual has pulp stones in one tooth it is likely that they have pulp stones in other teeth.

CLINICAL CONSIDERATIONS

Genetic, congenital, nutritional and traumatic factors that affect dentinogenesis exert that effect via the dental pulp. In

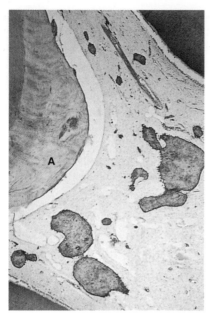

Fig. 10.39 Multiple free pulp stones present in the dental pulp and lacking dentine structure (false denticles). A = Dentine (H & E; × 20).

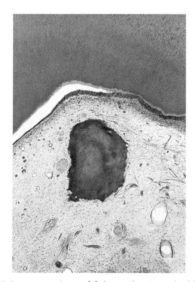

Fig. 10.40 High-power view of false pulp stone lacking dentinal structure (H & E; × 80).

the mature tooth, the pulp is the sense organ that mandates the use of anaesthesia during cavity preparation. It is the tissue that defends (or at least tries to defend) the integrity of the tooth in response to dental caries, attrition and trauma. Following pulp exposures and restorations it will, under the right conditions, form secondary dentine and maintain tooth vitality. When dental caries begins the pulp responds at a very early stage. Pulpal inflammation can often be detected when caries is limited to the enamel. On some occasions pulpal inflammation (pulpitis) is painful and induces a memorable experience for the patient, and sometimes a therapeutic challenge for the dentist. Pain from the dental pulp is difficult to localise and is commonly referred to other sites, either teeth or elsewhere. Sometimes pain in other sites is referred to the dental pulp (even angina). On many occasions pulpitis is painless and the dental pulp necroses. Necrotic pulp tissue can

induce inflammation and sepsis in the supporting tissues around the tooth with possibly serious sequelae. It is not known why pulpal inflammation on some occasions results in severe pain and on other occasions is silent.

The lack of sensitivity associated with older teeth, be it due to the increased thickness of dentine or the reduced innervation of the pulp, may allow, on some occasions, for the restorative treatment of teeth without anaesthesia.

Gingival recession may expose the opening of a lateral root canal, especially in the furcation area of cheek teeth, causing pain and the possible spread of infection into the pulp. Infection associated with periodontal disease may also affect the pulp and vice versa. The successful treatment of these endodontic–periodontic lesions is dependent on determining in which of the tissues the disease process originated.

If an uninfected pulp is exposed during cavity preparation in a tooth it can, if treated appropriately, repair and form a bridge of dentine over the exposure. New odontoblasts differentiate and lay down tertiary (reparative) dentine. Some materials, such as calcium hydroxide, seem to facilitate dentine bridge formation. Their effect may be more by their ability to protect the pulp and their biocompatibility rather than any direct stimulation of dentine producing cells. Other, more biologically active molecules, such as bone morphogenetic protein, TGF-β and some of the components of dentine matrix may have a direct effect on the differentiation and activation of hard tissue forming cells. These have not, as yet, been widely applied clinically. If the exposed pulp is infected or contaminated the likelihood of successful bridge formation is much reduced. It may, in the future, be possible to control infection and inflammation in the pulp. It may also be possible to replace or regenerate all or part of a diseased pulp that has been removed using biological matrices carrying growth factors and/or cultures of pulpal cells. Currently, the definitive treatment of the irreversibly diseased or necrotic pulp is to remove it and replace it with an inert root canal filling material.

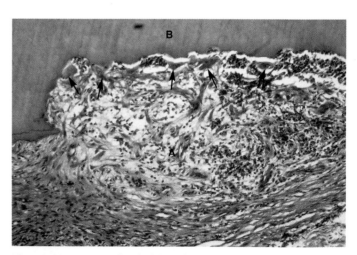

Fig. 10.41 Section of pulp (A) undergoing internal resorption. The odontoblast layer is lost as the pulp is replaced by a vascular granulation tissue. The dentine (B) is resorbed by large multinucleated odontoclast-like cells (arrows) (H & E; × 150). Courtesy of Dr J. Potts.

In certain instances, sometimes associated with trauma, the pulp becomes transformed into granulation tissue and the dentine commences to be resorbed internally at the pulp–dentine surface by odontoclast-like cells (Fig. 10.41). This condition is known as internal resorption of the pulp. If it proceeds far enough, the crown may have a pinkish colouration as the vascular granulation tissue is seen beneath the translucent enamel.

11 Cementum

Cementum is the thin layer of calcified tissue covering the dentine of the root (Fig. 11.1). It is one of the four tissues that support the tooth in the jaw (the periodontium), the others being the alveolar bone, the periodontal ligament and the gingivae. Although many of these periodontal tissues have been extensively studied, cementum remains the least known. Indeed, it is the least known of all the mineralised tissues in the body. For example, very little is known about the origin, differentiation and cell dynamics of the cementum-forming cell (the cementoblast).

Although restricted to the root in humans, cementum is present on the crowns of some mammals as an adaptation to a herbivorous diet. Cementum varies in thickness at different levels of the root. It is thickest at the root apex and in the interradicular areas of multirooted teeth, and thinnest cervically. The thickness cervically is 10–15 μm, and apically 50–200 μm (although it may exceed 600 μm).

Cementum is contiguous with the periodontal ligament on its outer surface and is firmly adherent to dentine on its deep surface. Its prime function is to give attachment to collagen fibres of the periodontal ligament. It therefore is a

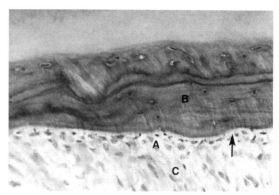

Fig. 11.2 The relationship between cementum (B), precementum (arrow), a layer of cementoblasts (A), and the periodontal ligament (C) (Decalcified section; H & E; × 200).

highly responsive mineralised tissue, maintaining the integrity of the root, helping to maintain the tooth in its functional position in the mouth, and being involved in tooth repair and regeneration.

Cementum is slowly formed throughout life and this allows for continual reattachment of the periodontal ligament fibres – some regard cementum as a calcified component of the ligament. Developmentally, cementum is said to be derived from the investing layer of the dental follicle. Like dentine, there is always a thin layer (3–5 μm) of uncalcified matrix on the surface of the cellular variety of cementum (see page 346). This layer of uncalcified matrix is called precementum (Fig. 11.2). Similar in chemical composition and physical properties to bone, cementum is, however, avascular and has no innervation. It is also less readily resorbed, a feature that is important for permitting orthodontic tooth movement. The reason for this feature is unknown but it may be related to:

- differences in physicochemical or biological properties between bone and cementum;
- the properties of the precementum;
- the increased density of Sharpey's fibres (particularly in acellular cementum);
- the proximity of epithelial cell rests to the root surface.

The arrangement of tissues at the **cement–enamel junction** is shown in Figs 11.3–11.5. In any single section of a tooth, three arrangements of the junction between cementum and enamel may be seen. Pattern 1, where the cementum overlaps the enamel for a short distance, is the predominant arrangement in 60% of sections. Pattern 2, where the cementum and enamel meet at a butt joint, occurs in 30% of sections. Pattern 3, where the cementum and enamel fail to meet and the dentine between them is exposed, occurs in 10% of sections. Although

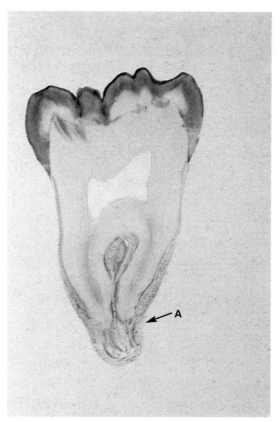

Fig. 11.1 The distribution of cementum (A) along the root of a tooth (Ground longitudinal section of a tooth; × 4).

one of these patterns may predominate in any individual tooth, all three patterns can be present.

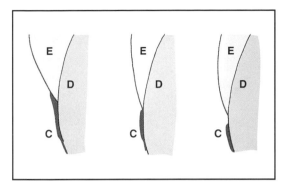

Fig. 11.3 Three patterns for the arrangement of the cement–enamel junction. C = Cementum; E = enamel; D = dentine. See text for further details.

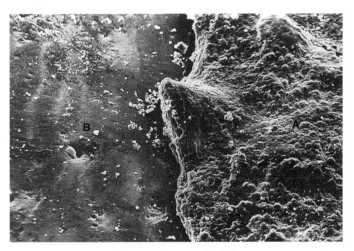

Fig. 11.4 Scanning electron micrograph of the cement–enamel junction where the cementum overlaps the enamel. A = Cementum; B = enamel (SEM; × 250).

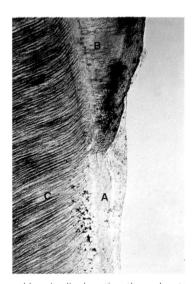

Fig. 11.5 Ground longitudinal section through a tooth to show cementum (A) overlapping enamel (B). C = Dentine (Ground section; × 80). Courtesy of Professor A.G.S. Lumsden.

PHYSICAL PROPERTIES

Cementum is pale yellow with a dull surface. It is softer than dentine. Permeability varies with age and the type of cementum, the cellular variety being more permeable. In general, cementum is more permeable than dentine. Like the other dental tissues, permeability decreases with age. The relative softness of cementum, combined with its thinness cervically, means that it is readily removed by abrasion when gingival recession exposes the root surface to the oral environment. Loss of cementum in such cases will expose dentine.

CHEMICAL PROPERTIES

Cementum contains on a wet-weight basis 65% inorganic material, 23% organic material and 12% water. By volume, the inorganic material comprises approximately 45%, organic material 33%, and water 22%. The degree of mineralisation varies in different parts of the tissue; some acellular zones may be more highly calcified than dentine. The principal inorganic component is hydroxyapatite, although other forms of calcium are present at higher levels than in enamel and dentine. The hydroxyapatite crystals are thin and plate-like and similar to those in bone. They are on average 55 nm wide and 8 nm thick. Their length varies, but values derived from sections cut with a diamond knife are underestimates due to shattering of the crystals along their length. As with enamel, the concentration of trace elements tends to be higher at the external surface. This, for example, is true of fluoride levels, which are also higher in acellular than in cellular cementum. The organic matrix is primarily collagen. The collagen is virtually all type I. In addition, the non-collagenous elements are assumed to be similar to those found in bone (see page 206). However, because of the difficulties of obtaining sufficient material for analysis, less information is available. Nevertheless, among the important molecules known to be present are bone sialoprotein, osteopontin and possibly other cementum-specific elements that are conjectured to be involved in periodontal reattachment and/or remineralisation.

CLASSIFICATION OF CEMENTUM

The various types of cementum encountered may be classified in three different ways: the presence or absence of cells, the nature and origin of the organic matrix and a combination of both.

Classification based on the presence or absence of cells – cellular and acellular cementum

Cellular cementum, as its name indicates, contains cells (cementocytes); acellular cementum does not. In the most common arrangement, acellular cementum covers the root adjacent to the dentine, whereas cellular cementum is found mainly in the apical area and overlying the acellular cementum (Fig. 11.6). Deviations from this arrangement are

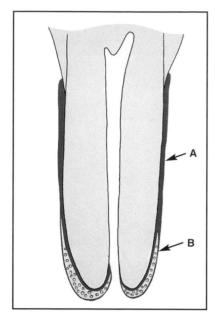

Fig. 11.6 The distribution of acellular (A) and cellular (B) cementum.

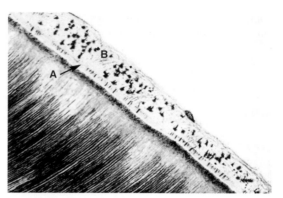

Fig. 11.8 Cellular cementum (B) overlying acellular cementum (A). Note the greater thickness of the cellular layer (Ground section; × 50).

common and sometimes several layers of each variant alternate. Being formed first, the acellular cementum is sometimes termed primary cementum and the subsequently formed cellular variety secondary cementum. Cellular cementum is especially common in interradicular areas.

Acellular cementum appears relatively structureless (Fig. 11.7). In the outer region of the radicular dentine, the granular layer (of Tomes) can be seen and outside this the hyaline layer (of Hopewell-Smith). These layers are also described on page 136. A dark line may be discerned between the hyaline layer and the acellular cementum; this may be related to the afibrillar cementum that is patchily present at this position. The usual arrangement at the apical region of the root is of a layer of cellular cementum overlying acellular cementum (Fig. 11.8). Many of the structural differences between cellular and acellular cementum are thought to be related to the faster rate of matrix formation for cellular cementum. Indeed, a major difference is that, as cellular

cementum develops, the formative cells (the cementoblasts) become embedded in the tissue as cementocytes. The different rates of cementum formation are also reflected in the presence of a precementum layer and in the more widely spaced incremental lines in cellular cementum.

Although the usual relationship between acellular and cellular cementum is for the cellular variety to overlie the acellular, the reverse may occur (Fig. 11.9). Furthermore, it is also common for the two variants of cementum to alternate (Fig. 11.10), probably representing variations in the rate of deposition.

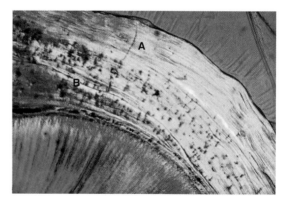

Fig. 11.9 Acellular cementum (A) overlying cellular cementum (B) (Ground section of the root; × 50).

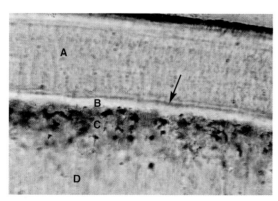

Fig. 11.7 The appearance of acellular cementum (A). B = Hyaline layer (of Hopewell-Smith); C = granular layer (of Tomes); D = root dentine. Note that the dark layer arrowed between the hyaline layer and the acellular cementum may be related to the afibrillar cementum patchily present at this position (Ground section; × 200).

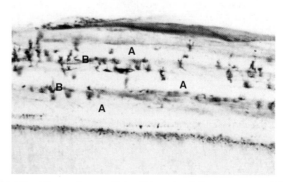

Fig. 11.10 Alternating acellular (A) and cellular cementum (B) (Ground section; × 60).

The spaces that the cementocytes occupy in cellular cementum are called **lacunae**, and the channels that their processes extend along are the **canaliculi** (Fig. 11.11; see also Fig. 11.2). Adjacent canaliculi are often connected, and the processes within them exhibit gap junctions. In ground sections (Fig. 11.11), the cellular contents are lost, air and debris filling the voids to give the dark appearance. In thicker layers of cellular cementum, it is highly probable that many of the lacunae do not contain vital cells. Compared with osteocytes in bone, cementocytes are more widely dispersed and more randomly arranged. In addition, their canaliculi are preferentially oriented towards the periodontal ligament, their chief source of nutrition. Unlike bone, the cementocytes are not arranged circumferentially around blood vessels in the form of osteons (Haversian systems). In decalcified sections (Fig. 11.2), the cellular contents of the lacunae are retained, albeit in a shrunken condition.

Fig. 11.12 illustrates the ultrastructural appearance of a cementocyte within a lacuna. Although derived from active cementoblasts, once they become embedded within the cementum matrix cementocytes become relatively inactive.

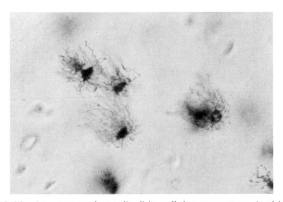

Fig. 11.11 Lacunae and canaliculi in cellular cementum. In this section, the preferential orientation of the lacunae indicates that the external surface is above and to the left (Ground section; × 500).

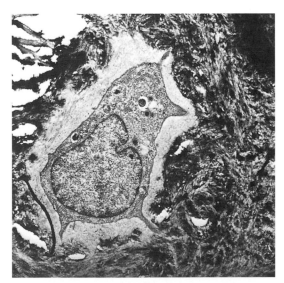

Fig. 11.12 TEM of a cementocyte within a lacuna. Note that the cementocyte processes here appear short only because they extend out of the plane of section (× 4500).

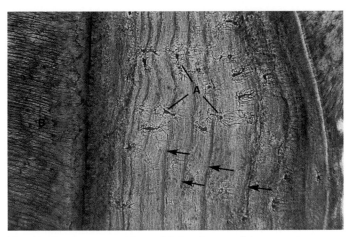

Fig. 11.13 Incremental lines of Salter (arrowed) in cementum. A = Cementocytes; B = dentine (Decalcified section; picrothionine; × 75). Courtesy of Professor M.M. Smith.

This is reflected in their ultrastructural appearance. Their cytoplasmic/nuclear ratio is low and they have sparse, if any, representation of the organelles responsible for energy production and for synthesis. Some unmineralised matrix may be seen in the perilacunar space. The cementocyte processes can extend for distances several times longer than the diameter of the cell body.

Cementum is deposited in an irregular rhythm, resulting in unevenly spaced **incremental lines** (of Salter; Fig. 11.13). Unlike enamel and dentine, the precise periodicity between the incremental lines is unknown, although there have been unsuccessful attempts to relate it to an annual cycle. In acellular cementum, incremental lines tend to be close together, thin and even. In the more rapidly formed cellular cementum, the lines are further apart, thicker, and more irregular. The appearance of incremental lines in cementum is mainly due to differences in the degree of mineralisation, but these must also reflect differences in composition of the underlying matrix since, as shown in Figure 11.13, the lines are readily visible in decalcified sections. Table 11.1 summarises differences between acellular and cellular cementum.

Classification based on the nature and origin of the organic matrix

Cementum derives its organic matrix from two sources: from the inserting Sharpey's fibres of the periodontal ligament, and from the cementoblasts. It is therefore possible to classify cementum according to the nature and origin of the fibrous matrix. When derived from the periodontal ligament, the fibres are referred to as the **extrinsic fibres**. These Sharpey's fibres continue into the cementum in the same direction as the principal fibres of the ligament (i.e. perpendicular or oblique to the root surface; see page 182). When derived from the cementoblasts, the fibres are referred to as **intrinsic fibres**. These run parallel to the root surface and approximately at right angles to the extrinsic fibres. Where both extrinsic and intrinsic fibres are present, the tissue may be termed **mixed fibre cementum**.

Table 11.1 *Summary of differences between acellular and cellular cementum*

Acellular cementum	Cellular cementum
No cells	Lacunae and canaliculi containing cementocytes and their processes
Border with dentine not clearly demarcated	Border with dentine clearly demarcated
Rate of development relatively slow	Rate of development relatively fast
Incremental lines relatively close together	Incremental lines relatively wide apart
Precementum layer virtually absent	Precementum layer present

Classification based on the presence or absence of cells and on the nature and origin of the organic matrix

This classification, which is becoming more widely used, contains a number of types of cementum. For human teeth, two main varieties of cementum are found – acellular extrinsic fibre cementum (AEFC) and cellular intrinsic fibre cementum (CIFC). AEFC is located mainly over the cervical half of the root and constitutes the bulk of cementum in some teeth (e.g. in premolars). AEFC is the first formed cementum (see pages 340–345) and layers attain a thickness of approximately 15 μm.

Acellular extrinsic fibre cementum (Fig. 11.14)

For this type of cementum all the collagen is derived as Sharpey's fibres from the periodontal ligament (the ground substance itself may be produced by the cementoblasts). This type of cementum corresponds with primary acellular cementum and therefore covers the cervical two-thirds of the root (Fig. 11.7). It is therefore formed slowly and the root surface is smooth (Fig. 11.4). The fibres are generally well mineralised. As shown in Fig.11.15, however, the extrinsic fibres seen in ground sections may have unmineralised cores. These may be lost during preparation of a ground section and replaced with air or debris. This results in the total internal reflection of transmitted light, giving the appearance of thin black lines.

Cellular intrinsic fibre cementum (Figs 11.16, 11.17)

This type of cementum is composed only of intrinsic fibres running parallel to the root surface. The absence of Sharpey's fibres means intrinsic fibre cementum has no role in tooth attachment. It may be found in patches in the apical region. It may be a temporary phase, with extrinsic fibres subsequently gaining a reattachment, or may represent a permanent region without attaching fibres. It generally corresponds to secondary cellular cementum and is found in the apical third of the root and in the interradicular areas. Although intrinsic fibre cementum is generally cellular due to the rapid speed of formation, sometimes intrinsic fibre cementum is formed more slowly and cells are not incorporated (**acellular intrinsic fibre cementum**).

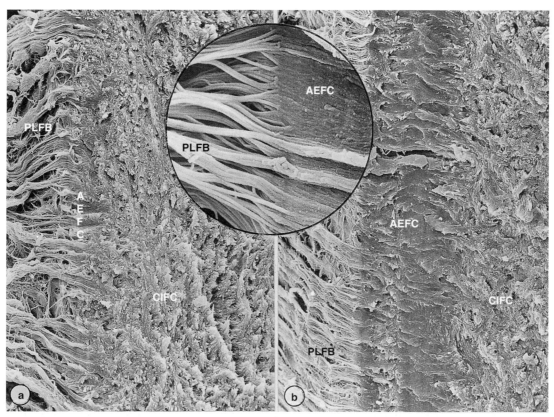

Fig. 11.14 SEMs of fractured surface of root illustrating acellular extrinsic fibre cementum (AEFC). PLFB = Inserting periodontal ligament fibre bundles; CIFC = underlying cellular intrinsic fibre cementum (a and b × 630; inset × 1650). Courtesy of Professor H.E. Schroeder and the editor of *Schweizer Monatsschrift für Zahnmedizin*.

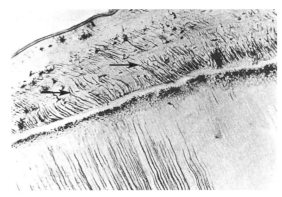

Fig. 11.15 Extrinsic fibres in ground sections. The arrows indicate that the core of the extrinsic fibre bundle has been lost during preparation of the ground section and replaced with air or debris (Ground section; × 100). Courtesy of Dr P.D.A. Owens.

Towards the root apex, and in the furcation areas of multi-rooted teeth, the acellular extrinsic fibre cementum and the cellular intrinsic fibre cementum commonly may be present in alternating layers known as **cellular mixed stratified** cementum (see Fig. 11.18).

Mixed-fibre cementum (Fig. 11.19)

For this third variety of cementum, the collagen fibres of the organic matrix are derived from both extrinsic fibres (from the periodontal ligament) and intrinsic fibres (from cementoblasts). The extrinsic and intrinsic fibres can be readily distinguished. First, the intrinsic fibres run between the extrinsic fibres with a

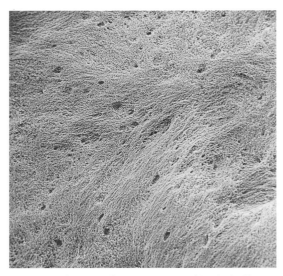

Fig. 11.16 SEM showing the appearance of intrinsic fibre cementum at the surface of the root apex. Note the absence of Sharpey's fibres and the parallel distribution of the bundles of mineralised intrinsic fibres (Anorganic preparation; × 150). Courtesy of Professor S.J. Jones.

different orientation. Indeed, the fewer the number of intrinsic fibres in mixed fibre cementum, the closer the extrinsic fibre bundles (Fig. 11.19). Second, the fibre bundles are of different sizes: the extrinsic fibres are ovoid or round bundles about 5–7 μm in diameter; the intrinsic fibres are 1–2 μm in diameter (Fig. 11.19).

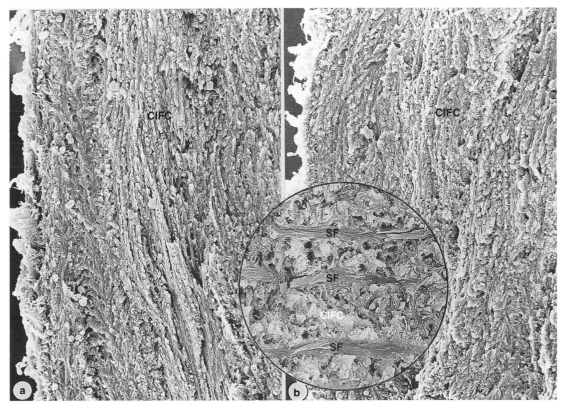

Fig. 11.17 SEMs of fractured surface of root showing the appearance of cellular intrinsic fibre cementum (CIFC). Note the absence of Sharpey's fibres and the parallel distribution of the bundles of mineralised intrinsic fibres (a and b × 470; inset × 1650). Courtesy of Professor H.E. Schroeder and the editor of *Schweizer Monatsschrift für Zahnmedizin*.

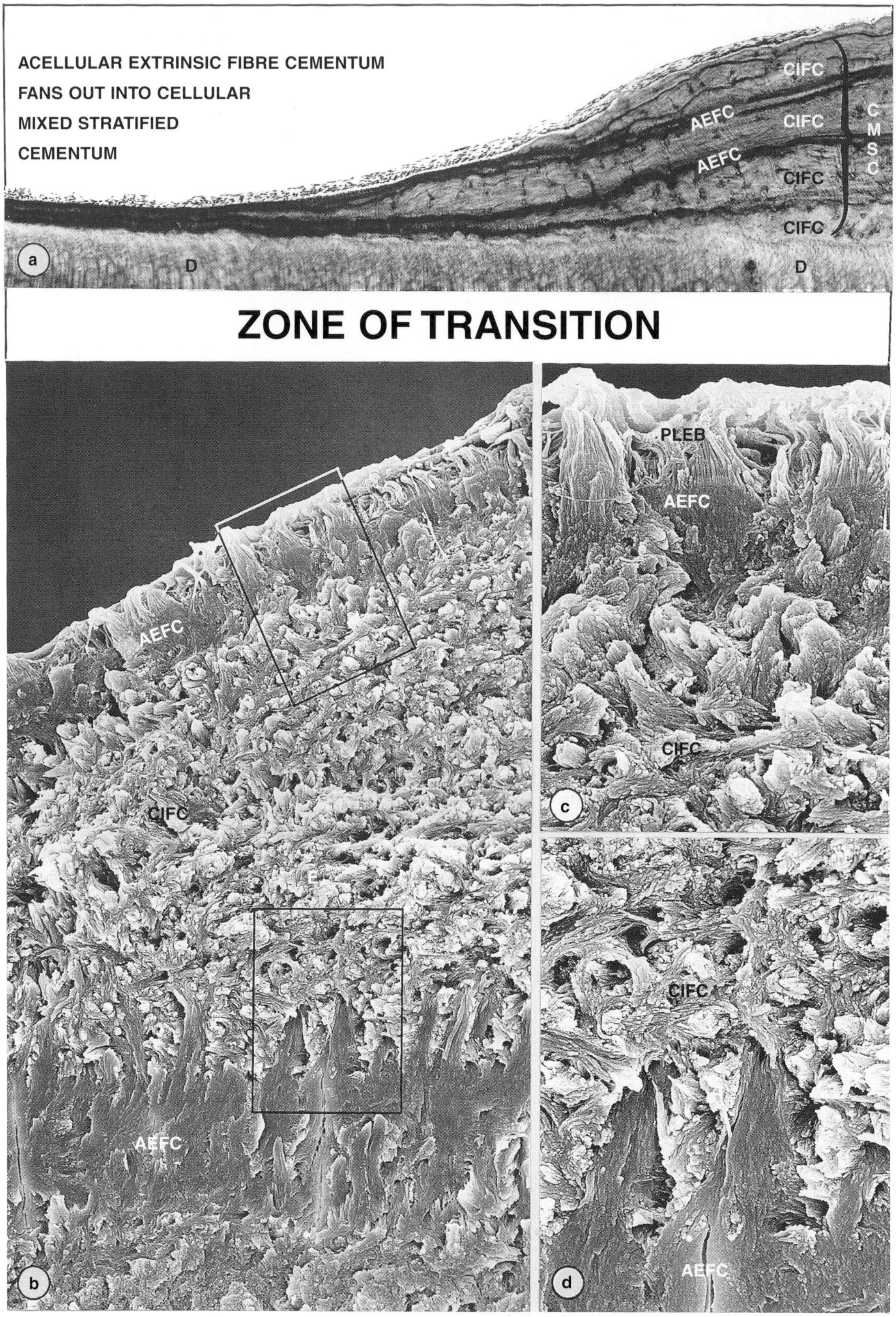

Fig. 11.18 (a) The appearance of mixed fibre cementum. A light micrograph to show the alternating distribution of acellular extrinsic fibre cementum (AEFC) and cellular intrinsic fibre cementum (CIFC), forming cellular mixed stratified cementum (CMSC). (Ground section; × 80). (b, c, d) SEMs illustrating mixed fibre cementum; (c) and (d) are highlighted areas provided by the boxes in (b). (SEM; (b) × 900; c and d × 2450). Courtesy of Professor H.E. Schroeder and the editor of *Schweizer Monatsschrift für Zahnmedizin*.

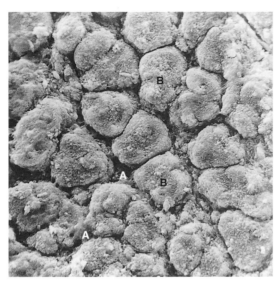

Fig. 11.19 SEM of the surface of a root showing the appearance of mixed fibre cementum. A = Mineralised intrinsic fibres (present here in small amounts); B = mineralised extrinsic fibres. Note the smaller dimensions of the intrinsic fibre bundles (Anorganic preparation; × 3000). Courtesy of Professor S.J. Jones.

cementum that contains no collagen fibres. This afibrillar cementum is sparsely distributed and consists of a well mineralised ground substance that may be of epithelial origin. Afibrillar cementum is a thin, acellular layer (difficult to identify at the light microscope level), which covers cervical enamel or

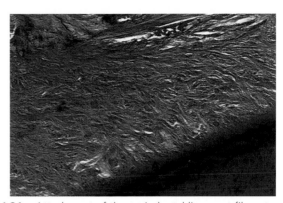

Fig. 11.21 Attachment of the periodontal ligament fibres to cementum. The fibres of the periodontal ligament (B) are seen to run into the organic matrix of precementum (A) (Decalcified section; Masson's blue trichrome; × 200).

If the formation rate is slow, the cementum may be termed **acellular mixed-fibre cementum** and is generally well mineralised. If the formation rate is fast, the cementum may be called **cellular mixed-fibre cementum** and the fibres are less well-mineralised (especially their cores).

Fig. 11.20 shows the fibre orientation in acellular and cellular cementum as seen in polarised light, the different colours reflecting different orientations of the collagen fibres. The acellular cementum contains primarily extrinsic fibres arranged perpendicular to the root surface. The overlying cellular cementum contains mainly intrinsic fibres running parallel to the root surface. Thus, there is a colour difference between the two layers.

Afibrillar cementum

The extrinsic, intrinsic and mixed fibre cementum types all contain collagen fibres. However, there is a further type of

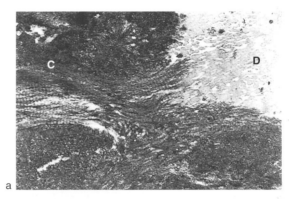

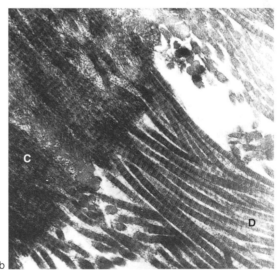

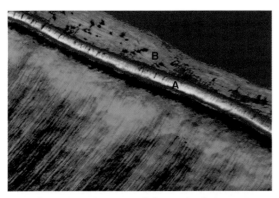

Fig. 11.20 Fibre orientation in acellular and cellular cementum. The root surface is seen in polarised light, the different colours reflecting different orientations of the collagen fibres. A = Acellular cementum; B = cellular cementum (Ground, longitudinal section; polarised light; × 50).

Fig. 11.22 Electronmicroscopic appearance of the insertion of Sharpey's fibres into cementum. (a) Ground section showing that the inserting collagen fibres darken as they enter the cementum due to their partial mineralisation. (b) Decalcified section showing the grouping of collagen into a bundle and collagen cross banding. C = Cementum; D = periodontal ligament (TEM; (A) × 8000; (B) × 15 000). Courtesy of Dr D.K. Whittaker.

intervenes between fibrillar cementum and dentine. Afibrillar cementum is thought to be formed at this site following the loss of the reduced enamel epithelium (see page 345).

ATTACHMENT OF THE PERIODONTAL LIGAMENT FIBRES TO CEMENTUM

The fibres of the periodontal ligament run into the organic matrix of precementum that is secreted by cementoblasts. Subsequent mineralisation of precementum will incorporate the extrinsic fibres as Sharpey's fibres into cementum (Figs 11.21, 11.22).

THE CEMENT–DENTINE JUNCTION

The nature of the cement–dentinal junction is of particular importance, being of interest biologically because it forms an interface (a 'fit') between two very different mineralised tissues that are developing contemporarily. It is also of clinical importance because of the processes involved in maintaining tooth function whilst repairing a diseased root surface.

It is often reported that an 'intermediate layer' (Fig. 11.23) exists between cementum and dentine and that this layer is involved in 'anchoring' the periodontal fibres to the dentine. A variety of names has been given to the 'intermediate layer' (including 'innermost cementum layer', 'superficial layer of root dentine' and 'intermediate cementum'). Indeed, it appears that the term has even been used to describe the hyaline layer of dentine (see page 136).

The intermediate layer is said to be characterised by wide, irregular branching spaces (Fig. 11.24) and is most commonly found in the apical region of cheek teeth. The spaces may interconnect with dentinal tubules. The nature and origin of the spaces is controversial; they may be related to entrapped epithelial cells (cell remnants containing filaments characteristic

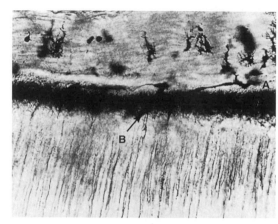

Fig. 11.24 Intermediate cementum (A) near the cement–dentine junction. B = Granular layer (Ground section; × 250). Courtesy of Dr P.D.A. Owens.

of epithelial cells have been described in this region). Alternatively, they may be enlarged terminals of dentinal tubules.

There appears to be marked species differences with respect to the intermediate layer. In rat molars, a distinct intermediate layer exists that is rich in the glycoproteins sialoprotein and osteopontin (both these glycoproteins being normally bone-related), although the role of these glycoproteins remains unclear. The origin of this layer in rat molars is also unclear, some believing that it is derived from the epithelial root sheath that lines the developing root (see page 340), while others claim that it is cementoblast-derived. Indeed, there are reports suggesting that, in humans, the region between the cementum and the root dentine contains enamel matrix protein and is a product of the epithelial root sheath. However, it has been claimed that, for many human teeth, the collagen within the AEFC layer intermingles with the dentine matrix, there is no sialoprotein and osteopontin, and there is no obvious zone between dentine and cementum.

Where an intermediate layer exists, it has been suggested that this functions as a permeability barrier, that it may be a precursor for cementogenesis, and that it is a precursor for cementogenesis in wound healing. These potential functions remain speculative. If, however, there is doubt about the very presence of an intermediate zone in human teeth then either human teeth do not require such functions (which is highly unlikely) or too much is being conjectured with too little experimental evidence.

The clinical significance of the interface between cementum and dentine relates to regeneration of the periodontium following periodontal surgery. Although a layer of cementum may regenerate, subsequent histological examination may show a 'space' between regenerated cementum and surface dentine, perhaps indicating an absence of a true union.

THE ULTRASTRUCTURAL APPEARANCE OF CEMENTUM

This varies with the level of the tissue examined. Near the periodontal surface (Fig. 11.25) cementum is not homogeneous, due to ongoing calcification and the presence of Sharpey's

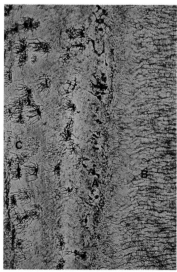

Fig. 11.23 Intermediate cementum (A). B = root dentine. C = cellular cementum (Demineralised section; picrothianine; × 75). Courtesy of Professor M.M. Smith.

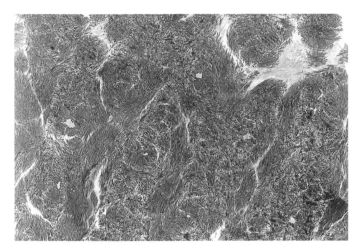

Fig. 11.25 Appearance of cementum near the periodontal surface (TEM; × 2000).

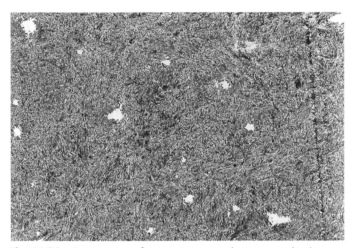

Fig. 11.26 Appearance of cementum near the cement–dentine junction (TEM; × 2000).

fibres. The calcification of precementum is probably initiated in the early phases by the presence of the underlying root dentine mineral, and continues on and around the collagen fibres (both those formed by the cementoblasts and those included as attachment fibres from the periodontal ligament). The outer part of the cementum, where Sharpey's fibres predominate, may be considered as calcified periodontal ligament. Unlike dentine, no calcospherites are present within precementum. At deeper levels (Fig. 11.26), closer to the cement–dentine junction, acellular cementum resembles peripheral dentine and a demarcation is often difficult to see. The small channels seen at this level may be canaliculi derived from more superficial cementocytes, but some may be the terminals of dentinal tubules that traverse the border between the two tissues.

RESORPTION AND REPAIR OF CEMENTUM

Although cementum is less susceptible to resorption than bone under the same pressures (e.g. with orthodontic loading), most roots of permanent teeth still show small, localised areas of resorption (Figs 11.27–11.29). The cause of this is not

known, but may be associated with microtrauma. The resorption is carried out by multinucleated odontoclasts (see page 351) and may continue into the root dentine.

Resorption deficiencies may be filled by deposition of mineralised tissue. Indeed, a line known as a reversal line may be seen separating the repair tissue from the normal underlying dental tissues (repair of cementum following a localised

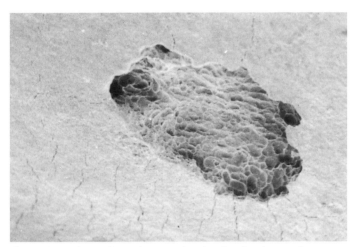

Fig. 11.27 The surface of a root showing localised area of resorption of cementum (SEM; × 250). Courtesy of Professor S.J. Jones.

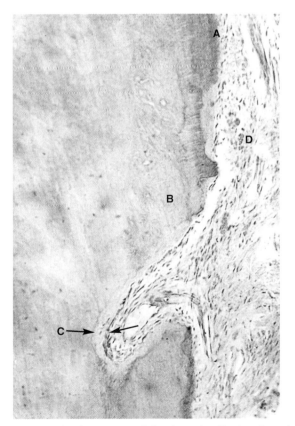

Fig. 11.28 Repair of cementum following a localised region of root resorption. A = Acellular cementum; B = root dentine; C = reversal line separating repair tissue from underlying dental tissues; D = periodontal ligament; arrows indicate cementoblasts depositing layer of precementum in resorption deficiency (Decalcified section of a root; H & E; × 90).

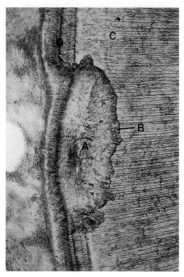

Fig. 11.29 Demineralised section of root showing infilled area of repair cementum (A). B = Reversal line; C = dentine; D = cementum (Picrothianine; × 75). Courtesy of Professor M.M. Smith.

region of root resorption is illustrated in Fig. 11.28). In this section, odontoclasts have resorbed through the thin layer of acellular cementum and penetrated into the root dentine. Repair is occurring and a layer of formative cells (cementoblasts) have deposited a thin layer of matrix (precementum) in the deficiency. An irregular, and dark-staining, reversal line separates the repair tissue from the underlying dental tissues. Fig. 11.29 shows an infilled area where dentine had been resorbed.

The repair tissue resembles cellular cementum. The formative cells have a similar ultrastructure to cementoblasts. Lines resembling incremental lines may be seen and there is a zone of uncalcified repair tissue homologous to precementum. However, differences can be noted between the repair tissue and cementum: the width of the uncalcified zone of reparative cementum (15 μm) is greater than that for precementum (5–10 μm); its degree of mineralisation is less (as judged by electron density); its crystals are smaller; and calcific globules are present, suggesting that mineralisation is not proceeding evenly.

These differences may be related to the speed of formation of the repair tissue. Where this is very slow, the repair tissue cannot be distinguished histologically, or in its mineralisation pattern, from primary cementum. However, where the repair tissue is formed rapidly (as in resorbing deciduous teeth), it closely resembles woven bone.

CLINICAL CONSIDERATIONS

Root fractures may, on some occasions, repair by the formation of a cemental callus. Unlike the callus that forms around fractured bone, the cemental callus does not usually remodel to the original dimensions of the tooth.

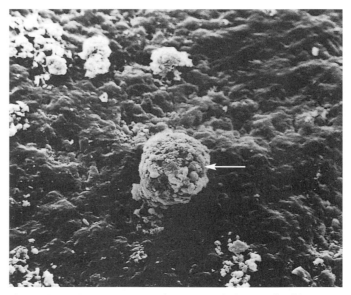

Fig. 11.30 SEM appearance of a cementicle (arrowed). This cementicle is attached to the root surface (× 1000).

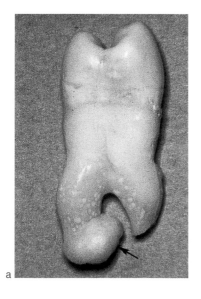

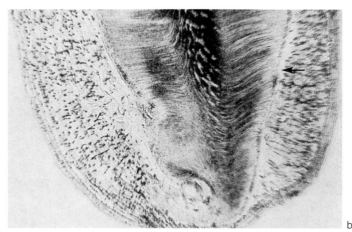

Fig. 11.31 (a) Hypercementosis at root apex (arrow). Courtesy of Dr J. Potts. (b) Ground section near the root apex showing hypercementosis. Arrow shows cement – dentine junction (× 25).

Cementicles (Fig. 11.30) are small, globular masses of cementum found in approximately 35% of human roots. They are not always attached to the cementum surface but may be located free in the periodontal ligament. Cementicles may result from microtrauma, when extra stress on the Sharpey's fibres causes a tear in the cementum. They are more common in the apical and middle third of the root and in root furcation areas.

Cementum continues to be deposited slowly throughout life, its thickness increasing about threefold between the ages of 16 and 70, although whether this proceeds in a linear manner is not known. Cementum may be formed at the root apex in much greater amounts as a result of compensatory tooth eruption in response to attrition (wear) at the occlusal surface.

Where there has been a history of chronic periapical inflammation, cementum formation may be substantial, giving rise to local hypercementosis (Fig. 11.31). This may cause problems during tooth extraction. Hypercementosis affecting all the teeth may be associated with Paget's disease.

Where the root canal exits at the apex of the tooth, cementum is deposited not only over the apex but also for a short distance (usually 0.5–1.5 mm) from the anatomical apex. This results in a narrowing of the canal at this point, the apical constriction. This represents the junction of the pulp and periodontal tissue (although there is no visible demarcation in the soft tissue). In clinical procedures of root canal therapy that call for the removal of a diseased or decayed pulp, this is the point to which the cleansing should be extended.

12 Periodontal ligament

The periodontal ligament is the dense fibrous connective tissue that occupies the periodontal space between the root of the tooth and the alveolus (Fig. 12.1). It is derived from the dental follicle (see page 293). Above the alveolar crest the periodontal ligament is continuous with the connective tissues of the gingiva; at the apical foramen it is continuous with the dental pulp. The continuity with the gingiva is important when considering the progression of periodontitis from gingivitis. The continuity with the pulp explains why inflammation from this dental tissue (often related to dental caries) spreads to involve the periodontal ligament and the other apical supporting tissues.

Although the average width of the periodontal space is said to be 0.2 mm, there is considerable variation both between teeth and within an individual tooth. The space has been described as hourglass in shape, being narrowest in the mid-root region, near the fulcrum about which the tooth moves when an orthodontic load (tipping load) is applied to the crown. The width of the periodontal space also varies according to the functional state of the periodontal tissues. The space

is reduced in non-functional and unerupted teeth and is increased in teeth subjected to heavy occlusal stress. With age, the periodontal space narrows slightly. The periodontal spaces of the permanent teeth are said to be narrower than those of the deciduous teeth.

Much research has been conducted in recent times into the structure, function and composition of the periodontal ligament, because the tissue is associated with important dental functions (in particular the mechanisms of tooth support and tooth eruption; see pages 201 and 352 respectively) and for clinical reasons. The tissue is involved with inflammatory periodontal disease (a common cause of tooth loss) and there is considerable interest in tissue reattachment following such disease. Furthermore, with the application of orthodontic loads, the periodontal tissues must adjust to permit tooth movements. Despite the amount of research undertaken, many of the important features of the periodontal ligament remain poorly understood and consequently there is much controversy.

Although we are only now beginning to understand the extent of specialisation of the tissue (see page 201), we still do not know why the periodontal ligament remains a soft connective tissue and does not calcify, even though it is enclosed by bone externally and cementum internally. Indeed, the periodontal ligament width is preserved over time and the alveolar bone rarely 'colonises' the periodontal space. It is evident that there must be some 'signalling systems' to accurately 'measure' and maintain the periodontal space. Failure of such a system is implicated in tooth ankylosis: that heat killing of periodontal cells induces ankylosis is some crude evidence that periodontal fibroblasts might regulate periodontal ligament width. More convincingly, periodontal cells can inhibit mineralised bone nodule formation by bone stromal cells and there is evidence to suggest that the block exerted by periodontal cells may be due to prostaglandin production. Recent work also indicates that bradykinin and thrombin can stimulate prostanoid synthesis by periodontal ligament cells. Contrariwise, periodontal ligament cells are capable of producing bone-like tissue *in vitro*, can form mineralised nodules and can express alkaline phosphatase. Indeed, alkaline phosphatase, an enzyme expressed by mineralised tissue forming cells, is expressed constitutively by periodontal ligament cells. That the ground substance may be implicated in preventing mineralisation may be deduced from *in vitro* experiments in which, following the administration of hyaluronidase, mineralisation can be produced in the remaining periodontal ligament connective tissue.

The periodontal ligament has the following functions:

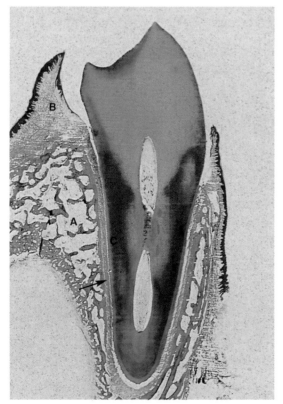

Fig. 12.1 The relationship of the periodontal ligament and the periodontal space (arrow) to the other tissues of the periodontium. A = Alveolar bone; B = gingiva; C = root of tooth lined by cementum (Decalcified, longitudinal section of a tooth *in situ*; H & E; × 4). Courtesy of Dr D.A. Lunt.

1. It is the tissue of attachment between the tooth and alveolar bone. It is thus responsible for resisting displacing forces (the tooth support mechanism) and for protecting the

dental tissues from damage caused by excessive occlusal loads (especially at the root apex).

2. It is responsible for the mechanisms whereby a tooth attains, and then maintains, its functional position. This includes the mechanisms of tooth eruption, tooth support (particularly the recovery response after loading), and drift.

3. Its cells form, maintain and repair alveolar bone and cementum.

4. Its mechanoreceptors are involved in the neurological control of mastication (see page 94 for reflex jaw activities).

The periodontal ligament has been likened to a fibrous joint (a gomphosis) and to periosteum. As will become apparent, however, such comparisons are not accurate (either from a structural or a functional point of view). In common with other dense fibrous connective tissues, the periodontal ligament consists of a stroma of fibres and ground substance containing cells, blood vessels and nerves.

FIBRES OF THE PERIODONTAL LIGAMENT

The connective tissue fibres are mainly collagenous (comprising well over 90% of the periodontal ligament fibres), but there may also be small amounts of oxytalan and reticulin fibres and, in some species, elastin fibres.

Collagen

The main types of collagen in the periodontal ligament are types I and III, and these are categorised as fibrous collagens. Most (more than 70%) of the periodontal collagen is type I collagen. This variety of collagen is the major protein component of most connective tissues (including bone and skin) and contains two identical $\alpha 1$ I chains and a chemically different $\alpha 2$ chain. It is low in hydroxylysine and glycosylated hydroxylsine. Unusually, however, the periodontal ligament is relatively rich in type III collagen (about 20%). This variety consists of three identical $\alpha 1$ III chains. It is high in hydroxyproline, low in hydroxylysine and contains cysteine. The function of type III collagen is not properly understood, although it is associated in other sites of the body with rapid turnover (e.g. granulation tissues and fetal connective tissue). Type III collagen is not localised to any specific region of the periodontal ligament but is covalently linked to type I collagen throughout the tissue. It is found in the periphery of Sharpey's fibre attachments into alveolar bone (see page 165). *In vitro* studies have shown that there is clonal heterogeneity for expression of type I and type III collagens and for fibronectin in periodontal ligament cell populations.

Small amounts of types V and VI collagens have been found in the periodontal ligament as well as traces of basement membrane collagens (types IV and VII) associated with epithelial cell rests (see page 194) and blood vessels. Although evident in all zones of the periodontal ligament in fully erupted teeth, type VI collagen is absent from the middle zone of erupting molars and from the tooth-related portion of the ligament of continuously growing incisors of rats (Fig. 12.2).

Recently it has been proposed that periodontal cells regulate the periodontal ligament's connective tissue architecture

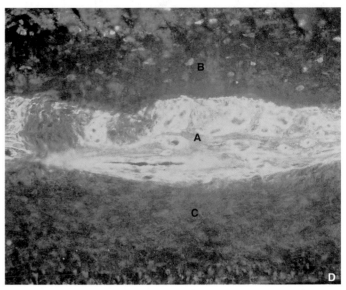

Fig. 12.2 Longitudinal cryosection of rat incisor periodontal ligament with immunofluorescent staining for type VI collagen showing strong positive yellow staining (A) towards the alveolar bone surface (B) with an absence of staining (C) in the ligament towards the tooth surface (D) (× 80). Courtesy of Professor P. Sloan and Mosby–Wolfe.

through expression of type XII collagen (Fig. 12.3). Type XII collagen is a non-fibrous collagen (known as a fibril-associated collagen) with interrupted helices. It may function by linking

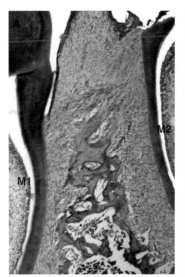 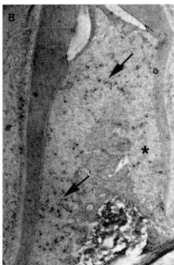

Fig. 12.3 The presence of type XII collagen within the periodontal ligament. (a) Developing periodontal ligament of maxillary first molar (MI) and second molar (M2) in a 25-day-old rat. In this specimen, the first molar has completed eruption and its periodontal ligament is more organized, whereas the second molar has not yet erupted. (b) *In situ* hybridisation of the S^{35}-labelled type XII collagen cDNA probe. The type XII collagen probe hybridised to fibroblasts in the periodontal ligament of the first molar (arrows). Fibroblasts in the second molar periodontal ligament (*) were less active in type XII collagen synthesis. It has been postulated that type XII collagen may contribute to the organisation of the mature and functional ligament collagen fibre architecture, which serves to resist unidirectional force. (Courtesy of Dr. Ichiro Nishimura, the UCLA Weintraub Center for Reconstructive Biotechnology.)

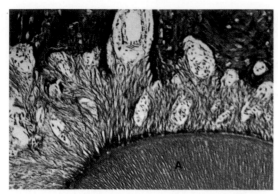

Fig. 12.4 Principal collagen fibres passing across the periodontal space from the root (A) to the alveolar bone (B). Note also the vascular nature of the periodontal ligament (Decalcified, transverse section through the periodontal ligament; Gomori's silver stain; × 250).

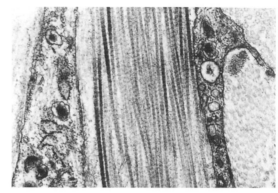

Fig. 12.6 High-power view of a fibroblast process enveloping a principal fibre. Note the individual collagen fibrils within the principal bundle sectioned longitudinally (TEM; × 10 000).

together other collagens. There is evidence to suggest that type XII collagen occurs within the periodontal ligament only when the ligament is fully functional.

Much of the collagen is gathered together to form bundles approximately 5 µm in diameter. These bundles are termed the principal fibres. They appear to be more numerous (but smaller) at their attachments to cementum than at the alveolar bone (see 12.19). Fig. 12.4 shows principal collagen fibres passing across the periodontal space from the root to the alveolar bone. The close association between the principal fibres and the fibroblasts of the periodontal ligament is shown in Figs 12.5 and 12.6. The fibroblasts are responsible for the synthesis and degradation of collagen. Cellular processes surround or envelop the fibre bundles; indeed, processes from adjacent cells are joined by intercellular contacts (see page 191) to form a cellular network. Many of the isolated islands of cytoplasm present in the section in Fig. 12.5 are cell processes from fibroblasts whose cell bodies are beyond the plane of section.

Within each collagen bundle, subunits of structure called collagen fibrils can be seen. The individual collagen fibrils

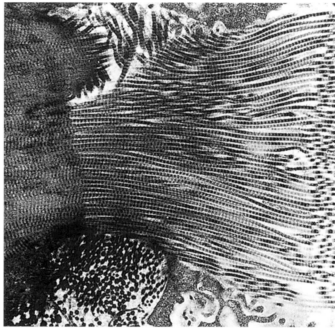

a

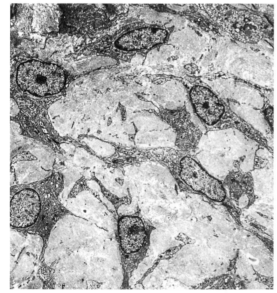

Fig. 12.5 TEM showing the close association between the principal fibres and the fibroblasts of the periodontal ligament (× 3000).

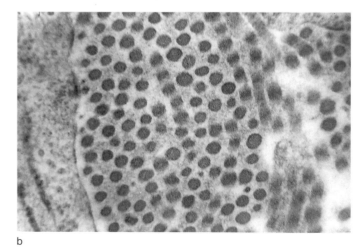

b

Fig. 12.7 High-power view of collagen fibrils within a principal fibre of the periodontal ligament. (a) Fibrils sectioned longitudinally; (b) fibrils sectioned transversely. The fibrils in longitudinal section display the banding characteristic of collagen. The fibrils in transverse section appear to be small and of uniform diameter (TEM; (a) × 16 000; (b) × 100 000).

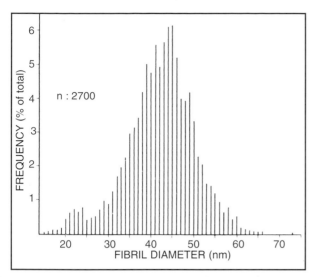

Fig. 12.8 Histogram showing the range of collagen fibril diameters in the periodontal ligament.

illustrated in Fig. 12.7(a) are sectioned longitudinally and show the classical banding characteristic of collagen. The collagen fibrils are formed by the packing together of individual tropocollagen molecules. The diameters of the collagen fibrils reflect the mechanical demands put upon the connective tissue. The collagen fibrils of the periodontal ligament are small and of uniform diameter (Fig. 12.7(b)). The histogram provided as Fig. 12.8 shows that, for the rat periodontal ligament, there is a sharply unimodal distribution of collagen fibrils (range ~20–70 nm) with a mode of approximately 42 nm. For humans, the mean is only slightly larger (50 nm). This confirms that the periodontal fibrils are small and of essentially uniform diameter. The pattern of distribution is reminiscent of collagen in connective tissues placed under compression and differs markedly from the bimodal distribution with large fibrils usually associated with tissues under tension (e.g. tendon). Recent research indicates that the distribution of periodontal

collagen alters neither with changes in periodontal function nor with age. The lack of change with age differs from many other fibrous connective tissues.

The principal collagen fibres show different orientations in different regions of the periodontal ligament (Figs 12.9– 12.13). They comprise: dentoalveolar crest fibres, horizontal fibres, oblique fibres, apical fibres and interradicular fibres. It has been usual to ascribe specific functions to each of the groups of principal fibres. For example, it has been suggested that the orientation of the oblique fibres shows that they form a suspensory ligament, which translates pressure on the tooth into tensional forces on the alveolar wall. However, no physiological evidence exists to support such a concept (see pages 201–203) and many of the structural features of the periodontal ligament (e.g. the collagen fibril diameters) suggest compression (see page 203).

Controversy exists concerning the extent of individual fibres across the width of the periodontal ligament. One view

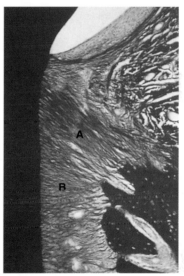

Fig. 12.10 The dentoalveolar crest fibres (A) and the horizontal fibres (B) of the periodontal ligament (Decalcified, longitudinal section through the ligament in the region of the alveolar crest; aldehyde Fuchsin and van Gieson; × 80).

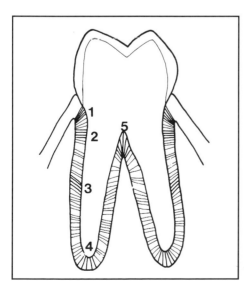

Fig. 12.9 The orientation of the principal fibres of the periodontal ligament seen in longitudinal section of a multirooted tooth: 1 = dentoalveolar crest fibres; 2 = horizontal fibres; 3 = oblique fibres; 4 = apical fibres; 5 = interradicular fibres.

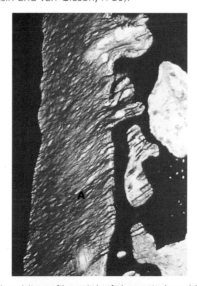

Fig. 12.11 The oblique fibres (A) of the periodontal ligament (Decalcified, longitudinal section; aldehyde Fuchsin and van Gieson; × 80).

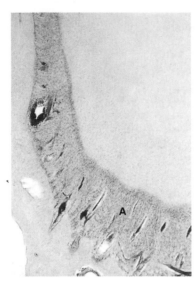

Fig. 12.12 The apical fibres (A) of the periodontal ligament (Decalcified, longitudinal section through the ligament in the region of the root apex; aldehyde Fuchsin and van Gieson; × 30).

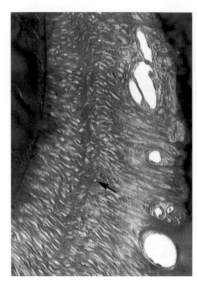

Fig. 12.14 Longitudinal section through the periodontal ligament producing an appearance of an intermediate plexus (arrowed) (Decalcified, longitudinal section; Alcian blue; × 200).

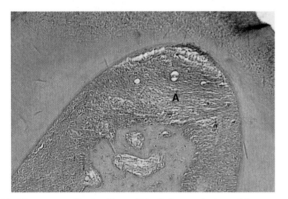

Fig. 12.13 Interradicular fibres (A) of the periodontal ligament (Decalcified, longitudinal section of the ligament in the region of a root bifurcation; orange green and light green; × 40). Courtesy of Dr R. O'Sullivan.

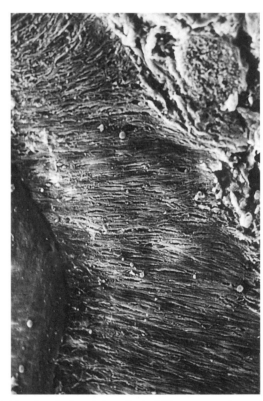

Fig. 12.15 Continuity of the principal fibres across the periodontal space seen in a periodontal ligament cut transversely (SEM; × 500). Courtesy of P. Sloan.

holds that there are distinct tooth-related and bone-related fibres, and that these intercalate near the middle of the ligament at an intermediate plexus (Fig. 12.14). However, recent evidence suggests that the fibres cross the entire width of the periodontal space but branch *en route* and join neighbouring fibres to form a complex three-dimensional network. While remodelling of fibres in the intermediate plexus provides a convenient model to explain how such axial tooth movements as eruption may be sustained, the plexus is usually seen only in longitudinal sections of continuously growing incisors (of rodents and lagomorphs): it is not seen in cross sections. Thus, the plexus is an artefact, probably related to the fact that the collagen fibres in the periodontal ligaments of continuously growing incisors are arranged mainly in the form of sheets rather than bundles. The continuity of the principal fibres across the periodontal space in teeth of non-continuous growth is displayed in Fig. 12.15. Here, no intermediate plexus can be seen, the fibres branching and joining with each other.

Despite the lack of histological evidence for an intermediate fibre plexus, it has been proposed that there is a 'zone of shear' – a site of remodelling during eruption. However, the location of this zone is in dispute. Some believe that it lies near the centre of the periodontal ligament, the relatively avascular, tooth-related part of the ligament moving with the erupting tooth. Studies using tritium-labelled proline have claimed that there is increased uptake in a zone in the mid-region of the periodontal ligament. However, other studies have been unable to support this, demonstrating uniform uptake of various labels over the whole width of the ligament. In contrast, counts of the number of intracellular collagen profiles in the periodontal fibroblasts (which indicate degenerating collagen: see page 190) indicate greater

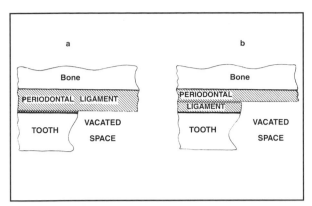

Fig. 12.16 The effects of root resection on the periodontal ligament and its significance to the 'zone of shear' and tissue remodelling. (a) The situation that would pertain if the zone of shear occurs centrally within the periodontal ligament – the tooth-related part of the ligament should move with the tooth, leaving behind the bone-related tissue only. (b) The whole width of the ligament is left behind the erupting tooth, indicating that the zone of shear is close to the tooth surface.

remodelling occurs in the centre of the tissue. The physiological significance of a central location for the zone of shear is thrown into doubt by experiments on the resected rodent incisor, which indicate that the zone of shear is close to the root surface (see Fig. 12.16). Root resection involves surgical removal of the growing base of the incisor. Because this tooth continues to erupt, it passes up the socket, leaving a space below its base. Accordingly, if the zone of shear occurs centrally within the periodontal ligament, the tooth-related part of the ligament should move with the tooth, leaving behind the bone- related tissue only. In fact, the whole width of the ligament is left behind the erupting tooth, indicating that the zone of shear is close to the tooth surface. This is further supported by experiments where lathyrogens – drugs that inhibit the formation of collagen cross links – are administered in the rodent diet: the lathyritic rat periodontal ligament is characterised by a longitudinal cleft down the ligament adjacent to the tooth surface.

The principal fibres of the periodontal ligament do not necessarily run a straight course as they pass from the region of the alveolar bone to the tooth. Indeed, they are said to be wavy, although it is not known whether the waviness is real or is an artefact of histological preparation. If real, it could have important implications for the biomechanical properties of the ligament and consequently the mechanism of tooth support (see pages 201–203). A specific type of waviness seen in collagenous tissues (including the periodontal ligament) is crimping. Collagen crimps are best seen under the polarising microscope (Fig. 12.17). The fibres are banded in polarised light, reflecting an underlying periodicity along the fibre. The period is about 16 μm and the angular deflection from the fibre axis in excess of 20°. It is important to realise that the banding does not rely on seeing shapes (waves in particular); the alternating dark and bright bands are evident in otherwise straight and smooth cylindrical fibres. Indeed, crimping can be displayed in a single teased-out collagen fibre from the periodontal ligament (Fig. 12.18) and the banding relates to the wavy course of the fibrils in the bundle. In functional

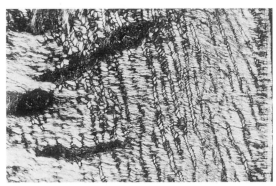

Fig. 12.17 Crimping of collagen in the periodontal ligament as viewed under polarised light. The fibres are seen to be banded between crossed polars, reflecting an underlying periodicity along the fibre (Transverse section of the central region of the rabbit incisor periodontal ligament; polarising optical micrograph; × 200). Courtesy of Professor P. Sloan.

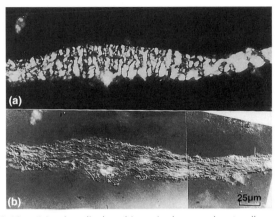

Fig. 12.18 Crimping displayed in a single teased-out collagen fibre from the periodontal ligament. (a) Polarising optical micrograph; (b) Nomarski differential interference contrast of same field as (a) (× 200). Courtesy of Dr L.J. Gathercole.

terms, it has been proposed that the crimp is gradually pulled out when the ligament is subjected to mechanical tension until it eventually disappears.

The principal fibres of the periodontal ligament that are embedded into cementum and the bone lining the tooth socket are termed **Sharpey's fibres** (Fig. 12.19). The principal fibres are more numerous but smaller at their attachments into cementum than at the alveolar bone. Under the electron microscope the mineralised parts of the Sharpey's fibres in alveolar bone (Fig. 12.20) appear as projecting stubs covered with mineral clusters. The occurrence of mineralisation at approximately right-angles to the long axes of the fibres may indicate that, in function, the fibres are subjected to tensional forces. The location and distribution of Sharpey's fibres from the periodontal collagen along the tooth socket is illustrated in Fig. 12.21. This diagram is conjectured from data obtained from a variety of species and suggests that the fibres near the alveolar crest show pronounced Sharpey's fibre insertions. Elsewhere, however, many of the principal fibres in the periodontal ligament do not insert into bone, but appear to terminate around the blood vessels of the ligament.

The rate of turnover of collagen within the periodontal ligament is faster than virtually all other connective tissues (half-

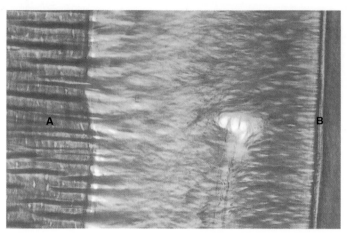

Fig. 12.19 The insertion of periodontal fibres into alveolar bone (A) and cementum (B). The horizontal lines in the bone and cementum represent the Sharpey's fibres (Decalcified section; aldehyde Fuchsin and van Gieson; × 250).

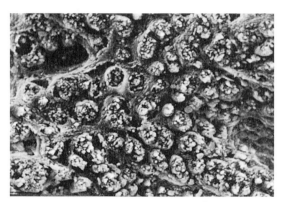

Fig. 12.20 SEM of Sharpey's fibres in the alveolar bone showing 'stub-like' appearance (× 300). Courtesy of Professor P. Sloan.

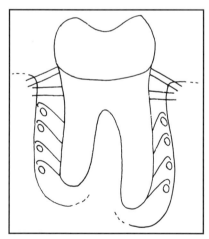

Fig. 12.21 The location and distribution of Sharpey's fibres from the periodontal collagen along the tooth socket.

life of collagen 3–23 days). The rate appears to vary in different parts of the same tooth, being highest towards the root apex. However, turnover seems to be relatively even across the width of the periodontal ligament, perhaps providing evidence against the existence of separate tooth-related and bone-related parts to the tissue (see pages 183–184). The explanation for

the high rate of turnover is not known, but it is reasonable to suppose that the high rate may relate to the considerable functional demands placed upon the tooth in terms of remodelling as a reaction to occlusal stress and to tooth movements. However, the ligaments of teeth subjected to greatly reduced masticatory loads do not show different rates of turnover from teeth subjected to normal loads. Furthermore, the turnover rate in teeth erupting very rapidly is no different from that in the ligaments of fully erupted teeth.

Recent studies indicate that measuring rates may not reflect total protein turnover and that there may be several protein pools having different turnover rates, each contributing to a different extent to overall protein turnover in the periodontal ligament. Indeed, control of matrix morphostasis may be more dependent on extracellular processing (e.g. fibrillogenesis, proteolysis) than upon initial rate of protein secretion. For example, far more collagen may be synthesised than is eventually secreted, the excess being degraded intracellularly without ever leaving the cell.

The high rate of turnover may also be reflected in the type of reducible cross link found in the periodontal collagen (i.e. dehydrodihydroxylysinonorleucine).

The possible role of the periodontal collagen in tooth support and tooth eruption is considered further on pages 201 and 352 respectively.

Oxytalan

Depending upon species, the periodontal ligament contains either oxytalan fibres or elastin fibres: in humans, it contains oxytalan fibres. In order to demonstrate periodontal oxytalan fibres at the light microscope level it is necessary to oxidise tissue sections strongly before staining with certain elastin stains. Unlike collagen, oxytalan fibres are not susceptible to acid hydrolysis. Although little is known about their composition, their ultrastructural characteristics suggest that they are immature elastin fibres (pre-elastin).

Oxytalan fibres are attached into the cementum of the tooth and course out into the periodontal ligament in various directions (Fig. 12.22), rarely being incorporated into bone. In the cervical region they follow the course of gingival and transseptal collagen fibres, but within the periodontal ligament proper they tend to be more longitudinally oriented, crossing the oblique fibre bundles more or less perpendicularly. In the outer part of the ligament, they are said to often terminate around blood vessels and nerves. Oxytalan fibres vary from 0.5 μm to 2.5 μm in diameter (as assessed with the light microscope) and constitute no more than about 3% of the extracellular fibre composition. The oxytalan fibre can be recognised at the ultrastructural level (Fig. 12.23) as a collection of unbanded fibrils arranged parallel to the long axis of the fibre. Each fibril is approximately 15 nm in diameter and an interfibrillar amorphous material is present in variable amounts. In cross section, the oxytalan fibre is oval and its dimensions are smaller than reported using the light microscope. They are thought to resemble pre-elastin in that, unlike mature elastin, there is no central amorphous core.

Fig 12.22 The course of oxytalan fibres (arrowed) (Decalcified, longitudinal section through the periodontal ligament; potassium monopersulphate, aldehyde fuchsin counterstained with van Gieson; (a) × 40; (b) × 120). Courtesy of Dr A.D. Beynon.

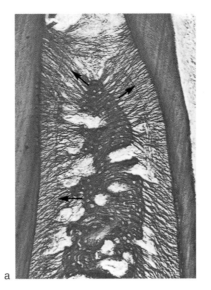
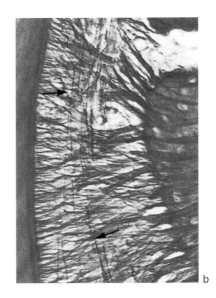

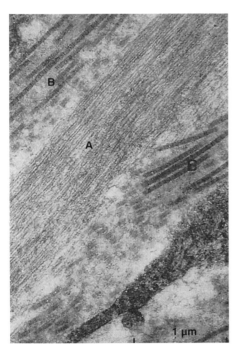

Fig. 12.23 TEM of an oxytalan fibre (A). B – collagen fibres (× 25 000).

The functions of the oxytalan fibres remain unknown and there is a paucity of experimental data. They are said to be thicker and more numerous in teeth that carry abnormally high loads, including abutment teeth for bridges and teeth being moved for orthodontic reasons. Thus, it appears that oxytalan may have a role in tooth support (perhaps also indicated by the relationship with the periodontal vasculature). However, experimental evidence shows that oxytalan fibres do not change with age or reduction in masticatory loading. Elastin fibres are restricted to the walls of the blood vessels, although in some animals (e.g. herbivores) they replace the oxytalan fibres. Reticulin fibres are related to basement membranes within the periodontal ligament (i.e. associated with blood vessels and epithelial cell rests) and are a variety of collagen.

Oxytalan microfibrils have a similar ultrastructure to the fibrils of fibronectin. In addition, they are stained strongly by immunohistochemical stains for fibronectin (Fig. 12.24). As fibronectin is important in fibroblast adhesion and migration, this would support the suggestion that oxytalan fibres aid fibroblast migration in the periodontal ligament.

GROUND SUBSTANCE OF THE PERIODONTAL LIGAMENT

Because of its relative inaccessibility and complex biochemical nature, little detailed information concerning this important component of the periodontal ligament is available. Although we are used to thinking of the ligament as a collagen-rich

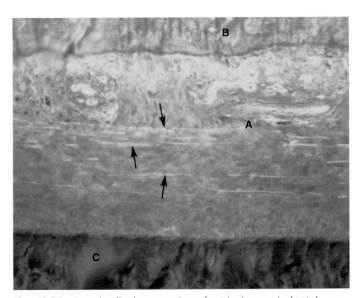

Fig. 12.24 Longitudinal cryosection of rat incisor periodontal ligament (A) with immunofluorescent staining for fibronectin showing positive staining (arrows) with the same longitudinal orientation as for oxytalan fibres. B = Alveolar bone; C = tooth (× 55). Courtesy of Professor P. Sloan and Mosby–Wolfe, London.

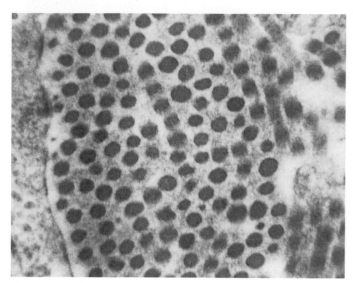

Fig. 12.25 Electron micrograph of the extracellular matrix of the periodontal ligament. About 60% by volume is ground substance (TEM; × 100 000).

stance in the periodontal ligament varies according to the developmental state of the tissue (Fig. 12.26) and according to location (Fig. 12.27). The data suggest that there is a marked change in the amount of hyaluronate as development proceeds from the dental follicle to the initial periodontal ligament, a trend that occurs during embryonic development of other connective tissues. Furthermore, a significant increase in the amount of proteoglycans occurs during eruption.

Much interest has been shown in a complex glycoprotein called fibronectin. This protein is thought to promote attachment of cells to the substratum, especially to collagen fibrils. Furthermore, as cells preferentially adhere to fibronectin, it may be involved in cell migration and orientation. Considering these functions together with the high rate of turnover in the periodontal ligament, it is not surprising that fibronectin may have considerable biological significance within the ligament. Immunofluorescent techniques at the light microscope level have revealed that fibronectin is uniformly distributed throughout the periodontal ligament in both erupting and fully erupted teeth. Ultrastructural studies have localised the glyco-

tissue, in reality it is a tissue rich in ground substance. Indeed, even the collagen fibre bundles are composed of about 60% ground substance by volume (Fig. 12.25).

The ground substance of the periodontal ligament consists mainly of hyaluronate glycosaminoglycans, proteoglycans and glycoproteins. The proteoglycans are compounds containing anionic polysaccharides (glycosaminoglycans) covalently attached to a protein core. Two proteoglycans have been isolated in the periodontal ligament: proteodermatan sulphate and a proteoglycan containing chondroitin sulphate/dermatan sulphate hybrids that has been designated PG1. All components of the periodontal ligament ground substance are presumed to be secreted by fibroblasts.

The ground substance is thought to have many important functions (ion and water binding and exchange, control of collagen fibrillogenesis and fibre orientation). Tissue fluid pressure is high in the periodontal ligament, about 10 mm Hg above atmospheric pressure, and the tissue fluid has been implicated in the tooth support and eruptive mechanisms (see page 355). Furthermore, the composition of the ground sub-

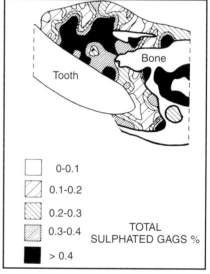

Fig. 12.27 Glycosaminoglycans (sulphated GAG) at different sites in the periodontal connective tissues (from sheep incisors). Courtesy of Professor J. Kirkham and the editor of *Archives of Oral Biology*.

Fig. 12.26 Glycosaminoglycans in the periodontal ligament at different stages of development (from bovine incisors). △ = Hyaluronate; □ = proteodermatan sulphate; ○ = PG1 proteoglycan. Group 1 specimens are of dental follicle. Group 2 is the initial stage of formation of the periodontal ligament. Sharpey's fibre attachments were discernible in Group 3. Groups 4 and 5 were for erupting teeth (the typical orientation of collagen fibres being first observed in Group 5). Group 6 specimens were from fully erupted teeth. HYP = Hydroxyproline, enabling determinations of ground substance components relative to collagen content. Courtesy of Dr C.H. Pearson and Pergamon Press.

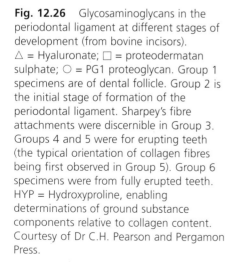
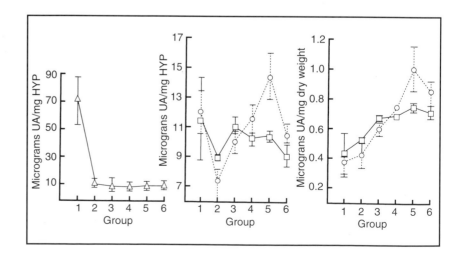

protein over collagen fibres and at certain sites on the cell–collagen interface. As loss of fibronectin has been observed during the terminal maturation of many connective matrices, its continued presence within the periodontal ligament may be indicative of the ligament retaining immature, fetal-like characteristics. Another glycoprotein (tenascin) has recently been identified in the periodontal ligament. Like fibronectin, tenascin is more characteristic of a fetal-like connective tissue than a fully 'mature' connective tissue. Unlike fibronectin, tenascin is not uniformly localised throughout the ligament but is concentrated adjacent to the alveolar bone and the cementum. The role of these glycoproteins in the functions of the periodontal ligament awaits clarification.

CELLS OF THE PERIODONTAL LIGAMENT

Although the predominant connective tissue cell within the periodontal ligament is the fibroblast, the tissue presents a heterogenous population (Fig. 12.28). Formative cells covering the surface of both cementum and alveolar bone (i.e. cementoblasts and osteoblasts) are considered part of the ligament and have a similar mesenchymal origin. Resorbing cells on the surface of bone and cementum are osteoclasts and cementoclasts; these are derived from a monocyte/macrophage lineage from the blood. In addition, the periodontal ligament contains undifferentiated mesenchymal cells, defence cells and epi-

thelial cells (rests of Malassez). The type and number of cells varies according to the functional state of the ligament.

Fibroblasts

The fibroblasts in the periodontal ligament are responsible for regeneration of the tooth support apparatus and have an essential role in the adaptive responses to mechanical loading of the tooth (including orthodontic loading). The periodontal ligament fibroblasts (Figs 12.29, 12.30) seem to have a variety of shapes with many fine cytoplasmic processes, although they are usually described as being fusiform. However, the overall shape can only be determined by consideration of the cell outlines in different planes. When this is done, the periodontal fibroblasts often appear as flattened, disc-shaped cells. Periodontal fibroblasts, being active cells, have low nuclear–cytoplasmic ratios, and each nucleus contains one or more prominent

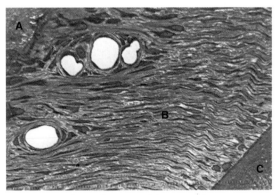

Fig. 12.29 A periodontal ligament (B) comprising numerous fibroblasts. A = Alveolar bone; C = cementum (Decalcified, longitudinal section through the periodontal ligament; Toluidine blue; × 300).

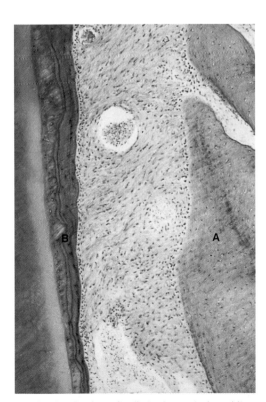

Fig. 12.28 The distribution of cells in the periodontal ligament. In addition to the numerous fibroblasts within the ligament, the surfaces of the alveolar bone (A) and cementum (B) are lined with osteoblasts and cementoblasts, indicating active deposition of bone and cementum in this specimen (Decalcified, longitudinal section through the periodontal ligament; H & E; × 80).

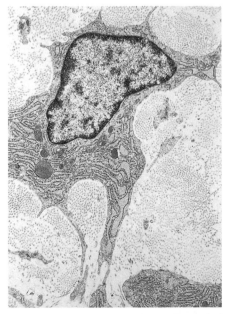

Fig. 12.30 Electronmicroscopic appearance of a periodontal fibroblast in vivo (TEM; × 4000).

nucleoli. The typical periodontal fibroblast is rich in the intracytoplasmic organelles associated with the synthesis and export of proteins: rough endoplasmic reticulum, Golgi apparatus and mitochondria (Fig. 12.30).

Much has been made of the possibility that the periodontal fibroblasts are motile–contractile cells, and that they are thereby capable of generating a force responsible for tooth eruption. Much of the evidence for migratory or contractile activities comes from research on the behaviour and appearance of periodontal fibroblasts *in vitro*. *In vitro*, periodontal fibroblasts can organise a fibrous network and can generate significant forces. However, the behaviour and appearance depends upon the method of culture. For example, cells cultured on plastic (Fig. 12.31) assume the properties of motile cells, are thin and highly polarised with respect to both shape and location of organelles. In particular, there are numerous microtubules and microfilaments (as stress fibres) that run along the length of the cell. Cells with these characteristics have not been seen in the periodontal ligament *in vivo*. Periodontal fibroblasts cultured on collagen gels (Fig. 12.32), during contraction of the gel, assume the appearance of myofibroblasts (see page 354), cells that have the properties of both fibroblasts and smooth muscle cells, and are found in contracting wounds. Myofibroblasts are characterised ultrastructurally by having polarity of shape, crenulated (folded) nuclei, and numerous microfilaments (as shown in Fig. 12.32). Adjacent cells contact by means of gap junctions. While periodontal fibroblasts *in vivo* may show occasional gap junctions (see Fig. 12.36b), they show no other features characteristic of myofibroblasts. Thus, although the evidence from *in vitro* studies suggests that the periodontal fibroblasts have the potential to be migratory or contractile cells, under normal functional conditions the cells are primarily involved in protein synthesis and secretion.

There is sufficient evidence, however, to show that there may be some localised movement of cells in the periodontal ligament *in vivo* and that the migration may be directed along the collagen fibres in an apicocoronal direction. Such migra-

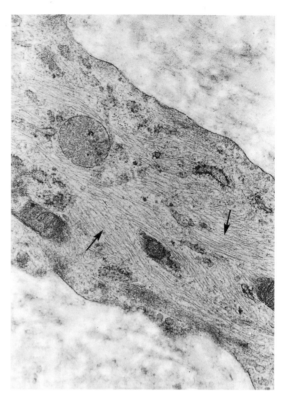

Fig. 12.32 The appearance of contractile periodontal fibroblasts cultured on collagen gels. Note the numerous microfilaments (arrows) (TEM; × 30 000). Courtesy of C.A. Shuttleworth.

tion is likely to be dependent on appropriate chemotactic stimuli. Evidence suggests that extracts from both bone and cementum have a potent chemotactic influence upon periodontal fibroblasts. The dependence of migratory behaviours upon the cytoskeleton and upon surface integrins has also been suggested. New populations of periodontal fibroblasts, osteoblasts and cementoblasts appear to arise from stem cells in the vicinity of blood vessels and then migrate to other regions of the ligament. However, how much the change in position of periodontal cells is due to active rather than passive movements (i.e. being carried with tooth movements) awaits clarification.

There is evidence that, in addition to synthesising and secreting proteins, the cells are responsible for collagen degradation. This contrasts with earlier views that degradation was essentially an extracellular event involving the activity of proteolytic enzymes such as collagenases. The main evidence indicating that the periodontal fibroblasts are also 'fibroclastic' is the presence of organelles termed intracellular collagen profiles (Figs 12.33, 12.34). These profiles show banded collagen fibrils within an elongated membrane-bound vacuole. It is thought that the intracellular collagen vacuoles are associated with the degradation of collagen that has been 'ingested' from the extracellular environment. The temporal sequence for intracellular digestion of collagen in the periodontal ligament is illustrated in Fig. 12.34. When a collagen fibril is first phagocytosed by the fibroblast, a banded fibril surrounded by an electron-lucent zone is seen. Subsequently, the banded fibrils are surrounded by an electron-dense zone. At this stage, the phagosome fuses with primary lysosomes to form a phagolysosome in which there is a gradual increase in electron density

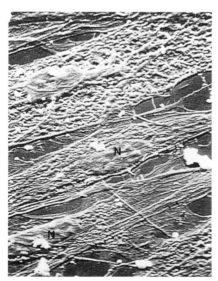

Fig. 12.31 The appearance of motile periodontal fibroblasts cultured on plastic. N = Nucleus (SEM; × 1200).

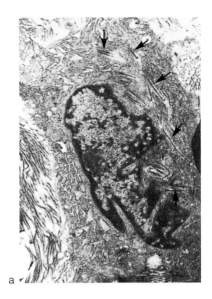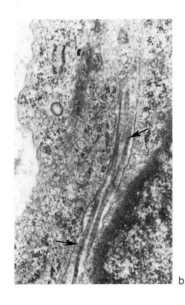

Fig. 12.33 (a) Periodontal fibroblast showing intracellular collagen profiles (arrowed) (TEM; × 5000) (b) Banded collagen fibrils (arrowed) seen within an elongated membrane-bound vacuole (TEM; × 25 000).

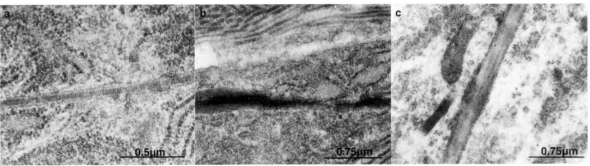

Fig. 12.34 The temporal sequence for intracellular digestion of collagen in the periodontal ligament. A, banded fibril surrounded by an electron-lucent zone. B, banded fibrils surrounded by an electron-dense zone. C, fibrils with indistinct banding surrounded by an electron-dense zone (TEM). Courtesy of Dr R.C. Shore and Moshy–Wolfe.

of the matrix. At the terminal stage the fibrils show indistinct banding and are surrounded by an electron-dense zone: enzymic degeneration of the fibril has proceeded to the point where the fibril loses its characteristic structure. The time taken to degrade collagen intracellularly is not known, although about 30 minutes has been suggested (a time similar to that required for synthesis).

It has been argued that the collagen profiles within periodontal fibroblasts are not truly intracellular and that the collagen merely lies in surface invaginations. If this were so, the degradation would still be an extracellular phenomenon. It has also been suggested that, because the periodontal fibroblasts may be synthesising collagen in excess of requirements, the profiles contain collagen that is being degraded without ever having been secreted extracellularly. Overall, however, the evidence suggests that the collagen is ingested from the extracellular compartment of the periodontal ligament and that the profiles are intracellular. Nevertheless, it is not known whether all periodontal fibroblasts are capable of phagocytosis.

The degradation of collagen may be expected to include both extracellular and intracellular events. Fibroblasts in the periodontal ligament secrete matrix metalloproteinase-1 (which degrades extracellular matrix collagen at physiological conditions) and can secrete tissue inhibitors of metalloproteinases (TIMPs). TIMPS are found in high concentrations at healthy periodontal sites.

Collagenase production and phagocytosis can be up-regulated after exposure to cytokines such as prostaglandin E2, IL-1 or lectin concanavalin A. Furthermore, because fibroblasts are induced to secrete prostaglandin when mechanical loads are applied, the periodontal fibroblasts may have 'intrinsic' mechanisms for remodelling the matrix. However, the precise role of collagenase in physiological remodelling awaits clarification as inhibition of its activity *in vitro* does not prevent the ingestion of collagen by fibroblasts.

The fibroblasts of the periodontal ligament have cilia and many intercellular contacts, a feature that is not particularly common in the fibroblasts of other fibrous connective tissues (intercellular contacts are a feature of fibroblasts in fetal-like connective tissues). Fig. 12.35 shows a cilium lying within an invagination of the cell membrane of a periodontal ligament fibroblast. The cilium differs from those seen in other cell types in that it contains no more than nine tubule doublets (compared to the usual '9 plus 2' configuration). The significance of the cilia in fibroblasts is unknown, although they may be associated with control of the cell cycle or inhibition of centriolar activity. The intercellular contacts (simplified desmosomes and gap junctions) between the fibroblasts of the periodontal ligament are shown in Fig. 12.36. The simplified desmosome is the most frequently seen of the contacts. There is little information concerning the

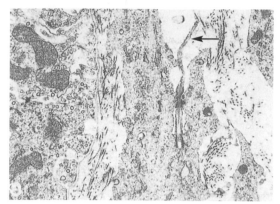

Fig. 12.35 A cilium (arrowed) lying within an invagination of the cell membrane of a periodontal ligament fibroblast (TEM; × 11 000).

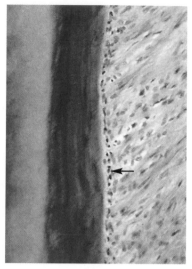

Fig. 12.37 A layer of cementoblasts (arrowed) lining the cementum (Decalcified, longitudinal section of periodontal ligament; H & E; × 160).

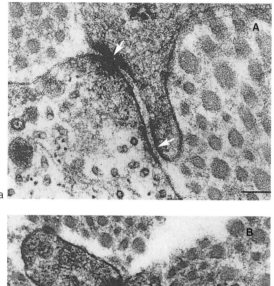

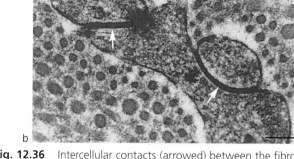

Fig. 12.36 Intercellular contacts (arrowed) between the fibroblasts of the periodontal ligament. A, simplified desmosome; B, gap junction (TEM; × 80 000).

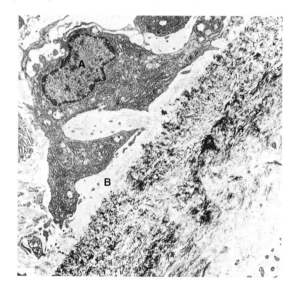

Fig. 12.38 A cementoblast (A) lining cementum. B = Precementum (TEM; × 3700).

functional significance of these organelles in the periodontal fibroblast.

Cementoblasts

The connective tissue cells of the periodontal ligament also include cementoblasts and cementoclasts, and osteoblasts and osteoclasts. Cementoblasts are the cement-forming cells lining the surface of cementum (Figs 12.37, 12.38). Cementoblasts are not as elongated as periodontal fibroblasts, being squat cuboidal cells. They are rich in cytoplasm and have large nuclei. Like fibroblasts, they contain all the intracytoplasmic organelles

necessary for protein synthesis and secretion. The nucleus of a cementoblast is distinctly vesicular, with one or more nucleoli. The appearance of a cementoblast will depend upon its degree of activity. Cells actively depositing acellular cementum do not have prominent cytoplasmic processes. However, cells depositing cellular cementum exhibit abundant basophilic cytoplasm and cytoplasmic processes, and their nuclei tend to be folded and irregularly shaped (see also pages 345–346).

Osteoblasts

Osteoblasts are the bone-forming cells lining the tooth socket (Fig. 12.39), closely resembling cementoblasts. The layer of osteoblasts is prominent only when there is active bone formation. Each osteoblast appears cuboidal and exhibits a basophilic cytoplasm that is related to the extensive endoplasmic reticulum within the cell. The prominent round nucleus tends to lie towards the basal end of the cell. A pale, juxtanuclear area indicates the site of the Golgi material. When bone is not forming, its surface is occupied by flattened, inactive bone-lining cells. Like the periodontal fibroblasts, active osteoblasts contain an extensive rough endoplasmic reticulum and numerous mitochondria and vesicles (Fig. 12.40) although their Golgi material appears more localised and extensive. Microfilaments are prominent beneath the cell membrane at the secreting surface. The cells contact one another by means of desmosomes and tight junctions. The cell surface adjacent to bone has many fine cytoplasmic processes, some of which contact underlying osteocytes by tight junctions to form part of a transport system throughout the bone (see also page 210).

Osteoclasts and cementoclasts

Osteoclasts and cementoclasts (or odontoclasts) are found in areas where bone and cementum are being resorbed. Recent evidence shows that these cells are actively involved in the resorption process. Osteoclasts and cementoclasts have the same cytoplasmic features. These cells are now known to arise from blood cells of the macrophage type. When osteoclasts resorb alveolar bone (Fig. 12.41) the surface of the alveolar bone shows resorption concavities termed Howship's lacunae, in which lie the osteoclasts. Osteoclasts show considerable variation in size and shape, ranging from small mononuclear cells to large multinuclear cells. The part of the cell that lies adjacent to bone often has a striated appearance, the so-called 'brush border' (Fig. 12.42). The brush border comprises many tightly packed microvilli which may be coated with fine, bristle-like structures. At the circumference of the brush border the plasma membrane tends to become smooth and the cytoplasm beneath it more dense. This modified annular zone may serve to limit the diffusion of hydrolytic enzymes, thereby creating a microenvironment in which resorption can take place. The osteoclast contains numerous mitochondria distributed

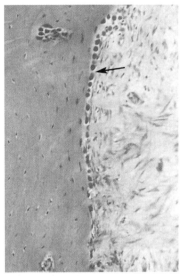

Fig. 12.39   A layer of osteoblasts (arrowed) lining the alveolar bone (Decalcified, longitudinal section of periodontal ligament, H & E; × 230).

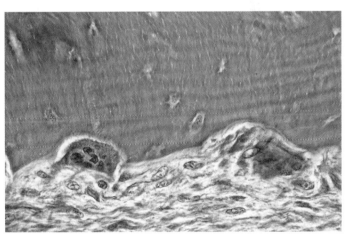

Fig. 12.41   Resorbing alveolar bone and the osteoclast. Resorption concavities termed Howship's lacunae in which lie osteoclasts are arrowed (Decalcified, longitudinal section of the periodontal ligament; H & E; × 250). Courtesy of Professor M.M. Smith.

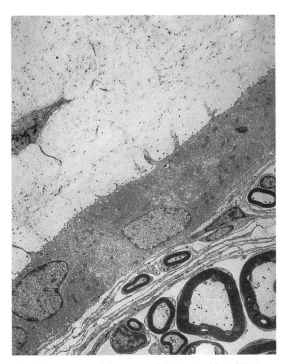

Fig. 12.40   Ultrastructural features of the osteoblast (TEM; Decalcified section. × 6000).

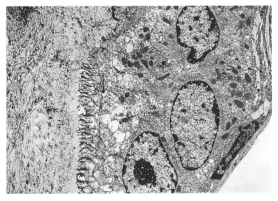

Fig. 12.42   Ultrastructural features of a multinucleated osteoclast. A = Brush border (TEM; × 3000). Courtesy of Dr R.C. Shore and Mosby–Wolfe.

throughout the cytoplasm, except for the region immediately beneath the brush border. The rough endoplasmic reticulum is less conspicuous than in osteoblasts, but Golgi material is prominent (especially in juxtanuclear areas). Most of the remaining cytoplasm contains large numbers of vesicles of different sizes and types; some contain acid phosphatase (see Fig. 13.16).

Epithelial cells

Aggregations of epithelial cell rests, the rests of Malassez (Fig. 12.43), are a normal feature of the periodontal ligament. They are said to be the remains of the developmental epithelial root sheath of Hertwig (see page 336). Epithelial rests can be distinguished from adjacent fibroblasts by the close packing of their cuboidal cells and their tendency to stain more deeply. The rests lie about 25 μm from the cementum surface. Differ-

ences have been observed in the distribution of epithelial cells according to site and age: during the first and second decades they are most prevalent in the apical zone; between the third and seventh decades the majority are located cervically in the gingiva above the alveolar crest. This might imply that they have a slow rate of turnover, which might be related to the presence of receptors for epidermal growth factor. That the cell rests are epithelial in origin is indicated by using immuno-fluorescent techniques for the detection of cytokeratins (Fig. 12.44).

In cross section, the epithelial cells appear cluster-like (Fig. 12.45), though tangential or serial sections show a network of interconnecting strands parallel to the long axis of the root (Fig. 12.46).

The ultrastructural appearance of the epithelial cell rests is illustrated in Fig. 12.47. The cluster arrangement of the cells is reminiscent of a duct-like structure. The cells are separated from the surrounding connective tissue by a basal lamina. The nucleus of each cell is prominent and often shows invaginations. The scanty cytoplasm is characterised by the presence of tonofibrils, some of which insert into the desmosomes that are frequently found between adjacent cells, and into hemi-desmosomes between the cells and the basal lamina. Tight junctions are also found between the cells. Mitochondria are distributed throughout the cytoplasm, while the rough endoplasmic reticulum and Golgi material are poorly developed. A primary cilium is often present, although its function is not understood. Histochemical and electron microscope studies

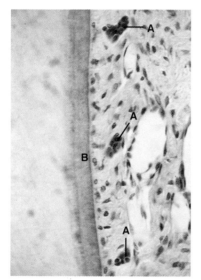

Fig. 12.43 The position of the epithelial rests (A) close to the cementum (B) (Decalcified section through periodontal ligament; H & E; × 240).

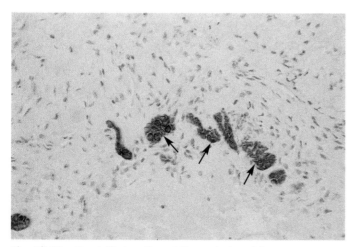

Fig. 12.44 Decalcified section of the periodontal ligament, showing positive brown staining for simple cytokeratins in epithelial cell rests (arrowed) (Immunohistochemistry; × 300). Courtesy of Dr A.E. Barrett.

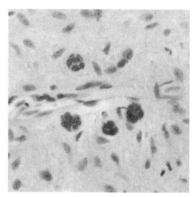

Fig. 12.45 Cluster-like appearance of epithelial rests (Decalcified section through periodontal ligament; H & E; × 250).

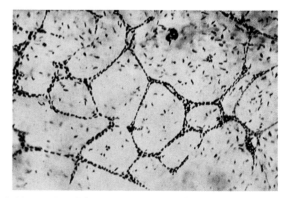

Fig. 12.46 Tangential section through the epithelial rests, showing a network appearance (Iron haematoxylin; × 60).

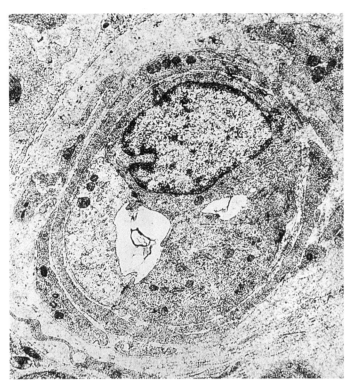

Fig. 12.47 Ultrastructural appearance of the epithelial cell rest (TEM; × 6100).

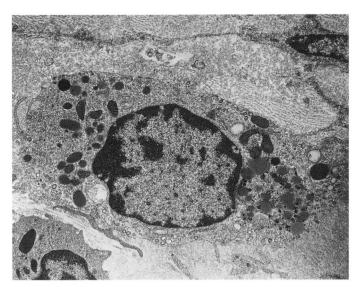

Fig. 12.48 Ultrastructural features of a macrophage (TEM; × 6000).

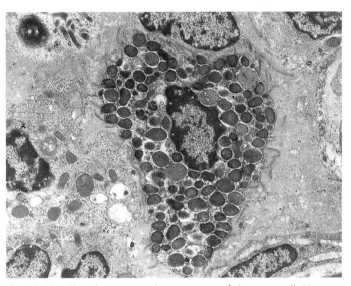

Fig. 12.49 The ultrastructural appearance of the mast cell. Note the numerous dense membrane-bound vesicles (TEM; × 5000).

reveal little activity in the epithelial cells, and cell turnover is slow (they can, however, be readily cultured), although they may proliferate to form cysts or tumours if appropriately stimulated (e.g. by chronic inflammation). Following orthodontic movement, there is no regeneration of the epithelial rests, although there is regeneration of connective tissue on the compression side. There is some evidence that secretory products from the epithelial cell rests could direct cellular events during cementogenesis and might inhibit cementogenesis in the mature tooth. *In vitro*, the cell rests are capable of phagocytosing collagen and synthesising metalloproteinases and prostaglandins.

Defence cells

Defence cells within the periodontal ligament include macrophages, mast cells and eosinophils. These are similar to defence cells in other connective tissues.

Macrophages make up about 4% of the periodontal ligament cell population (Fig. 12.48) and are responsible for phagocytosing particulate matter and invading organisms and synthesising a range of molecules with important functions such as interferon (the antiviral factor), prostaglandins and factors that enhance the growth of fibroblasts and endothelial cells. Macrophages are derived from blood monocytes. Their structure depends upon their site of activity. The resting macrophage differs from the fibroblast in that there is a paucity of rough endoplasmic reticulum, there are thin, finger-like projections from the cell surface, and many lysosomes and other membrane-bound vesicles of varying density. When active, macrophages have many mitochondria and vesicles and may possess many branching processes.

Mast cells (Fig. 12.49) are often associated with blood vessels. They show a large number of intracytoplasmic granules (which explains the intense staining reaction with basic analine dyes for light microscopy). The granules are dense, membrane-bound vesicles of varying sizes. Other cytoplasmic organelles are relatively sparse. When the cell is stimulated it degranulates. Numerous functions have been ascribed to the mast cell, including the production of histamine, heparin, and factors associated with anaphylaxis.

Eosinophils (Fig. 12.50) are only occasionally seen in the normal periodontal ligament. Characteristically they possess granules (peroxisomes) that consist of one or more crystalloid structures. The cells are capable of phagocytosis.

The various cells of the periodontal ligament are capable of synthesising and releasing bioactive molecules such as cytokines, growth factors and cell adhesion molecules. These are important when considering the biology of the tissues. Many

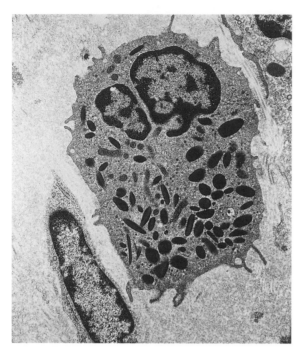

Fig. 12.50 The ultrastructural features of an eosinophil. Note the characteristic granules (peroxisomes) (TEM; × 2500).

of these substances are upregulated during orthodontic tooth movement.

CELL KINETICS IN THE PERIODONTAL LIGAMENT

The actual mechanisms that contribute to the development of cellular lineages in the periodontal ligament are unknown and the cellular hierarchies in fibroblast populations of adult mammalian periodontal tissues are poorly understood, in part due to the lack of clear-cut phenotypic markers. Nevertheless, some reports suggest that there is significant morphological heterogeneity among periodontal cells. For example, there are said to be varying nuclear sizes (perhaps related to different capacities for undergoing cell division), a feature that has been claimed to provide a system for identifying the various cells in the osteoblast lineage. Other quantitative electron microscopy studies, however, indicate that the cells are remarkably homogeneous. Furthermore, morphological diversity is not itself indicative of functional heterogeneity.

Periodontal fibroblasts comprise a renewal cell system in steady-state and the progenitors can generate multiple cell types of more differentiated, specialised cells. Renewal systems are characterised by a balance between newly generated cells and cells lost by apoptosis and migration out of the tissue.

Progenitor cell populations of the periodontal ligament are located adjacent to the blood vessels near the surface of the alveolar bone and in the contiguous endosteal spaces. At the blood vessels some of the cells exhibit the classical features of stem cells – small size, responsiveness to stimulating factors and slow cycle time. Grafting experiments suggest that the tooth-related part of the ligament also contains cementoblast precursors (that have no paravascular association) whilst the bone-related part contains osteoblast precursors. Tritiated thymidine injections show that mitotic cells appear at paravascular sites and then migrate towards the bone surface. In addition, cells from the vascular channels within alveolar bone migrate towards the periodontal ligament. It has also been reported that there is a significant migration of periodontal cells to the surface of the alveolar bone with orthodontic tooth movement.

In normal periodontal ligament, the rate of cell generation (mitotic index) is modest (0.5–3%; the higher level has been found in the central part of the periodontal ligament where there is the least cell density). Such variation may be related to diurnal periodicity, or to location within the ligament, as well as to individual variation. As for other periodontal tissues, there is a reduction of the mitotic index with age, although this rate is relatively rapid for a soft connective tissue. Cell mitosis and cell differentiation increase markedly with wounding or after the application of orthodontic loads.

As osteoblasts and cementoblasts of the periodontal ligament become incorporated into alveolar bone and cellular cementum, replacement cells must be provided within the ligament to permit osteogenesis and cementogenesis to continue. A major question concerns whether periodontal fibroblasts, cementoblasts and osteoblasts all arise from a common precursor or whether each cell type has its own specific precursor cell. Although progenitor cells can be identified by their ability to incorporate tritium-labelled thymidine, little is known about their origin and life cycle. One of the problems of answering this question is the lack of specific markers to distinguish fibroblasts, osteoblasts and cementoblasts (and their precursors). However, progress is being made and the combined use of markers such as type I and III collagens (present in periodontal fibroblasts), bone sialoprotein and osteocalcin (present in cementoblasts and osteoblasts) receptors to epidermal growth factor (present in periodontal fibroblasts and possibly osteoblasts) may help alleviate the problem.

Dividing cells are located predominantly paravascularly and migrate towards the bone and cementum surfaces. During normal physiological orthodontic loading and wounding it has been reported that there is a relatively low mitotic index. However, orthodontic pressure and injury may recruit progenitors that are distinctly different cell types (osteoblastic versus fibroblastic respectively).

The presence of binding sites for epidermal growth factor (EGF) on periodontal fibroblasts is said to have an important role in their differentiation. Recently, it has been shown that numerous receptors for epidermal growth factor (EGF-Rs) are expressed on the cells of the periodontal ligament, particularly for fibroblasts, paravascular cells and pre-osteoblasts. However, they are not expressed on fully differentiated cementoblasts and osteoblasts. Such observations have led to the hypothesis that the fibroblast phenotype in the periodontal ligament requires the continued expression of EGR-Rs and that they inhibit their differentiation into mineralised tissue-forming cells. When exposed to EGF, periodontal fibroblasts showed slightly increased mitogenic and chemotactic responses

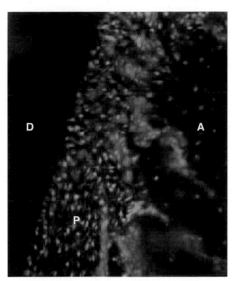

Fig. 12.51 Labelling for apoptosis within the periodontal ligament using the TUNEL technique. D = Root dentine of a rat second molar in an aged animal; P = periodontal ligament showing many positively labelled green apoptotic cells (such cells are absent in the non-aged tissue); A = Alveolar bone (TUNEL fluoresecent micrograph; × 120). Courtesy of J.M. Pycroft.

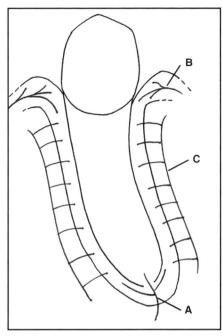

Fig. 12.52 The blood supply to the periodontal ligament. A = Arteries from dental pulp; B = arteries from gingion; C = arteries from alveolar bone.

but decreased collagen synthesis. It has also been reported that platelet-derived growth factor (-AB and -BB) and insulin-like growth factor-I have potent mitogenic and chemotactic effects on the cells of the periodontal ligament. Furthermore, platelet-derived growth factor stimulates collagen synthesis. In contrast, transforming growth factor (TGF-β) had only slight chemotactic effects and inhibited mitogenic responses.

In contrast to periodontal ligament fibroblasts, gingival fibroblasts belong to two progenitor cell populations: one with limited proliferative capacity, the other having extensive self-renewal capacity. These differences are considered further on page 241.

Apoptosis (programmed cell death) is not a common feature in the mature connective tissues of the periodontal ligament. In the aged animal, however, many of the cells are apoptotic (Fig. 12.51) and this is supported by immunocytochemical studies that show a reduced level of focal adhesions in the cells of the aged tissues.

Upregulation of the enzyme focal adhesion kinase within the periodontal ligament is seen during a phase of maximum eruption of the tooth (particularly at the root base) and this feature is associated with upregulation of proliferating cell-nuclear antigen.

BLOOD VESSELS AND NERVES OF THE PERIODONTAL LIGAMENT

Blood supply

The rich blood supply to the periodontal ligament is derived from the appropriate superior and inferior alveolar arteries, although arteries from the gingiva (such as the lingual and palatine arteries) may also be involved (Fig. 12.52). The arteries

supplying the periodontal ligament are not primarily derived from those entering the pulp at the apex of the tooth, but from a series of perforation arteries passing through the alveolar bone. The dual source of the main arterial supply allows the periodontal ligament to function following removal of the root apex as a result of various endodontic treatments.

The major vessels of the periodontal ligament lie between the principal fibre bundles, close to the wall of the alveolus

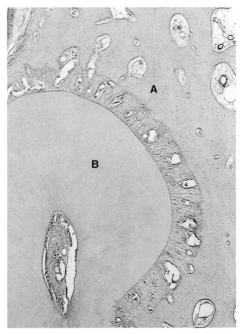

Fig. 12.53 Transverse section through a periodontal ligament to show blood vessels lying close to alveolar bone. A = Alveolar bone; B = dentine (van Gieson; × 30).

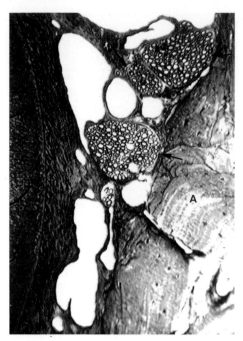

Fig. 12.54 Semithin section of periodontal ligament showing large bood volume in the periodontal space. Nerve bundles are arrowed. A = Aveolar bone; B = dentine (Toluidine blue; × 100).

(Fig. 12.53). They have an average diameter of 20 μm. The vessels branch and anastomose to form a capillary plexus around the teeth. Semithin sections of periodontal ligament show that the blood vessels are seen as large spaces (Fig. 12.54). Indeed, the volume of the periodontal space occupied by blood vessels and by blood may be so great that we should perhaps think of the periodontal ligament as a 'blood space' as much as a 'connective tissue'!

Specialised features of the vasculature of the periodontal ligament vasculature are a crevicular plexus of capillary loops and the presence of large numbers of fenestrations in the capillaries. A crevicular plexus of capillary loops (Fig. 12.55) completely encircles the tooth within the connective tissue beneath the region of the gingival crevice. Each loop consists of one or two thin (8–10 μm in diameter) capillary ascending limbs and one or two postcapillary sized venules. The crevicular capillary loops are separated from other more marginally situated loops in the gingival surface by a distinct gap and arise from a circular plexus, which is composed of 1–4 inter-communicating vessels (6–30 μm in diameter) lying at the level of the junctional epithelium. The circular plexus anastomoses with both the gingival and periodontal ligament vessels. Species differences may occur in the pattern of the vasculature, which may also be affected by inflammation. More complex glomerular-like structures have also been described. The functional significance of the complex vasculature in this region is not fully understood, although it may be related to the provision of a dentogingival seal. It may provide a means for

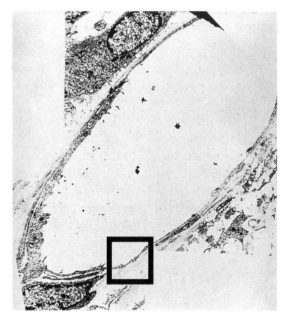

Fig. 12.56 Fenestrated capillaries within the periodontal ligament. Note the thinning of the endothelium in the boxed area, where fenestrations are present (TEM; × 10 000).

Fig. 12.55 A crevicular plexus of capillary loops (A). B = Capillary loops in the gingival surface; C = circular plexus; arrow indicates gap between crevicular and circular plexuses (SEM of vascular cast; × 80). Courtesy of Professor M.R. Sims.

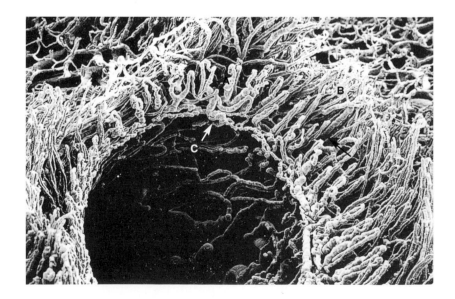

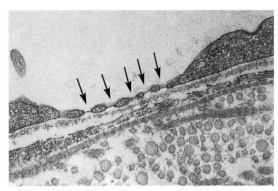

Fig. 12.57   Fenestrated capillaries within the periodontal ligament. This is a higher power view of the boxed area shown in Fig. 12.57. Arrows indicate the fenestrations (TEM; × 35 000).

blood flow reversal and rapid redistribution of the blood under varying occlusal loads and as a reaction to pathological stimuli.

Fenestration of capillaries within the periodontal ligament (Figs 12.56, 12.57) is unusual because fibrous connective tissues usually have continuous capillaries. The presence of fenestrated capillaries in large numbers (up to $40 \times 10^6/mm^3$ of tissue) is therefore a specialised feature of the periodontal ligament. Fenestrated capillary beds differ from continuous capillary beds in that the diffusion and filtration capacities are greatly increased. It is possible that the fenestrations are related to the high metabolic requirements of the periodontal ligament (high rate of turnover). Experimental evidence suggests that the number of fenestrations also relates to the stage of eruption.

The veins within the periodontal ligament do not usually accompany the arteries. Instead, they pass through the alveolar walls into intraalveolar venous networks. Anastomoses with veins in the gingiva also occur. A dense venous network is particularly prominent around the apex of the alveolus.

Innervation

The nerve fibres supplying the periodontal ligament are functionally of two types: sensory and autonomic. The sensory fibres are associated with nociception and mechanoreception. The autonomic fibres are associated mainly with the supply of the periodontal blood vessels. Compared with other dense fibrous connective tissues, the periodontal ligament is well innervated (Fig. 12.58).

The nerve fibres entering the periodontal ligament are derived from two sources. Some nerve bundles enter near the root apex and pass up through the periodontal ligament; others enter the middle and cervical portions of the ligament as finer branches through openings in the alveolar walls.

Periodontal nerve fibres are both myelinated and unmyelinated. The myelinated fibres are on average about 5 μm in diameter (although some are as large as 15 μm) and are sensory fibres only. The unmyelinated fibres are about 0.5 μm in diameter and are both sensory and autonomic.

At the light microscope level, a plethora of forms that are assumed to represent nerve endings have been described within the periodontal ligament. These forms vary from simple free endings to more elaborate arborising structures, although they still only mediate two sensory modalities – pain or pressure.

Most attention has been paid to the periodontal mechanoreceptors. The discharge of afferent impulses from mechanoreceptors has been recorded from single nerve fibres dissected free from the inferior alveolar nerve in animals. The discharge appears to vary according to the direction and amplitude of

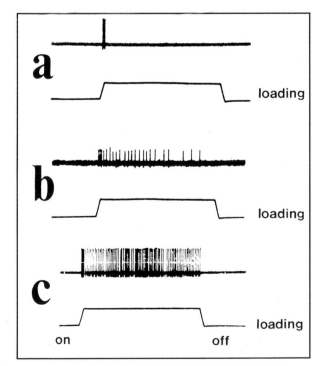

Fig. 12.59   The responses of three periodontal ligament mechanoreceptors to suprathreshold ramp-plateau stimuli of 1N (duration 3 s; rise time 50 ms). a = Rapidly adapting response; b = intermediate adapting response; c = slowly adapting response. The receptors were located in the same tooth: a, 1.5 mm; b, 3.0 mm; c, 5.5 mm from the fulcrum. Courtesy of Professor R.W.A. Linden.

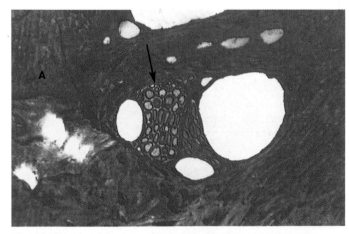

Fig. 12.58   The rich nerve supply (arrow) to the periodontal ligament. A = Alveolar bone. (Decalcified, transverse section through a tooth and its periodontal ligament; Toluidine blue; × 150).

the displacing force. Periodontal mechanoreceptors exhibit directional sensitivity in that they respond maximally to a force applied to the crown of the tooth in one particular direction. Their conduction velocities place them within the Aβ group of fibres. The response characteristics can vary from slowly adapting through to rapidly adapting fibres (Fig. 12.59). The question arises as to whether the slowly adapting, intermediate adapting and rapidly adapting mechanoreceptors are truly different types of receptor. Where it has been possible to examine histologically nerve endings that have been physiologically characterised, it seems that the endings of the mechanoreceptors are all similar, being unencapsulated Ruffini-like terminals. Furthermore, the response characteristics (i.e. whether slowly or rapidly adapting) are dependent upon the position of the ending within the ligament relative to the position of loading.

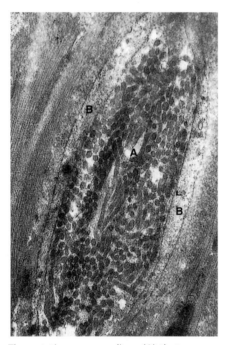

Fig. 12.60 The putative nerve endings (A) that may represent Ruffini-like mechanoreceptors in the periodontal ligament. B = Ensheathing Schwann-type cell. Note the large number of mitochondria (TEM; × 5700).

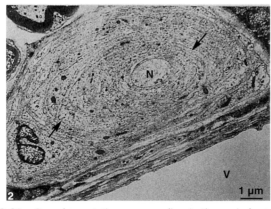

Fig. 12.61 Complex putative nerve ending in the periodontal ligament. Arrow indicates numerous circularly arranged cell processes; N = nerve terminal; V = blood vessel (TEM; × 4500).

Putative nerve endings, which may represent mechanoreceptors, are characterised by the very large concentrations of mitochondria in the unmyelinated terminations of myelinated nerves (Fig. 12.60). The surrounding process of the ensheathing Schwann-type cell is noteworthy and this type of ending is regarded as being akin to a Ruffini-like nerve terminal. Even more complex putative nerve endings have very occasionally been observed within the periodontal ligament (Fig. 12.61). These are characterised by numerous circularly arranged cell processes surrounding a central structure containing microfilaments, microtubules and mitochondria. This central structure is thought to represent a nerve terminal. The morphology of this lamellated structure is reminiscent of cutaneous mechanoreceptors of the Paccinian type. However, because of their rarity, their significance in the periodontal ligament is unknown.

It has been suggested that about 75% of mechanoreceptors within the periodontal ligament have their cell bodies in the trigeminal ganglion while the remaining 25% of cell bodies lie in the mesencephalic nucleus.

The cell bodies of the ensheathing Schwann-type cells contain rough endoplasmic reticulum and the nucleus may be indented (Fig. 12.62). Numerous vesicles may be observed within, and forming on, both the inner and outer surfaces of the ensheathing cells. These vesicles may be associated with rapid transport of materials to and from the nerve terminal. The collagen in the immediate vicinity of the nerve ending appears to be arranged in a lamellar pattern.

Little is known about pain fibres within the periodontal ligament, but it is presumed that, as elsewhere in the body, they are represented by fine, unmyelinated fibres terminating

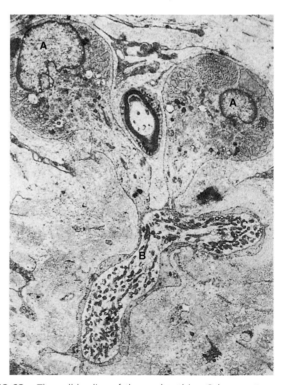

Fig. 12.62 The cell bodies of the ensheathing Schwann-type cells. A = Indented nuclei; B = mitochondria-rich nerve terminal (TEM; × 5000).

as free nerve endings. A similar lack of information exists concerning the fine (0.2–1 µm diameter) autonomic fibres. These fibres are important in the control of regional blood flow, having vasoconstrictor activity. Thus, experiments affecting the sympathetic system are seen to produce changes in tooth position.

As for the pulp, sensory nerve endings in the periodontal ligament can release neuropeptides such as substance P, vasoactive intestinal peptide and calcitonin gene-related peptide. These substances can have widespread effects on blood vessels and cells and must have an important, but as yet undetermined, role in the biology of the ligament. Many of them are upregulated during orthodontic tooth movement.

THE PERIODONTAL LIGAMENT AS A SPECIALISED CONNECTIVE TISSUE

Although the periodontal ligament has the same components as other soft, fibrous connective tissues (i.e. it is composed essentially of an unmineralised collagen and proteoglycan stroma in which are found connective tissue cells), it has the following features that, in combination, provide a specialised tissue.

- The principal collagen fibres have a characteristic orientation.
- The types (and amounts) of collagen (types I and III) and the variety of collagen cross links are unlike those found within most other adult fibrous connective tissues.
- In some species, a pre-elastin-like fibre (oxytalan) is present within the periodontal ligament.
- The rate of turnover of the periodontal ligament is very fast.
- The periodontal ligament is remarkably cellular and rich in ground substance.
- The type of proteoglycan in the periodontal ligament (PG1) is specific to this tissue.
- The tissue hydrostatic pressure may be high.
- The periodontal ligament fibroblasts have features unusual for fibroblasts in adult fibrous connective tissues (e.g. many intercellular contacts, cilia).
- The periodontal ligament has cells concerned with the formation of dental tissues.
- The periodontal ligament has a rich vascular and nerve supply.
- The capillaries within the periodontal ligament are fenestrated.

However, the mere listing of these specialised characteristics does not permit inference of the role of these features in the function and pathobiology of the tissue. To do this, we need to discover whether there are structural and/or biochemical analogues for the periodontal ligament elsewhere in the body.

Initially, an analogue for the periodontal ligament was sought in mature (adult) fibrous connective tissues with known mechanical demands (i.e. connective tissue placed under either tension or compression). However, such comparisons showed that the periodontal ligament had some characteristics of a tissue under tension and others suggestive of compression (see pages 202–203). More recently, it has been shown that the periodontal ligament resembles immature, fetal-like connective tissues.

The periodontal ligament and fetal connective tissues (mesenchyme) have the following common features:

- High rates of turnover.
- Sharp, unimodal size/frequency distributions of small collagen fibrils.
- Significant amounts of type III collagen.
- The major reducible cross link is the collagen dehydro-dihydroxylisinonorleucine.
- Changes in collagen fibrils with lathyrogens.
- Large volumes of ground substance.
- High content of glucoronate-rich proteoglycans.
- High contents of the glycoproteins tenascin and fibronectin.
- Presence of pre-elastin fibres (oxytalan in the periodontal ligament).
- High cellularity, the fibroblast-like cells passing numerous intercellular contacts.
- Similar biomechanical properties.

The functional significance of the periodontal ligament being fetal-like relates to the fact that the structural, ultrastructural and biochemical features of the tissue do not depend primarily upon mechanical demands. Indeed, the high rates of turnover may have a greater role in determining the characteristics of the periodontal ligament.

The fetal-like characteristics of the periodontal ligament also may aid our understanding of inflammatory periodontal disease. First, it is well known that processes involved in wound healing in fetal connective tissues differ markedly from those in adult tissues; consequently, our understanding of repair/periodontal reattachment may benefit from an appreciation of the mode of repair of fetal wounds. Second, it has been proposed that periodontal defects produced by inflammatory periodontal disease may be corrected by grafting of connective tissues. At present, adult-type connective tissues have been tried with varying success. Perhaps grafting of fetal-like connective tissues may be more appropriate.

THE TOOTH SUPPORT MECHANISM

The tooth support mechanism describes the manner whereby the periodontal ligament resists the axially directed intrusive loads that occur during biting.

It is still frequently stated that the periodontal ligament behaves as a 'suspensory ligament' during masticatory loading. Accordingly, loads on the tissue are dissipated to the alveolar bone primarily through the oblique principal fibres of the ligament, which, being placed in tension, are analogous to the guy-ropes of a tent. On release of the load there is elastic recoil of the tissue, which enables the tooth to recover its resting position. The essentially elastic responses of the periodontal ligament during both loading and recovery imply that the tissue obeys Hooke's Law. However, tooth mobility studies, surgical studies and morphological and biochemical studies have provided evidence against the notion that the periodontal ligament is a suspensory ligament.

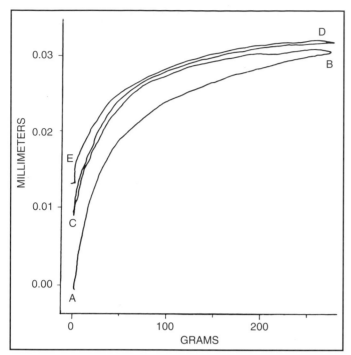

Fig. 12.63 Axial load/mobility curve for a human maxillary incisor to show hysteresis. A = Initial position of tooth; B = position at peak force on the first application of load; C = return point on removal of load; D = position at peak force on second application; E = return point after second removal of load. Note the lack of straight-line relationship between load and displacement (expected for elastic responses) and also that successive loads and recovery cycles pass along different paths (i.e. there are hysteresis loops). Courtesy of Professor G.W. Parffit and the editor of *Journal of Dental Research*.

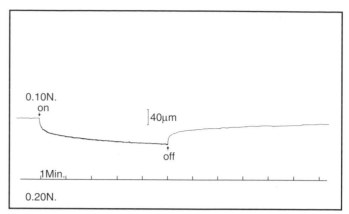

Fig. 12.64 The viscoelastic responses of a tooth observed with an axially directed intrusive load. This is a pen recorder race of tooth position which shows the effect of applying a load and then sustaining the load for a period of 5 minutes. Note the time dependency of the response, which is biphasic. The first phase is an elastic phase, the more gradual second phase is indicative of the property of creep (i.e. a viscous phase. The recovery responses are also biphasic and suggestive of viscoelasticity. Courtesy of Professor B.S. Moxham and Dr A. Coehlo and the editor of *Archives of Oral Biology*.

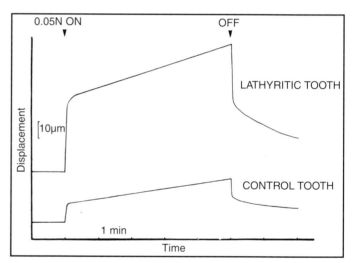

Fig. 12.65 The effects of lathyrogens on tooth support. This experiment assesses the effects of the drug on axially directed extrusive loads. Note the significant increase in mobility for the tooth in the lathyritic animal, which suggests a role for the periodontal collagen in tooth support. However, the precise mechanism of action remains elusive since the patterns of mobility are the same for normal and lathyritic animals. Courtesy of the editor of *Archives of Oral Biology*.

Physiological tooth mobility studies provide information concerning the basic biomechanical properties of the periodontal ligament. They rely upon analysis of the patterns of mobility when loading teeth whose periodontal tissues have not been altered experimentally. These studies show that the ligament: does not obey Hooke's law during loading and recovery (Fig. 12.63), shows the property of hysteresis (Fig. 12.63), and exhibits responses whose time dependency suggests that the tissue has viscoelastic properties (Fig. 12.64). Furthermore, the patterns of loading are not dependent on the direction of the load relative to the orientation of the principal fibres in the periodontal ligament and, for loads of similar magnitude, the amount of displacement for an axially directed intrusive load is greater than for an extrusive load.

Experimental tooth mobility studies rely upon investigating the effects on the patterns of mobility obtained following alterations to a specific component of the periodontal ligament. Experiments with lathyrogens (drugs which specifically inhibit the formation of collagen cross links and disrupt the fibrous network of the periodontal ligament; Fig. 12.65), with vasoactive drugs and following surgical disruption of the periodontal ligament indicate that both the periodontal collagen fibres and the periodontal vasculature are involved in tooth support.

In experiments where the apical half of the periodontal ligament was removed and the tooth loaded to assess the effects on its mobility no effects were observed; consequently it was argued that the ligament did not behave as a compressive structure because it was presumed that only the tissue around the root apex could behave in this manner. Subsequent experiments performed to assess the role of tension in the more cervically situated principal fibres of the ligament have shown that the periodontal ligament around the alveolar crest could also be removed without major changes in tooth mobility. These experiments therefore do not provide definitive evidence for or against tension or compression in the periodontal ligament but do suggest that, even where there is marked trauma to a region of the ligament, the remaining tissue can still perform a supporting function in the short term.

Some morphological evidence suggesting that the periodontal collagen is placed in tension during masticatory loading comes from study of the Sharpey's fibre attachments and from the collagen crimps. As mentioned previously (see page 185), the Sharpey's fibres appear as mineralised stubs projecting into the periodontal ligament from the wall of the alveolus. The occurrence of mineralisation at approximately right-angles to the long axes of the fibres has been adduced as evidence that the fibres are under tension. However, even if this were the case, the distribution of Sharpey's fibres along the alveolus indicates that they are limited mainly to the region of the alveolar crest (see Fig. 12.21). The crimping of collagen in the periodontal ligament was described on page 185. Evidence from connective tissue elsewhere in the body (particularly from tendons) suggests that the crimps are involved in the initial stages of loading, allowing some degree of movement before the tissue is placed under tension.

Morphological and biochemical comparisons between the periodontal ligament and other connective tissues known to be under tension or compression have been undertaken to throw some light on the role of the periodontal ligament in tooth support. This has been undertaken on the assumption that the structure of a connective tissue is dictated by the mechanical demands placed upon it. Table 12.1 shows the results of such a comparison. Whereas some features of the periodontal ligament suggest a tensional mode of activity, many of the features indicate a compressive mode. Indeed, experiments involving relatively long-term changes in the mechanical demands placed upon the tissue (e.g. pinning a tooth to completely prevent tooth movements) produced no major changes in the structure of the periodontal ligament and provided evidence for the view that the ligament is not as affected by the mechanical demands placed upon it as tissues elsewhere in the body.

Recent biochemical analysis of the proteoglycans within the periodontal ligament and under different loading regimes shows

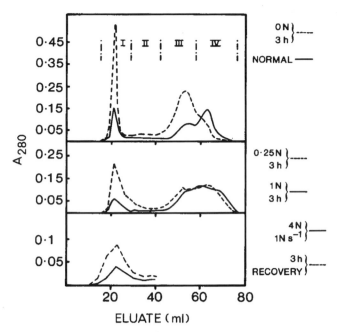

Fig. 12.66 Molecular size profiles of periodontal ligament proteoglycans following various degrees of intrusive loadings of macaque monkey teeth. Top = High-molecular-weight fraction (peak I) increased when the periodontal ligament is undisturbed for 3 hours; middle = decrease in peak I size between 0.25 N and 1 N loads; bottom = further decrease in peak I size with 4 N loads followed by an increase during a 3-hour undisturbed recovery phase. Courtesy of Professor C. Embery and the editor of *Archives of Oral Biology*.

that the degree of aggregation/disaggregation of the ground substance may have a role in tooth support (Fig. 12.66). Where teeth are unloaded for a period of 3 hours, a high-molecular-weight fraction within the periodontal ligament is greatly increased. On the other hand, with loads between 0.25 N and 1 N, this fraction is greatly reduced. Loads of 4 N are associated with a further decrease, followed by an increase during a 3-hour undisturbed recovery phase.

There is thus evidence that the collagen fibres, vasculature and ground substance of the periodontal ligament are all involved in tooth support. Consequently, the mechanism of tooth support should not be regarded as a property of a single component of the periodontal ligament, but as a function of the tissue as a whole.

CLINICAL CONSIDERATIONS

The most important clinical condition affecting the periodontal ligament is chronic inflammatory periodontal disease, when toxic products released by dental plaque (and the host's defence mechanisms) result in the destruction and loss of periodontal ligament tissue and adjacent alveolar bone. Such a process results in the formation of a deeper periodontal pocket and the vicious circle continues. The loss of attachment tissue will expose the root of the tooth in the mouth, increasing tooth mobility, and the tooth may eventually be

Table 12.1 *Relationship betwen the ultrastructural features of the periodontal ligament and mechanical properties*

Features of the periodontal ligament suggesting tension	Features of the periodontal ligament suggesting compression
Sharpey's fibre structure (Fig. 12.20)	Small collagen fibril diameters (Fig. 12.7)
The flattened, disc shape of the fibroblasts	Unimodal collagen size/ frequency distribution (Fig. 12.8)
Dermatan sulphate-rich composition of ground substance (page 188)	Distribution of Sharpey's fibres to socket (Fig. 12.21)
	Smooth surface of fibroblast membrane
	Large amounts of ground substance (page 188)

lost. When faced with such a condition, the dental surgeon may have two aims in mind: to repair the existing condition so that the disease process progresses no further (usually involving surgical removal of diseased tissue) and to regenerate the lost tissues, restore the bone and periodontal ligament to their original form, and reattach new periodontal ligament fibres to the tooth and bone. One common problem following surgery is that the junctional epithelium proliferates rapidly downwards to cover the root surface, which will prevent periodontal ligament fibres from attaching to cementum.

Following periodontal surgery with the removal of diseased tissue and various methods of conditioning the root surface to make it more likely to reattach periodontal ligament fibres (e.g. root planing, citric acid etching), a blood clot will form. It is obvious that the connective tissue of the wound may be re-populated from either the gingiva growing down or the periodontal ligament growing up. There is a body of opinion that believes that the best result is achieved when most of the wound is repopulated by cells of the existing periodontal ligament. Although both tissues may appear to be similar they differ in a number of features, which may be important to the final outcome (see page 241). For this reason, a particular surgical technique may be adopted to exclude the gingival tissues from the deeper part of the wound by placing some sort of tissue barrier over the alveolar crest to obtain 'guided tissue regeneration'.

We have also indicated that bioactive molecules such as growth factors and cytokines may be important during the induction of periodontal cells (osteoblasts, cementoblasts and fibroblasts) and bone itself. Such bioactive molecules (e.g. bone morphogenetic protein) have been placed in suitable carriers within wounds and have been claimed to help regenerate the periodontal tissues (bone, cementum and periodontal ligament).

In the process of cementogenesis (see Chapter 25), enamel proteins may have an important role during the early stages. Evidence is accumulating that the application of such proteins to the root surface may be an aid to periodontal regeneration (see page 348).

Important changes take place within the periodontal ligament with orthodontic loading. Should such a load act perpendicularly to the longitudinal axis of the tooth, wide areas or pressure on one side of the root and corresponding areas of tension on the other side are produced. Only if the force is placed near the centre of the root (through its centre of resistance) could a translation (or bodily) movement of the tooth be produced, with essentially uniform distribution of pressures on one side of the root and of tension on the other. However, tipping can easily occur as a result of the application of an orthodontic load, the point of rotation depending on the site of force application, the shape of the tooth, and the nature of the periodontal tissues supporting the tooth. The result is that crown and root tip in opposite directions, producing pressure and tension zones on either side of the root and a varying distribution of stress such that the load is concentrated in localised areas of the periodontal ligament. In such areas the fibrous part of the periodontal ligament will differ where the tooth is pressed against the alveolar wall and where it is drawn away from it.

On the side under tension, the periodontal space will become wider where the tooth is drawn away from the alveolar bone following the application of a continuous orthodontic load. Bundles of fibres are stretched and the alveolar crest is pulled in the same direction. There is an increase in connective tissue cell number, particularly near the socket wall. The periodontal fibroblasts appear spindle-shaped, although the cells near the alveolar wall appear more spherical. The blood vessels also appear to be distended. Osteoid tissue is deposited on the socket wall and, where the fibrous bundles are thick, new bone appears to be deposited along them. If the bundles are thin, a more uniform layer is deposited along the root surface. Calcification in the deeper layers of the osteoid starts shortly afterwards, while the superficial part remains uncalcified. New Sharpey's fibres are secreted simultaneously with new bone deposition. As the fibroblasts migrate with the bone, they may deposit either entirely new Sharpey's fibres or new fibrils, which are incorporated into existing fibres. While part of the newly synthesised collagen will be incorporated into the new osteoid, some will be incorporated into the periodontal ligament, perhaps associated with the increase in width on the tension side. Lengthening of fibres also seems to occur by incorporation of new fibrils into existing fibres (even at some distance from alveolar bone wall). On the side under pressure, the periodontal space becomes narrower and the crest of the alveolar bone is slightly deformed. Resorption of the alveolar bone surface occurs on the side towards which the tooth is moving by means of osteoclasts. Vascular activity is low and few leukocytes and macrophages are seen. Changes on the pressure side can be categorised broadly into 'direct resorption', where the pressure is relatively light, and 'hyalinisation', where the pressure is large enough to produce degenerative changes. With 'direct resorption', osteoclastic activity is evident; with 'hyalinisation', osteoclasts are absent: there is oedema and obliteration of the blood vessels within the periodontal ligament. Degenerative changes in the fibroblasts are also seen. The term 'hyalinisation' comes from the 'glassy' appearance of the periodontal ligament in routine histological specimens.

13 Alveolar bone

The part of the maxilla or mandible that supports and protects the teeth is known as alveolar bone. An arbitrary boundary at the level of the root apices of the teeth separates the alveolar processes from the body of the mandible (Fig. 13.1) or the maxilla. Like bone in other sites, alveolar bone functions as a mineralised supporting tissue, giving attachment to muscles, providing a framework for bone marrow, and acting as a reservoir for ions (especially calcium). Apart from its obvious strength, one of the most important biological properties of bone is its 'plasticity', allowing it to remodel according to the functional demands placed upon it. Alveolar bone is dependent on the presence of teeth for its development and maintenance. Where teeth are congenitally absent (as in anodontia), alveolar bone is poorly developed. Alveolar bone requires functional stimuli to maintain bone mass (see also page 218). Thus, following tooth extraction, it atrophies.

CLASSIFICATION OF BONE

Bone may classified in several ways. Developmentally, there is **endochondral bone** (where bone is preceded by a cartilaginous model which is eventually replaced by bone and marrow by a process termed endochondral ossification) and **intramembranous bone** (where bone forms directly within a vascular fibrous membrane). Histologically, mature bone

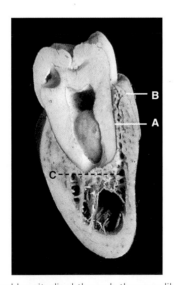

Fig. 13.1 Ground longitudinal through the mandible showing the alveolar bone. A = Inner layer of compact alveolar bone lining the tooth socket wall; B = outer alveolar plate of compact bone (note the spongy bone lying between the two plates of alveolar bone); C = arbitrary boundary between the alveolar bone and the body of the jaw. Courtesy of the Royal College of Surgeons of England.

may be categorised as **compact** (cortical) or **cancellous** (spongy) according to its density. As the names suggest, compact bone forms a dense, solid mass, while in spongy bone there is a lattice arrangement of the individual bony trabeculae that surround soft tissue. Internally, a thin layer of compact bone lines the tooth socket and gives attachment to the principal fibres of the periodontal ligament. Externally, on the buccal/ labial and lingual/palatal surfaces, are thicker layers of compact bone, forming the external and internal alveolar plates. Between these plates of compact bone are variable amounts of spongy bone, depending on site (Fig. 13.1; see also page 12). In the first-formed bone, the collagen fibres have a more variable diameter and a more irregular orientation, giving the bone a matted appearance, compared with **adult lamellar bone**, when viewed in polarised light. This bone, termed **woven bone**, has larger, more numerous cells that comprise about 30% of the volume of the tissue (compared with about 2% for adult bone). It is formed more rapidly and has a higher turnover rate. Woven bone is also seen initially at sites of fracture repair or in healing tooth sockets.

One of the most important properties of bone concerns its ability to continuously remodel and adapt to changing functional situations. This relates to the different types of bone cells, some having the property to form bone (osteoblasts) or to detect the mechanical stresses and strains to which the bone is subjected (osteoblasts and osteocytes), whilst others have the capacity to resorb bone (osteoclasts). Although bone under mechanical load will remodel, cementum is less readily resorbed than bone under similar loads, which allows for orthodontic tooth movement.

GROSS MORPHOLOGY OF ALVEOLAR BONE

The alveolar, tooth-bearing portion of the jaws is composed of outer and inner alveolar plates. The individual sockets are separated by plates of bone termed the interdental septa, while the roots of multirooted teeth are divided by interradicular septa (Fig. 13.2). The compact layer of bone lining the tooth socket has been given various names. It has been referred to as the cribriform plate, reflecting the sieve-like appearance produced by the numerous vascular canals (Volkmann's canals) passing from the alveolar bone into the periodontal ligament (Figs 13.3, 13.4); it has also been called bundle bone because numerous bundles of Sharpey's fibres pass into it from the periodontal ligament. In clinical radiographs, the bone lining the alveolus commonly appears as a dense white line and is given the name lamina dura (see page 54), which is often used synonymously for the cribriform plate (although, paradoxically

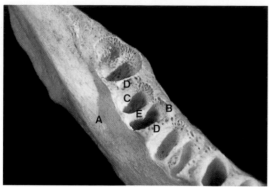

Fig. 13.2 Mandible with teeth removed to demonstrate the components of alveolar bone. A = Outer alveolar plate; B = inner alveolar plate; C = cribriform plate lining the socket wall; D = interdental septum; E = interradicular septum.

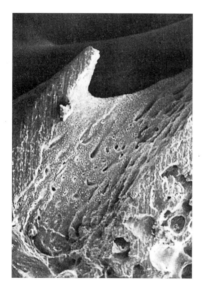

Fig. 13.3 A tooth socket showing the cribriform nature of the cribriform plate (SEM; × 5). Courtesy of Professor P. Sloan.

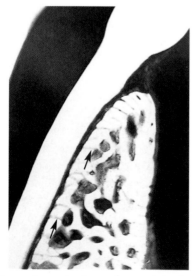

Fig. 13.4 Microradiograph of vascular canals in the cribriform plate (arrowed). Note the spongy bone lying in the central part of the alveolar bone. (× 7).

they are almost etymological opposites). The radio-opaque appearance might give the false impression that it is more dense than adjacent bone. However, the radiographic appearance derives from the beam passing tangentially through the socket wall and relates to the quantity of bone the beam passes through and not to any greater degree of mineralisation than adjacent bone. Superimposition also obscures the Volkmann's canals. The cribriform plate varies in thickness from 0.1 to 0.5 mm. The external alveolar plate is usually about 1.5–3 mm thick over posterior teeth but is highly variable around anterior teeth, depending on tooth position and inclination. The gross morphology and radiographic appearance of the alveolus and tooth sockets are described on pages 10–13 and 52–54.

CHEMICAL PROPERTIES OF BONE

Bone is a mineralised connective tissue. About 60% of its wet weight is inorganic material, about 25% organic material and about 15% water. By volume, about 36% is inorganic, 36% is organic and 28% is water. The mineral phase is carbonated hydroxyapatite, in the form of needle-like crystallites or thin plates about 50 nm wide, up to 8 nm thick and of variable length distributed both within the spaces between and on the surfaces of the collagen fibrils. Although contributing little to the weight of bone, the cells, through their capacity for osteosynthesis and resorption, have a pivotal role in the maintenance of the matrix.

Organic matrix

The organic matrix of bone is about 90% collagen. Most can be regarded as intrinsic collagen secreted by osteoblasts. However, collagen inserted as Sharpey's fibres can be considered as extrinsic collagen formed by adjacent fibroblasts. The dominant collagen in bone is type I, although small amounts of type III may be present, particularly in immature or healing bone. Mutation in the genes encoding the constituent peptides of the collagen type I triple helix are clinically important and may give rise to the inherited conditions of osteogenesis imperfecta and dentinogenesis imperfecta.

Non-collagenous proteins

The non-collagenous proteins, which are a heterogeneous group of about 200 proteins, collectively comprise the remaining 10% of the total organic content of bone matrix. Most are endogenous proteins produced by the bone cells, whilst some, like albumin, are derived from other sources such as the blood and become incorporated into the bone matrix during osteosynthesis. One group of non-collagenous proteins is the proteoglycans. In bone, these incorporate chondroitin sulphate and heparan sulphate glycosaminoglycans and are mainly in the form of decorin and biglycan. Other components are represented by molecules such as the glycoproteins osteonectin, osteopontin (bone sialoprotein), bone sialoprotein II, thrombospondin, osteocalcin and fibronectin. Osteonectin accounts for about 2% of the total protein. The biological function of individual glycoproteins awaits clarification. Some are presumably involved in the initial, formative aspects of bone, whilst others may play a role following their release during bone resorption. As the proteoglycans bind to collagen, they may help regulate collagen fibril diameters and may play a role in mineralisation. Osteonectin, for example, has the ability to bind calcium, suggesting a role in mineralisation. Osteopontin, osteonectin and fibronectin are termed RGD-containing proteins as they have a specific amino acid sequence arginine–glycine–aspartic acid (Arg–Gly–Asp), which has important implications for the attachment of cells to the bone matrix. Osteocalcin (also termed Gla protein as it contains the amino acid γ–carboxy glutamic acid) is a calcium-binding protein synthesised only by osteoblasts and odontoblasts. This specificity means that recognition of osteocalcin in a cell characterises that cell as being of an osteoblastic or odontoblastic lineage.

Bone contains exogenously derived proteins that may circulate in the blood and become locked up in the bone matrix itself. It is a rich source of cytokines (such as interleukin, tumour necrosis factor and colony-stimulating factors) and growth factors (such as transforming growth factors, fibroblast growth factors, platelet-derived growth factors and insulin-like growth factors) produced by a variety of cells associated with bone. Such molecules have important biological activity in the life cycle of bone cells. When present within the bone itself they are inactive but may become mobilised when bone is being resorbed by osteoclasts. They may then play a determining role on the pattern of subsequent bone activity. Bone morphogenetic proteins (BMPs), of which eight have been identified (BMP-1 to BMP-8), are also represented in bone. They are part of the TGF-β superfamily (apart from BMP-1) and have the ability to induce bone to form by their ability to influence the movement, cell division and differentiation of stem and osteoprogenitor cells. BMPs, either directly or indirectly using demineralised bone, are currently being assessed for use clinically as a method for inducing bone formation.

HISTOLOGY OF BONE

Osteoid

Any surface where active bone formation is occurring will be covered by a layer of newly deposited unmineralised bone matrix called osteoid (see Fig. 13.8). This layer is analagous to predentine. The molecular ingredients of osteoid are secreted by the osteoblasts that form a well defined layer at its surface. Osteoid has a thickness of approximately 5–10 μm before reaching a level of maturity conducive to mineralisation. The mineralising front is relatively linear at the light microscope level, unlike that of dentine, which may reveal a calcospheritic pattern. In routine light microscopic demineralised sections, osteoid will stain differently from that of the matrix associated with mineralised bone indicating that, at the mineralising front, biochemical changes take place within the matrix to enable mineralisation to occur; some molecules may be added, others are degraded. Osteoid consists of type I collagen fibres arranged more or less parallel to bone surface, embedded in a complex ground substance of proteoglycans, glycoproteins and other protein molecules. The biochemical changes occurring at the mineralising front are poorly understood. When alveolar bone is first formed, initial mineralisation may be controlled by osteoblasts from whose cell membrane matrix vesicles are budded off into the osteoid, within which the first crystals are formed. The cell membrane around these first crystals breaks down to form the seed around which further mineralisation can occur by epitaxy. A similar process of initial mineralisation seems to occur in dentine (see pages 326–327). However, whereas certain molecules involved in the mineralisation process may bypass the predentine by being transported via the odontoblast process directly to the mineralising front, this would not appear possible in osteoid. There is a lag phase of about 10 days before the deeper layer of the osteoid has matured sufficiently to undergo mineralisation. This clearly involves biochemical changes within the organic matrix and accounts for the different staining properties seen in demineralised sections of bone between the osteoid and the rest of the bone matrix, the latter staining more darkly (see Fig. 13.8).

Bone organisation

Bone is deposited in layers, or lamellae, each lamella being about 5 μm thick. In compact bone the lamellae are arranged in two major patterns. At external (periosteal) and internal (endosteal) surfaces they are arranged in parallel layers completely surrounding the bony surfaces as circumferential lamellae. Deep to the circumferential lamellae, the lamellae are arranged as small concentric layers around a central vascular canal. The vascular (Haversian) canal, together with

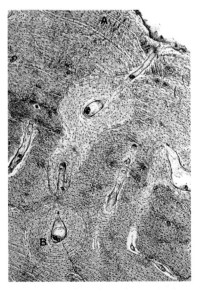

Fig. 13.5 Horizontal ground section of alveolar bone showing circumferential lamellae (A) and Haversian systems (B) where a central vascular canal is surrounded by concentrically arranged bony lamella (× 80).

the concentric lamellae, is known as an **Haversian system** or **osteon** (Fig. 13.5). There may be between 4 and 20 concentric lamellae within each Haversian system, the number being limited by the ability of nutrients to diffuse from the central vessel to the cells in the outermost lamella. A cement line of mineralised matrix delineates the Haversian system. The collagen fibres within each lamella spiral along the length of the lamella but have different orientations to those in the adjacent lamella. This change in orientation can be demonstrated by viewing bone in polarised light (Fig. 13.6). The longitudinally running Haversian canals are connected by a series of horizontal ones (interconnecting canals). In adult bone, as a result of remodelling, fragments of previous Haversian

systems may be present (the interstitial lamellae; Fig. 13.7), which can contain old remnants of circumferential lamellae as well as osteonal remnants (Fig. 13.7). This causes confusion to the uninformed, who may misinterpret relocated Sharpey's fibres (which originally were in the circumferential lamellar bone but are now embedded deep within the bone in isolated islands amongst osteones) as 'unusual coarse fibres'. This is a common feature in growth with active cortical drift.

In spongy bone the lamellae are apposed to each other to form trabeculae about 50 μm thick. The trabeculae are not arranged randomly but aligned along lines of stress so as best to withstand the forces applied to the bone while adding minimally to mass. The trabeculae surround the marrow spaces from which they derive their nutrition and only infrequently are seen to possess Haversian canals. In young bone the marrow is red and haemopoietic. It contains stem cells of both the fibroblastic/mesenchymal type (capable of giving rise to fibroblasts, osteoblasts, adipocytes, chondroblasts and myoblasts) and blood cell lineage (capable of giving rise to osteoclasts). In old bone, the marrow is yellow, with loss of haemopoietic potential and increased accumulation of fat cells.

In the body as a whole, about 85% of bone is of the cortical variety while about 15% is spongy. However, these figures are likely to vary according to site and age. Although it only occupies a small percentage of bone volume, spongy bone has a far higher turnover rate than cortical bone: cortical bone is said to remodel about 3% of its mass each year, while spongy bone remodels about 25%. The cortical bone functions mainly in a mechanical/protective role, while the spongy bone has a more metabolic function.

CELL TYPES IN BONE

Several cell types are responsible for the synthesis, maintenance

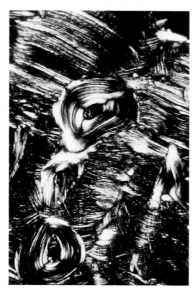

Fig. 13.6 Same section as Fig. 13.5, viewed in polarised light. The alternating black and white bands indicate the different orientations of collagen in adjacent lamellae. Note the characteristic 'X' superimposed on the Haversian system (× 80).

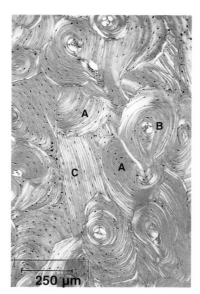

Fig. 13.7 Horizontal ground section of bone showing interstitial lamella (A), Haversian system surrounding a central canal (B) and original circumferential lamella lying deep within the bone following remodelling (C) (× 60). Courtesy of Professor M. Smith.

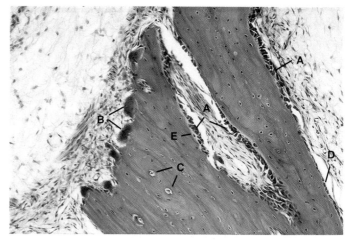

Fig. 13.8 Horizontal section of bone demonstrating a layer of osteoblasts (A) lining a surface where active bone formation is occurring (as indicated by the presence of a pale staining layer of osteoid), some large multinucleated osteoclasts (B) lying against Howships lacunae in a region of bone undergoing resorption, and large numbers of osteocytes (C) lying embedded within the bone matrix itself. D = Bone-lining cells; E = pale-staining osteoid layer (Decalcified section; H & E; × 80). Courtesy of Dr T.R. Arnett.

and resorption of bone (Fig. 13.8). These can be regarded as belonging to two main families, one mesenchymal and the other haemopoietic. The osteoblasts, osteocytes, and bone lining cells are derived from a mesenchymal (or ectomesenchymal) stem cell. These stem cells reside in the bone marrow and in a region of proliferating cells adjacent to the osteoblast layer in the periosteum. In the periodontal ligament and other bone-forming tissues the osteogenic precursors may be associated with small blood vessels. The osteoclasts, however, belong to a different lineage. They form part of the haemopoietic system, being derived from the mononuclear/phagocyte system (including monocytes and macrophages).

Osteoblasts

Osteoblasts are specialised fibroblast-like cells of mesenchymal origin. A cuboidal layer of these cells is prominent on a bone surface where there is active bone formation (Fig. 13.9). Unlike cartilage, which grows interstitially, bone can be deposited (or resorbed) only at surfaces. However, these surfaces are widespread and include the periosteal and endosteal surfaces, the linings of the Haversian canals and the surfaces of bony trabeculae in spongy bone. Active osteoblasts appear cuboidal and exhibit a basophilic cytoplasm that is related to the extensive endoplasmic reticulum within the cells. The cells are polarised and the prominent, round nucleus tends to lie towards the basal end. A pale, juxtanuclear area indicates the site of

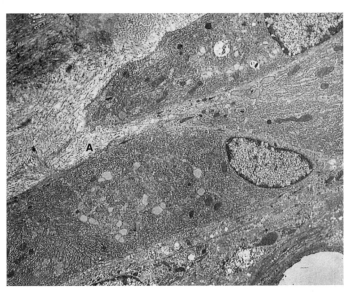

Fig. 13.10   Electron microscopic appearance of an active osteoblast. The cell contains an extensive rough endoplasmic reticulum and a conspicuous and localised Golgi apparatus (B), and is connected to adjacent cells by cell contacts. The cell surface adjacent to the demineralised bone (A) has many fine cytoplasmic processes, some of which contact underlying osteocytes. The flattened cell (C) immediately adjacent to the osteoblasts may represent an osteoprogenitor cell (× 6000).

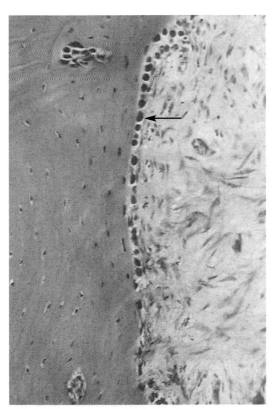

Fig. 13.9   Alveolar bone at the periodontal ligament surface showing a layer of osteoblasts (arrowed). Sharpey fibres are seen passing into the bone and there is a pale-staining osteoid layer. Within the bone itself are seen osteocytes, which, in routine demineralised sections do not exhibit obvious canaliculi (Decalcified section; H & E; × 400).

the Golgi complex. Numerous cell contacts are seen between the cell membranes of adjacent cells. At the ultrastructural level, active osteoblasts (like periodontal fibroblasts) contain rough endoplasmic reticulum (which is even more extensive and arranged in parallel stacks) and numerous mitochondria and vesicles; the Golgi complex is localised and extensive (Fig. 13.10).

The cells contact one another by means of adherens and gap junctions. These are functionally connected to micro-filaments and enzymes (such as protein kinases) associated with intracellular secondary messenger systems. This complex arrangement provides for intercellular adhesion and cell–cell communication, helping to ensure that the osteoblast layer completely covers the osteoid surface and that the osteoblasts function in a co-ordinated manner.

The osteoblast secretes the organic matrix of bone, which initially is represented by an unmineralised layer known as osteoid, about 5–10 μm thick (Figs 13.8, 13.9). The intrinsic collagen fibrils lie parallel to the bone surface. At the surface of alveolar bone adjacent to the periodontal ligament, extrinsic Sharpey's fibres pass into the osteoid layer more perpendicularly (Fig. 13.9). About 15% of osteoblasts become embedded in the organic matrix as osteocytes.

The osteoblast secretes the various endogenous components of the bone matrix. Some, such as collagen type I, are widely distributed and not unique to osteoblasts. Others are specific to cells of the osteoblast lineage and provide useful markers of the osteoblast phenotype. These include osteocalcin and the recently described osteoblast transcription factor, cbfa-1. Alkaline phosphatase activity, although not entirely specific to bone, is easy to identify and is a reliable indicator of osteoblastic differentiation.

In addition to its obvious involvement in bone formation, the osteoblast has a controlling influence in activating the bone-resorbing cells, the osteoclasts. It is a source of factors involved in this process (such as colony-stimulating factors, prostaglandins and the recently described protein osteoprotegerin ligand). The osteoblast, and not the osteoclast, contains receptors for parathyroid hormone and regulates the osteoclastic response to this hormone (see page 213).

Osteocytes

Osteocytes are the cells lying within the bone itself and are 'entrapped' osteoblasts. There are about 25 000 osteocytes per cubic millimetre of bone. In preparing ground sections of bone, the osteocytes themselves are lost, but the spaces or lacunae they occupy are filled with air or cell debris and appear black in routine transmitted light sections (Fig. 13.11). The lacunae are regularly distributed, and many fine canals called canaliculi radiate from them in all directions. The canaliculi allow the diffusion of substances through the bone. Numerous cell processes from the osteocytes run in the canaliculi in all direc-

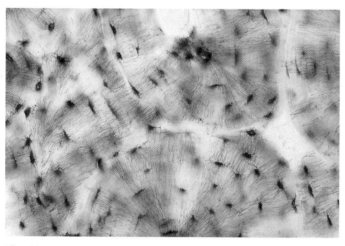

Fig. 13.11 Ground section of part of a Haversian system cut horizontally to show osteocyte lacunae and associated canaliculi (× 200).

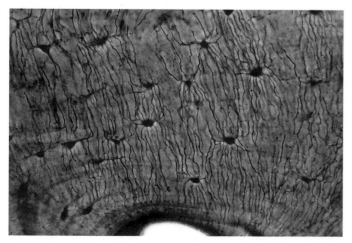

Fig. 13.12 Demineralised section of bone perfused with picrothionine to visualise the osteocyte lacunae and canaliculi (× 280). Courtesy of Professor M.M. Smith.

tions. The canaliculi of osteocytes are preferentially oriented, more being directed perpendicularly to the bone surface than parallel to it. Unlike cementocytes (see page 170), only those osteocytes close to the cement line have more canaliculi directed towards the bone surface than away from it. Osteocytes also differ from cementocytes in that they are more regularly distributed. In routine demineralised sections the osteocytes are retained, but the canaliculi are little in evidence. However, the canaliculi can be visualised in demineralised sections if perfused with a stain such as picrothionine (Fig. 13.12). Recent studies have shown that it is possible to isolate and culture osteocytes, which retain their characteristic morphology (Fig. 13.13).

As a result of their widespread distribution and interconnections osteocytes are obvious candidates to detect stresses induced in bone and are therefore regarded as the main mechanoreceptors of bone.

As they are derived from osteoblasts, it is not surprising that osteocytes share many common markers, such as osteopontin, osteocalcin, osteonectin, fibronectin and parathormone and oestrogen receptors. However, one or two antibodies appear to be specific, but the epitopes they recognise have yet to be fully characterised.

At the ultrastructural level, the appearance of the osteocyte may vary according to its position in relation to the surface layer. Osteocytes newly incorporated into bone matrix from the osteoblast layer have a high organelle content similar to osteoblasts. However, as they become more deeply situated with continued bone formation, they appear to be less active. The cell is then seen to have a nucleus and thin ring of cytoplasm containing few organelles, reflecting the decreased cellular activity (Fig. 13.14). Numerous slender processes from the osteocyte extend into canaliculi in the matrix. The processes of one cell are joined to those of another by gap junctions, which allow cell-to-cell communication and co-ordination of activity. In this feature they differ from chondrocytes, which, lacking processes, are isolated. A pericellular space (which might represent a shrinkage artefact) is usually seen to intervene between the cell membrane and the surrounding bone and contains unmineralised matrix and a few collagen fibrils. Osteocytes are also in communication with osteoblasts at the surface.

Bone-lining cells

When bone surfaces are neither in the formative nor resorptive phase, the bone surface is completely lined by a layer of flattened cells termed bone-lining cells (Fig. 13.8). These show little sign of synthetic activity as evidenced by their organelle content. They are regarded as postproliferative osteoblasts. By covering the surface of bone, they protect it from any resorptive activity from osteoclasts. They may also be reactivated to form osteoblasts.

Osteoprogenitor cells

In order to generate the osteoblasts throughout life, a stem-cell population is required. The stem cells have the ability to

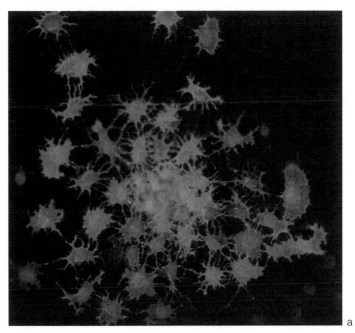

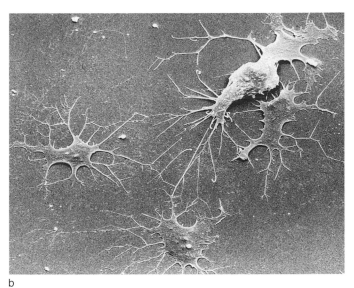

b

a

Fig. 13.13 Osteocytes in tissue culture. (a) A group of osteocytes isolated from bone and maintained for 24 hours in tissue culture on glass. The cytoplasm (green fluorescence) has been stained with an osteocyte-specific monoclonal antibody (OB7.3) while the nuclei have been stained using a blue fluorescence. A small number of osteoblasts (negative for the green osteotype-specific antibody but with a blue-staining nucleus) can also be seen (× 350). (b) SEM of cultured osteocytes. The cells were characterised by their positive staining with an osteocyte-specific antibody (OB7.3). Like osteocytes *in vivo*, the cells have long, slender, often branched cell processes by which they have contacted those of adjacent cells during culture (× 1000). Courtesy of Doctors P.J. Nijweide and A. van der Plas and the editor of *Bone and Mineral Research*.

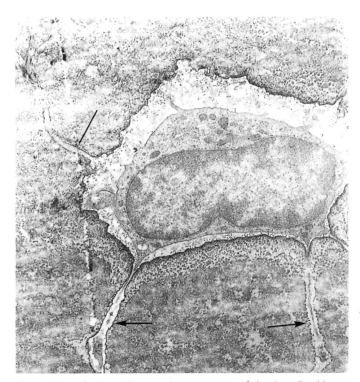

Fig. 13.14 Electron microscopic appearance of demineralised bone showing an osteocyte. The cell has few organelles and possesses cell processes (arrowed) extending into canaliculi. A pericellular space is seen between the cell membrane and the wall of the lacuna and is probably related to a shrinkage artefact (× 5300).

maintain their numbers throughout life. When a stem cell divides, one of the daughter cells remains as a stem cell, while the other can differentiate into another cell type. This property of self-renewal is a unique property of stem cells. In the case of alveolar bone, the cells that eventually give rise to osteoblasts are termed osteoprogenitor cells and reside in the layer of cells beneath the osteoblast layer in the periosteal region, in the periodontal ligament, or in the marrow spaces. Initially, they are fibroblast-like cells, with an elongated nucleus and few organelles (Fig. 13.10). Their life cycle may involve up to about eight cell divisions before reaching the osteoblast stage. There is a gradual acquirement of osteoblast-like features associated with an ordered increase in gene expression. Initially, genes related to cell growth are expressed (such as *c-myc*, *c-fos* and *cbfa 1*), followed by genes related to osteoblast products such as type I collagen, fibronectin, some growth factors and alkaline phosphatase. Finally, genes are expressed related to products associated with mineralisation (such as osteocalcin and osteopontin).

Osteoclasts

Osteoclasts are the cells responsible for bone resorption. They are derived from haemopoietic cells of the monocyte/macrophage lineage by fusion of mononuclear precursors, giving rise to multinucleated cells. Resorbing surfaces of alveolar bone show resorption concavities (Howship's lacunae), in which lie the multinucleated osteoclasts (Fig. 13.15). The cells can show considerable variation in size and shape, ranging from smaller mononuclear cells to very large cells. There is evidence to indicate that large osteoclasts (containing many nuclei) resorb more bone than small osteoclasts (containing few nuclei). Characteristically, osteoclasts may be up to 100 μm in diameter and have on average 10–20 nuclei. In actively resorbing osteoclasts, the cells are highly polarised. That part of the cell that lies adjacent to bone, and where resorption is occurring, often has a foamy, striated appearance at the light microscope level (the so-called 'ruffled border'). A useful marker for osteoclasts is tartrate-resistant acid phosphatase (Fig. 13.16), although the precise function of this enzyme is unknown. Tissue culture studies indicate that osteoclasts are highly motile, although the cells will resorb only when attached to bone (Fig. 13.17). Evidence from the 'snail tracks' on bone surfaces suggests that osteoclasts also move across the bone *in vivo*. Osteoclasts are recruited only when required; there is consequently no significant reservoir of inactive osteoclasts. The lifespan of osteoclasts is not known with any certainty, although it is thought to be about 10–14 days. Different nuclei within the osteoclast are often of different ages. There is evidence of apoptosis (programmed cell death) of its nuclei. Indeed, as the administration of oestrogens and bisphosphonates induces apoptosis, this may help explain the

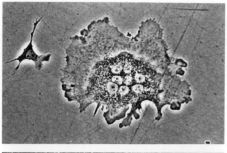

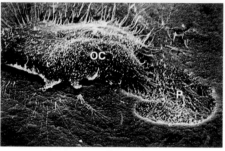

Fig. 13.17 Osteoclasts in tissue culture: (a) phase contrast; (b) SEM. The osteoclast (OC) has moved away from an area of resorption (R) in which collagen fibrils have been exposed following removal of mineral (× 700). Courtesy of Dr T.R. Arnett.

use of such materials in combating osteoporosis and other diseases characterised by loss of bone. The possibility exists that additional fusion of new cells may prolong the activity of osteoclasts.

At the ultrastructural level, the ruffled border is composed of many tightly packed microvilli adjacent to the bone surface. This border provides a large surface area for the resorptive process. At the circumference of the ruffled border, the plasma membrane tends to become smooth and the cytoplasm beneath it contains numerous contractile actin microfilaments (surrounded by two vinculin rings) (Fig. 13.18). It has been suggested that this modified annular zone (also referred to as

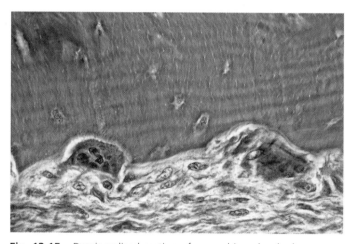

Fig. 13.15 Demineralised section of a resorbing alveolar bone showing two osteoclasts lying in Howship's lacunae (× 350). Courtesy of Professor M.M. Smith.

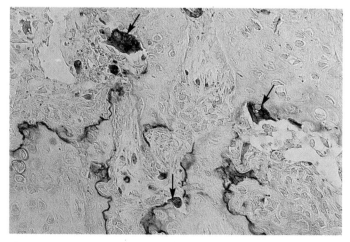

Fig. 13.16 Demineralised section of bone showing osteoclasts staining positively (red) for tartrate-resistant acid phosphatase (arrows) (× 240). Courtesy of Dr A Grigoriadis.

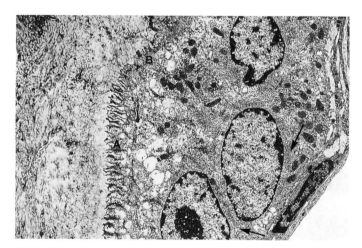

Fig. 13.18 Electron microscopic appearance of demineralised bone showing part of an osteoclast. The brush border (A) comprises numerous microvilli adjacent to the bone surface. At the circumference of the brush border the annular zone (B) contains numerous microfilaments. There are numerous vesicles and mitochondria and three nuclei are evident (× 3600).

the clear zone) may serve to attach the cell very closely to the surface of the bone. This provides a 'sealing zone' and thus creates an isolated microenvironment in which resorption can take place without diffusion of the hydrolytic enzymes produced by the cell into adjacent tissue. A distinguishing feature of osteoclasts is the presence of receptors for calcitonin. Administration of calcitonin inhibits bone resorption by, among other things, blocking the formation of actin rings employed in cell attachment.

The osteoclast contains many pleomorphic mitochondria distributed throughout the cytoplasm (except for the region immediately beneath the ruffled border). The rough endoplasmic reticulum is less conspicuous than in osteoblasts, but Golgi material is prominent (especially in juxtanuclear areas). Most of the remaining cytoplasm contains large numbers of vesicles of different sizes and types, some containing lysosomal enzymes (e.g. cysteine proteinases).

The attachment of the osteoclast cell membrane to the bone matrix at the sealing zone is due to the presence of cell membrane proteins known as integrins (especially $\alpha v\beta 3$). These integrins bind to specific amino acid sequences present in proteins of the bone matrix, namely Arg–Gly–Asp (RGD). Interference with the formation of such integrins or the administration of competing synthetic peptides will inhibit bone resorption.

Once the osteoclast has been activated against the bone surface, bone resorption occurs in two stages. Initially, the mineral phase is removed and later the organic matrix. To provide a low pH, the osteoclast secretes protons across the ruffled border by means of an ATP dependent proton pump: the enzyme carbonic anhydrase II, which is involved in generating protons by catabolising the reaction of carbon dioxide with water to form carbonic acid. The acidic microenvironment in the forming resorption lacuna dissolves the mineral crystals in bone and exposes the organic matrix. The organic matrix is then degraded by neutral matrix metalloproteinases (MMPs) and cysteine proteinases. As the name suggests, neutral MMPs function at higher pH ranges. Such enzymes include interstitial collagenases, gelatinases and stromelysins. It is not known how much of this organic degradation takes place extracellularly and how much intracellularly. Compared with the fibroblasts of the periodontal ligament (see Fig. 12.34), intracellular collagen profiles have hardly ever been reported present in osteoclasts.

BONE RESORPTION–FORMATION COUPLING

There is clearly a close relationship between bone deposition and bone resorption. During the growing phase of a child, the amount of deposition exceeds that of resorption, giving an increase in bone mass. During the adult phase, the amount of bone deposition is equivalent to that of bone resorption and bone mass is more or less constant. In old age, the amount of bone deposition is generally less than that of bone resorption and there is an overall decrease in bone mass. In postmeno-

pausal women particularly this loss may be sufficient to lead to the clinical condition of osteoporosis.

Many of the factors that result in bone resorption are known to have no direct effect on osteoclasts, but act indirectly through osteoblasts. Most of the receptors to bioactive molecules that cause bone resorption are present on osteoblasts (e.g. receptors to PTH and PTHrP). Indeed, the main receptor found in osteoclasts is related to calcitonin. There are several mechanisms whereby osteoblasts might promote bone resorption:

- By the local release of substances such as cytokines and growth factors (e.g. macrophage colony-stimulating factor, osteoprotegerin and interleukins), osteoblasts could stimulate the production of osteoclasts.
- By releasing enzymes (such as MMPs) to degrade the unmineralised osteoid layer covering forming bone, osteoblasts could help expose mineralised matrix on which osteoclasts could attach and commence resorption.
- By bioactive molecules present within bone (e.g. cytokines, BMPs, TGF-β) that could be activated as a result of osteoclastic bone resorption and subsequently have an effect on remodelling.

Reversal lines mark the position where bone activity changes from resorption to deposition. Such lines are darkly stained and irregular in outline, being composed of a series of concavities that were once the sites of the resorptive Howship's lacunae. They may be seen to contain the enzyme acid phosphatase (Fig.13.19).

Radiographic techniques readily demonstrate that bone is continually remodelling to adapt to the different functional regimes impinging on it. In this context, newly formed bone is less dense (and therefore more radiolucent) than mature bone (Figs 13.20, 13.21). As mentioned previously, spongy bone remodels about 25% of its mass each year, compared to only 3% for cortical bone. On account of collagen degradation occurring during bone resorption, analysis of its special cross

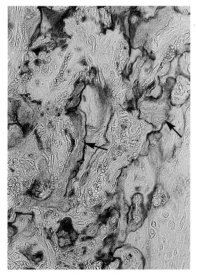

Fig. 13.19 Portion of bone showing the scalloped outline of a reversal line staining positively (red) for acid phosphatase (arrows) (× 100). Courtesy of Dr A. Grigoriadis.

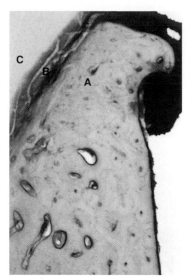

Fig. 13.20 Ground longitudinal section of alveolar bone at the alveolar crest. A = Alveolar bone; B = periodontal space; C = root (× 16). Courtesy of R.V. Hawkins.

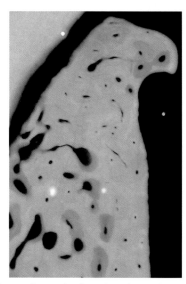

Fig. 13.21 Microradiograph of section shown in Fig. 13.15. The varying densities of alveolar bone indicate its active remodelling, the darker, radiolucent areas being most recently formed and less mineralised. Courtesy of R.V. Hawkins.

links retained in urine (pyridinoline fragments) is used clinically as a marker to indicate rates of bone remodelling.

There are a considerable number of factors that can influence bone remodelling. The complexity of the topic is illustrated by the fact that certain reagents can produce opposite effects, depending on concentration. Synergism must also be taken into account. Some of the more common factors are listed in Table 13.1.

SCANNING ELECTRON MICROSCOPE APPEARANCES OF BONE SURFACES

Scanning electron microscopy provides a useful technique for visualising the appearance of large areas of bone surfaces at

Table 13.1 *Factors affecting bone resorption and formation, directly and indirectly (Courtesy of Dr T.R. Arnett)*

	Resorption	Formation
Systemic hormones		
PTH	+	+/−
$1,25(OH)_2D_3$	+	+/−
Calcitonin	−	?+
Sex steroids	−	+/−
Glucocorticoids	+	+/−
Growth hormone		+
Thyroid hormone	+	+/−
Cytokines growth factors		
Prostaglandins	+/−	+
Interleukin 1	+	+
Tumour necrosis factor	+	?+
Interferon Y	−	−
Insulin-like growth factors		+
Macrophage colony stimulating factor	+	
Epidermal growth factor	+	?
Transforming growth factor	+/−	+
Bone morphogenic proteins	?	+
Platelet-derived growth factor	+	?+
Fibroblast growth factor		+/−
Vasoactive intestinal peptide	+	
PTH-related peptide	+	+/−
Osteoprotegerin ligand	+	
Osteoprotegerin	−	
Calcitonin gene-related peptide	−	
Miscellaneous agents		
Immobilisation, weightlessness	+	−
Stress/exercise	+/−	+
Protons	+	?−
Calcium	−	+
Phosphate	+	+
Fluoride	−	+
Bisphosphonates	−	
Alcohol/tobacco	+	−

+ Direct effect; − indirect effect

high magnification. Cells and the organic material in any covering osteoid layer are removed by substances such as sodium hypochlorite, producing an anorganic preparation and revealing the underlying mineralised or mineralising surface layer.

An alveolar bone surface on which bone formation is occurring is characterised by the presence of numerous small, calcified nodules within and around collagen fibrils. Sharpey's fibres may be encountered as small, dark, circular areas and larger ovoid areas represent lacunae occupied in vivo by osteocytes becoming entombed in bone (Fig. 13.22). If the forming alveolar bone surface is rendered only partially anorganic, the smallest calcified nodules of bone may be seen depositing on the intrinsic collagen fibrils, and the orientation of the collagen parallel to the bone surface is also visualised (Fig. 13.23).

An alveolar bone surface on which bone resorption is occurring is characterised by the presence of Howship's resorption lacunae (Fig. 13.24). If a periosteal surface is examined,

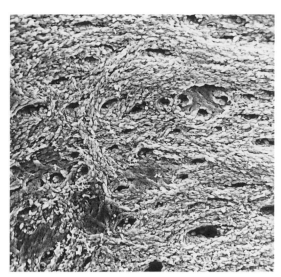

Fig. 13.22   SEM appearance of alveolar bone surface where bone formation is occurring, characterised by numerous small calcific nodules in partly mineralised intrinsic collagen, masking the underlying collagen fibrils. The larger dark elongated areas represent the lacunae of osteoblasts becoming entombed as osteocytes, while the smaller circular dark areas represent the unmineralised cores of the Sharpey's fibres (Anorganic preparation; × 550). Courtesy of Professor S.J. Jones.

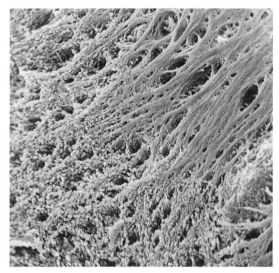

Fig. 13.23   SEM appearance of alveolar bone surface where bone formation is occurring, as evidenced by the numerous small nodules in the lower and left part of the field. However, the surface has been rendered only partly anorganic to show the collagen fibres of the extracellular matrix (Partial anorganic preparation; × 550). Courtesy of Professor S.J. Jones.

there may be no Sharpey's fibres present. In addition to localised, pit-like resorption lacunae bone may also exhibit longer 'snail-track' resorption lacunae. In contrast to a periosteal surface, the appearance of an area of resorption in bundle bone (periodontal surface) shows the presence of Sharpey's fibres in the resorbing areas (Fig. 13.25).

When neither bone deposition nor resorption is occurring the surface of the bone is described as a resting surface. The resting surface may be characterised by projections marking the sites of extrinsic mineralised Sharpey's fibres, separated by

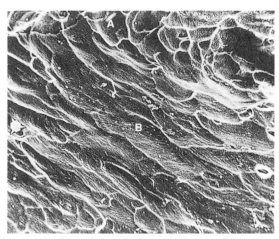

Fig. 13.24   SEM of periosteal surface of bone (lacking Sharpey's fibres) undergoing resorption. In addition to pit-like resorption lacunae (A), elongated 'snail-track' resorption lacunae are evident (B) (Anorganic preparation; × 300). Courtesy of Professor S.J. Jones.

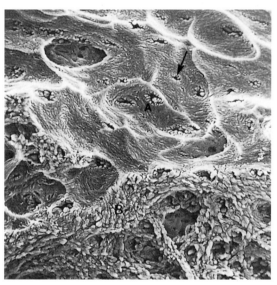

Fig. 13.25   SEM of alveoar bone surface contrasting the appearance of an area of bone resorption (A) with an adjacent area of bone formation (B). Note the presence of Sharpey's fibres with unmineralised cores in the resorbing areas (arrowed) (Anorganic preparation; × 300). Courtesy of Professor S.J. Jones.

smooth areas containing intrinsic mineralised collagen fibres. This contrasts with the granular appearance of the mineral of the intrinsic fibres of any adjacent forming surface (Fig. 13.26).

SHARPEY'S FIBRES

In addition to intrinsic fibres secreted by osteoblasts, which are aligned parallel to the bone surface, alveolar bone contains extrinsic Sharpey fibres that enter bone perpendicular to the surface (Fig. 13.27). Extrinsic fibres, inserting into the cribriform plate as Sharpey's fibres, are derived from the principal fibres of the periodontal ligament. Most Sharpey's fibres appear in the cervical portion (alveolar crest region) of the

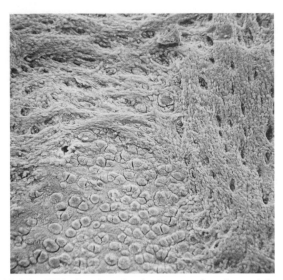

Fig. 13.26 SEM of resting alveolar bone surface (lower left part of field) characterised by projections marking the sites of mineralised extrinsic Sharpey's fibres separated by smooth areas. This contrasts with the granular appearance of the forming bone surface in the upper right part of the field, where the Sharpey's fibres are seen as holes (Anorganic preparation; × 500). Courtesy of Professor S.J. Jones.

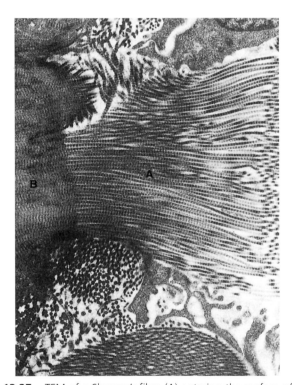

Fig. 13.27 TEM of a Sharpey's fibre (A) entering the surface of alveolar bone (B). Note the periodicity evident on the collagen fibrils (Decalcified section; × 10 500).

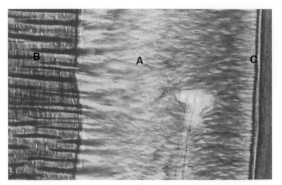

Fig. 13.28 Section of a root of a tooth showing Sharpey's fibres from the periodontal ligament (A) entering alveolar bone (B). The Sharpey's fibres in bone are seen to be thicker, but less numerous, than those entering the cementum on the tooth surface (C) (Decalcified section; aldehyde Fuschin and van Gieson; × 250). Courtesy of Professor S.J. Jones.

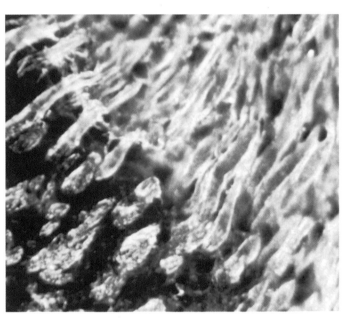

Fig. 13.29 Sharpey's fibre insertion from the periodontal ligament (A) into alveolar bone (B), showing peripheral staining of inserting collagen bundles with immunofluorescent stain for collagen type III. (× 350) Courtesy of Professor P. Sloan and Mosby-Wolfe, London.

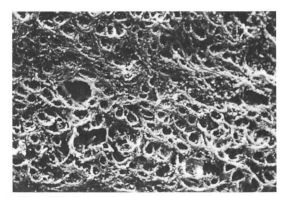

Fig. 13.30 SEM of Sharpey's fibres in alveolar bone with unmineralised centres, which are removed by the hypochlorite used to prepare this anorganic specimen (× 300). Courtesy of Professor P. Sloan.

cribriform plate. Sharpey's fibres in bone are less numerous, but thicker than those at the cementum surface (Fig. 13.28). There is evidence that traces of type III collagen are found at the periphery of Sharpey's fibres (Fig. 13.29). Because of the attachments of numerous bundles of collagen fibres, the cribriform plate has also been called bundle bone. Bundle bone usually comprises thin lamellae running parallel to each other and to the root surface (see Fig. 13.34).

Scanning electron micrographs of anorganic preparations of the periodontal surfaces of alveolar bone show that the

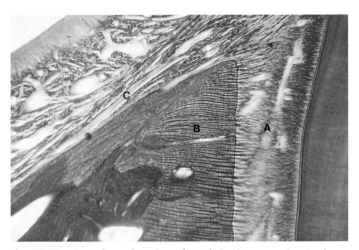

Fig. 13.33 Buccolingual section of tooth *in situ* appearing to show Sharpey's fibres (arrows) passing from the periodontal ligament (A) through the compact alveolar bone (B) in the cervical region to reach the lamina propria of the attached gingiva (C) (Decalcified longitudinal section; van Gieson; × 80). Courtesy of Professor S.J. Jones.

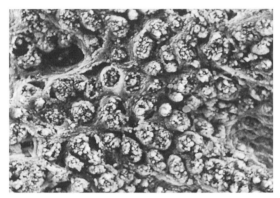

Fig. 13.31 SEM of Sharpey's fibres in alveolar bone which are mineralised beyond the surface of the bone and remain as small, calcified projections into the periodontal ligament (Anorganic preparation; × 300). Courtesy of Professor P. Sloan.

Sharpey's fibres may have two main appearances, depending upon the degree of mineralisation. In one, the embedded fibres may remain unmineralised at their centres, and removal of their organic material results in a series of hollow centres (Fig. 13.30). Conversely, the inserting fibres may be fully mineralised and project beyond the surface of the bone as small, calcified prominences into the periodontal ligament (Fig. 13.31).

In the cervical part of the interdental septum, where the bone type is mainly compact, Sharpey's fibres entering the bone in the mesiodistal plane may pass straight through to become continuous with similar fibres from the root of the adjacent tooth. These are called transalveolar fibres (Fig.13.32). A similar pattern exists in the interradicular bone, although in this situation the fibres link roots of the same tooth. Transalveolar fibres also pass through the entire thickness of the alveolar bone in the buccal and lingual planes, intermingling with the overlying periosteum or with the lamina propria of the gingiva (Fig. 13.33). However, where the alveolar bone is cancellous no transalveolar fibres are seen.

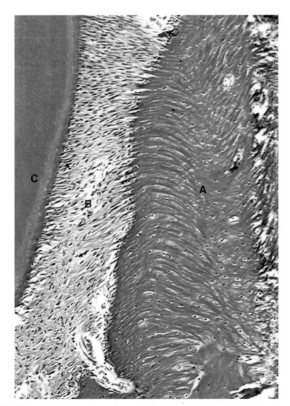

Fig. 13.32 Mesiodistal section of interdental bone (A), showing Sharpey's fibres from the periodontal ligament (B) appearing to pass more or less completely through the full thickness of bone between two adjacent teeth. C = Root. (Decalcified longitudinal section; Masson's trichrome; × 100).

STRUCTURAL LINES IN BONE

Bone is laid down rhythmically, which results in the formation of regular parallel lines that, because they are formed in periods of relative quiescence, are termed resting lines. Such resting lines differ biochemically from adjacent bone. These lines are prominent in bundle bone on the distal surface of the socket wall during physiological mesial drift of the teeth (Fig. 13. 34). Bone will also contain reversal lines, representing the site of change from bone resorption to bone deposition (see page 213). Such reversal lines will show evidence of a scalloped outline, reflecting the position of Howships lacunae (Figs 13.18, 13.35).

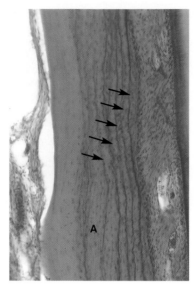

Fig. 13.34 Alveolar bone (A) on the distal wall of a tooth socket undergoing mesial drift, showing many vertical resting lines (arrows) due to rhythmic deposition of bone with periods of quiescence, (H & E; × 40).

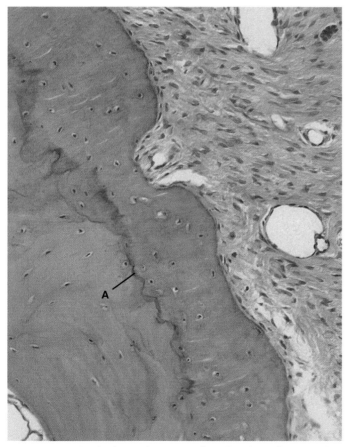

Fig. 13.35 Alveolar bone showing scalloped outline of a reversal line (A) (H & E; × 250).

CLINICAL CONSIDERATIONS

Because maintenance of bone mass is dependent on suitable functional stimuli, alveolar bone will atrophy when functional loads are decreased. Thus, following tooth extraction, alveolar bone will resorb unless the remaining ridge is loaded. Even the placement of a denture over the remaining alveolar ridge will help retard bone loss. The ability of alveolar bone to remodel throughout life allows teeth to be repositioned during orthodontic treatment.

As fractures involving the face are among the most common type of bone fractures encountered, an understanding of the principles involved in bone healing is essential in the clinical situation. Similarly, after tooth extraction, the empty socket will fill in with bone. In the wound, stem cells and osteoprogenitor cells will be stimulated and eventually give rise to osteoblasts, this process involving cell–matrix interactions. The initial immature (woven) bone will be remodelled to form mature, fine-fibred bone. Future developments of strategies to improve healing may be through the supplementation of osteoprogenitor cells or bioactive substances such as bone morphogenetic proteins. The rate of fracture repair appears to slow down with age, the precise reason for which remains to be clarified: it may be that there is a reduction in the number of stem cells in bone with age. An approach to speed up fracture repair in older patients is to isolate some stem cells from the patient's bone, culture them to increase their numbers and then seed them in a suitable framework which is then placed in the fracture site.

Alveolar bone will be resorbed in the presence of inflammation. This is most commonly associated with periodontal disease and periapical abscesses. Among important bioactive molecules implicated in this resorption process are cytokines and prostaglandins, as well as protons (as inflamed tissue is generally acidic).

Apart from inflammation, conditions exist where the normal balance between bone formation and bone resorption is disturbed. For example, osteopetrosis is a heterogeneous disorder characterised by impaired osteoclast function. In one type there is a deficiency of the enzyme carbonic anhydrase type II and, although bone formation occurs, the defective osteoclasts lose their ability to resorb bone. The bone of such patients therefore becomes increasingly thickened. An analogous condition in rodents prevents teeth from erupting due to the inability of bone overlying erupting teeth to resorb. The cause of one such condition is a lack of production of colony stimulating factor. If the missing factor is replaced, osteoclasts can be switched on to resorb alveolar bone and the teeth can then erupt. Osteoporosis is a bone disorder characterised by a low bone mass. It particularly affects trabecular bone and this predisposes bones to fractures as, once lost, it cannot be replaced. Sites notably prone to such fractures include the neck of the femur and the lumbar vertebrae. Osteoporosis is of less importance for the jaws, which have comparatively small amounts of cancellous bone. It can be age-related and particularly affects postmenopausal women. The precise cause of osteoporosis is not known although a number of factors including sex hormone deficiency, lack of mechanical loading and glucocorticoid excess, have been identified. Bone loss generally can be prevented or reduced by exercise, hormone-replacement therapy and the administration of calcium supplements and other drugs such as bisphosphonates.

Another important clinical area where a knowledge of bone biology is important concerns the field of implantology. Whereas a foreign material placed into bone is normally regarded as 'non-self' and becomes surrounded by a fibrous capsule, some materials allow for a direct structural union. When inserted into the jaw to provide the basis of support for a tooth, denture or orthodontic appliance, this union between the dental implant and adjacent living bone is termed osseo-integration. The materials most used are based on titanium or chrome–cobalt alloys. A narrow interface (20–40 nm) between the bone and implant contains non-collagenous bone matrix proteins such as osteopontin and bone sialoprotein. The successful long-term retention of an implant will depend on (apart from careful surgical technique to ensure minimum trauma at the implant site and absence of excessive micro-motion following implantation) factors related to the implant (such as the shape, topography, composition and surface chemistry, with particular reference to the formation of an oxidised layer) and the host response (the formation of a blood clot in which the necessary factors for successful osteogenesis are present, such as cytokines, growth factors, costeoprogenitor cells). The bone immediately adjacent to the implant to a depth of 1 mm will necrose and be remodelled and replaced by new bone, a period of about 17 weeks being required for the establishment of a suitable viable bone interface with the implant. From a knowledge of basic bone biology, implants are being used that are coated with materials thought likely to encourage osseointegration, such as cell-adhesion molecules and hydroxyapatite crystals.

14 Oral mucosa

Whereas the skin is dry and provides the covering for the external surface of the body, the alimentary tract is lined with a moist mucosa (mucous membrane). The mucosa is specialised in each region of the alimentary tract, but the basic pattern of an epithelium with an underlying connective tissue (the lamina propria) is maintained and is analogous to the epidermis and dermis of the skin respectively. In many regions, a third layer (the submucosa) is found between the lamina propria and the underlying bone (palate) or muscle (cheeks and lips).

The oral mucosa shows specialisations that allow it to fulfil several roles:

- It is protective mechanically against both compressive and shearing forces.
- It provides a barrier to microorganisms, toxins and various antigens.
- It has a role in immunological defence, both humoral and cell-mediated.
- Minor glands within the oral mucosa provide lubrication and buffering as well as secretion of some antibodies.
- The mucosa is richly innervated, providing input for touch, proprioception, pain and taste.

Two distinct layers are readily recognised in the oral mucosa for all regions of the mouth (Fig. 14.1). The outer layer is a stratified squamous epithelium that in areas subjected to masticatory forces (e.g. gingiva, palate and dorsum of tongue) is keratinised. The epithelium is derived embryologically from either ectoderm or endoderm. Beneath the epithelium is the connective tissue, comprising the lamina propria. The sub-

mucosa consists of a looser connective tissue containing fat deposits and glands. Larger nerves and blood vessels run in the submucosa. The boundary between the connective tissues of the lamina propria and the submucosa is often indistinct.

The oral mucosa may be classified into three types: masticatory, lining and specialised mucosa. Masticatory mucosa is found where there is high compression and friction and is characterised by a keratinised or parakeratinised epithelium and a thick lamina propria, which is usually bound down directly and tightly to underlying bone (mucoperiosteum). Masticatory mucosa covers the hard palate and oral surface of the gingiva. Lining mucosa is not subject to high levels of friction, but must be mobile and distensible. It is non-keratinised, has a loose lamina propria, and covers the mucosa of the cheeks, lips, alveolus, dentogingival region, floor of mouth, ventral surface of tongue and soft palate. The dorsum of the tongue is a specialised region of gustatory mucosa.

THE EPITHELIUM

Several layers of cells of distinct morphologies may be recognised in the stratified squamous epithelium lining the oral cavity (Fig. 14.2). A variety of terms have been used to identify the layers, the more common being:

- stratum germinativum (or stratum basale)
- stratum spinosum (or prickle cell layer)
- stratum granulosum (or granular layer)
- stratum corneum (the keratinised or cornified layer).

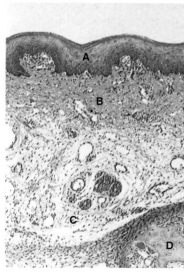

Fig. 14.1 Section showing regions of oral mucosa. A = Stratified squamous epithelium; B = lamina propria; C = submucosa; D = bone (Masson's trichrome; × 35).

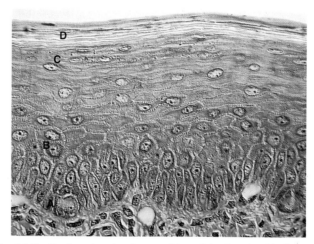

Fig. 14.2 Section showing layers of keratinised oral epithelium. A = Stratum germinativum (basal layer); B = stratum spinosum (prickle cell layer); C = stratum granulosum (granular layer); D = stratum corneum (keratinised or cornified layer) (× 180).

Unlike skin, the oral mucosa does not have a stratum lucidum (clear layer) between the stratum granulosum and stratum corneum.

The different layers of the oral epithelium represent a progressive maturation process. Cells from the most superficial layer (i.e. the stratum corneum) are continuously being shed and replaced from below. Turnover time is fastest in the region of the junctional and sulcular epithelia (about 5 days), which are located immediately adjacent to the tooth surface. This is probably about twice as fast as that seen in lining mucosa such as the cheek. Turnover time in masticatory mucosa appears to be a little slower than that in non-masticatory (lining) mucosa.

Stratum germinativum

The stratum germinativum is the single cell layer adjacent to the lamina propria (and demarcated from it by a basal lamina; (see page 229). It consists of cuboidal cells, which, containing progenitor cells, give rise to the cells in the epithelial layers

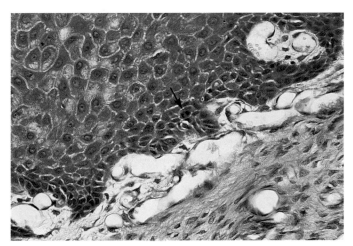

Fig. 14.3 Section of oral epithelium showing a mitotic figure (arrow) near basal layer (H & E; × 200). Courtesy of Dr R. O'Sullivan.

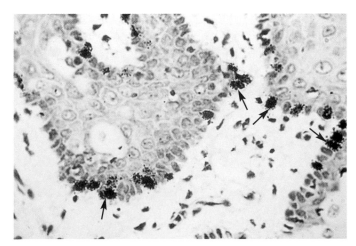

Fig. 14.4 Autoradiograph of oral epithelium using tritiated thymidine to reveal mitotic cells in the basal layer via presence of black granules (arrows) (Background stain H & E; × 200). Courtesy of Dr D. Adams.

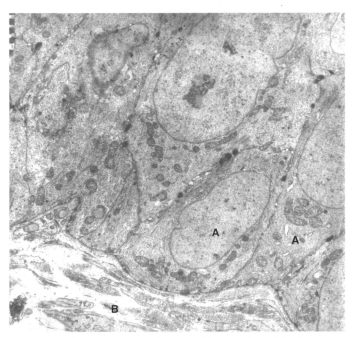

Fig. 14.5 Electron micrograph of basal layer of keratinised stratified squamous epithelium. The cells (A) are undifferentiated, contain various intracellular organelles such as mitochondria, free ribosomes and microfilaments and rest on a basal lamina. B = lamina propria (× 4000). Courtesy of Professor M. Smith.

above. Cells from the stratum germinativum are the progenitors. Whether all the cells are stem cells is uncertain. There are indications that germinative cells are heterogeneous and that only a minority are true stem cells, the remainder being committed 'transit' cells undergoing a limited number of amplifying divisions before succumbing to terminal differentiation. Mitosis occurs only in this layer. Mitotic figures can occasionally be seen with routine staining (Fig. 14.3). However, they are clearly in evidence when using autoradiography (Fig. 14.4). Daughter cells pass towards the surface and, during the process of maturation, take on the appearance characteristic of the various layers.

The cells of the stratum germinativum are the least differentiated within the oral epithelium and this is reflected in their ultrastructural appearance, where they are seen to contain the usual variety of organelles, including a nucleolus, mitochondria, ribosomes, Golgi material, and tonofilaments and desmosomes (Fig. 14.5). The stem cells within the stratum germinativum are thought to lie in the epithelial ridges that project into the lamina propria. Maturing cells are believed to produce growth inhibitors that restrict further cell division by negative feedback. The precise mechanism of inhibitor release is not known but, as the mitotic rate shows diurnal variation, systemic factors may be implicated. There is also evidence for a role for polypeptide growth factors (e.g. epidermal growth factor, transforming growth factor α) in promoting proliferation and possibly differentiation.

It is not known what triggers differentiation, but it does not appear to be simply a matter of displacement away from the basal layer as tissue culture studies indicate that, if cells are prevented from migrating away from the basal lamina, differentiation still occurs. Rather, the onset of differentiation seems to change the adhesive properties of the cell and leads to its 'expulsion' from the stratum germinativum.

Non-keratinocytes may be found in the stratum germinativum (see pages 226–229).

Stratum spinosum

Above the stratum germinativum, round or ovoid cells form a layer several cells thick called the stratum spinosum (Fig. 14.2). These cells show the first stages of maturation, being larger and rounder than those in the stratum germinativum. The transition from stratum germinativum to stratum spinosum is characterised by the appearance of new cytokeratin types (see pages 224–225). They contribute to the formation of the tonofilaments, which become thicker and more conspicuous. Involucrin (the soluble precursor protein of the cornified envelope eventually found in the cornified layer) appears first in the stratum spinosum. There is a progressive decrease in synthetic activity through the layer.

In the upper part of the stratum spinosum appear small, intracellular membrane-coating granules (Odland bodies) that are rich in phospholipids. These granules are approximately 0.25 μm in length and, in keratinised epithelium, consist of a series of parallel lamellae. They probably originate from the Golgi apparatus. In the more superficial layers of the stratum spinosum the granules come to lie close to the cell membrane.

Within the stratum spinosum desmosomes increase in number and become more obvious than in the stratum germinativum (Figs 14.6, 14.7). The slight shrinkage that occurs in most histological preparations causes the cells to separate at all points where desmosomes do not anchor them together. This gives the cells their 'spiny' appearance.

The term 'parabasal' is used to refer to the deepest layer of cells of the stratum spinosum that lie next to the stratum germinativum. They may show features similar to that of the

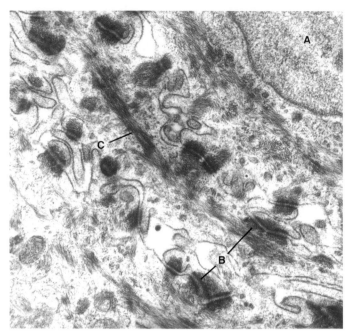

Fig. 14.7 Electron micrograph of the prickle cell layer. A = Nucleus; B = desmosome surrounded by inserting tonofilaments; C = tonofilaments of keratin (× 20 000). Courtesy of Professor M.M. Smith.

stratum germinativum in that they may be elongated and undergo cell proliferation.

Stratum granulosum

The cells of the stratum granulosum (Fig. 14.2) show a further increase in maturation compared with those of the strata germinativum and spinosum. Many organelles are reduced or lost, such that the cytoplasm is predominantly occupied by the tonofilaments and tonofibrils. The cells are larger and flatter (Figs 14.8, 14.9), but most significantly now contain large numbers of small granules called keratohyaline granules (Fig. 14.10). These contain the precursor to filaggrin (profilaggrin). The granules are 0.5–1.0 μm in length and form the matrix in

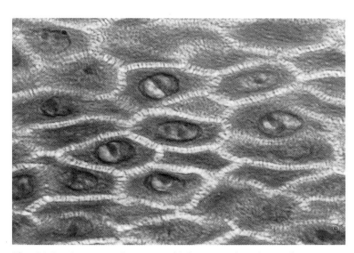

Fig. 14.6 Stratum spinosum at high power showing 'spiky' desmosomes connecting adjacent cells (H & E; × 1000). Courtesy of Professor M.M Smith.

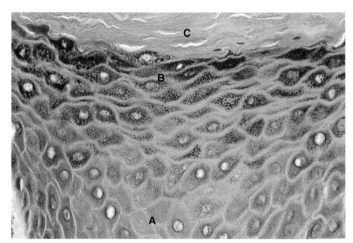

Fig. 14.8 Section showing upper part of stratum spinosum (A), the stratum granulosum (B) and the stratum corneum (C). Note the granular nature of the cells in the granular layer (H & E; × 350). Courtesy of Professor M.M. Smith.

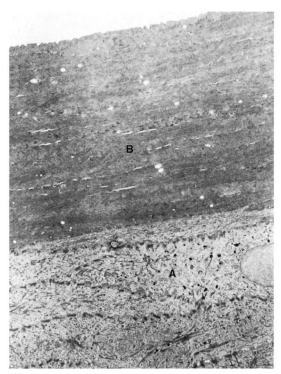

Fig. 14.9 Electron micrograph showing granular (A) and keratinised (B) layers. Within the cells of the granular layer can be seen the keratohyalin granules, while the cells of the keratin layer lack nuclei and other organelles (× 2800). Courtesy of Profesor C.A. Squier.

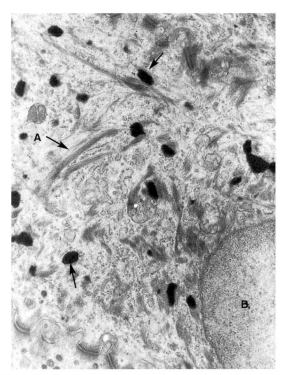

Fig. 14.10 Higher power electron micrograph of cell of granular layer. A = Tonofibril; B = nucleus. Keratohyalin granule arrowed (× 12 000). Courtesy of Professor C.A. Squier.

which the tonofilaments are embedded. The membrane-coating granules discharge into the extracellular space. This is associated with the development of a barrier in the epithelium that limits the movement of substances between the cells.

Stratum corneum

In keratinised epithelium the final stage in the maturation of the epithelial cells is the loss of all organelles (including nuclei and keratohyaline granules) (Figs 14.8, 14.9, 14.11). Indeed, the cells of the stratum corneum become filled entirely with closely packed tonofilaments surrounded by the matrix protein filaggrin. This mixture of proteins is collectively called keratin. The cells of the stratum corneum may be termed epithelial squames; it is these cells that are shed (the process of desquamation), necessitating the constant turnover of epithelial cells. Desmosomes weaken and disappear to allow for this desquamation.

The stratum corneum provides the mechanical protective function to the mucosa. It varies in thickness (up to 20 cells) and is thicker for the oral mucosa than for most areas of skin (except for the palms of the hands and the soles of the feet). In some areas such as the gingiva the nuclei may be retained, although small and shrunken. These cells are described as parakeratinised (in contrast to the more usual orthokeratinised cells without nuclei) (Fig. 14.12).

In the cornified layer involucrin becomes cross-linked (by the enzyme transglutaminase) to form a thin (10 nm), highly resistant, electron-dense, cornified envelope just beneath the plasma membrane. The trigger for this is probably cell death and the influx of calcium ions. The keratin is also strongly cross-linked by disulphide bonds, contributing to the mechanical and chemical resistance of the layer.

In lining epithelium the epithelial cells are non-keratinised at the surface (Fig. 14.13). Ultrastructurally, the surface layers differ from the cells of keratinised epithelia in that they show less developed and dispersed tonofilaments and lack keratohyaline granules. There are also more organelles in the surface layers than in keratinised cells, although there are still considerably fewer than in the stratum germinativum. Above the

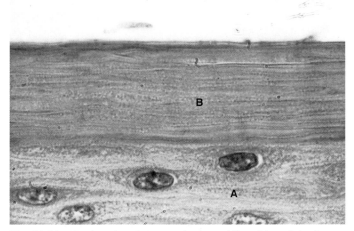

Fig. 14.11 Section showing granular layer (A) and keratinised layers (B) (H & E; × 1000). Courtesy of Dr D. Adams.

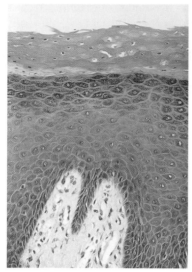

Fig. 14.12 Section of parakeratinised oral epithelium from the gingiva. The superficial layer stains more heavily for keratin but nuclei are retained (H & E; × 100). Courtesy of Dr A.W. Barrett.

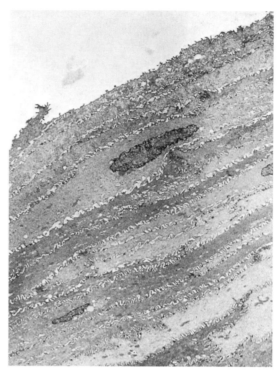

Fig. 14.14 Electronmicrograph of surface layers in non-keratinised lining epithelium. Note the retention of nuclei (× 2000). Courtesy of Professor C.A. Squier.

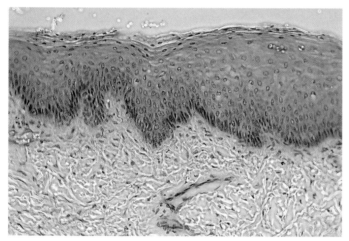

Fig. 14.13 Section of lining oral epithelium from the alveolar mucosa. There is an absence of keratin in the superfical layer. (H & E; × 80). Courtesy of Professor M.M. Smith.

stratum spinosum, the layers are not as clearly defined as in a keratinised epithelium. The outer layers are usually termed the stratum intermedium and the stratum superficiale. Nuclei persist within the surface layers (Fig. 14.14).

CYTOKERATINS

In epithelial cells the cytoskeleton is composed of micro-filaments, microtubules and intermediate filaments. Micro-filaments are approximately 4–6 nm in diameter and have a molecular weight of the order of 43 kDa. By contrast, micro-tubules are 25 nm in diameter with a molecular weight of 55 kDa. Although intermediate in terms of diameter (7–11 nm), the intermediate filaments have a molecular weight ranging from 40 kDa to as high as 200 kDa. In contrast with microfilaments and microtubules, which are ubiquitous proteins, intermediate filaments have a high degree of tissue

specificity. Six major classes of intermediate filaments have been identified, including the cytokeratins (CK), which have a high specificity for epithelial cells. 'Moll' numbers were assigned to the CK proteins, which are the products of two gene families and which translate into at least 20 CK polypeptides. The products of each CK gene family are divided into the neutral or basic type II CK (numbered 1–8) and the acidic type I CK (numbered 9–20). They occur in pairs. The type I CK is the smaller of each pair, ranging between 40–56.5 kDa and always about 8 kDa smaller than its type II counterpart, which has a molecular weight 53–67 kDa.

CK expression conforms to several 'rules', each epithelial cell expressing at least one CK pair comprising one type I and one type II. The ultimate CK phenotype reflects the differen-tiation pathway the cell has followed. Because they are only expressed in simple epithelia, such as ductal luminal cells, CKs 7, 8 and 18 are designated 'simple'. The best-characterised CKs associated with epithelial stratification are pairs 5 and 14, 4 and 13, 1 and 10.

Within epithelial cells CK filaments function as components of the cytoskeleton and cell contacts (desmosomes and hemidesmosomes). However, the physiological reason for the large number of CKs remains obscure. Some insight into their functional significance can be obtained from analysis of con-genital or experimental CK abnormalities. For example, in some forms of epidermolysis bullosa (a group of mucocutaneous lesions, all of which produce subepithelial blistering) there is a mutant form of CK14. Some CKs may be important in main-taining the metabolic homeostasis of the cell.

Apart from their structural role in the cytoskeleton, there is evidence for other roles for CKs, possibly related to their location. For example, CK14 is most strongly positive in the stratum germinativum. The fact that CK14-positive basal cells in palatal and lingual epithelium synthesise neurogenic peptides may be related to the innervation of the superficial oral mucosa. This view is supported by work which showed that denervation of rodent taste buds causes loss of CK expression and is consistent with a possible role for CK in signal transduction.

Major distribution patterns of cytokeratins in oral epithelium (Table 14.1)

CK5 and 14 are usually restricted to the basal and parabasal layers (Fig. 14.15), although CK14 may also be expressed by suprabasal keratinocytes. CK 1 and 10 (or CK 2 and 11) are characteristically found in the suprabasal layers of masticatory mucosa and are associated with terminal differentiation and keratinisation (Fig. 14.16). The keratin layer itself is negative. In lining mucosa, the suprabasal keratinocytes stain primarily for CK4 and 13 rather than the CK1 and 13 found in masticatory mucosa (Fig. 14.17). There is variable expression of other cytokeratins. CK6 and 16 are associated with rapid turnover epithelia. CK19 may also be a marker for basal keratinocytes in lining mucosa, but reports concerning its presence are inconsistent. Variations in the CK distribution of non-keratinised oral epithelium at different anatomical sites have been reported. The epithelium lining the ventral surface of the tongue may be distinguished from other lining oral epithelium by its increased expression of CKs 5, 6 and 14. However, most unusual is the epithelium covering the soft palate, which apparently expresses the simple cytokeratins (CK7, 8 and 18) as well as high levels of CK19.

Table 14.1 *Distribution of cytokeratins in human stratified squamous epithelium (SSE)*

	CK pair	
	Type I, acidic, low M_R	Type II, basic, high M_R
Suprabasal, keratinised SSE	1, 2 and 3	10 and 11
Cornea	3	12
Suprabasal, non-keratinised SSE	4	13
Basal keratinocytes (all SSE)	5	14
Hyperproliferative epithelia	6	16
Simple epithelia	8	18
Some simple epithelia, pilosebaceous tracts, basal cell carcinomas	?	17
Basal keratinocytes in non-keratinised SSE, some simple or 'plastic' epithelia (e.g. odontogenic)	?	19

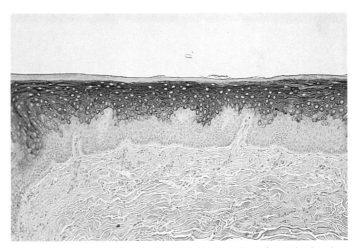

Fig. 14.16 Section of orthokeratinised epithelium from the hard palate stained for cytokeratin 10, showing positive suprabasal staining (brown) (Streptavidin biotinylated immunoperoxidase stain; × 50). Courtesy of Dr A.W. Barrett.

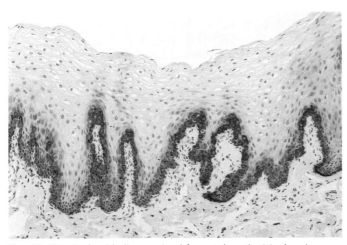

Fig. 14.15 Oral epithelium stained for cytokeratin 14, showing positive staining (purple) restricted to the basal cell layer (Streptavidin-biotinylated immunoperoxidase alkaline phosphatase stain; × 100). Courtesy of Dr A.W. Barrett.

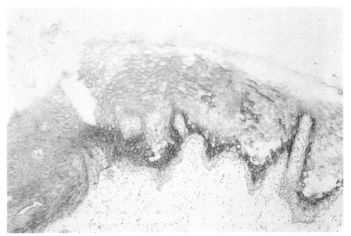

Fig. 14.17 Section of non-keratinised epithelium from the cheek stained for cytokeratin 4, showing positive staining (brown) throughout except for the basal layer (Streptavidin biotinylated immunoperoxidase stain; × 60). Courtesy of Dr A.W. Barrett.

FACTORS CONTROLLING ORAL EPITHELIAL PHENOTYPE

In reviewing the nature of the oral epithelium, it has been shown that regional specificity exists throughout life, even though there is a continuous and rapid replacement of the components. This poses questions as to the nature of the factor(s) determining such specificity. The specificity may be considered as being the result of extrinsic inductive stimuli from the underlying lamina propria or an intrinsic property of the basal layer of the epithelium. Knowledge of the underlying mechanisms has clinical relevance as, following surgical removal of the dentogingival tissues, the three distinctive epithelia of the oral gingiva, sulcular epithelium and junctional epithelium do regenerate, presumably from the remaining oral gingival epithelium. Furthermore, conditions exist where non-keratinised zones of epithelia are encountered in regions of masticatory epithelia and treatment may be geared towards attempting to replace these zones with the appropriate keratinised epithelium.

As regards the view that specificity is the result of epithelial/mesenchymal interactions, this has been well established during tooth development (see page 297). The role of mesenchyme in determining the phenotype of the overlying epithelium, and its ability to maintain this property and therefore redirect patterns of epithelial morphogenesis in the adult, has been investigated by a number of researchers using classical methods in which portions of oral mucosa were transplanted to different regions or were separated into their epithelial and connective tissue components and then homo- and heterotypically recombined and transplanted. Such studies support the view that the underlying lamina propria is primarily responsible for the specificity of the overlying epithelia, in terms of both morphology and CK content. Thus, lining oral epithelium combined with lamina propria from masticatory mucosa took on the features of a masticatory mucosa, whilst masticatory epithelium combined with lamina propria from lining mucosa modulated to lining epithelium. Such modulation does not appear to require a vital lamina propria as a similar effect was seen even after the connective tissue was frozen. These fundamental changes are not only seen in subcutaneous sites in animal experiments but they have also been reported in clinical situations. Deep connective tissue, however, was not able to facilitate such changes.

Although there is considerable evidence for the importance of the underlying mesenchyme in specifying the form and phenotype of the overlying epithelium, both during development and in the adult, there is also evidence for some regionally related variations in the competence of epithelia to respond to these influences.

NON-KERATINOCYTES

As many as 10% of the cells in the oral epithelium are non-keratinocytes, and include melanocytes, Langerhans cells and Merkel cells. All lack the tonofilaments and desmosomes characteristic of keratinocytes (except for the Merkel cells). Non-keratinocytes may appear as clear cells in sections stained routinely with haematoxylin and eosin (Fig. 14.18). Lacking the typical cytokeratins associated with normal keratinocytes, they remain unstained in sections of epithelium stained for CK (Fig. 14.19). Some non-keratinocytes are inflammatory cells that have migrated through the epithelium (e.g. lymphocytes).

Melanocytes

Melanocytes are pigment-producing cells located in the stratum germinativum. They are derived from the neural crest and are present in the skin at about 8 weeks of intrauterine life. Once located in the epithelium, they are assumed to be long lived but with some powers of self-replication and are seen to divide *in vitro*. Melanocytes have long processes that extend in several directions and across several epithelial layers. As suggested by their name, melanocytes produce the pigment melanin, using the enzyme tyrosinase (which is lacking in albinos). They can be identified by special staining (Fig. 14.20).

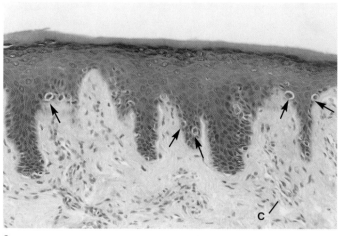

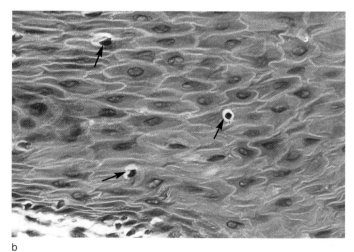

a   b

Fig. 14.18 (a) Section of red zone of lip showing clear cells (arrowed) in the basal layer, representing mainly melanocytes (× 80). (b) Clear cells in the upper layers of the epithelium (arrowed), mainly representing Langerhans cells (H & E; × 350). (b) Courtesy of Professor M.M. Smith.

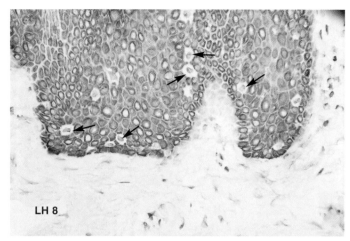

Fig. 14.19 Basal region of oral epithelium stained for cytokeratin 14 (brown) and illustrating clear cells (arrows) lacking cytokeratin and representing mainly melanocytes (× 200). Courtesy of Professor P. Morgan.

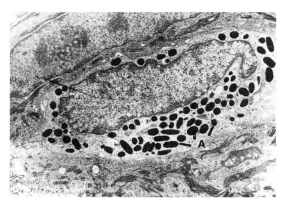

Fig. 14.21 Electronmicrograph of a melanocyte packed with melanosomes (A) (× 60 000). Courtesy of Professor C.A. Squier.

of the cells (rather than the absolute number), the size of the melanosomes, the number and degree of dispersion of the melanosomes, the degree of melanisation of the melanosomes and the rate of degradation of the pigment.

Langerhans cells

Langerhans cells are dendritic cells situated in the layers above the stratum germinativum. They are derived from bone marrow precursors and leave the bloodstream to enter the lamina propria, before penetrating the basal lamina to reach the epithelium. Such migration may relate to certain chemokines released by keratinocytes with surface receptors on the Langerhans cells. Langerhans cells act as part of the immune system as antigen-presenting cells. They express Ia antigens and Fc receptors and move back and forth from the epithelium via dermal lymphatics to local lymph nodes. They play an important role in skin in producing contact hypersensitivity reactions, in anti-tumour immunity and in graft rejection; they also react as propagators of HIV-1 transmission to T cells. The cells may be localised due to the presence of ATPase on the cell membrane (Fig. 14.22).

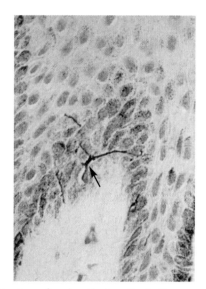

Fig. 14.20 Section of oral epithelium illustrating a melanocyte (arrowed) (Masson's Fontana stain; × 280). Courtesy of Professor I. Mackenzie.

Ultrastructurally, in addition to mitochondria, endoplasmic reticulum and Golgi complex, the cytoplasm of melanocytes characteristically contains pigment that is packaged in small granules termed melanosomes (Fig. 14.21). The long processes of the melanocyte extend between adjacent keratinocytes and each melanocyte establishes contact with about 30–40 keratinocytes. Indeed, keratinocytes release numerous mediators that are essential for normal melanocyte function. As the melanosomes mature under the activity of tyrosinase, their content of melanin increases. The pigment is passed to adjacent keratinocytes (and hair cortex cells) as the tips of the dendrites are actively phagocytosed by the keratinocytes. Melanin pigmentation is usually not pronounced in the buccal mucosa, tongue, hard palate or gingiva.

The number of melanocytes varies in different regions, but the difference in the degree of pigmentation between races is the result of a combination of the size and degree of branching

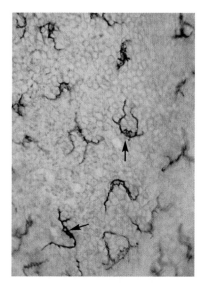

Fig. 14.22 Section of superficial layers of oral epithelium showing Langerhans cells (arrowed) (Lead capture staining for ATPase; × 200). Courtesy of Professor I. Mackenzie.

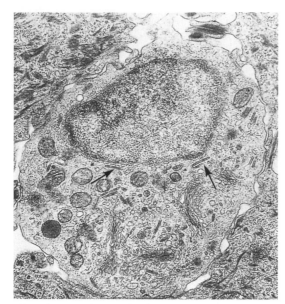

Fig. 14.23 Electronmicrograph of Langerhans cell showing the characteristic Birbeck granules (arrows) (× 15 000). Courtesy of Dr N.G. El-Labban.

Ultrastructurally, the Langerhans cell contains characteristic, trilaminar, rod-shaped granules called Birbeck granules (Fig. 14.23). Foreign antigens penetrate the superficial layers and bind to dendritic antigen-presenting cells such as Langerhans cells, which stimulate helper T lymphocytes, and Granstein cells, which stimulate specific suppressor T lymphocytes. T cells also receive a signal in the form of a cytokine (interleukin-1) from both keratinocytes and dendritic cells, then secrete a lymphokine (interleukin-2) that causes the proliferation of T cells.

Merkel cells

The Merkel cell is found in the stratum germinativum, often closely apposed to nerve fibres. It is thought to act as a receptor and is derived from the neural crest. As they contain CK filaments, Merkel cells can be identified by immunohistochemical techniques using antibodies for CK 8/18 and 20 (Fig. 14.24).

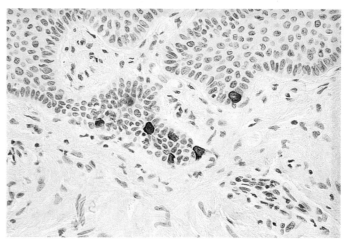

Fig. 14.24 Section showing Merkel cells in basal layer of epithelium staining positively (brown) for cytokeratin18 (Streptavidin-biotinylated immunoperoxidase stain; × 200). Courtesy of Dr W.A. Barrett.

Fig. 14.25 Electron micrograph of Merkel cell. Note the indented nucleus and nuclear rodlet. The cytoplasm contains numerous characteristic dense granules 80–180 nm in diameter (× 16 000). Courtesy of Dr S-Y. Chen.

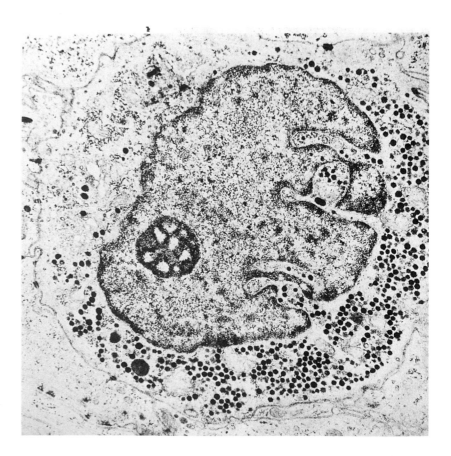

Merkel cells are common in masticatory epithelia such as gingiva and generally absent from lining mucosa such as the buccal mucosa.

Ultrastructurally, the nucleus of the Merkel cell is often deeply invaginated and may contain a characteristic rodlet (Fig. 14.25). The cytoplasm contains numerous mitochondria, abundant free ribosomes, and a collection of electron-dense granules (80–180 nm in diameter), the function of which is unknown. In addition, there are many small vesicles in the region adjacent to the nerve terminal. Desmosomes are associated with the cell membrane. Free nerve endings not associated with a Merkel cell are also found within the epithelium. These are nociceptors.

LAMINA PROPRIA

The connective tissue underlying the oral epithelium can be described as having two layers: a superficial, papillary layer between the epithelial ridges, in which the collagen fibres are thin and loosely arranged; and, beneath this, a deep, reticular layer dominated by thick, parallel bundles of collagen fibres.

The fibroblasts of the lamina propria are typical of those found in loose connective tissues. In outline their shape varies, a number appearing spindle-shaped. They contain the full complement of synthetic organelles consistent with their role in the continuous production and secretion of extracellular fibres and ground substance for the lamina propria (Fig. 14.26).

The extracellular matrix of the lamina propria contains collagen fibres (about 90% Type I, about 8% Type III, plus small amounts of the non-fibrous forms of collagen) and elastin fibres (the ratio depending on site). Oxytalan fibres have also been described in this site. The ground substance of the lamina propria consists of a hydrated gel of proteoglycans and glycoproteins. As with all general connective tissues, the

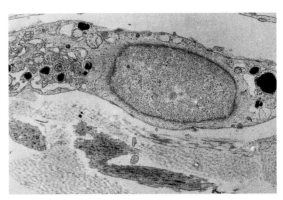

Fig. 14.27 Electron micrograph of macrophage in lamina propria. It contains many lysosomes but little endoplasmic reticulum (× 10 000). Courtesy of Professor C.A. Squires.

usual defence cells will occur. Macrophages are seen in the lamina propria. In their fixed, inactive stage, they are known as histiocytes and are difficult to distinguish from fibroblasts. They have a smaller, darker nucleus than fibroblasts and contain lysosomes but little endoplasmic reticulum (Fig. 14.27). As well as having a phagocytic role, macrophages act as antigen-presenting cells. Mast cells are mononuclear, spherical or elliptical in shape, and contain histamine and heparin intracellular granules (see page 195). They play a role in vascular homeostasis, in inflammation, in cell-mediated immunity and are responsible for anaphylactic (type 1) hypersensitivity. Lymphocytes are also found in small numbers in healthy mucosa, but increase dramatically in inflammation.

EPITHELIAL–CONNECTIVE TISSUE INTERFACE

A complex arrangement links epithelial and connective tissue components of the oral mucosa. In the light microscope, a layer 1–2 μm thick is seen on the lamina propria side of the junction. This is termed the basement membrane. In the electron microscope, the layer appears much thinner and is then termed the **basal lamina**. The thicker appearance in the light microscope is probably due to the inclusion of some of the sub-epithelial collagen fibres, which in this region have staining properties similar to those of the basal lamina.

Ultrastructurally, the basal lamina is found to consist of a complex of fibrils and ground substance (Fig. 14.28). Two zones are seen.

- The electron-lucent lamina lucida is 20–40 nm thick and lies immediately under the epithelium.
- The thicker (20–120 nm) lamina densa is deep to this.

The lamina lucida consists of a glycoprotein called laminin that cements non-fibrillar type IV collagen in the lamina densa to the epithelial cells. The lamina densa consists of type IV collagen coated on each side by a glycosaminoglycan – heparan sulphate. Thick collagen fibrils attach onto the lamina densa with finer fibrils running though these to link the whole complex mechanically to the connective tissue. Fibronectin has sometimes been found in the lamina densa

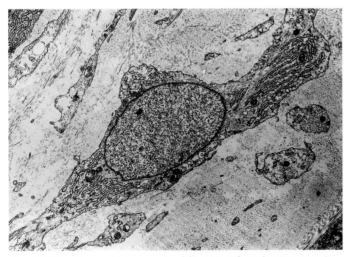

Fig. 14.26 Electron micrograph of fibroblast from lamina propria. The cell contains a full complement of all the intracellular organelles associated with collagen synthesis. Note the conspicuous rough endoplasmic reticulum (× 11 000). Courtesy of Professor C.A. Squiers.

Fig. 14.28 Electron micrograph showing appearance of basal lamina (× 34 000). Courtesy of Professor C.A. Squires.

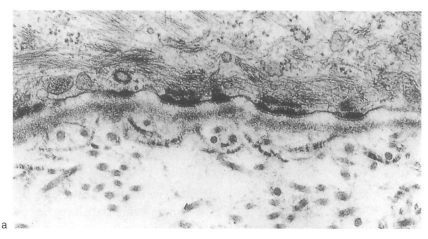

a

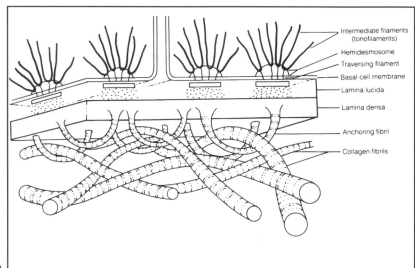

Intermediate filaments (tonofilaments)
Hemidesmosome
Traversing filament
Basal cell membrane
Lamina lucida
Lamina densa
Anchoring fibril
Collagen fibrils

b

and may play a role in adhering fibroblasts and proteoglycans to it. The cell side of the basal lamina consists of hemidesmosomes.

The basal lamina provides mechanical adhesion between the oral epithelium and the lamina propria, acts as a molecular barrier and plays a role in the response to tissue injury. All the major products of the basal lamina appear to be synthesised by the epithelial cells.

REGIONAL VARIATIONS IN THE STRUCTURE OF THE ORAL MUCOSA

In different parts of the mouth, the mucosa has different roles and experiences different degrees and types of stress during mastication, speech and facial expression. As a consequence, the structure of the oral mucosa varies in terms of the thickness of the epithelium, the degree of keratinisation, the complexity of the connective tissue–epithelium interface, the composition of the lamina propria, and the presence or absence of the submucosa.

There are three types of oral mucosa: masticatory, lining, and specialised mucosa. **Masticatory mucosa** is found where there is high compression and friction, and is characterised by

a keratinised epithelium and a thick lamina propria. The mucosa of the gingiva and palate is masticatory, the bulk of which is bound down directly and tightly to underlying bone (mucoperiosteum), except for the region at the side of the palate where a submucosa is present. **Lining mucosa** is not subject to high levels of friction but must be mobile and distensible. It is thus non-keratinised and has a loose lamina propria. Within the lamina propria, the collagen fibres are arranged as a network to allow free movement, and the elastic fibres allow recoil to prevent the mucosa being chewed. Commonly, lining mucosa also has a submucosa. The lips, cheeks, alveolus, floor of the mouth, ventral surface of the tongue and soft palate have a lining mucosa. Two areas of **specialised mucosa** occur: the specialised gustatory mucosa of the dorsum of the tongue and where the vermilion zone forms a transition between the skin and the oral mucosa.

Regional variations of the oral mucosa are summarised in Table 14.2.

The lip

The lip has skin on its outer surface and labial mucosa on its inner surface. Between these two tissues lies the vermilion zone (also known as the red or transitional zone of the lip) (Fig. 14.29). The lips have striated muscles in their core that

Table 14.2 *Principal features and regional variations of the oral mucosa*

Region	Epithelium		Lamina propria		Submucosa		Type of mucosa
	Thickness	Keratinisation	Papillae	Fibre types	Density	Attachment	
Labial and buccal mucosa	Thick	Non-keratinised	Short and irregular	Collagen and some elastic fibres	Dense	Firmly to under-lying muscle	Lining
Vermilion (red) zone of lip	Thin	Keratinised	Long and narrow	Collagen and some elastic fibres	Dense	Firmly to under-lying muscle	Specialised
Alveolar mucosa	Thin	Non-keratinised	Short or absent	Many elastic fibres	Loose	Loose attachment to periosteum	Lining
Attached gingiva	Thick	Keratinised and parakeratinised	Long and narrow	Dense collagen firmly attached to underlying periosteum	No distinct submucosa		Masticatory
Floor of mouth	Thin	Non-keratinised	Short and broad	Collagen and some elastic fibres	Loose	Loose attachment to underlying muscle	Lining
Ventral surface of tongue	Thin	Non-keratinised	Short and numerous	Collagen and some elastic fibres	Not very distinct layer; attached to underlying muscle		Lining
Dorsum of tongue (anterior two-thirds)	Thick	Primarily keratinised	Long	Collagen and some elastic fibres	Not very distinct layer; attached to underlying muscle		Specialised gustatory
Dorsum of tongue (posterior one-third)	Variable	Generally non-keratinised	Short or absent	Collagen and some elastic fibres	Not very distinct layer; attached to underlying muscle		Lining gustatory
Hard palate	Thick	Keratinised	Long	Dense collagen in submucosa laterally, but lamina propria firmly bound to periosteum without submucosa in midline			Masticatory
Soft palate	Thick	Non-keratinised	Short	Many elastic fibres	Loose	Loose attachment to underlying tissues	Lining

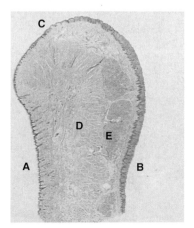

Fig. 14.29 Transverse section of the lip. A = Skin on external surface; B = labial mucosa on inner surface; C = vermilion (red) zone; D = striated muscles of orbicularis oris; E = minor salivary glands (H & E; × 2). Courtesy of S. Kariyawasam.

are part of the muscles of facial expression. Substantial amounts of minor mucous salivary glands are present in the submucosa beneath the oral mucosa.

The skin on the outer surface of the lip shows all the features of skin elsewhere (Fig. 14.30). A keratinised layer of epidermis lies on a bed of connective tissue, the dermis. The border between epidermis and dermis in this area is not markedly folded. The connective tissue contains sweat glands; sebaceous glands and the bases of hair follicles pass through the epithelium. The epidermis is, in fact, continuous around the bases of the follicles and is responsible for producing the keratin of which the hair is formed. Sebaceous glands drain either into the hair follicles or occasionally directly onto the skin surface.

Vermilion zone

The vermilion zone lacks the appendages of skin. However, very occasional sebaceous glands may be found, especially at

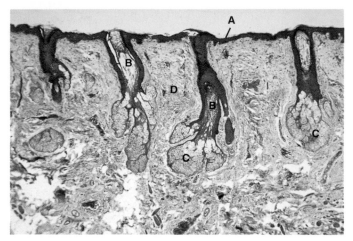

Fig. 14.30 Section of skin of lip. A = Keratinised epidermis; B = shaft of hair; C = sebaceous gland; D = dermis (Masson's trichrome; × 30).

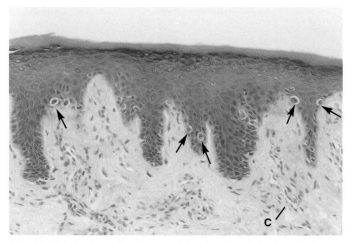

Fig. 14.31 Section of red zone of lip. A = Keratinised epithelium; B = lamina propria. Note the folded interface between epithelium and lamina propria bringing blood vessels (C) close to the surface (× 80).

the angles of the mouth. As the vermilion zone also lacks mucous glands, it requires constant moistening with saliva by the tongue to prevent drying. The epithelium of the vermilion zone is keratinised, but thin and translucent. The connective tissue papillae of the lamina propria are relatively long and narrow, and contain capillary loops (Fig. 14.31). The proximity of these vessels to the surface, combined with the translucency of the epithelium, gives the surface a red appearance – hence its name. This red appearance is a human characteristic. The junctional region between the vermilion zone and the oral mucosa is sometimes known as the intermediate zone and is parakeratinised. In infants this becomes thickened and forms the suckling pad.

Labial mucosa

The inner surface of the lip, the labial mucosa is covered by a relatively thick, non-keratinised epithelium. The lamina propria is also wide but the papillae are short and irregular. A submucosa containing many minor salivary glands is present

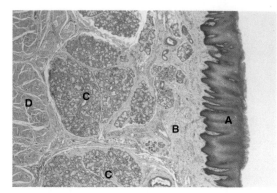

Fig. 14.32 Section of labial mucosa. A = Non-keratinised oral epithelium; B = lamina propria; C = minor salivary gland in submucosa; D = fibres of orbicularis oris (H & E; × 15). Courtesy of S. Kariyawasam.

(Fig. 14.32). Strands of dense connective tissue bind the mucosa down to the underlying orbicularis oris muscle.

The cheek

The buccal mucosa lining the cheeks is, like the labial mucosa, a lining mucosa. The epithelium is non-keratinised and the lamina propria is dense with short, irregular papillae. A submucosa is present with many minor salivary glands, beneath which lie fibres of the buccinator muscle (Fig. 14.33). Sometimes, along a line coincident with the occlusal plane, the epithelium becomes keratinised, forming a white line (the linea alba). Sebaceous glands are sometimes present and seem to become more obvious after puberty in the male and after menopause in the female, when they appear as small yellow patches. These patches are termed Fordyce spots (see page 3). The role, if any, of sebaceous glands in this location is unknown, although it is important to differentiate them from pathological changes.

The gingiva and alveolar mucosa

The **gingiva** is that portion of the oral mucosa that surrounds, and is attached to, the teeth and the alveolar bone. It has two recognised regions (Fig. 14.34). The main com-

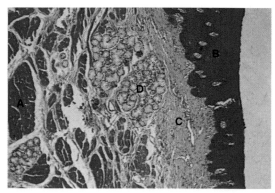

Fig. 14.33 Section of buccal mucosa. B = Non-keratinised oral epithelium; B = lamina propria; C = minor salivary gland in submucosa; A = fibres of buccinator muscle (H & E; × 15).

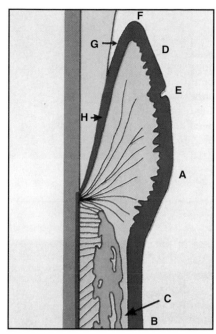

Fig. 14.34 Diagrammatic representation of gingiva. A = Attached gingiva; B = alveolar mucosa; C = submucosa associated with alveolar mucosa; D = free gingiva; E = free gingival groove; F = gingival margin; G = gingival sulcus; H = junctional epithelium.

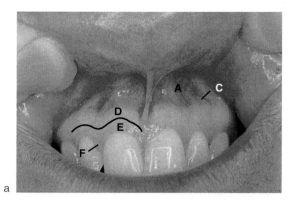

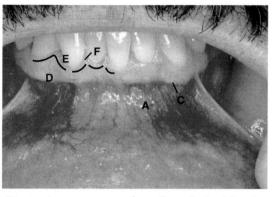

Fig. 14.35 *In vivo* appearance of maxillary gingiva (a) and mandibular gingiva (b). A = Alveolar mucosa; C = mucogingival junction; D = attached gingiva; E = free gingiva; F = interdental papilla.

ponent is the attached gingiva, which is directly bound down to the underlying alveolar bone and tooth. Coronal to the attached gingiva is the free gingiva, which is the narrow rim of mucosa that is not bound down to underlying hard tissue. Its junction with the attached gingiva is sometimes demarcated by a shallow groove, the free gingival groove. Its coronal limit is the gingival margin. The unattached region between the free gingiva and the tooth is the gingival sulcus. The region apical to this, where the gingiva is bound to the underlying tooth, is the junctional epithelium.

Apically, the attached gingiva is demarcated from the alveolar mucosa (which is loosely attached to the lower part of the alveolar bone) by the mucogingival junction, which normally lies 3–5 mm below the level of the alveolar crest. The height of the gingiva above this junction is about 4–6 mm. The alveolar mucosa has a submucosa.

The appearance of the gingiva and alveolar mucosa in the maxilla and mandible *in vivo* is seen in Fig. 14.35. The alveolar mucosa lines the lower part of the alveolus and is reflected over the buccal and labial sulcus to meet the buccal and labial mucosa respectively. It has a loose submucosa that allows for wide degrees of movement. The submucosa on its deep aspect is firmly attached to the underlying periosteum. The mucogingival junction (or health line) demarcates the boundary between attached gingiva and alveolar mucosa. The difference in appearance between the alveolar mucosa and the attached gingiva is due to differences in keratinisation and translucency. The alveolar mucosa epithelium is translucent and the blood vessels lie superficially. Small blood vessels are clearly seen. The junction may be scalloped, paralleling the contours of the gingival margin. The free gingival groove that separates the attached gingiva from the free gingiva is apparent in

about 40% of teeth. It follows the contours of the cement–enamel junction. The groove may be produced by the bundles of principal collagen fibres that run from the cervical cementum to the gingiva, or the groove might correspond to a heavy epithelial ridge. When present, the free gingival groove lies approximately at the level of the cement–enamel junction. Healthy attached gingiva often shows surface stippling, which corresponds to sites of intersecting epithelial ridges. In some cases, when the free gingival groove is absent, an irregularly aligned line of stipples marks the junction between attached and free gingiva. The free gingiva is smooth. The widths of both the free and attached gingivae vary regionally. The interdental papilla is that part of the gingiva which fills the space between the teeth. Its shape in three dimensions, and its histological appearance, depend on the shape and nature of contact between the adjacent teeth.

On the palatal surface of the maxillary teeth, there is no alveolar mucosa. Here, the attached gingiva merges with the palatal mucosa, with no clearly demarcated boundary (see Fig. 1.10).

The **alveolar mucosa** comprises a thin, non-keratinised epithelium overlying a lamina propria that shows poorly developed dermal papillae. Underlying blood vessels lie near the surface (Fig. 14.36). The extensive submucosa houses many minor mucous salivary glands and, near the vestibular sulcus, is loosely attached with numerous elastin fibres, allowing for free movement. Where it adjoins the attached gingiva the alveolar mucosa is thicker than elsewhere (and commonly thicker than the adjacent keratinised epithelium). The demarcation between keratinised and non-keratinised epithelium (the mucogingival junction) is well defined and submucosal vessels and glands are limited to the alveolar mucosa (Fig. 14.37).

The mucosa of the **attached gingiva on its external surface** (oral gingival epithelium) is a masticatory mucosa (Figs 14.37, 14.38). It is keratinised, but the degree and extent vary considerably between and within individuals. Orthokeratinisation is the norm in mucosa unimpeded by inflammation; however, as much as 75% of the surface may be parakeratinised (i.e. the surface shows a strong pink stain with haematoxylin and eosin stain, as for keratin but nuclei are

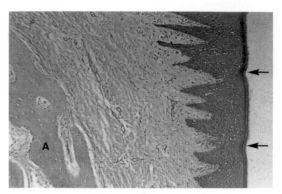

Fig. 14.38 Section of the attached gingiva. The epithelium is a keratinised stratified squamous epithelium. The lamina propria is dense and relatively avascular and the interface with the epithelium is highly folded. The lamina propria is directly attached to the underlying alveolar bone (A), forming a mucoperiosteum. Arrows indicate surface stippling. (H & E; × 75).

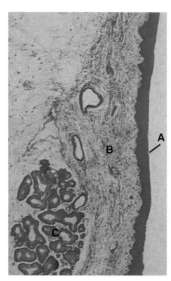

Fig. 14.36 Section of alveolar mucosa. A = Non-keratinised oral epithelium; B = lamina propria; C = minor salivary gland in submucosa (H & E; × 15).

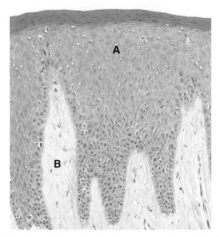

Fig. 14.39 Section of the gingival mucosa. The epithelium (A) is parakeratinised with nuclei being retained in the superficial keratinised layer. B = Lamina propria (H & E; × 100). Courtesy of Dr A.E. Barrett.

retained in the surface layer – Fig. 14.39) and as much as 10% non-keratinised. Papillation is variable, the papillae often being aligned in rows (especially at the margin). As little as 0.08 mm may separate the tips of some papillae from the surface. The surface is stippled, the stipples arising from intersecting epithelial ridges. There is no submucosa, the lamina propria being bound directly to bone forming a mucoperiosteum (Figs 14.37, 14.38).

The mucosa of the **free gingiva** is indistinguishable from that of the attached gingiva (Fig. 14.40), but may be demarcated from it by the free gingival groove (or a line of stipples). The gingival margin marks the boundary with the **gingival sulcus**. In germ-free animals, and in strictly healthy, plaque-free gingivae, the sulcus is absent and the gingival margin corresponds to the coronal extent of the junctional epithelium. In clinically healthy mouths, the clinical sulcus is 0.5–2.0 mm deep. Sulci deeper than 3 mm (measured clinically) are generally accepted as diseased and are described as 'periodontal pockets'. In routine decalcified sections, the enamel will be lost, but its position must be envisaged in order to appreciate

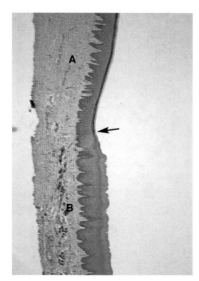

Fig. 14.37 Section of the attached gingiva (A) and alveolar mucosa stripped off from underlying bone. The arrow points to the sharp demarcation site of the mucogingival junction. Note the keratinised epithelium covering the attached gingiva, the non-keratinised epithelium covering the alveolar mucosa and the numerous blood vessels in the alveolar mucosa (Papanicolaou stain; × 20). Courtesy of Professor C.A. Squires.

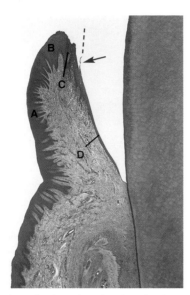

Fig. 14.40 Demineralised section showing the dentogingival junction. The outline of the original enamel surface is indicated by the broken black line. A = Region of attached gingiva covered by masticatory epithelium; B = region of free gingiva covered externally by masticatory epithelium; C = non-keratinised crevicular epithelium; D = non-keratinised junctional epithelium. Note the tag of enamel cuticle (arrow) that helps to delineate the oral sulcular epithelium from the junctional epithelium. (H & E; × 30). Courtesy of Professor H.E. Schroeder.

the approximate position of the gingival sulcus and thus distinguish between the sulcular (crevicular) epithelium, which faces the gingival sulcus, and the junctional epithelium, which is in direct contact with the enamel surface at the base of the sulcus (Fig. 14.40).

The epithelium on the inner surface of the gingiva constitutes the **sulcular epithelium** (oral sulcular epithelium) and the junctional epithelium. These form the so-called gingival cuff at the site where the oral mucosa meets the tooth. Histologically, the sulcular epithelium may be distinguished from the junctional epithelium by having a more folded interface with the underlying connective tissue. In addition, tags of an enamel cuticle may be seen at the interface between the two epithelia (Figs 14.40, 14.41). The two epithelia can also be distinguished by their different cytokeratin profiles. As is to be expected, the superficial layers of the sulcular epithelium stain positive for CK4, typical of lining epithelium. However, unusually, junctional epithelium not only lacks CK4 (even though it can be considered a lining mucosa) but characteristically expresses the basal keratinocyte markers CK5, 14 and 19 throughout all its layers (Fig. 14.42), indicating it is a non-differentiating tissue. This CK profile is similar to that of the reduced enamel epithelium from which it is derived.

The gingival sulcus (Figs 14.34, 14.40) is bounded by the gingival margin above and the junctional epithelium below. The epithelium is non-keratinised and thinner, but otherwise similar to the epithelium of the attached gingiva. The sulcular epithelium merges with the junctional epithelium and a distinct boundary is not usually seen. Externally, the base of the sulcus corresponds approximately with the free gingival groove when present.

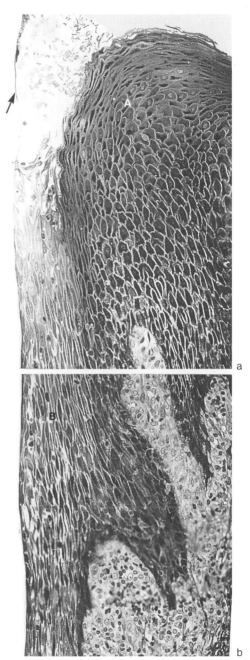

Fig. 14.41 Section of gingiva showing the crevicular epithelium (A) and the upper portion of the junctional epithelium (B). At this site the junctional epithelium may be 15–30 cells thick. Note the tag of enamel cuticle (arrow) helping to delineate the two types of epithelia (× 200) Courtesy of Professor H.E. Schroeder.

The **junctional epithelium** is an epithelial collar that surrounds the tooth and extends from the region of the cement–enamel junction to the bottom of the gingival sulcus (Figs 14.40–14.43). It may extend for up to 2 mm. Coronally the junctional epithelium may be 15–30 cells thick (up to 100 μm – Fig. 14.41), whilst apically it narrows to only 1–3 cells thick. It consists of two zones: a single cell layer of cuboidal cells (the stratum germinativum) overlying several layers of flattened cells equivalent to a stratum spinosum. There is no stratum granulosum or corneum. The junctional epithelium has a high rate of turnover (in the order of 5–6 days) and many cells

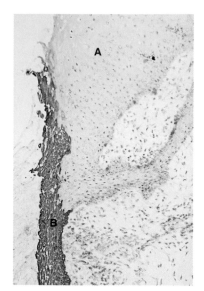

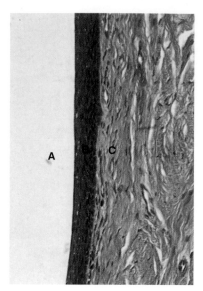

Fig. 14.42 Demineralised section of gingiva showing sulcular (A) and junctional epithelium (B) staining for cytokeratin 19. The junctional epithelium stains positively (brown) (× 150). Courtesy of Professor P. Morgan.

Fig. 14.43 Demineralised section of gingiva showing non-keratinised stratified squamous epithelium forming junctional epithelium (B). Note the smooth interface with the underlying lamina propria (C). A = Enamel space (H & E; × 150).

are exfoliated coronally. It is initially derived from the rapidly replaced reduced enamel epithelium (probably from the stratum intermedium component of that tissue) and this may explain why its cytokeratin profile resembles odontogenic epithelium rather than the lining stratified squamous epithelium typical of oral mucosa (see Fig. 14.42). The cells of the stratum germinativum rest on a typical lamina propria, which shows many capillaries and appears to be more cellular than other parts of the gingiva. The connective tissue interface is smooth (Fig. 14.43).

The principal features of the junctional epithelium are shown diagrammatically in Fig. 14.44. The cells of the junctional epithelium immediately adjacent to the tooth attach themselves to the tooth in the same way as cells of the stratum germinativum elsewhere attach themselves to the lamina propria (by hemidesmosomes within the cell and a basal lamina

produced by the cell beyond the cell). The combination of the hemidesmosomes and basal lamina is known as the attachment apparatus or epithelial attachment. The basal lamina in contact with the tooth is termed the internal basal lamina. On the other surface of the junctional epithelium in contact with the lamina propria is the normal basal lamina (the external basal lamina). The junctional epithelium is therefore unique in having two basal laminae. Like epithelial cells elsewhere, the cells of the junctional epithelium are joined by desmosomes and gap junctions; tight junctions are rare. However, the desmosomes are fewer in number, and this is correlated with larger intercellular spaces that may comprise up to 5% of the volume of the tissue. This has profound clinical significance because not only crevicular fluid but also defence cells can pass across the junctional epithelium (Fig. 14.45). Indeed, even healthy gingival tissue may exhibit neutrophils in the

Fig. 14.44 Diagrammatic representation of junctional epithelium.

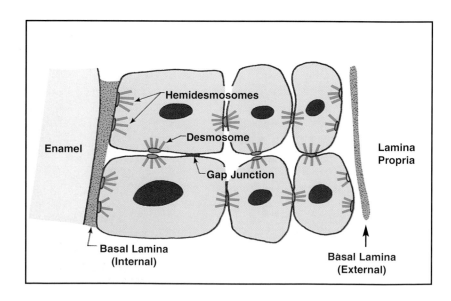

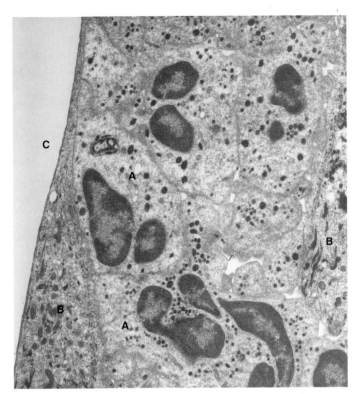

Fig. 14.45 Electronmicrograph of demineralised section of junctional epithelium showing defence cells (leukocytes, A) migrating through junctional epithelial cells (B). C = Enamel space (× 10 000). Courtesy of Professor M. Smith.

intercellular spaces, indicative of its protective role. The lack of membrane-coating granules (see page 222) may also assist the permeability of the cell layer. The turnover rate for cells of the junctional epithelium is the highest of any oral mucosa (perhaps of the order of 5–6 days). There is also evidence for a high turnover rate for the internal basal lamina.

Ultrastructural examination of junctional epithelial cells interfacing with enamel will show that the attachment of the cell to the enamel is mediated by hemidesmosomes and a basal lamina (Fig. 14.46). The internal basal lamina, as elsewhere, is seen to contain two zones: an electron-lucent zone adjacent to the cell and an electron-dense layer against the tooth surface. The pattern of a lamina densa and lamina lucida is apparently not as clear as in other basal laminae, the lamina densa not always being clearly delineated, but the combined thickness is similar (100–140 nm). The internal basal lamina also differs from the external basal lamina in lacking type IV collagen and anchoring fibrils. It is therefore not surprising that the composition of the internal basal lamina differs from the external in lacking laminin. The basement membrane seen in light microscopy adjacent to the connective tissue would appear much thicker due to a reticular component derived from the connective tissue (which is not discernible in an electronmicrograph). The hemidesmosomes consist of thickenings of the inner leaflet of the plasma membrane (called the attachment plaque). Opposite the attachment plaque at the enamel surface there is a peripheral dense line comparable to that seen in the lamina lucida of the basal lamina between epithelium and connective tissue.

The nature of the adhesive mechanisms associated with the cells of the gingiva has been studied by observing the distribution of the integrin $\alpha6\beta4$. As this transmembrane receptor glycoprotein is a component of hemidesmosomes, it is present in both basal laminae of the junctional epithelium (compared with the crevicular epithelium where it is only found in the single basal lamina). However, the $\alpha6$ component is also associated with all the remaining cells of the junctional epithelium, allowing these cells to be distinguished from those of the crevicular epithelium that lack the $\alpha6$ component. This, together with the distribution of CK19, implies a difference in adhesive mechanisms within the junctional and crevicular epithelia.

Fig. 14.46 Electronmicrograph of demineralised section of part of junctional epithelial cell adjacent to enamel space (A). B = Lamina lucida and lamina densa of basal lamina; C = Golgi complex; arrows indicate hemidesmosomes (× 70 000). Courtesy of Professor J.V. Soames.

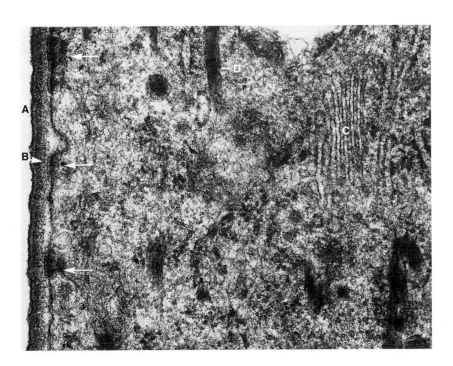

In addition, as the components of the basal lamina must also be synthesised, transported and secreted by these cells, the cytoplasm of the cells contains numerous free ribosomes, cisternae of rough endoplasmic reticulum and a prominent Golgi complex (Fig. 14.46). As the junctional epithelium is non-masticatory, there is an absence of both membrane-coating granules and keratohyaline granules, and few cytokeratin filaments are present.

An element not visible in decalcified preparations is the **enamel cuticle** (see pages 120–122). This cuticle is a non-mineralised structure interposed between the junctional epithelium and the underlying hard tissue. It varies in extent and is not always present. When present, it is patchy and most prominent when filling depressions in the calcified surface. The cuticle is ultrastucturally amorphous and biochemically distinct from the basal lamina. It is probably proteinaceous and may be derived from serum.

The length of the junctional epithelium attached to the enamel surface varies according to the stage of eruption (see Fig. 26.6). When the tooth first erupts into the oral cavity, most of the enamel will be covered by junctional epithelium. By the time the tooth reaches the occlusal plane, about one-quarter of the enamel surface is still coverered by junctional epithelium. Eventually it will come to lie close to the cement–enamel junction (Figs 14.40, 14.47). In older patients with exposure of the roots the junctional epithelium proliferates apically and, as a consequence, may establish a firm union with the surface of the cementum (Fig. 14.48), also via a basal lamina

(Fig. 14.49). When this occurs, and in the absence of obvious periodontal inflammatory disease, the question arises as to whether it is a physiological age change (passive eruption) or whether, as there must have been some associated loss of collagen fibres at the cervix of the tooth to allow for epithelial proliferation apically, it is the result of a disease process.

The lamina propria associated with the junctional epithelium has a rich blood supply and is the obvious source of gingival crevicular fluid.

The **dentogingival junction** seals the underlying connective tissue of the periodontium from the oral environment.

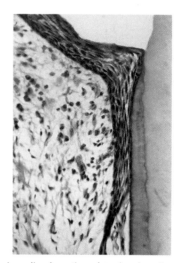

Fig. 14.48 Demineralised section showing junctional epithelium (A) having proliferated rootwards to lie on cemental surface of root (B). C = Enamel space; D = dentine. (H & E; × 120). Courtesy of Dr D. Adams.

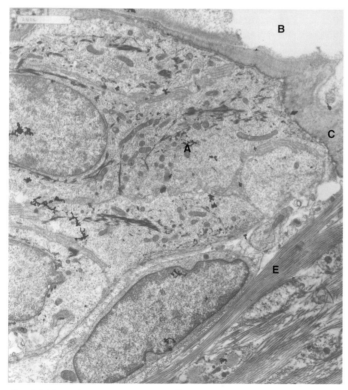

Fig. 14.47 Electronmicrograph of demineralised section showing the apical limit of the junctional epithelial cells (A) at the cement–enamel junction. B = Enamel space; C = cementum; D = basal lamina; E = collagen fibre of gingiva (× 2 500). Courtesy of Professor M. Smith.

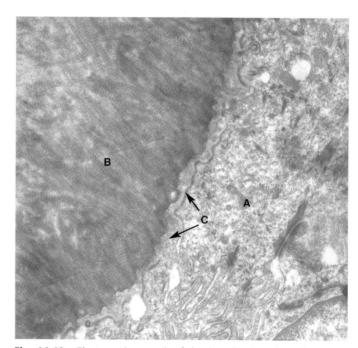

Fig. 14.49 Electronmicrograph of demineralised section of junctional epithelium (A), which has proliferated rootwards to lie on cementum (B), the collagen fibrils of which are evident. The epithelial cells are attached to the cementum by a basal lamina/cuticle (C) (× 20 000). Courtesy of Professor M. Smith.

The strength of the seal is thought to be dependent not only upon the attachment of the junctional epithelium to the tooth but also upon the pressure exerted by the fibres and tissue fluid of the underlying connective tissue. The weakness of the dentogingival junction derives from its situation, the enamel being a non-shedding surface, allowing persistent bacterial colonisation. The epithelium provides less resistance to passage of toxic products emanating from the consequent bacterial accumulation. The junctional epithelium is permeable. Indeed, tissue fluid and cells (as well as experimental substances such as dyes, carbon particles and horseradish peroxidase) pass readily through the epithelium from the connective tissue into the sulcus. This is known as **gingival crevicular fluid** (GCF). The permeability of the junctional epithelium may be related to the presence of particularly wide intercellular spaces. GCF contains material of low molecular weight and is said to pass continuously from the subepithelial tissue into the gingival crevice. Other oral epithelial surfaces do not show such exudation of tissue fluid. As GCF contains gamma globulins and polymorphonucleocytes, it has been suggested that the immunological and phagocytic properties of the fluid are important in the defence mechanism of the gingival junction. It is thought by some, however, that fluid only passes into the crevice as a response to pathological stimuli and is absent from perfectly healthy gingiva. Recent investigations suggest that the composition of the GCF provides an indicator of the state of health of the underlying periodontium and may indeed enable the development of a diagnostic marker for the severity of inflammatory periodontal disease.

The turnover of the junctional epithelium is rapid. The epithelial cells migrate in a coronal direction, to be shed into the oral cavity via the gingival crevice. The continual breakdown and reformation of lamina densa, hemidesmosomes and desmosomes allows cells to alter their relationship as they migrate through the junctional epithelium. The rate of turnover is dependent on the demands placed upon the tissue and appears to be directly related to the degree of inflammation. Following the surgical removal of the gingiva, a new junctional epithelium rapidly forms that has all the original characteristics. As the newly reformed dentogingival junction can have been derived only from the gingival epithelium (which is keratinised), it can be assumed that proliferating epithelial cells from this surface are modified by underlying connective tissue cells closer to the tooth surface to express a different phenotype (see pages 226).

The **interdental gingiva** is the part of the gingiva between adjacent teeth. The shape and arrangement of the gingival tissues between the teeth depend on the shape of the contact between the teeth (although free and attached gingivae are always present). The interdental gingiva occupies the space between the teeth and conforms to its shape. From the buccal or lingual aspects, the interdental gingiva has a wedge-shaped appearance (Fig. 14.35). Between the anterior teeth (which contact only at a small point), it would appear similarly 'pointed' when viewed in a buccolingual plane. In the posterior cheek teeth, which have a broader area of contact, the appearance from the buccal or lingual side would show the typical wedge shape (Fig. 14.50) but across its buccolingual plane there are two peaks on the buccal and lingual aspects with a curved depression between them (the **interdental col**), where they fill the contour around the contact point (Fig. 14.51).

The epithelium of the col is continuous with the junctional epithelium on each side. It is similarly non-keratinised and initially derived from the reduced enamel epithelium. Its epithelium is thin and, as the region is not easy to keep plaque-free, inflammatory cells may be seen infiltrating the underlying lamina propria (Fig. 14.52). When teeth are spaced, the col does not exist and an often very flat gingiva is seen, which is covered by a keratinised epithelium.

The **lamina propria of the gingiva** contains dense bundles of collagen whose functions include support of the free gingiva, binding of the attached gingiva to the alveolar bone and tooth, and linkage of teeth one to another. These principal fibre groups have been given names based upon their orientation and attachments, although whether they always exist

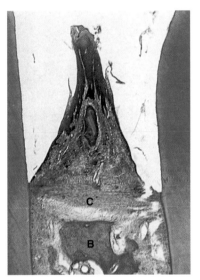

Fig. 14.50 Demineralised section showing the interdental gingiva (A) between two cheek teeth in the anteroposterior plane. B = Alveolar crest; C = transseptal group of gingival fibres; (H & E; × 20).

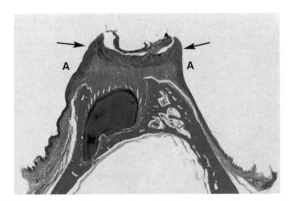

Fig. 14.51 Demineralised section of the interdental papilla cut in the buccolingual plane between two cheek teeth showing the 'interdental col'. The buccal and lingual margins (arrows) of the attached gingiva externally (A) are raised above the central concavity of the col, whose margin passes below the contact points of the teeth (H & E; × 4).

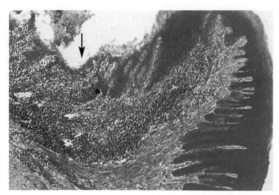

Fig. 14.52 Higher-power view of the thin, non-keratinised epithelium of the interdental col (arrow). There is a substantial infiltrate of inflammatory cells in the area (H & E; × 40).

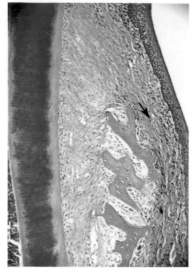

Fig. 14.54 Demineralised section showing direction of dentogingival fibres (arrowed) passing over the alveolar crest (A) and inserting into the lamina propria of the attached gingiva (B). C = Root of tooth; D = periodontal ligament (Masson's trichrome; × 80).

as such discrete and definable groups is debatable (Fig. 14.53). Their main function is to provide support for the gingiva against the tooth and alveolar bone surface, resisting masticatory loads.

Dentogingival fibres arise from the root surface above the alveolar crest and radiate to insert into the lamina propria of the gingiva. The most superficial fibres lie beneath the sulcular epithelium, a middle group lies almost horizontally and the deepest group courses between the gingiva and the alveolar bone (Fig. 14.54).

Longitudinal fibres extend for long distances within the free gingiva, some possibly for the whole length of the arch.

Circular fibres encircle each tooth within the marginal and interdental gingiva. Some attach to cementum, some to alveolar bone. Some cross interdentally to join the fibre group of the adjacent tooth.

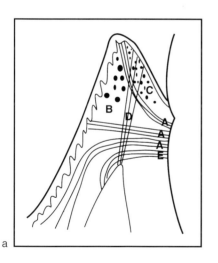

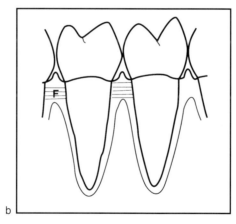

Fig. 14.53 Diagram showing arrangement of principal collagen fibre groups in the lamina propria of the gingiva. (a) = Buccolingual section; (b) = mesiodistal section; (c) = horizontal section; (d) = buccolingual section along interdental col. A = Dentogingival fibres; B = longitudinal fibres; C = circular fibres; D = alveologingival fibres; E = dentoperiosteal fibres; F = transseptal fibres; G = semicircular fibres; H = transgingival fibres; I = interdental fibres; J = vertical fibres.

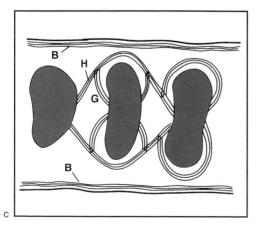

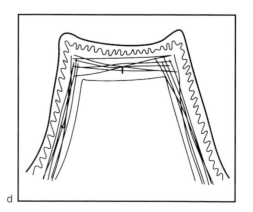

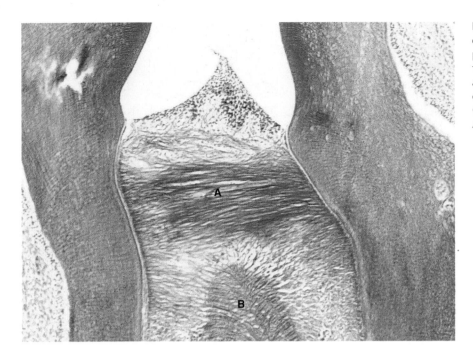

Fig. 14.55 Decalcified section of two cheek teeth sectioned in the anteroposterior plane showing transseptal fibres (A) passing from the cementum of one tooth over the alveolar crest (B) to attach into the cementum of the adjacent tooth (von Gieson; × 140). Courtesy of Dr M.E. Atkinson.

Alveologingival fibres run from the crest of the alveolar bone and interdental septum, radiating coronally into the overlying lamina propria of the gingiva.

Dentoperiosteal fibres occur only in labial/buccal and lingual gingiva. They arise from cementum and pass over the alveolar crest to insert into the periostium.

Transseptal fibres pass horizontally from the root of one tooth, above the alveolar crest, to be inserted into the root of the adjacent tooth (Figs 14.50, 14.55). Such fibres provide an anatomical basis for linking all the teeth in the dentition. They have been implicated in the mechanism of mesial drift (page 362).

Semicircular fibres emanate from cementum near the cement–enamel junction, cross the free marginal gingiva, and insert into a similar position on the opposite side of the tooth.

Transgingival fibres reinforce the circular and semicircular fibres. The fibres arise from the cervical cementum and extend into the marginal gingiva of the adjacent tooth, merging with the circular fibres.

Interdental fibres pass through the coronal portion of the interdental gingiva in the buccolingual direction, connecting buccal and lingual papillae.

Vertical fibres arise in alveolar mucosa or attached gingiva and pass coronally towards the marginal gingiva and interdental papilla.

The lamina propria of the gingiva has properties that distinguish it from the connective tissue of the periodontal ligament (see Chapter 12). For example, the fibroblasts lack alkaline phosphatase, have less contractile proteins, and can release more prostaglandin in response to histamine. The extracellular matrix has less ground substance, less type III collagen, is hyaluronan-rich and has a lower turnover rate. Such differences in properties may be relevant when considering periodontal regeneration (see pages 203–204).

The vasculature of the lamina propria of the gingiva is very rich and forms two plexuses, one beneath the oral gingival epithelium, the other beneath the oral sulcular epithelium.

These plexuses allow the tissues to respond very quickly to stimuli. Each dermal papilla of the lamina propria beneath the oral gingival epithelium possesses an ascending arterial loop and a descending venous loop, between which lies a terminal capillary loop. Beneath the junctional epithelium lies a complex vascular plexus comprising postcapillary venules. From this region is derived the gingival crevicular fluid. Specialisations also allow for the rapid passage of cells and molecules across the junctional epithelium.

The palate

Hard palate

The mucosa of the hard palate is a typical masticatory mucosa with a keratinised (or parakeratinised) epithelium (Fig. 14.56). In much of the central region there is no submucosa and the dense lamina propria binds down directly to bone

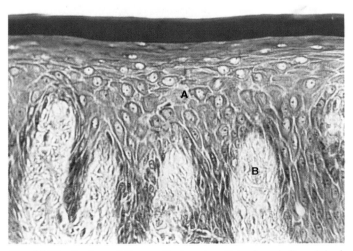

Fig. 14.56 Section of the masticatory keratinised epithelium (A) of the hard palate. Note the highly folded interface with the lamina propria (B) (H & E; × 250). Courtesy of Dr D. Adams.

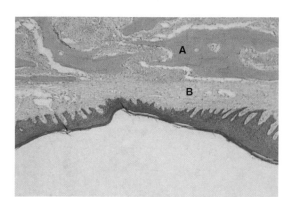

Fig. 14.57 Demineralised section of the hard palate. The keratinised epithelium exhibits deep epithelial rete. The dense lamina propria (B) is attached to the bone of the hard palate (A) in the absence of a submucosa, forming a mucoperiosteum (H & E; × 20).

(mucoperiosteum; Fig. 14.57). The same arrangement is seen in much of the attached gingiva (see Fig. 14.38). Where the palate joins the alveolus, a submucosa is present and contains the main neurovascular bundles. There are also minor mucous glands (predominantly posteriorly) that open onto the surface by ducts (Fig. 14.58) and adipose tissue (predominantly anteriorly).

While the oral surface of the hard palate is lined by masticatory epithelium, the nasal surface of the hard palate is lined by a respiratory mucosa (Fig. 14.59). The respiratory mucosa consists of ciliated columnar epithelial cells with many goblet cells (Fig. 14.60). The ciliated cells contain 'simple' cytokeratin types (i.e. 7, 8 and 18). In addition, there are proliferative basal cells characterised by cytokeratin types 5 and 14. Beneath the respiratory epithelium there is a vascular submucosa containing minor glands of both the mucous and serous types.

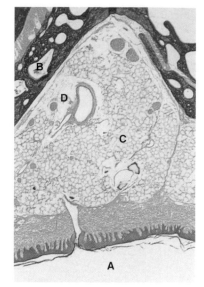

Fig. 14.58 Demineralised section of posterior part of the hard palate at its junction with the alveolar process showing the presence of a submucosa (C) containing minor mucous salivary glands with ducts (arrow) opening onto the surface. A = Oral cavity; B = bone. Note the masticatory mucosa lining the surface (Masson's trichrome; × 15).

Soft palate

The mucosa covering the oral surface of the soft palate is a non-keratinised lining mucosa (Fig. 14.61). Thus, the connective tissue papillae are short and broad. The lamina propria contains many elastic fibres and its collagen bundles are relatively thin. There is a broad submucosa containing many small mucous glands. The submucosa attaches into the palatal muscles. The nasal surface of the soft palate is lined by a respiratory mucosa of ciliated columnar epithelium.

Fig. 14.59 Demineralised section of the hard palate showing the oral surface (A) lined by masticatory epithelium and the nasal surface (B) lined by a respiratory epithelium. C = Bone of hard palate; D = duct from mucous gland opening onto surface (H & E; × 110). Courtesy of Dr M.E. Atkinson.

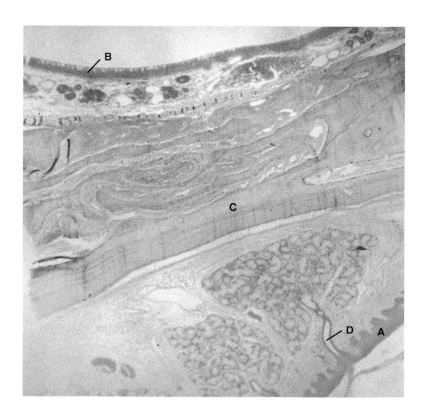

Fig. 14.60 Section of nasal surface of hard palate from Fig. 14.59. A = Ciliated columnar epithelium; B = goblet cell; C = minor gland; arrow indicates basal cell in epithelium (H & E; × 500). Courtesy of Dr M.E. Atkinson.

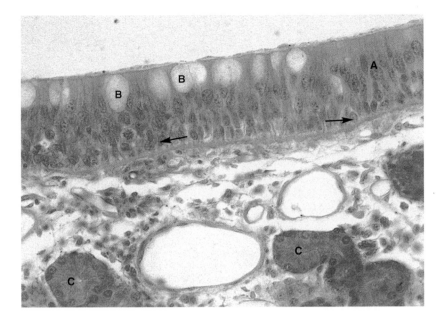

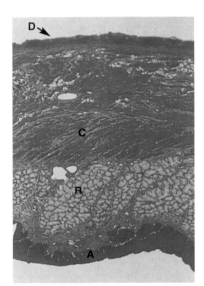

Fig. 14.61 Section of soft palate showing the oral surface being covered by a non-keratinised lining mucosa (A). Numerous minor salivary glands lie in the submucosa (B), beneath which is seen the palatal musculature (C). The nasal surface is lined by a pseudostratified ciliated columnar epithelium. (H & E; × 20).

The tongue and the floor of the mouth

The ventral surface of the tongue and the floor of the mouth are covered by typical lining mucosa (Fig. 14.62). There is little wear and tear but a need for considerable mobility. The epithelium is thin, non-keratinised and shows short papillae. The submucosa is extensive on the floor of the mouth but indistinct (if not absent) on the ventral surface of the tongue where the mucosa binds down to the tongue muscles. The thinness of the epithelium and the vascularity of the connective tissue make this a route by which some drugs can rapidly reach the blood stream.

An indistinct groove, the sulcus terminalis (see Fig. 1.15) divides the tongue into an anterior two-thirds (palatal surface) and a posterior one-third (pharyngeal surface). The anterior two-thirds of the tongue is covered with numerous papillae,

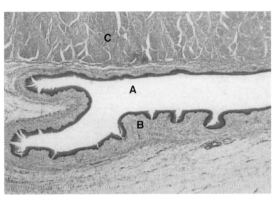

Fig. 14.62 Section showing the ventral surface of the tongue (A) and floor of mouth (B) being lined by non-keratinised lining epithelium. The submucosa in the floor of the mouth is indistinct, the thin lamina propria being bound to the underlying tongue musculature (C). (H & E; × 20).

which can be classified into four types: filiform, fungiform, foliate and circumvallate papillae (see Figs 1.16–1.18). The posterior one-third of the tongue is studded with small lymphatic nodules (or follicles). In addition to its mechanical functions, the tongue has important sensory functions (particularly taste) and is regarded as a specialised mucosa.

The mucosa on the dorsum of the anterior two-thirds of the tongue is classified as a masticatory mucosa as a large part of it is covered by the numerous keratinised (or parakeratinised) **filiform papillae** (Fig. 14.63). The overlying stratified squamous epithelium is keratinised and forms hair-like tufts, although the regions between the papillae are non-keratinised (Fig. 14.64). Each filiform papilla consists of a central core of lamina propria with smaller, secondary papillae branching from it. The filiform papillae are highly abrasive during mastication when the bolus is compressed against the palate.

The simplest model of homeostasis in stratified epithelia is that all basal epithelial cells divide in a fairly homogeneous manner, and that increased basal cell 'pressure' generated by dividing cells results in an upward random migration of

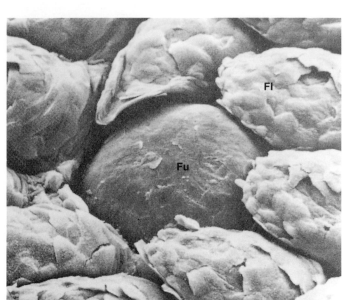

Fig. 14.63 Scanning electron micrograph showing filiform papillae (Fi) surrounding a fungiform papilla (Fu) (× 90). Courtesy of S. Franey.

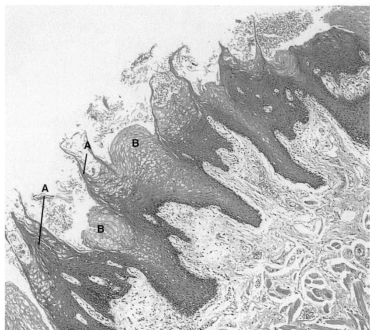

Fig. 14.64 Section showing dorsum of anterior two-thirds of tongue covered by keratinised filiform papillae (A) with non-keratinised regions between (B) (H & E; × 35). Courtesy of Professor P. Morgan.

keratinocytes destined for desquamation. However, it is now clear that many renewing tissues (including oral epithelium) are organised in a much more complicated way, as reference to the mouse filiform papilla shows (Fig. 14.65(a)). Each mouse filiform papilla comprises several columns of cells around a central connective tissue core. The anterior column is two cells wide and has well defined boundaries that result from the difference in cell size and differentiation on either side of each boundary. The posterior column of 16–20 cells piled one on top of another gradually inclines as cells move upwards so that the top cell desquamates backwards (towards the pharynx). The buttress column appears to fill in the rear of the papilla

structure to 'buttress' the posterior column. Note the maturity of basal cells over the apex of the connective tissue core and the method used to number individual cell positions within each column.

A schematic representation of column boundaries and cell migration patterns in the mouse filiform papilla is shown in Fig. 14.65(b). The stem cell population is at position 1, next to column boundaries. As cells move bodily along the basement membrane their capacity for proliferation decreases so that by

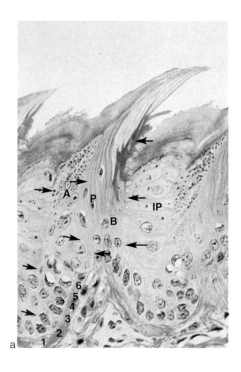

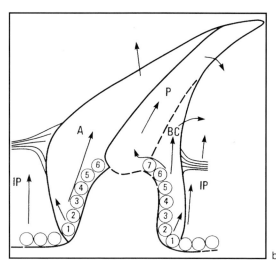

Fig. 14.65 (a) Section of mouse filiform papilla; (b) schematic representation of column boundaries and cell migration patterns. A = Anterior column; B = buttress column; IP = interpapillary epithelium; P = posterior column (Masson's trichrome × 120). Courtesy of Professor W.J. Hume.

the time they reach the highest cell position number, they are postmitotic, differentiating cells. This model implies that, because of rapid desquamation of cells, 4–5 cells per day in the posterior column are the stem cells. There is some suprabasal migration in the anterior column in addition to migration along the basement membrane. The posterior column is derived from lateral cell migration and the buttress column from suprabasal migration from the stem cell population at the rear of the papilla. Thus, each of these columns is one cell wide whereas the anterior column is two cells wide.

Fungiform papillae are found as isolated, elevated mushroom-shaped papillae scattered between the filiform papillae and are approximately 150–400 μm in diameter (Fig. 14.63). They are covered by a relatively thin epithelium that may or may not be keratinised and have a vascular core of lamina propria. Taste buds may be found found on the surface (Figs 14.66, 14.67).

Foliate papillae may be present as one or two longitudunal clefts at the side of the posterior part of the tongue (see Fig. 1.18). Taste buds may be found within the non-keratinised epithelium of these papillae (Fig. 14.68).

Circumvallate papillae are large and rounded. They are surrounded by a trench-like feature and do not project beyond the normal surface level of the tongue (see Figs 1.15, 14.69, 14.70). The circumvallate papilla is generally covered by a non-keratinised epithelium. Taste buds predominate on the internal wall of the trench in the epithelium. Small serous glands (of Von Ebner) empty into the base of the trench (Fig. 14.71). Groups of mucous glands are also seen within the muscle of the tongue, particularly in the posterior part, and these are unencapsulated.

Fig. 14.66 (a) Section of fungiform papilla on dorsal surface of anterior part of tongue showing taste buds (arrowed). The papilla is keratinised (H & E; × 120). (b) High-power view of surface of fungiform papilla seen in (a), showing taste buds (arrow) (× 240). Courtesy of Professor P. Morgan.

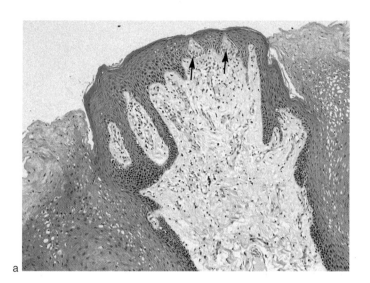

a

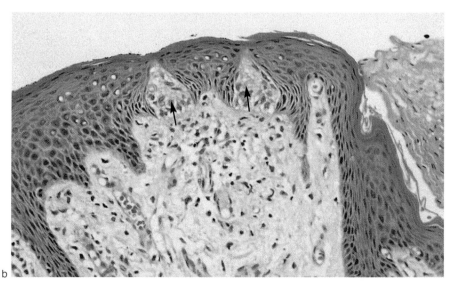

b

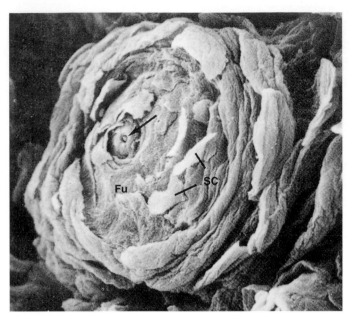

Fig. 14.67 Scanning electron micrograph of fungiform papilla (Fu) showing opening of taste bud on surface (arrow) (× 175). Courtesy of S. Franey.

The **taste bud**, the special chemoreceptive organ responsible for taste, is located within the epithelium particularly around the walls of the circumvallate papillae (Figs 14.70, 14.72), but also in small numbers on the upper surface of fungiform papillae, in the lateral walls of foliate papillae, in the mucosa of the soft palate and in the epiglottis. Two types of cell are present in the taste bud: the supporting cell and the taste cell. A small pore opens from the surface into the taste bud (Fig. 14.69).

At the ultrastructural level the cells of the taste bud are clearly demarcated from the adjacent epithelial cells (Fig. 14.73). The morphology of a taste bud may vary according to species and site. Four distinct cell types have been described: the relatively undifferentiated type IV cells are distinguished by their basal position and the presence of intermediate filaments; type I cells have a dark appearance, while types II and III cells are lighter. Types I and Ill cells may form synapses with intrageminal nerves. The taste bud is separated from the underlying connective tissue by a basal lamina.

The collection of lymphoid follicles on the posterior one-third of the tongue is collectively known as the **lingual tonsil** and forms a component of Waldeyer's ring, which protects the opening into the pharynx (with the palatine tonsil, and the tubal and pharyngeal tonsils within the nasopharynx). The follicles are deep crypts lined with epithelium and containing a mass of lymphoid material (Fig. 14.74). The follicles usually open onto the surface of the tongue. The mucosa in this region also contains many mucous glands. Some small mucous glands also occasionally occur at the margin and tip of the anterior two-thirds of the tongue.

Simple cytokeratins are expressed by taste buds: most are positive for CK7, 8 and 19, with fewer expressing CK18.

CLINICAL CONSIDERATIONS

In pathological situations, the cytokeratin profiles of, and differences between, masticatory and lining epithelium may be altered: CK1 (or 2) and 10 (or 11) in the former and CK4 and 13 in the latter. However, some masticatory epithelium may show a reduction in, or even disappearance of, CK1 and 10 and an increased expression of CK4 and 13. This feature has been related to the presence of an underlying gingival inflammation (which may also produce CK19 expression in basal and parabasal layers).

It was quickly recognised that there was potential to exploit the epithelial specificity of cytokeratins in diagnostic histopathology, principally in the determination of origin of poorly differentiated neoplasms. A further possibility was that dysplastic lesions would 'declare' themselves by an alteration in

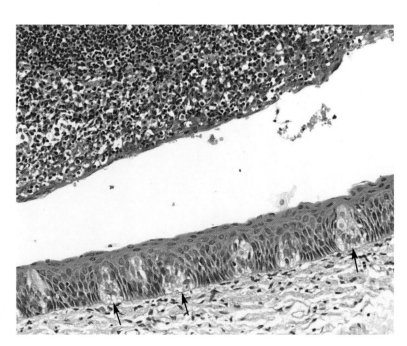

Fig. 14.68 Section of foliate papilla showing taste buds (arrowed). Note the adjacent lymphoid material characteristic of the posterior part of the tongue (× 200).

Fig. 14.69 Scanning electron micrograph showing a circumvallate papilla (CP), surrounded by a trench (arrow). OTB = Opening pore of taste bud (× 80). Courtesy of S. Franey.

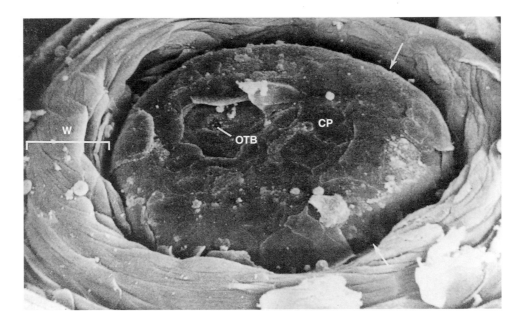

cytokeratin profiles, thus enabling those with invasive potential to be identified early. In terms of the latter, these hopes have not yet reached fruition, but pancytokeratin antibodies to determine whether an anaplastic neoplasm is, for example, a poorly differentiated carcinoma or a lymphoma are now in widespread use. It to be remembered, however, that some malignancies are too poorly differentiated to synthesise intermediate filaments, and other cell types (e.g. endothelial and mesenchymal cells) may contain cytokeratins, as may other malignant cell lineages which are expressing other abnormal phenotypes.

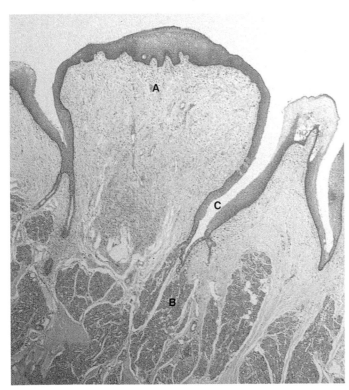

Fig. 14.70 Section of circumvallate papilla (A). Serous glands (B) of von Ebner empty via ducts into the base of the trench (C) surrounding the papilla, which is not raised above the surface of the tongue. D = Muscle of tongue; arrow shows taste buds (H & E; × 35). Courtesy of Professor P. Morgan.

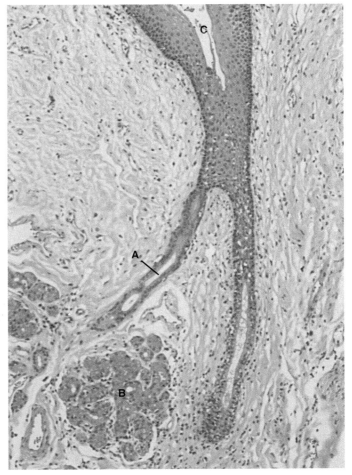

Fig. 14.71 Section of base of circumvallate papilla showing duct (A) from serous gland (B) emptying into the base of the trench (C) (H & E; × 130). Courtesy of Professor P. Morgan.

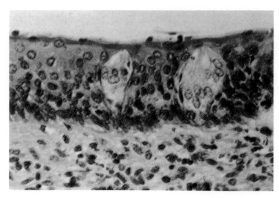

Fig. 14.72 Section of wall of circumvallate papilla showing two pale barrel-shaped areas representing two taste buds (Masson's trichrome; × 300).

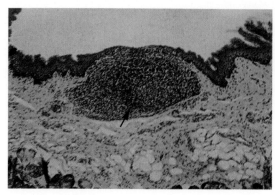

Fig. 14.74 Section of dorsal surface of posterior one-third of tongue containing a lymphoid follicle (arrow). This part of the tongue is covered by a non-keratinised lining epithelium (H & E; × 40).

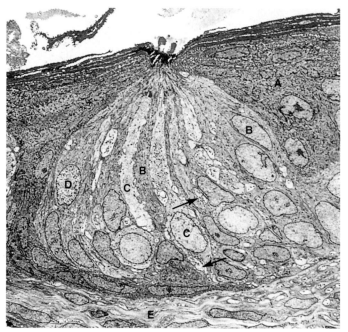

Fig. 14.73 Electron micrograph of a taste bud. A = Epithelial cells adjacent to taste bud; B = darker type I cells; C = lighter type II cell; D = lighter type III cell; E = underlying connective tissue; F = taste pore; arrows indicate where type I and type III cells form synapses with intragemmal nerves (× 11 000). Courtesy of Doctors S.M. Royer and J.C. Kinnamon.

A knowledge of the cytokeratins present in various epithelia has also been applied in determining the origin of cysts within the jaws, based on the assumption that cysts arising from odontogenic epithelium show similar expression of keratins, but differ from cysts originating from epithelium of non-odontogenic origin. This assumption appears to be correct and allows us to distinguish odontogenic cysts from nasopalatine and epidermoid cysts. In the case of inflammatory dental cysts, some authors believe epithelial cell rests are transformed and become positive for CK13, although retaining characteristics of odontogenic epithelium (CK5 and 19).

The gingiva does not scar on wounding. This is a property that has been documented for wound healing in the fetus. That oral connective tissues (e.g. the periodontal ligament) may be fetal-like has been described on page 201. Thus, the gingival connective tissues might also be akin to fetal mesenchyme.

15 The temporomandibular joint

The temporomandibular joint (TMJ) is the synovial articulation between the mandible and the cranium (the temporal bone). Being a synovial joint, it allows considerable movement and has a joint cavity filled with synovial fluid. The synovial membrane that secretes the synovial fluid lines the internal surface of the joint capsule.

Unlike most other synovial joints, the temporomandibular joint space is divided into two joint cavities (upper and lower) by an intra-articular disc (Fig. 15.1). In addition, the articular surfaces are not composed of hyaline cartilage but of fibrous tissue (reflecting the joint's intramembranous development; see page 285). The gross anatomy of the temporomandibular joint is described on pages 58–62.

ARTICULAR SURFACES OF THE TEMPOROMANDIBULAR JOINT

Four distinct layers have been described covering the bony head of the condyle (Fig. 15.2).

1. The most superficial layer forms the articular surface and is composed of fibrous tissue. Although most of the fibres are collagenous, some elastin fibres are also present. The collagen fibres comprising its uppermost component are arranged parallel to the surface and, when viewed between crossed polars in a polarising microscope, shows alternating light and dark bands that indicate that the fibres are wavy or crimped (Fig. 15.3). In the deeper layer, fibres run more

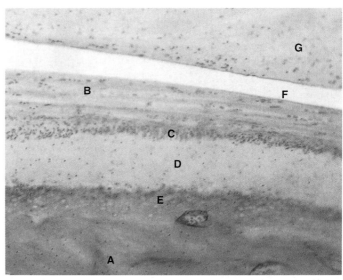

Fig. 15.2 Articular surface of adult condyle showing the four main layers covering the bone. A = Bone of condylar head; B = fibrous articular surface zone; C = cellular rich zone; D = fibrocartilagenous zone; E = zone of calcified cartilage; F = lower joint space; G = intra-articular disc (H & E; × 100).

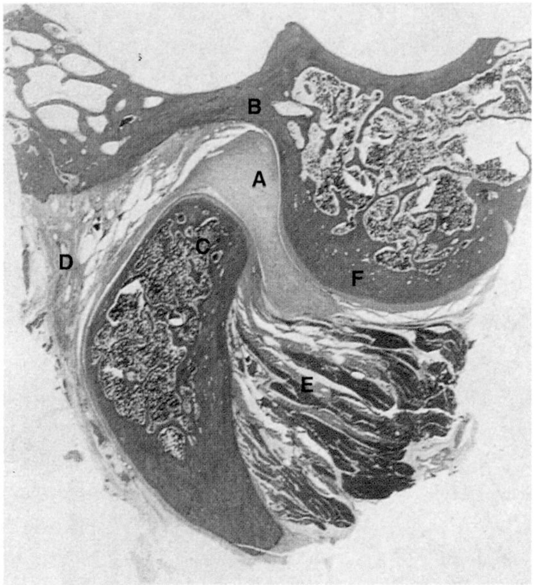

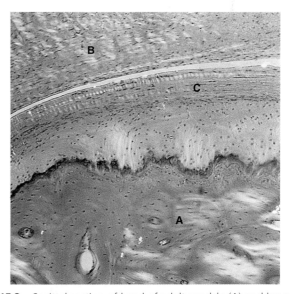

Fig. 15.1 Low-power sagittal section showing general distribution of tissues of the temporomandibular joint. A = Intra-articular disc; B = mandibular (glenoid) fossa; C = condyle of mandible; D = capsule of joint; E = lateral pterygoid muscle; F = articular eminence (H & E; × 3). Courtesy of S. Kariyawasam.

Fig. 15.3 Sagittal section of head of adult condyle (A) and lower part of intra-articular disc (B), viewed in partial polarised light. The alternating dark and light bands seen in the fibrous articular layer of the condyle (C) are indicative of the collagen being crimped. Crimping is also evident in the disc. Note the bony surface is composed of compact bone (× 77). Courtesy of Professor M.M. Smith.

vertically. Fibroblasts/fibrocytes within the surface layer are sparsely distributed.

2. Beneath the articular surface layer is a more cellular zone in which proliferation occurs, providing a source of cells to replenish adjacent layers.

3. Beneath the cell-rich zone is another fibrous layer that can have a variable appearance. However, as a number of the cells are rounded, and have an appearance reminiscent of cartilage-like cells, the layer has been described as a fibro-cartilaginous layer.

4. Immediately covering the bone is a thin zone of calcified cartilage, distinguished from the bone by its different staining properties. This calcified cartilage is a remnant of the secondary condylar cartilage (see page 285).

The articular surface covering the mandibular fossa of the temporal bone is similar to that of the condyle. Although generally thinner, it thickens as it passes over the articular eminence. It also shows crimping of the superficial collagen fibres.

THE INTRA-ARTICULAR DISC

The gross anatomy of the intra-articular disc has been described on pages 61–62. The disc is composed of dense collagenous fibrous tissue. In the thinner, central region of the disc the collagen fibres run mainly in an anteroposterior direction. In the thicker anterior and posterior portions, however, prominent fibre bundles also run transversely with a mediolateral orientation, as well as running superoinferiorly, giving the fibres a much more convoluted appearance (Fig. 15.4). At the periphery of the disc, the collagen fibre bundles are arranged circumferentially. When viewed in polarised light, the collagen fibres show alternating dark and light bands, indicating that they are wavy or crimped (Figs 15.3, 15.5). Using specialised interference microscopy, the crimped nature of the collagen can be visualised directly (Fig. 15.6). The periodicity of the

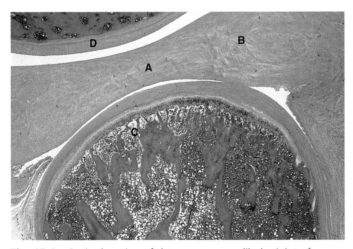

Fig. 15.4 Sagittal section of the temporomandibular joint of a child showing the collagen fibres of the central portion of the intra-articular disc (A) being more regularly aligned than at the periphery (B). Compare with Fig. 15.3, and note the larger marrow spaces and the lack of a layer of compact bone at the surface of the condyle (C). D = Articular surface of mandibular fossa (× 5). Courtesy of Professor M.M. Smith.

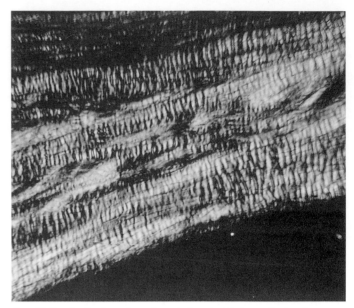

Fig. 15.5 Sagittal section of central part of intra-articular disc viewed in polarised light. The banded appearance indicates the collagen is crimped (× 100). Courtesy of the editor of *Archives of Oral Biology*.

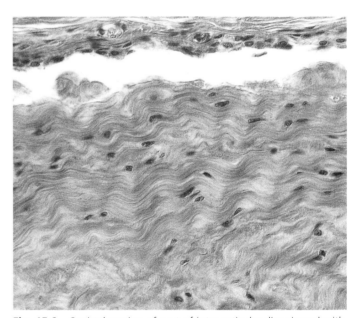

Fig. 15.6 Sagittal section of part of intra-articular disc viewed with interference microscopy to directly demonstrate the crimped nature of the collagen fibres (× 300). Courtesy of the editor of *Archives of Oral Biology*.

crimping is of the order of 15–20 μm. Such crimping is seen in a wide variety of animal tissues and is unlikely to be the result of a fixation artefact as it is evident even in fresh, unfixed material. As the presence of collagen crimps in other sites (such as ligaments) has been shown to be an important component in determining the biomechanical properties of the connective tissue, the presence of significant crimping in the intra-articular disc and the articular surfaces of the TMJ is an important factor when considering the functioning of the joint. One might infer that crimping in the intra-articular disc is indicative of tensional loads. Ultrastructural studies suggest that collagen fibril diameters tend to be small (about 45 nm) and unimodal, which is a pattern often associated with connective tissues subjected to compression. However, regional and species differences may exist, as fibrils with larger diameters and a wider distribution have also been reported, being more typically associated with a connective tissue subjected to tension (such as a ligament) (see page 203).

The fibres within the intra-articular disc are principally composed of type I collagen and comprise about 80% (dry weight) of the disc. Small amounts of type III collagen are also present throughout the disc. The apparent presence of localised areas of fibrocartilage (see below) would also account for the claimed presence of small amounts of type II collagen. Elastin fibres are also present in the intra-articular disc and are said to decrease with age. The ground substance of the disc comprises about 5% of its dry weight. About two-thirds of the glycosaminoglycan is chondroitin sulphate and about one-third is dermatan sulphate, with additional traces of hyaluronan and heparan sulphate. As chondroitin sulphate is also the major glycosaminoglycan present in cartilage, its presence in the intra-articular disc suggests that the disc is subjected to compressional loads.

Cells in the intra-articular disc are more numerous at the time of birth (Fig. 15.7), and become more sparsely distributed in the adult (Fig. 15.8). Although the precise shape of the cells can only ultimately be determined by three-dimensional reconstruction, the cells show an outline varying between flattened and rounded, with many having a rounded appearance. At the ultrastructural level the cells show moderate amounts of endoplasmic reticulum, indicating that they are actively synthesising and secreting protein. The cells also exhibit considerable quantities of intermediate filaments (Fig. 15.9). The cell membrane of most cells lies adjacent to the collagen fibrils of the extracellular matrix. A question arises as to the terminology used for these cells of the articular disc: since the rate of turnover within the intra-articular disc is presently unknown, we cannot be clear as to whether the cells should be referred to as fibroblasts or fibrocytes. However, the not insignificant amounts of rough

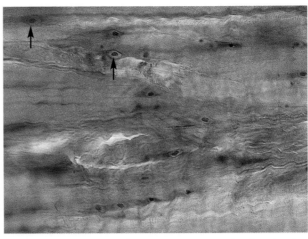

Fig. 15.8 Sagittal section of an adult intra-articular disc showing the sparse distribution of cells compared with Fig. 15.7. Note the rounded cartilage-like appearance of some cells (arrow) (H & E; × 150).

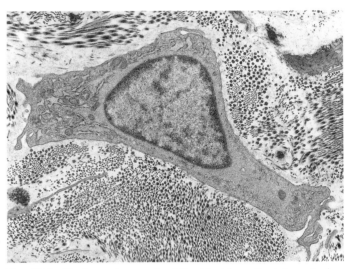

Fig. 15.9 Electron micrograph of fibroblast from the intra-articular disc. The left part of the cell contains rough endoplasmic reticulum; surrounding the nucleus and projecting into the right side of the cell is a clear zone containing microfilamentous material. The extracellular matrix shows transversely sectioned collagen fibrils (× 8000). Courtesy of the editor of *European Journal of Orthodontics*.

endoplasmic reticulum suggest that the term fibroblast would not be inappropriate.

Owing to the rounded appearance of islands of cells described in some discs at the light microscope level, which is reminiscent of cartilage cells lying in lacunae, some have described these tissue areas of the intra-articular disc as being fibrocartilaginous. In support of this are the facts that the interface between the cell and the lacunae stains with substances such as alcian blue and toluidine blue (revealing cartilage-like glycosaminoglycans) and that type II collagen has been identified by immunocytochemistry around the cell in some species. Such a change appears to be related to age. A characteristic of true cartilage-like cells is the presence at the ultrastructural level of a pericellular matrix intervening between the cell membrane and the adjacent type I collagen fibrils of the extracellular matrix. This pericellular matrix

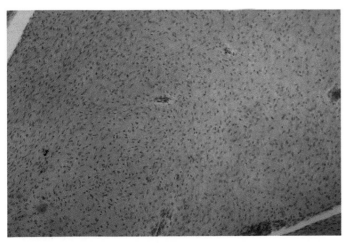

Fig. 15.7 Sagittal section of the intra-articular disc of a neonate showing the presence of numerous fibroblasts (H & E; × 100). Courtesy of Professor M.M. Smith.

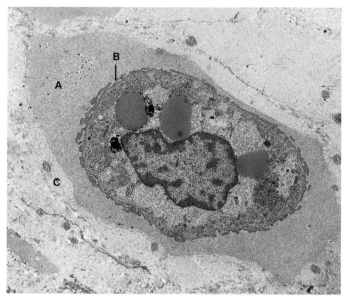

Fig. 15.10 Electron micrograph of cell from an adult marmoset intra-articular disc. Note the presence of a pericellular matrix (A) between the cell membrane (B) and the collagen fibrils of the extracellular matrix (C) (× 6000). Courtesy of the editor of *Archives of Oral Biology.*

contains microfilamentous material. Such cells have been identified to date in the intra-articular discs of older specimens of the rat and marmoset (Fig. 15.10), but have yet to be confirmed in the healthy discs of humans. Unlike the cells in hyaline cartilage, but like cells in fibrocartilage from other sites (e.g. at the insertion of tendons), cells in the intra-articular disc lack a pericellular capsule at the periphery of the pericellular matrix. Some, however, regard the presence of chondrocytes in the intra-articular disc as a pathological change.

The bulk of the intra-articular disc is avascular (Figs 15.4, 15.8) and it may derive its nutrition by diffusion from the synovial fluid. Blood vessels are localised to the periphery of the disc. However, posteriorly in the bilaminar zone where the disc divides into superior and inferior lamellae (see pages 61–62), the region of the superior lamella possesses numerous blood vascular spaces (Fig. 15.11). As the tendon of the lateral pterygoid muscle pulls the disc forwards during jaw opening, blood flows into the back part of the disc to fill the space behind the migrating condyle. The volume of this retrodiscal tissue appears to increase four to five times as a result of venous engorgement as the jaw is opened. This venous engorgement is not the result of the tissue having erectile properties, but more the result of continuity with the pterygoid venous plexus lying medial to the condyle. As the mandibular condyle moves backwards during jaw closure, blood leaves the retrodiscal tissues. Elastic tissue in the superior lamella has been regarded by some authors as providing elastic recoil, aiding the backward movement of the disc during jaw closure. Others believe that the return of the disc is entirely passive. The inferior lamella is relatively avascular and inelastic.

SYNOVIAL MEMBRANE

The synovial membrane lines the inner surface of the fibrous capsule of the temporomandibular joint and the margins of articular disc (Fig. 15.12). It obviously does not cover the articular surfaces. The synovial membrane consists of a layer of flattened endothelial-like cells resting on a vascular layer. The cells comprising the superficial layer are of two types: a macrophage-like cell type, which is phagocytic, and a fibroblast-like cell. The synovial membrane may be folded at rest, these folds flattening out during movements of the joint. With age, the number and size of the projections increase.

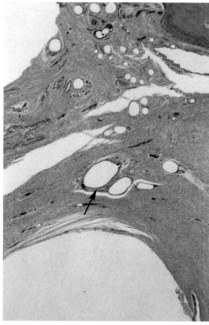

Fig. 15.11 Section of the superior lamella of the intra-articular disc showing considerable vascularity (arrowed) compared with the rest of the disc, which is relatively avascular (H & E; × 14).

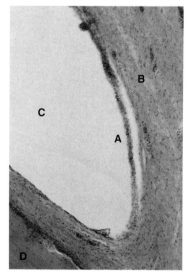

Fig. 15.12 Section showing the synovial membrane (A) lining the margins of the inferior joint cavity (C). B = Articular disc; D = condyle. (H & E; × 60).

The synovial membrane secretes the synovial fluid that occupies the joint cavities. The inferior joint cavity contains about 1 ml of synovial fluid, while the slightly larger superior joint cavity contains a little more. Synovial fluid lubricates the joint and may have nutritive functions. Important components of the synovial fluid are the proteoglycans that aid lubrication. Hyaluronan can also bind to fibronectin to maintain surface non-adherence. At rest, the hydrostatic pressure of the synovial fluid has been reported as being subatmospheric, but is greatly elevated during mastication.

The synovial membrane shows high metabolic activity and has considerable powers of regeneration.

THE CONDYLE OF A CHILD

The histological appearance of the mandibular condyle varies according to age. This is due to the presence of the secondary condylar cartilage. This cartilage appears initially at about the tenth week of intrauterine life and remains as a zone of proliferating cartilage until about the latter half of the second decade of life.

Like that of the adult, the condyle of a child is lined by a layer of fibrous tissue, beneath which is a proliferative layer of undifferentiated cells that shows more activity. Cells from this proliferative layer divide to give rise to fibroblast-like cells, which subsequently differentiate into chondrocytes, which form the secondary condylar cartilage (Fig. 15.13). The chondrocytes hypertrophy at the site of endochondral ossification. In brief, the process involves mineralisation of the cartilage matrix and subsequent degeneration of the chondrocytes. Part of the calcified cartilage is resorbed by large multinucleated osteoclasts. Subsequently, bone-forming cells, the osteoblasts, deposit woven bone around the template of calcified cartilage. Eventually, this area will be remodelled to produce mature bone. Unlike the chondrocytes in a typical growth plate, the chondrocytes of the condylar cartilage are not aligned into columns. The possible role of the condylar cartilage in growth of the mandible is contro-

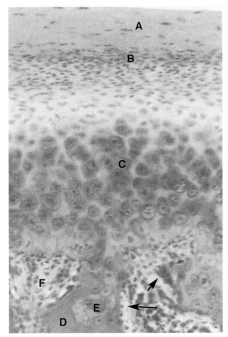

Fig. 15.13   Section through the condyle of a child. A = Fibrous articular layer; B = cell-rich proliferative layer; C = hypertrophic chondrocytes of the secondary condylar cartilage; D = woven bone being deposited around a template of calcified cartilage (E); F = marrow space; small arrow = multinucleated osteoclast; large arrow = osteoblast layer depositing bone on calcified cartilage (× 130). Courtesy of Dr D.A. Luke.

versial and is discussed on page 288. The condyle of the young child is not lined by a distinct layer of compact bone as is that of the adult (compare Figs 15.3 and 15.4).

THE SPHENO-OCCIPITAL SYNCHONDROSIS

The spheno-occipital synchondrosis, an example of a primary cartilage, is described here to provide a comparison between a

Fig. 15.14   Section through the spheno-occipital synchondrosis. Chondrocytes aligned in columns at each end of the cartilage (arrows). The reddish zones at both sides indicate the sites of endochondral ossification. Note the large amounts of extracellular matrix compared with that seen in Fig. 15.13.

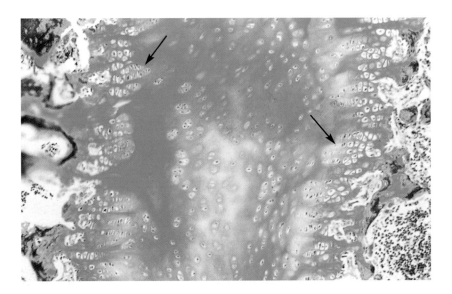

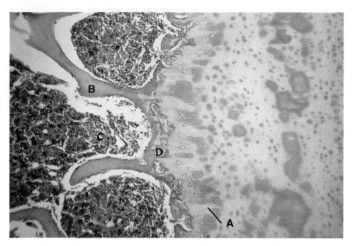

Fig. 15.15 Section at one surface of the spheno-occipital synchondrosis showing the alignment of chondrocytes into columns (A). B = bone; C = marrow space; D = endochondral ossification front (× 80). Courtesy of Dr M.E. Atkinson.

primary cartilage and a secondary cartilage, as exemplified by the condylar cartilage. Developmentally, the primary cartilage appears first to map out the shape of the future bone. In the case of the condylar cartilage, the ramus has already formed in membrane before this secondary cartilage appears. Primary cartilages have inherent growth potential, as is evidenced when they are transferred to tissue culture. The condylar cartilage has little intrinsic growth potential when placed in tissue culture. In the synchondrosis, proliferative zones lie on either side of the central region of the cartilage, and proliferation involves cartilage cells. This contrasts with the condylar cartilage, where it is undifferentiated fibroblast-like cells that undergo proliferation. In the synchondrosis, the chondrocytes are aligned in columns in the direction of growth on both sides of the cartilage and undergo endochondral ossification

(Figs 15.14, 15.15): there is also considerable production of extracellular matrix, which, together with the original proliferation, is responsible for providing the growth force. In the secondary condylar cartilage, however, there is far less production of extracellular matrix and there is no alignment of the hypertrophic chondrocytes into columns. This might relate to the ability of the secondary cartilage to produce some growth in more than one direction. In the case of an epiphyseal growth plate (as opposed to a synchondrosis), columns of cartilage cells are produced only on one side of the cartilage.

CLINICAL CONSIDERATIONS

Like other synovial joints, the temporomandibular joint is subjected to similar inflammatory and degenerative conditions, such as rheumatoid and osteoarthritis. In addition, the intra-articular disc may be displaced (especially anteromedially) in a condition referred to as internal derangement, with associated pain, clicking and restriction of mandibular movement (see page 62). In this condition, degenerative changes are seen in the disc with subsequent changes in its shape. With antero-medial displacement, the posterior part of the disc may end up between the bony articular surfaces and receive abnormal loading which results in a loss of its normal loosely textured structure. The disc may eventually become perforated. Degenerative changes are also seen on the bony articular surfaces. There may be a loss of proteoglycans, which, together with an increased water content, may affect the biomechanical properties of the tissues. Animal experiments involving gross changes to occlusion have resulted in changes in tissues of the temporomandibular joint. Similarly, experimental removal of the intra-articular disc results in degenerative changes in the mandibular condyle.

16 Salivary glands

Salivary glands are compound, tubuloacinar, merocrine, exocrine glands whose ducts open into the oral cavity. The term compound refers to the fact that a salivary gland has more than one tubule entering the main duct; tubuloacinar describes the morphology of the secreting cells; merocrine indicates that only the secretion of the cell is released; exocrine describes a gland that secretes fluid onto a free surface.

Secretion of saliva is a reflex function emanating from salivary centres that is dependent on afferent stimulation (e.g. taste and mastication) and involves complex integration from higher centres. Species differences exist, which accounts for some of the controversy surrounding this topic.

Saliva is over 99% water, yet the very small amount of additional inorganic and organic compounds (such as proteins, glycoproteins and enzymes) allows it to perform many important functions. Its major role is related to the production of mucin, which acts as a lubricant during mastication, swallowing and speech. The mucous film protects the mucosa and keeps it moist. Saliva brings substances into solution so that they can be tasted. It also limits the activity of bacteria by preventing their aggregation and by the presence of antibacterial substances such as lysozyme. Saliva contains minerals and acts as a buffer; both features help to maintain the integrity of the dental enamel. Epidermal growth factor is produced by the submandibular gland and is involved in wound healing and (together with mucin) gastro-oesophageal epithelial integrity. Immunoglobulins (lgA) are produced by plasma cells within the stroma of the salivary glands and secreted into saliva to function as part of a widespread mucosal immune system that also includes lymphoid tissue in the gut and bronchi. A polysaccharide-hydrolysing enzyme (amylase) is present in saliva to aid digestion. Also present in saliva are kallikrein and blood group substances.

The varied functions of saliva can be taken for granted and it is only when salivary production and flow is disrupted that its true importance to the general well-being of the individual is realised: with an ageing population this is of potential clinical importance (see pages 267–268).

Salivary glands consist of two main elements: the glandular secretory tissue (the parenchyma) and the supporting connective tissue (the stroma). From the stroma of the capsule surrounding and protecting the gland pass septa that subdivide the gland into major lobes; lobes are further subdivided into lobules. Each lobe contains numerous secretory units consisting of clusters of grape-like structures (the acini) positioned around a lumen (Fig. 16.1). A secretory acinus may be serous, mucous or mixed. Serous acini can be distinguished from mucous acini according to the nature of the secretion produced and, in structural terms, the morphology of their secretory

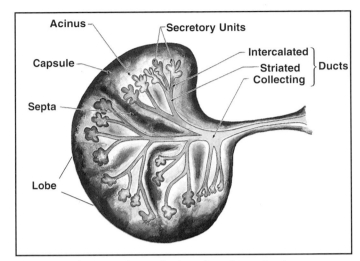

Fig. 16.1   The general organisation of a salivary gland.

granules. The acinus, via its lumen, empties into an intercalated duct lined with cuboidal epithelium, which in turn joins a larger striated duct formed of columnar cells. Both the intercalated and striated ducts are intralobular and affect the composition of the secretion passing through them. Plasma cells (which secrete the immunoglobulins) are found in the stroma of the gland around the intralobular ducts. The striated ducts empty into the relatively inert collecting ducts, which carry the saliva to the mucosal surface and which may be lined near their termination by a layer of stratified squamous epithelial cells. The collecting ducts are interlobular. The connective tissue septa carry the blood and nerve supply into the parenchyma. Apart from fibroblasts and collagen, the connective tissue also contains fat cells. With age, there is a decrease in the volume of the secretory cells and an increase in the connective tissue components, especially the number of fat cells. Unlike endocrine glands, whose secretion is controlled by the activity of hormones, the secretion of saliva by the salivary glands is under the control of the autonomic nervous system.

The acini of the parenchyma are responsible for the production of the primary secretion. Saliva is the product of an active secretory process and is not an ultrafiltrate of blood. The serous cells produce a watery proteinaceous fluid and are the source of amylase. The secretory product of mucous cells contains proteins linked to a greater amount of carbohydrate, forming a more viscous, mucin-rich product. Both serous and mucous cells are arranged as acini, although groups of mucous cells may have a more tubular form. Acini may contain either serous or mucous cells, or may be mixed. When mixed, the serous cells have been traditionally described as forming a cap or demilune outside the mucous cells (Fig. 16.2), although the results of recent studies have challenged this view (see page

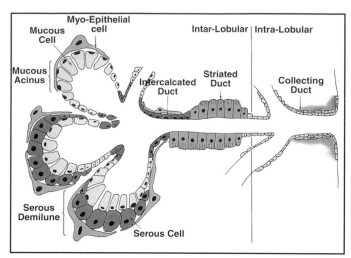

Fig. 16.2 The secretory and ductal elements in a mixed salivary gland. However, as discussed later, the serous demilunes are artefacts of preparation.

264). Around the acini, contractile cells with several processes are present and represent the myoepithelial (basket) cells.

Salivary glands may be classified according to size (major and minor) and/or the types of secretion (mucous, serous or mixed). The three, paired, major salivary glands are the parotid, the submandibular and the sublingual glands. The numerous minor salivary glands are scattered throughout the oral mucosa and include the labial, buccal, palatoglossal, palatal and lingual glands. Salivary glands are not present in the gingiva or the dorsum of the anterior two-thirds of the tongue.

There is a low level of secretion of saliva throughout the day, with periodic large additions from the major glands (e.g. at meal times). With an average salivary flow rate of 0.3 ml/min, it has been calculated that 500–750 ml of saliva is secreted each day (with about 90% derived from the major salivary glands). A very small contribution to the pooled saliva is derived from gingival fluid (see page 239). The sublingual gland and the minor salivary glands spontaneously secrete saliva, but the bulk of this secretion is nerve-mediated. The parotid and submandibular glands do not secrete saliva spontaneously and their secretion is entirely nerve-mediated. Thus, during anaesthesia, secretion ceases almost entirely.

METHODS OF SALIVARY SECRETION

There are two methods of protein secretion involved in salivary acini. In the first and main pathway, the cells store, and then secrete, protein by a process of stored granule exocytosis upon receipt of a signal (Fig. 16.3); the time taken from synthesis to exocytosis is at least 3.5 hours. As it has been found that some proteins (e.g. kallikrein) can be secreted within about half an hour of synthesis, irrespective of whether the cells are being stimulated, a second pathway must also be involved. For this pathway, cells do not store the protein but secrete it continuously by a vesicular mechanism, vesicles travelling directly from the Golgi complex to the plasma membrane (Fig. 16.4). Whereas some proteins pass in this

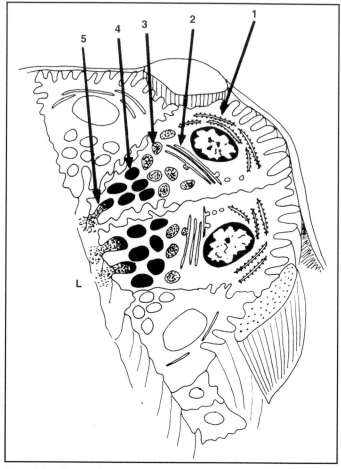

Fig. 16.3 The pathway in secretory protein synthesis, storage and stimulated exocytosis. 1 = Protein synthesis in the rough endoplasmic reticulum; 2 = transport via the Golgi complex to the trans-face; 3 = initial storage within immature granules; 4 = concentration of secretory proteins in mature storage granules; 5 = exocytosis of stored proteins into the lumen of the acinus. Courtesy of Dr G. Procter and Karger Press.

way into the lumina, others may pass in the opposite direction to reach the interstitial tissue where they can gain access to the blood. In the latter context, the salivary glands should not be considered endocrine glands in the conventional sense, but any movement of molecules into the blood may contribute to widespread effects if they are not inactivated. This second pathway has been termed a *constitutive pathway*, to indicate that some proteins may be secreted as they are synthesised. In addition, there is also transcytosis, whereby substances such as IgA, that are present in the interstitial tissue, pass across the cell from the basolateral to the apical membrane (Fig. 16.4). How such transcytosis interacts with the other vesicular pathways described and whether it is responsible for the delivery of other non-salivary cell proteins into saliva is unclear.

PAROTID GLAND

Serous cells

The parotid gland is the largest of the salivary glands. It is enclosed within a well defined capsule, the parotid capsule (see page 70). The acini of the gland are serous, although mucous cells have occasionally been reported. The cells have a

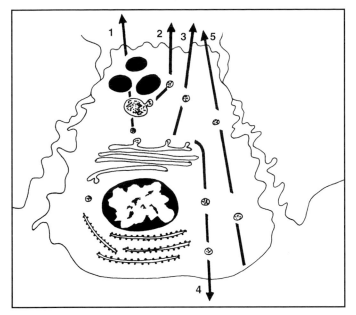

Fig. 16.4 The vesicular protein secretory pathways likely to be operating in parotid acinar cells. 1 = Storage granule pathway; 2 = constitutive-like pathway; 3 = constitutive pathway to the apical membrane; 4 = constitutive pathway to the basolateral membrane; 5 = transcytosis from the basolateral to the apical membrane. Courtesy of Dr G. Procter and the Karger Press.

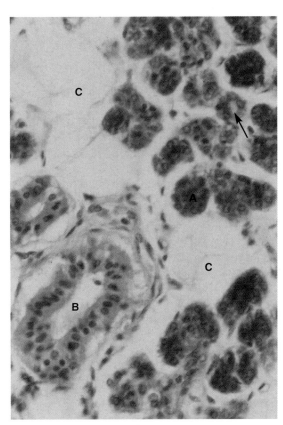

Fig. 16.6 Darkly staining serous acini of parotid gland (A). The narrow lumen of an acinus is arrowed. B = striated duct with nuclei centrally positioned within the cells; C = fat cells (H & E; × 400). Courtesy of S. Franey.

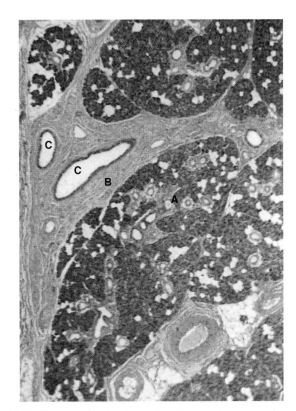

Fig. 16.5 The parotid gland showing the secretory parenchyma (A) being divided into lobules by the paler staining septa of the stromal connective tissue (B). C = Collecting ducts (H & E × 36). Courtesy of Dr E.H. Batten.

characteristic granular appearance with routine haematoxylin and eosin staining (Fig. 16.5). Connective tissue septa can be seen subdividing the secretory parenchyma into lobes and then lobules. The connective tissue contains blood vessels, nerves and collecting ducts. The lumina of the acini are very narrow, unless distended by the accumulation of secretions (Fig. 16.6). The prominent nuclei are round and located in the basal third of the cell, which is basophilic (due to the presence of rough endoplasmic reticulum). The granular appearance of the serous acinar cell results from the numerous refractile granules in the luminal portion of the cell (adjacent to the lumen). Intercalated ducts pass from the acini and open into striated ducts, which are well represented in the parotid gland.

The ultrastructural appearance of a serous acinus is illustrated in Fig. 16.7. The cells have a wedge-shaped outline and surround the central lumen. The basal part of each serous cell is delineated from the surrounding connective tissue by a basal lamina. This region of the cell contains the nucleus and rough endoplasmic reticulum and capillaries are seen in close approximation to this surface. The luminal part of the cell contains dense, round zymogen granules. Many narrow canaliculi run between the cells and join the lumen. Both the canaliculi and the lumen are lined by short microvilli. Adjacent cell membranes contact at desmosomes, gap junctions and tight junctions.

Over 99% of saliva is water, which passes both across the cell membrane (transcellularly) and between adjacent cells

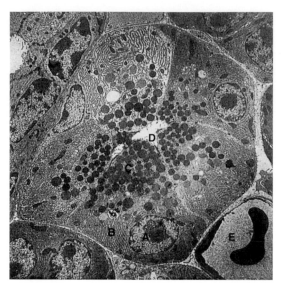

Fig. 16.7 Electron micrograph of serous acinus. A = Nucleus in basal part of cell; B = rough endoplasmic reticulum; C = zymogen granules in luminal part of cell; D = central lumen; E = capillary (× 2000). Courtesy of P.F. Heap.

(paracellularly) as a result of chloride secretion into the lumen. The proteinaceous components are packaged in granules for release into the luminal system by exocytosis at the luminal surface of the cells. For this reason, the cells are highly polarised. Like proteins in other cells, those in the serous cells of the parotid gland are assembled by the ribosomes of the rough endoplasmic reticulum, move into the cisternae of the endoplasmic reticulum and from there to the Golgi complex. Here the proteins are glycosylated and released in vacuoles that become secretory granules. Initially, the immature granules are of pale electron density, but as they move to the luminal plasma membrane they become more electron-dense (Fig.

16.8). Following this maturation period, the granules are discharged by exocytosis when required. Mitochondria within the cell supply the energy for the synthetic and secretory process.

The appearance of serous cells will clearly vary with the levels of secretory activity. Following the synthesis of secretory products, resting (unstimulated) serous cells will contain numerous zymogen granules in the luminal parts of their cytoplasm (Fig. 16.9). With reflex stimulation of salivary flow during mastication at mealtimes, the number of granules will be severely depleted after being discharged into the lumen by exocytosis (Fig. 16.10).

Both parasympathetic and sympathetic fibres innervate the acini and act collaboratively in the production of saliva during feeding. The main neurotransmitter for parasympathetic nerves is acetylcholine and that for sympathetic nerves is noradrenaline. In addition to these substances, each axon contains arrays of neuropeptides (such as vasoactive intestinal polypeptide, substance P, calcitonin gene-related peptide). These neuropeptides are not necessarily uniform for each type of nerve, nor are all present within every nerve of the same type. Embryologically, the transmitters are likely to influence the genetic expression of the glandular cells and, conversely, the cell types are likely to influence the neuropeptides in the axons innervating them. Some nerve endings occur beneath the basal lamina in direct contact with the plasma membrane (hypolemmal), while others remain outside the basal lamina (epilemmal) (Figs 16.11–16.13). Endings of either type

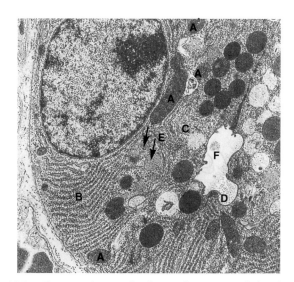

Fig. 16.8 Electron micrograph of part of a serous cell showing secretory pathway. A = Mitochondria; B = rough endoplasmic reticulum; C = secretory granules; D = site of discharge of granule by exocytosis into lumen; E = Golgi material; F = lumen of acinus. Note the granules are initially pale (arrow), but become more electron dense as they mature (× 6700). Courtesy of P.F. Heap.

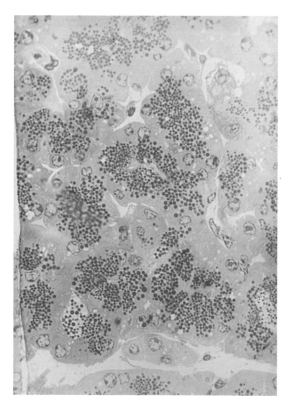

Fig. 16.9 Following synthesis of secretory products, resting (unstimulated) serous cells contain numerous zymogen granules in the distal parts of their cytoplasm (Toluidine blue; × 600). Courtesy of P.F. Heap.

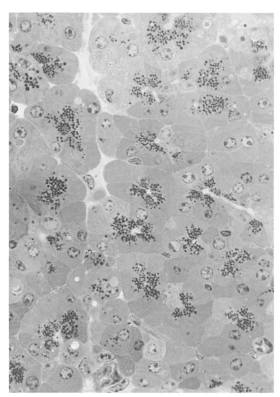

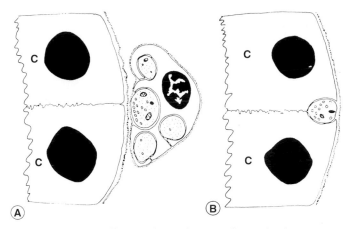

Fig. 16.11 Neuro-effector relationships in salivary glands. A = Epilemmal; B = hypolemmal; C = parenchymal cells. Courtesy of Professor J.R. Garrett and Karger Press.

Fig. 16.10 Soon after stimulation, the zymogen granules are depleted after being discharged into the lumen of the acini by exocytosis (compare with Fig. 16.7) (Toluidine blue; × 600). Courtesy of Mr P.F. Heap.

probably affect the cell if transmitter vesicles are present. In electron micrographs, the conventional neurotransmitters are contained in small vesicles while the neuropeptides are contained in larger, dense-cored vesicles (Fig. 16.14). Parasympathetic drive causes fluid formation by the secretory units; sympathetic drive usually increases the output of

preformed components from the cells. Both pathways cause contraction of the myoepithelial cells, which helps direct fluid from the acinar lumen out along the duct system.

The duct system

The smallest (and most distal) of the ducts is the intercalated duct. This leads from the serous acini into the striated duct and is usually compressed between the acini (Fig. 16.15). It is lined by cuboidal epithelial cells. The nuclei in the duct cells appear prominent, owing to the relatively scanty cytoplasm. At the ultrastructural level, intercalated ducts are seen to consist of a simple cuboidal epithelial tube. Both luminal and basal surfaces of the duct cells are smooth and desmosomes unite adjacent cells (Fig. 16.16). The cells have occasional granules and only small amounts of the organelles normally associated with protein synthesis. It is not known whether the duct cells

Fig. 16.12 Electron micrograph showing the Schwann cell nucleus (A) of an epilemmal nerve fibre in association with a parotid acinus cell (B). C = Adrenergic axon; D = two cholinergic axons; E = basal lamina of acinus. Note the small translucent vesicles and the dense-cored vesicles (with neuropeptides) in the axons (× 14 000). Courtesy of Professor J.R. Garrett and the editor of *Archives of Oral Biology*.

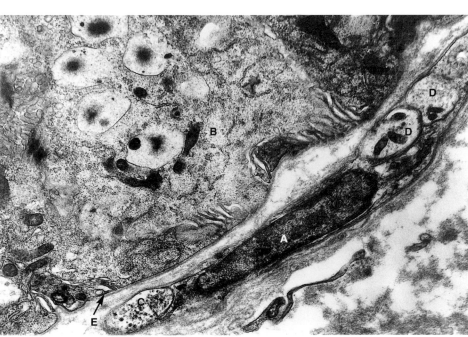

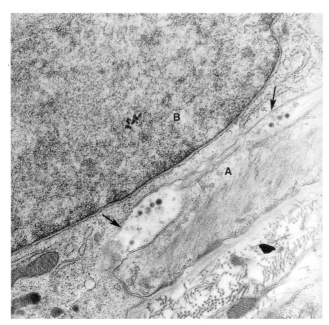

Fig. 16.13 Electron micrograph of submandibular gland showing hypolemmal axons (arrowed) containing mainly large dense-cored vesicles, and lying between a myoepithelial cell (A) and a central acinar cell (B) (× 15 000). Courtesy of Professor J.R. Garrett and the editor of *Microscopy Research and Technique*.

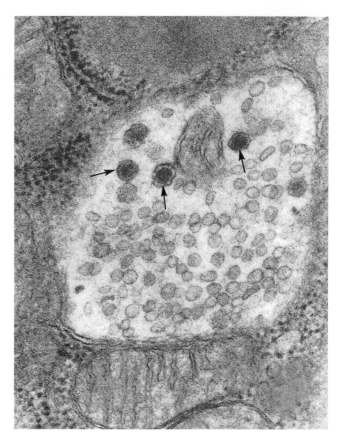

Fig. 16.14 Electron micrograph of terminal part of a hypolemmal parasympathetic axon showing small agranular vesicles (which would contain acetylcholine) and larger dense-cored granular vesicles (arrow) containing neuropeptides (× 60 000). Courtesy of Professor J.R. Garrett and the editor of *Microscopy Research and Technique*.

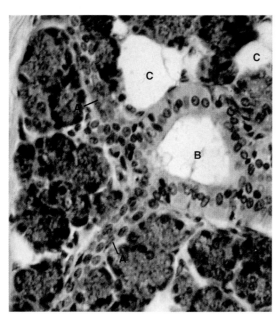

Fig. 16.15 Parotid gland showing compressed intercalated ducts (A) leading from serous acini and into the striated duct (B). Note the cuboidal epithelial cells lining the intercalated ducts have prominent nuclei due to their scanty cytoplasm. The nuclei in the striated ducts are more centrally positioned within the cells (H & E; × 360). Courtesy of Dr E.H. Batten.

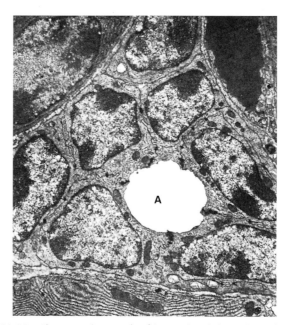

Fig. 16.16 Electron micrograph of intercalated duct. The cuboidal lining cells of the duct (A) possess only small amounts of the intracellular organelles associated with protein synthesis. The cells are united by desmosomes and both the luminal and basal surfaces are smooth (× 5700). Courtesy of P.F. Heap.

have any role in modifying the electrolyte composition of the secretion: they might act as stem cells and be able to differentiate into secretory, myoepithelial or striated duct cells. Several acini drain into each intercalated duct. In the parotid gland, intercalated ducts are characteristically long, narrow and branching.

The striated ducts form a much longer and more active component of the duct system than the intercalated ducts. The cells of the striated ducts have a large amount of cytoplasm and a large, spherical, centrally positioned nucleus that makes them easy to identify in the interlobular septa (Figs 16.6, 16.15). The cells of the striated duct are highly polarised. Their luminal surfaces have short microvilli. The duct's basal (abluminal) surface, adjacent to the basal lamina separating it from the adjacent connective tissue, shows numerous striations in the light microscope. Ultrastructurally, the striations correspond to multiple infoldings of the plasma membrane at the base of the cell (Fig. 16.17). Vertically aligned

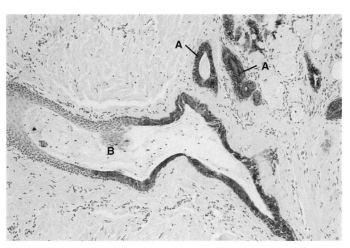

Fig. 16.18 Striated ducts staining positive (brown) for cytokeratin 8 and 18 using immunohistochemical techniques (A), typical of the type of cytokeratin intermediate filaments associated with simple ducts. The early part of a collecting duct also stains positively, but this is lost as the duct becomes stratified near the surface (B) (× 80). Courtesy of Dr A.W. Barrett.

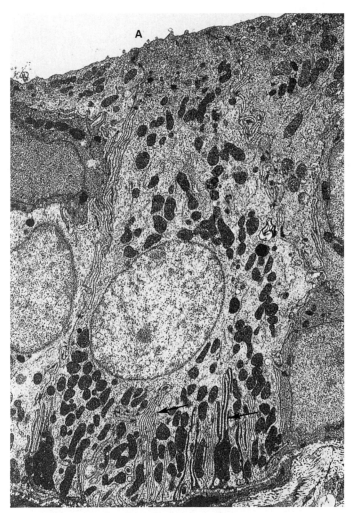

Fig. 16.17 Electron micrograph of striated duct cells. The nucleus is centrally positioned within the cell due to the large amount of cytoplasmic material. Adjacent cell membranes are intertwined in a complex pattern and united by numerous desmosomes. Note the multiple infoldings of the plasma membrane at the base of the cell (arrowed) between which are packed numerous mitochondria. A = Lumen surface of duct (× 12 000). Courtesy of P.F. Heap.

mitochondria are packed between the infoldings. Adjacent cells are intertwined in a complex pattern and anchored together by desmosomes. This large surface area, supplied with high levels of energy, is clearly involved in active transport. The striated ducts are the site of electrolyte reabsorption (especially of sodium and chloride) and secretion (potassium and bicarbonate). As this reabsorption is against a concentration gradient, it requires substantial amounts of energy. The effect on the material in the lumen is to convert an isotonic or slightly hypertonic fluid (with concentrations similar to those in the plasma) into a hypotonic fluid. The cells of the striated duct exhibit small secretory granules on the luminal side containing epidermal growth factor and kallikrein. The granules are less abundant in humans than in many other species and less abundant in the parotid than in the submandibular gland.

The single-layered epithelium comprising the striated (and intercalated) ducts contains only the simple cytokeratin Intermediate filaments 8 and 18 (and possibly 19) (Fig. 16.18).

The striated duct leads into the collecting duct (Fig. 16.19). In addition to the columnar layer (which now lacks striations), the collecting duct may have a layer of basal cells. As it enlarges, the main parotid duct appears like many excretory passages and contains two layers: the mucosa and the outer connective tissue adventitia. Near its termination the lining of the main duct may become stratified as it merges with the stratified squamous epithelium of the surface oral epithelium. When stratified, the duct epithelium contains keratin intermediate filament types typical of stratified epithelium in the oral mucosa (see pages 224–225).

Myoepithelial cells

Myoepithelial cells lie between the basal lamina and the basal membranes of the acinar secretory cells and the intercalated duct cells. Myoepithelial cells around acini are dendritic cells,

Fig. 16.19 A collecting duct (A) in the parotid gland. As illustrated here, the duct may have two layers of cells (H & E; × 60).

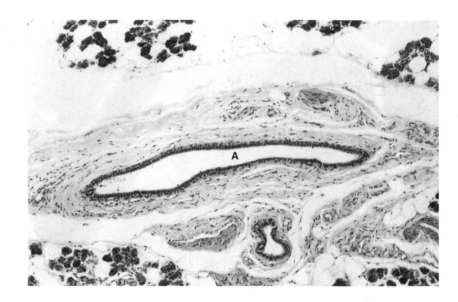

consisting of a stellate-shaped body containing the nucleus and a number of tapering processes radiating from it. A different arrangement exists around the intercalated ducts, where the myoepithelial cells are elongated, run longitudinally along the duct and have few, short, processes. Around the acini, the processes lie in gutters on the surface of the secretory cells so the outline of the acinus remains smooth; around the intercalated ducts, the cells lie more superficially and produce a bulge in the outline of the duct. Although salivary myoepithelial cells in some species stain positively for alkaline phosphatase, those in humans do not. Myoepithelial cells contract as a result of activity of both parasympathetic and

sympathetic stimulation, supporting the view that the two autonomic divisions act in concert, not in conflict.

Ultrastructurally, the nucleus tends to be flattened and intracellular organelles associated with protein synthesis are not particularly abundant. However, the cell contains numerous contractile actin microfilaments 4–8 μm in diameter (Figs 16.13, 16.20). Myoepithelial cells have desmosomal attachments with underlying parenchymal cells, gap junctions and hemidesmosomal attachments with the basal lamina, the last suggesting that some of their activity is transmitted via the basal lamina. Myoepithelial cells (and the basal cells of double-layered ducts) also contain

Fig. 16.20 Electron micrograph showing a myoepithelial cell (A) with a dendritic process (B) surrounding some serous cells (C). Bundles of contractile myofilaments (arrowed) are evident in the process. Note also the variable appearance and density of the secretory granules in the serous cells (× 6500). Courtesy of Dr J.D. Harrison.

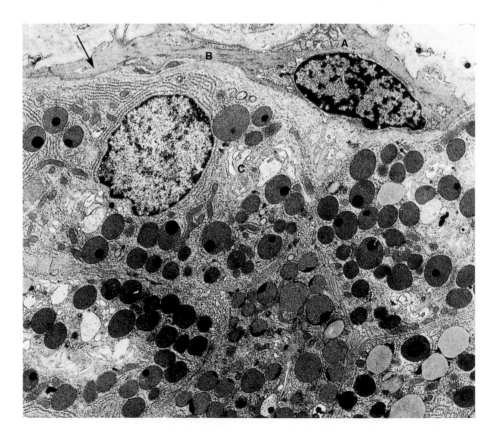

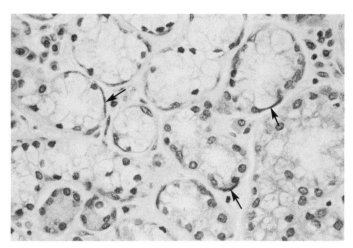

Fig. 16.21 Myoepithelial cells staining positively (brown) for the antibody to cytokeratin 14 using immunohistochemical techniques (arrows) (× 240). Courtesy of Dr A.W. Barrett.

cytokeratin intermediate filament 14 (Fig. 16.21) and contractile actin filaments (Fig. 16.22), which can be used to help identify them using immunocytochemistry. The presence of cytokeratin confirms the epithelial origin of the myoepithelial cell. Pinocytotic vesicles and dense attachment areas are associated with that part of the plasma membrane of the myoepithelial cell covered by the basal lamina.

The precise functional role of myoepithelial cells in salivary secretion awaits clarification. However, functional studies clearly indicate that myoepithelial activity can

- accelerate the initial outflow of saliva;
- reduce luminal volume;
- contribute to the secretory pressure;
- support the underlying parenchyma and reduce back permeation of fluid;
- help salivary flow to overcome increases in peripheral resistance – but if this is excessive it may lead to sialectatic damage of striated ducts, thereby increasing overall permeability.

Other possible functions include assistance for some parenchymal cells to expel their contents and a milking effect on any

underlying extracellular fluid, assisting passage via parenchymal tight junctions.

SUBMANDIBULAR GLAND

The second largest of the salivary glands, the submandibular gland, produces a mixed mucous–serous secretion. Serous acini appear to outnumber mucous acini by at least 7:3. The gland has a well formed connective tissue capsule. Much of the submandibular gland contains serous acini that appear similar to those in the parotid gland.

Mucous cells

In routine microscopy, the collections of mucous acini within the submandibular gland are readily distinguished in the resting gland from the darker staining and granular serous acini because the mucous acini are paler since their mucinous content does not readily take up routine stains, or is lost during preparation. In addition, their nuclei tend to be

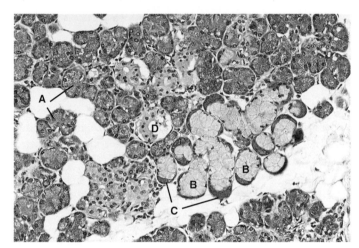

Fig. 16.23 Submandibular gland showing darker serous (A) and lighter mucous (B) acini. The nuclei of the mucous cells are compressed against the basal aspect of the cell. In addition, a crescent-shaped collection of serous cells forming a serous demilune is seen (C). D = Striated duct (H & E; × 120). Courtesy of Professor P. Morgan.

Fig. 16.22 Myoepithelial cells and their numerous dendritic processes staining positively (green) for antibody to F-actin (bodipy-phallacidin) around secretory acini (stained red with ethidium homodimer 1). (a) Submandibur gland; (b) sublingual gland; × 1000. Courtesy of Dr Y. Satoh.

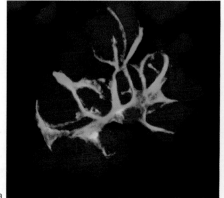

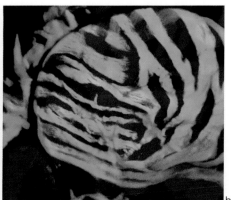

a

b

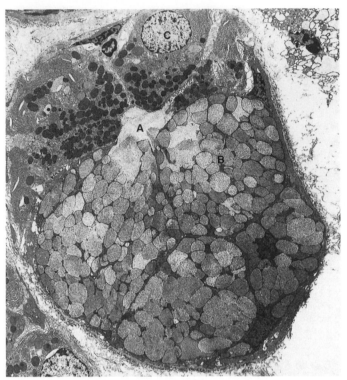

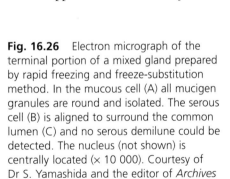

Fig. 16.24 An electron micrograph of the submandibular gland showing serous cells (C) forming a serous demilune capping a mucous acinus (B). A = Lumen (TEM; × 1600). Courtesy of Dr J.D. Harrison.

compressed into the basal part of the cell. Small, crescent-shaped collections of serous cells may be found in routine sections at the most distal ends of the mucous acini; these are referred to as serous demilunes (Figs 16.23, 16.24). In contrast to their appearance in haematoxylin and eosin-stained sections,

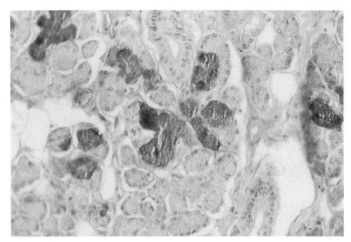

Fig. 16.25 Submandibular gland with mucous acini stained brown/purple with periodic acid–Schiff stain while the serous cells, lacking mucosubstance, take up the yellow counterstain (tartrazine and iron haematoxylin) (× 250). Courtesy of S. Franey.

mucous acini can be specifically differentiated from serous cells by staining with alcian blue or PAS (periodic acid–Schiff) (Fig. 16.25).

The traditional, and widely held, view relating to the disposition of serous demilunes and the ultrastructural morphology of the mucous cell has recently been challenged: it has been shown to be the result of an artefact of preparation. Using methods of rapid freezing and freeze-substitution to obtain minimal distortion and dimensional changes during fixation, it has now been demonstrated that all the serous cells align with mucous cells to surround a common lumen, leaving no demilune structure (Fig. 16.26) whereas samples fixed by conventional methods resulted in distended mucous cells that displaced the serous cells towards the basal portion of the

Fig. 16.26 Electron micrograph of the terminal portion of a mixed gland prepared by rapid freezing and freeze-substitution method. In the mucous cell (A) all mucigen granules are round and isolated. The serous cell (B) is aligned to surround the common lumen (C) and no serous demilune could be detected. The nucleus (not shown) is centrally located (× 10 000). Courtesy of Dr S. Yamashida and the editor of *Archives of Histology and Cytology.*

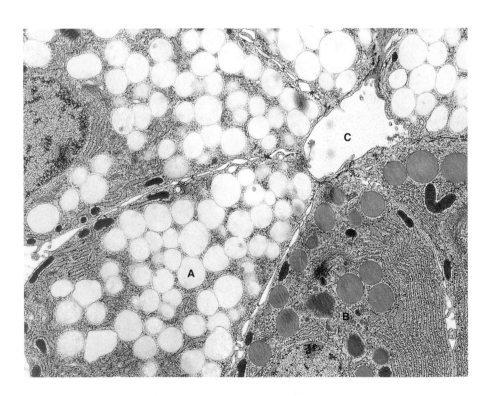

Fig. 16.27 Electron micrograph of the terminal portion of a mixed gland prepared by conventional immersion fixation in glutaraldehyde. Secretory granules of mucous cells (A) are irregular in size due to coalescence by the disruption of limiting membranes. Serous cells (B) are compressed by the distended mucous cells towards the peripheral portion of the acinus, forming the demilune structure (× 5500). Courtesy of Dr S. Yamashida and the editor of *Archives of Histology and Cytology*.

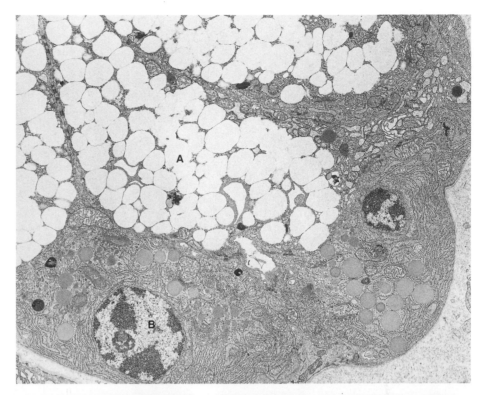

Fig. 16.28 Computer reconstruction of a terminal portion of the submandibular gland showing mucous (purple) and serous (red) cells and luminal space (green). (a) In the upper diagram, following rapid freezing, a surface view indicates that the terminal portion consists of mucous and serous cells distributed not only at the most fundal portion of the acinus but also in the portion nearest the duct. In the lower diagram, the mucous cells have been deleted from the above reconstruction to show more clearly the relation of the serous cells to the luminal space. All serous cells prepared by the rapid freezing method are found to have a direct connection with the luminal space. (b) In the upper diagram, following conventional immersion fixation, the acinus illustrated is found to be branched and serous cells appear attached to the outer wall of the acinus formed by mucous cells. In the lower diagram, the mucous cells have been deleted from the above reconstruction to show more clearly the relation of the serous cells to the luminal space. The serous cells are found to be disconnected from the luminal space, giving a floating appearance. Courtesy of Dr S. Yamashida and the editor of *Archives of Histology and Cytology*.

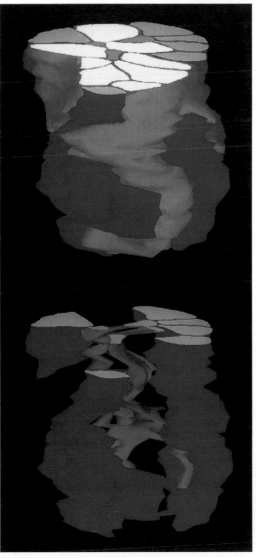

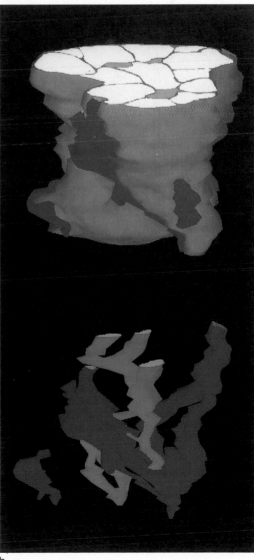

a

b

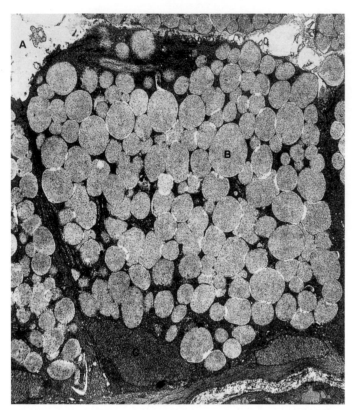

Fig. 16.29 Electron micrograph of mucous cell using conventional immersion fixation leading to swelling of the mucigen granules. The cell illustrated is in a late secretory phase with numerous granules (B) of irregular size (due to coalescence by the disruption of limiting membranes) occupying most of the cell and compressing the organelles and nucleus (C) to the periphery. The granules will discharge into the lumen (A) by exocytosis (TEM; × 5000). Courtesy of P.F. Heap.

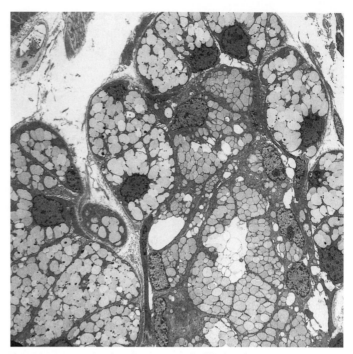

Fig. 16.30 Unstimulated mucous cells filled with secretory granules; consequently their nuclei are compressed into the basal parts of the cells (Conventional immersion fixation) (TEM; × 1000).

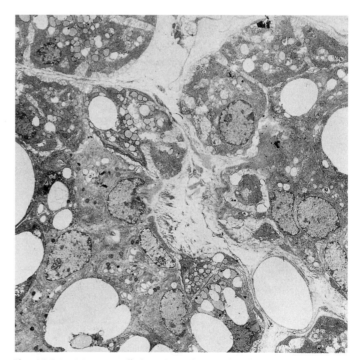

Fig. 16.31 Mucous cells in a recently stimulated submandibular gland. The mucous cells have lost their secretory granules and consequently their nuclei are more prominent (TEM; × 1000).

acinus to form the demilune structure (Fig. 16.27). This has been confirmed using three-dimensional reconstruction techniques (Fig. 16.28). In addition, the distension caused by mucous granules within each cell results in a flattening and displacement of the nucleus into the basal cytoplasm. (This feature is further illustrated in Fig. 16.29.)

The mucous cell can be readily distinguished from the serous cell at the ultrastructural level. In the early stages of synthesis of its secretory products, large amounts of rough endoplasmic reticulum are present in mucous cells together with a few mucous droplets. Compared with serous cells, mucous cells have a more conspicuous Golgi apparatus (because of the greater amount of carbohydrate that is added to the secretory protein). At a later phase of its secretory cycle, the mucous cell exhibits numerous round and isolated secretory granules which are readily distinguished from those of serous cells by their pale appearance (Fig. 16.26). The nuclei of mucous cells are round and centrally located. This account of the ultrastructure of the mucous cell contains two features that distinguish it from accounts derived using conventional immersion fixation. In conventional fixation there is distension of the mucous granules, which show discontinuous limiting membranes and coalescence to form irregularly sized granules and the nucleus

is flattened and displaced into the basal part of the cell (Fig. 16.29).

Like the serous cell, the granules discharge into the lumen by exocytosis. The depletion in granule content of mucous cells in the recently stimulated and unstimulated cells is illustrated ultrastucturally in Figs 16.30 and 16.31.

Division of salivary acini into serous and mucous types in routine sections stained with haematoxylin and eosin is clear cut. Ultrastructural and histochemical methods do not contribute further to the ease of identification. However, morphological variations among secretory granules of the same type of cell have been found in secretory acini (as well as ductal cells). Variation is greatest in serous cells (Fig. 16.20). A possible explanation is that one type of cell may be able to produce a range of secretory products, packaging them variously into secretory granules and thus creating different appearances.

The ductal cells of the submandibular gland are similar to those of the parotid. The intercalated ducts are, however, much shorter, and may be difficult to locate in routine light microscopy, while the striated ducts are longer and more obvious.

SUBLINGUAL GLAND

The human sublingual gland is not a single unit like the parotid and submandibular glands, but is made up of one large segment (the major sublingual gland) and a group of 8–30 mixed, minor salivary glands, each having its own duct system emptying into the sublingual fold (see Fig. 1.13). The major sublingual gland is a mixed gland but with a preponderance of mucous elements.

With routine staining at the light microscope level, the sublingual gland is seen to consist of many groups of pale-staining mucous cells (Fig. 16.32). While there are some serous acini, most serous cells are contained in serous demilunes around mucous acini or tubules in routinely fixed material (Fig. 16.33) (but see pages 263–264: as described for the submandibular gland, these demilunes are now thought to be preparation artefacts).

The duct system is much less well developed than in the other major salivary glands and striated ducts are lacking. The

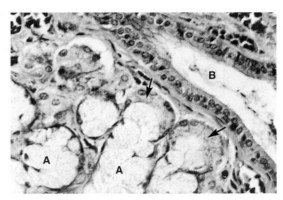

Fig. 16.33 Sublingual gland showing mucous acini or tubules (A) and serous demilunes (arrowed). B = Collecting duct.

initial duct segments are similar to intercalated ducts elsewhere but are short. The next larger ductal element, while being rich in mitochondria, lacks the basal striations that characterise striated ducts. This may be related to the formation of a sodium-rich saliva. Only part of the sublingual gland drains into a main collecting duct, the remainder draining independently through many smaller ducts.

MINOR SALIVARY GLANDS

The minor salivary glands are classified by their anatomical location: buccal, labial, palatal, palatoglossal and lingual. They are primarily mucous. Labial and buccal glands are illustrated on page 232. The palatoglossal glands are located in the region of the pharyngeal isthmus. The palatal glands lie in both the soft and hard palate (Figs 14.60, 16.34). The anterior lingual glands are embedded within muscle near the ventral surface of the tongue, and have short ducts opening near the lingual frenulum. The posterior glands are located in the root of the tongue. Both groups are mucous. The von Ebner glands

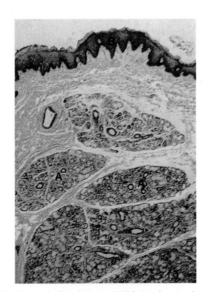

Fig. 16.32 Sublingual gland tissue (A) lying beneath the oral mucosa (B). Note the preponderance of pale-staining mucous cells (Masson's trichrome; × 25).

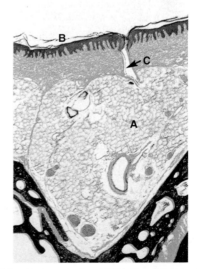

Fig. 16.34 Minor mucous gland (A) in hard palate. B = Keratinised masticatory mucosa; C = collecting duct of gland opening on to surface (Masson's trichrome; demineralised section; × 15).

empty into the trench of the circumvallate papillae and are serous (see Figs 14.70, 14.71).

CLINICAL CONSIDERATIONS

Older patients frequently complain of a dry mouth (xerostomia), with all the unpleasant symptoms one might expect from a consideration of the important functions of saliva. This was once thought to be a reflection of decreased salivary production associated with the ageing process. However, this does not always appear to be the case, in many patients it being more likely that the decreased salivary production reflects increased use of medication (many drugs depress salivary production sometimes centrally as well as peripherally – with unstimulated salivary flow rates falling from approximately 0.3 ml/min to less than half this value).

Loss of salivary tissue is also a consequence of radiotherapy treatment for certain tumours in the region of the jaws or of Sjögren's syndrome, where there is invasion and destruction of the parenchyma by lymphoid tissue. As saliva is important in the maintenance of oral health, decreased secretion from the salivary glands results in an increased incidence in oral conditions such as periodontal disease, dental caries and candidal infections ('thrush'). Partial relief may be obtained by the frequent administration of artificial salivas.

17 Development of the face

During early development (4 weeks *in utero*) the primitive oral cavity (stomodeum) is bounded by five **facial swellings**, produced by proliferating zones of mesenchyme lying beneath the surface ectoderm (Fig. 17.1). These are the frontonasal, mandibular and maxillary processes. The **frontonasal process** lies above, the two **mandibular processes** lie below, and the two **maxillary processes** are located at the sides. The maxillary and mandibular processes are derived from the first branchial arches. The facial processes are demarcated by grooves that, in the course of normal development, become flattened out by the proliferative and migratory activity of the underlying mesenchyme.

At this early stage of development a membrane (the **oropharyngeal membrane**) separates the primitive oral cavity from the developing pharynx. The oropharyngeal membrane is bilaminar, being composed of an outer ectodermal layer and an inner endodermal layer. This membrane soon breaks down to establish continuity between the ectodermally lined oral cavity and the endodermally lined pharynx. Although not detectable in the adult, the demarcation zone between mucosa derived from ectoderm and endoderm corresponds to a region lying just behind the third permanent molar tooth.

In a 5-week-old embryo (Fig. 17.2), localised thickenings of ectoderm give rise to the **nasal** and **optic placodes**. These placodes will form the olfactory epithelium and the lenses of the eyes respectively. The nasal placodes sink into the underlying mesenchyme, forming two blind-ended **nasal pits** (the primitive nasal cavities). Proliferation of mesenchyme from the frontonasal process around the openings of the nasal pits produces the **medial** and **lateral nasal processes**. The nasal pits continue to deepen until eventually they approach the roof of the primitive oral cavity, being partitioned from it by **oronasal membranes**. By the end of the fifth week, these membranes rupture to produce communications between the

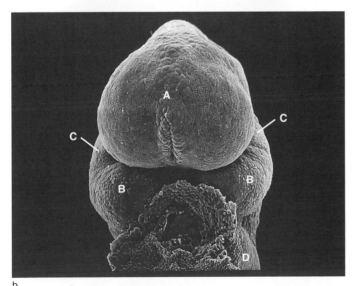

Fig. 17.1 (a) Model of a face of a 4-week-old human embryo (frontal aspect) (b) SEM of the face at an equivalent 4-week stage in the rat (frontal aspect). A = Frontonasal process; B = mandibular processes; C = maxillary processes; D = pericardial swelling. Courtesy of Professor A.G.S. Lumsden.

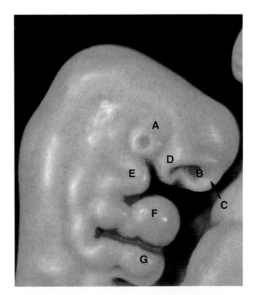

Fig. 17.2 Model of a face of a 5-week-old human embryo (lateral aspect). A = Optic placode; B = nasal pit; C = medial nasal process; D = lateral nasal process; E = maxillary process; F = mandibular process; G = second branchial arch.

269

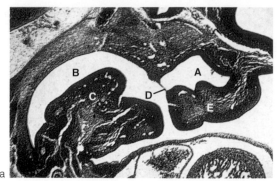

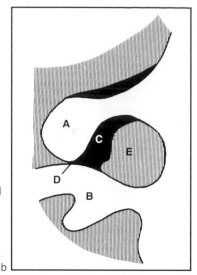

Fig. 17.3 (a) Sagittal section through the developing nasal (A) and oral (B) cavities to illustrate the nasal fin (C). D = Oronasal membrane; E = maxillary isthmus; F = developing tongue ((a) Toluidine blue; × 30). Courtesy of Dr D.A. Luke. (b) Diagram with similar labelling.

developing nasal and oral cavities. Before the oronasal membrane ruptures, a sheet of epithelium (the **nasal fin**) may be seen in front of each nasal pit. The nasal fin does not, as was once thought, form an epithelial partition between the maxillary and medial nasal processes. A bridge of mesenchyme, the **maxillary isthmus**, joins the two processes in front of the nasal fin. Fig. 17.3 shows a sagittal section through the developing nasal and oral cavities and the positions of the nasal fin, the oronasal membrane and the maxillary isthmus at the end of the fifth week of development. The nasal fin is eventually incorporated into either the walls of the nasal pit or the oronasal membrane. However, should the fin become enlarged, it may constitute a line of weakness between the mesenchyme of the maxillary and medial nasal processes and eventually lead to a cleft in this region.

In the 6-week-old embryo (Fig. 17.4), the two mandibular processes fuse in the midline to form the tissues of the lower jaw. Rarely, persistence of a midline groove in this region produces a mandibular cleft. The mandibular processes and maxillary processes meet at the angle of the mouth, thus defining its outline. Disturbances in this development may give rise to macrostomia (enlarged oral orifice), microstomia (small oral orifice) or, rarely, to an astomia (lack of an oral orifice). From the corners of the mouth the maxillary processes grow inwards beneath the lateral nasal processes and towards the medial nasal processes of the upper lip (Fig. 17.4b). Between the merging maxillary and the lateral nasal processes lie the **naso-optic furrows**. From each furrow a solid ectodermal rod of cells sinks below the surface and canalises to form the nasolacrimal duct. Persistence of the naso-optic furrow may produce an oblique facial cleft (see Fig. 17.7).

Two differing accounts have been given for the development of the upper lip. One view suggests that the maxillary processes overgrow the medial nasal processes to meet in the midline

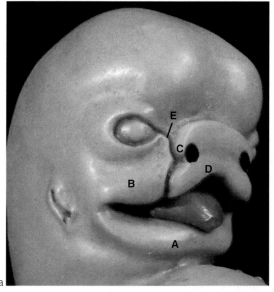

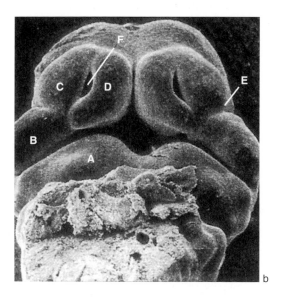

Fig. 17.4 (a) Model of a face of a 6-week-old human embryo (lateral aspect). A = Mandibular process; B = maxillary process; C = lateral nasal process; D = medial nasal process; E = naso-optic furrow. (b) SEM of developing rat upper jaw and lip at an equivalent stage to 6 weeks showing the merging maxillary and medial nasal processes. Inset courtesy of Professor A.G.S. Lumsden.

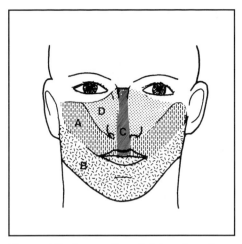

Fig. 17.5 The contributions to the adult face from the embryonic facial processes. A = Maxillary process; B = mandibular process; C = medial nasal process; D = lateral nasal process.

and thus contribute all the tissue for the upper lip. This is based upon an appreciation of the innervation of the fully formed upper lip (i.e. the infraorbital branch of the maxillary division of the trigeminal nerve), the maxillary processes being supplied by the maxillary nerve and the frontonasal process by the ophthalmic nerve. Alternatively, it has been suggested that the maxillary processes meet the medial nasal processes without such overgrowth, the middle third of the upper lip being derived from the frontonasal process. While histological evidence favours the latter explanation, at present little is known about the behaviour of the mesenchyme of the facial processes after the initial fusion, thereby not excluding the possibility of subsequent migration of tissue derived from the maxillary processes towards the midline. The possible contributions to the adult face from the embryonic facial processes (based upon the suggestion that the middle third of the upper lip is derived from the frontonasal process) are described in Fig. 17.5. The facial derivatives shown are therefore at odds with the sensory distribution of the adult face, because (as previously mentioned) the fully developed lip is supplied only by the maxillary divi-

sion of the trigeminal nerve and has no contribution from the ophthalmic division. Note that the facial muscles are derived from the mesenchyme of the second branchial arch, and are therefore innervated by the facial nerve.

Fusion of the facial processes ultimately produces the region known as the 'intermaxillary segment'. It is from this area that the primary palate will develop (see page 273).

The cells that make up the mesenchyme of the facial primordia are derived from two main sources: connective tissue cells migrating from the neural crest and muscle cells from the paraxial mesenchyme. Further development involves the four fundamental mechanisms that underlie all embryonic development: growth, morphogenesis, cell differentiation and pattern formation. The last mechanism leads to the spatial ordering of cell differentiation. Present research into the development of the face is geared towards understanding the basis of all these mechanisms.

The size of the cell populations is of key importance and is likely to be controlled, at least in part, by growth factors. These may also be of significance in the epithelial–mesenchymal interactions known to induce cartilage, bone and tooth differentiation within facial primordia. Pattern formation in developing limbs is controlled by vitamin A derivatives (retinoids), which form morphogenetic gradients within the limb bud. While such gradients have not yet been demonstrated in the face, a similar mechanism seems likely, as the facial primordia are sensitive to exogenous retinoic acid and the mesenchymal cells contain specific retinoic acid receptors.

Quantitative electron microscopic studies (Fig. 17.6) show that, at the time of fusion of the facial processes, there is a marked increase in the number of small projections/processes from the mesenchymal cells. This change is consistent with reports that changes within the epithelial cells occur and may be related to intercellular signalling between the mesenchymal cells at the time of fusion of the upper lip, just before the onset of major histogenic events.

It is worth noting that the brain and facial mesenchyme have been shown to express particular genes at key times in their development. These 'homeobox genes' were discovered in

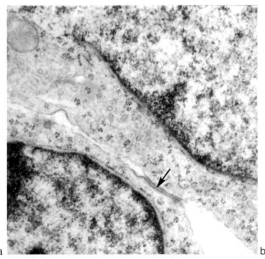
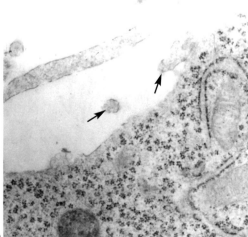

Fig. 17.6 Electron micrographs of the mesenchyme within the maxillary facial processes (TEM; × 15 000). Courtesy of D. Symons. (a) Shows cell junction (arrow). (b) Shows small cell processes (arrows).

embryos of the fruit fly *Drosophila* and are responsible for the spatial organisation of the developing *Drosophila* embryo. Similar genes are expected to be of major importance in mammalian development and are the subject of intensive research.

'Sonic hedgehog' is a protein switched on by retinoic acid, which along with fibroblast growth factor (FGF), has been located in the ectoderm of the frontonasal and maxillary processes in chick embryos. Their function is unclear, but it is possible that Sonic hedgehog may act as an organiser of morphogenesis, whereas FGF may be involved in the stimu-lation of the mesenchyme of the facial processes to produce growth.

CLINICAL CONSIDERATIONS

Failure of fusion of the maxillary and medial nasal processes produces the common congenital malformation of cleft lip, which may be unilateral or bilateral. Failure of the medial nasal processes to merge may be responsible for the formation of median cleft lip (Figs 17.7–17.9).

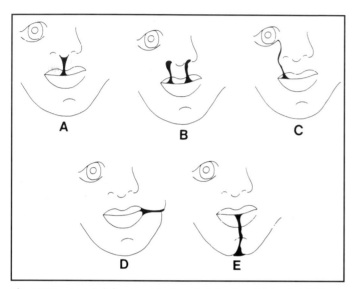

Fig. 17.7 Facial clefts. A = Median cleft lip; B = bilateral cleft lip; C = oblique facial cleft; D = lateral facial cleft; E = median mandibular cleft.

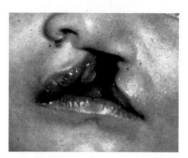

Fig. 17.8 Unilateral cleft lip.

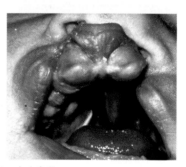

Fig. 17.9 Bilateral cleft lip.

18 Development of the palate

The definitive palate (or secondary palate) appears in the human fetus between the sixth and eighth weeks of intrauterine life. Palatogenesis is a complex event and is often disturbed, producing the congenital defect known as cleft palate. Consequently, the events and mechanisms responsible for the development of the palate have been much studied, although some controversy remains.

By the sixth week of development (Fig. 18.1), the primitive nasal cavities are separated by a primary nasal septum and are partitioned from the primitive oral cavity by a **primary palate**. Both the primary nasal septum and the primary palate are derived from the frontonasal process. The stomodeal chamber is divided at this stage into the small primitive oral cavity

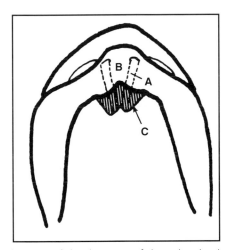

Fig. 18.1 The state of development of the palate by the sixth week of intrauterine life. A = Primitive nasal cavities; B = primary nasal septum; C = primary palate.

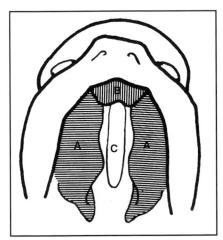

Fig. 18.2 The development of the palate during the sixth week of intrauterine life. A = Lateral palatal shelves; B = primary palate; C = secondary nasal septum.

beneath the primary palate and the relatively large oronasal cavity behind the primary palate. As shown in Fig. 18.2, during the sixth week of development, two lateral palatal shelves develop behind the primary palate from the maxillary processes. A secondary nasal septum grows down from the roof of the stomodeum behind the primary nasal septum, thus dividing the nasal part of the oronasal cavity into two. It seems that the mesenchyme within the palatal shelves originates from the neural crest.

During the seventh week of development the oral part of the oronasal cavity becomes completely filled by the developing tongue (Fig. 18.3). Growth of the palatal shelves continues such that they come to lie vertically. Two peaks of DNA synthesis occur as the palatal shelves are formed: during initial shelf outgrowth and during vertical shelf elongation. The reason for mammalian shelves forming with a vertical orientation is unknown. It has been suggested that the potential space in the oronasal cavity is insufficient because of the evolution of a large tongue in mammals.

During the eighth week of development (Fig. 18.4), the stomodeum enlarges, the tongue 'drops' and the vertically inclined palatal shelves become horizontal. It has been suggested that the descent of the tongue is related to mandibular growth and/or a change in the shape of the tongue. On becoming horizontal, the palatal shelves contact each other (and the secondary nasal septum) in the midline to form the definitive or secondary palate. The shelves contact the primary palate anteriorly so that the oronasal cavity becomes subdivided into its constituent oral and nasal cavities (Fig. 18.5). After contact, the medial edge epithelia of the two shelves fuse to form a midline epithelial seam. Subsequently this degenerates so that mesenchymal continuity is established across the now intact and horizontal secondary palate. Fusion of the palatal processes is complete by the twelfth week of development. Behind the

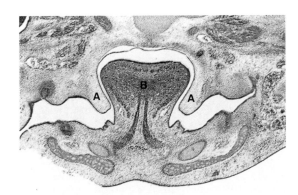

Fig. 18.3 Coronal section through the developing head during the seventh week of development showing the palatal shelves (A). B = Developing tongue (Masson's trichrome; × 30).

273

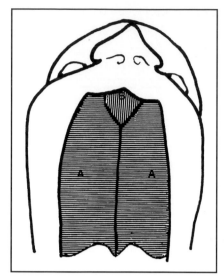

Fig. 18.4 The state of development of the palate during the eighth week of intrauterine life. A = Palatal shelves; B = primary palate.

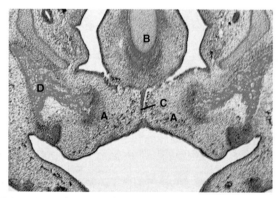

Fig. 18.5 Coronal section through developing oronasal regions following contact of the palatal shelves (A) and secondary nasal septum (B). C = Midline epithelial seam; D = developing bone of maxilla (Masson's trichrome; × 30).

secondary nasal septum the palatal shelves fuse to form the soft palate and uvula.

Clefts of the palate, like those of the lip, are multifactorial malformations, involving both genetic (polygenic) and environmental factors. Clefts may result from disturbances of any of the processes involved during palatogenesis (i.e. from defective palatal shelf growth; delayed shelf elevation or failure of elevation; defective shelf fusion or lack of degeneration of the midline epithelial seam; or failure of mesenchymal consolidation and/or differentiation). Recent research on palatogenesis has concentrated on two main events: palatal shelf elevation and the initial stage of fusion of the shelves.

PALATAL SHELF ELEVATION

Several mechanisms have been proposed to account for the rapid movement of the palatal shelves from the vertical to the horizontal position. Although it was once thought that extrinsic forces might be responsible (e.g. forces derived from the tongue

or jaw movements), research has primarily focused on the search for a force intrinsic to the palatal shelf. It has been proposed that the intrinsic shelf elevation force might develop as a result of hydration of 'ground substance' components (principally hyaluronan) in the shelf mesenchyme, or as a result of mesenchymal cell activity. The intrinsic shelf elevating force might be multifactorial, although there is as yet no experimental evidence to support what otherwise might be considered this common-sense view.

The changing amounts of glycosaminoglycans (GAG) during development of the anterior (presumptive hard) and posterior (presumptive soft) palates are illustrated in Fig. 18.6. Stage A occurs immediately before shelf elevation, stage B immediately after shelf elevation, stage C is the stage of shelf fusion and early histogenesis and stage D represents a stage of marked histogenesis after fusion. The most significant changes occur after elevation; during the time of elevation there are no differences between the anterior and posterior regions of the shelves even though, in the species studied in Fig. 18.6 (the rat), the posterior region of the shelf does not elevate but grows initially

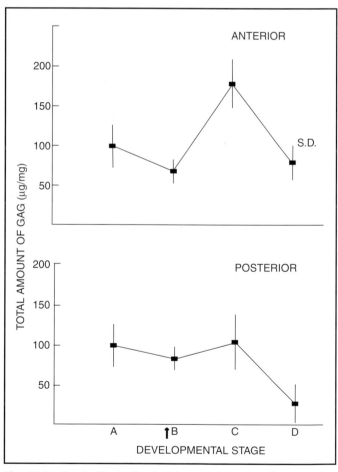

Fig. 18.6 Graphs illustrating the changing amounts of glycosaminoglycans (GAG) during development of the anterior (presumptive hard) and posterior (presumptive soft) palates. Stage A before shelf elevation; stage B after shelf elevation; stage C during shelf fusion and early histogenesis; stage D a stage of marked histogenesis after fusion. Arrow indicates time of shelf elevation. Courtesy of Dr G.D. Singh and the editor of *Archives of Oral Biology*.

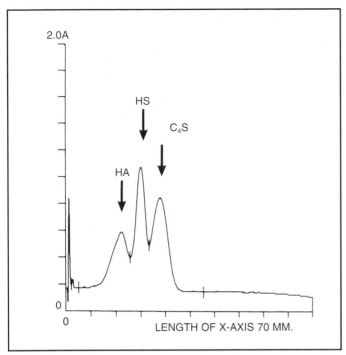

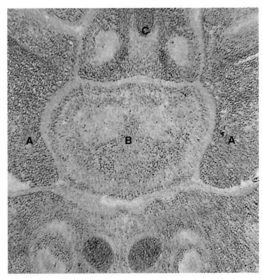

Fig. 18.8 Coronal section through a vertical (pre-elevation) palatal shelf (A) stained using the hyaluronectin/anti-hyaluronectin technique. Positive brown staining shows presence of hyaluronan in shelf mesenchyme. B = Tongue; C = nasal septum (× 30).

Fig. 18.7 Densiometric scan of electrophoretograms showing the GAGs within the palatal shelves *in vivo*. HA = Hyaluronan; HS = heparan sulphate; C₄S = chondroitin 4-sulphate. Courtesy of Dr G.D. Singh and the editor of *Archives of Oral Biology*.

with a horizontal disposition. Three GAG types are found *in vivo*: hyaluronan (HA), heparan sulphate (HS) and chondroitin 4-sulphate (C4S) (Fig. 18.7). If palatal shelves are cultured *in vitro*, dermatan sulphate is also present, highlighting the difficulties of extrapolating from the findings of tissue culture to the *in vivo* situation.

A section through a vertical (pre-elevation) palatal shelf (A) stained using the hyaluronectin/anti-hyaluronectin technique is shown in Fig. 18.8. Note the intense staining for hyaluronan within the palatal shelf mesenchyme. It has been proposed that hyaluronan is a GAG involved in shelf elevation because it is a highly electrostatically charged, open-coil molecule capable of binding up to 10 times its own weight in water. The

changing concentrations of hyaluronan within the anterior and posterior regions of palatal shelves are illustrated in Fig. 18.9. The stages of palatogenesis (A–D) are the same as those described in Fig. 18.6. Note that, statistically, there is significantly more hyaluronan in the shelves immediately before elevation than immediately after; however, the data does not agree with some reports that there is less hyaluronan posteriorly than anteriorly, and again the pattern of change in hyaluronan is similar both anteriorly and posteriorly even though the posterior region does not undergo elevation to reach the horizontal.

More recent studies have revealed the presence during palatogenesis of enzymes associated with hyaluronan synthesis, of a cell-surface receptor associated with hyaluronan, of the hyaluronan binding extracellular matrix components versican and hyaluronectin, and of hyaluronan binding sites (Fig. 18.10). Furthermore, using an organ-culture system (Figs 18.11–18.14), agents that alter hyaluronan content or size, that disrupt

Fig. 18.9 Graphs showing the changing concentrations of hyaluronan within the anterior and posterior regions of palatal shelves. A–D: stages of palatogenesis described in Fig. 18.6. Courtesy of Dr G.D. Singh and the editor of *Archives of Oral Biology*.

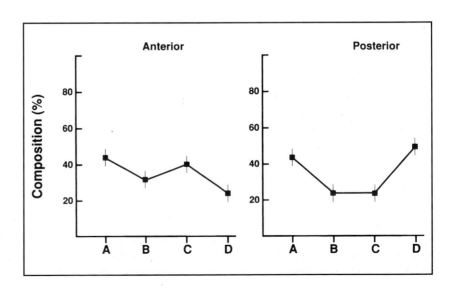

Fig. 18.10 The palatal shelves before (a) and after (b–d) elevation showing the presence of binding for the glycosaminoglycan hyaluronan (white label) using CD44 antibody immunohistochemistry. A = Palatal shelves (Fluorescent immunohistochemistry; × 80). Courtesy of S. Thomas, R. Hall and B.J. Moxham.

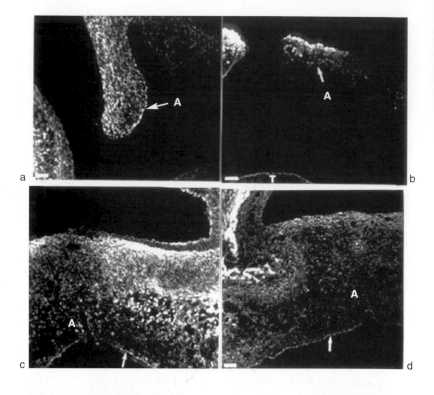

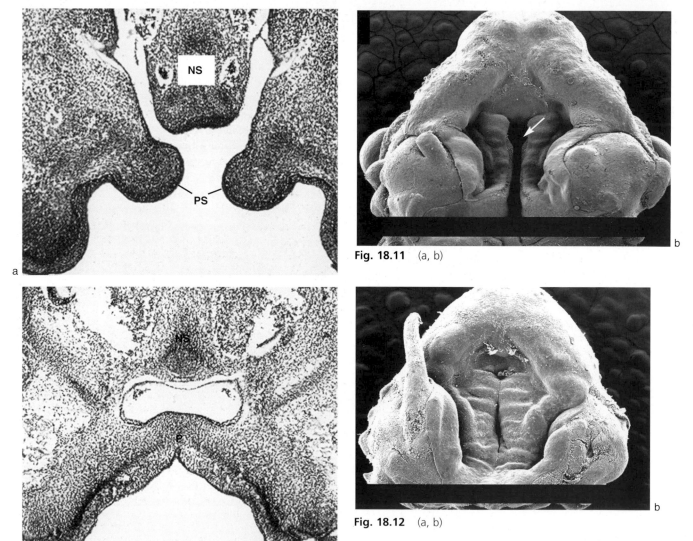

Fig. 18.11 (a, b)

Fig. 18.12 (a, b)

Fig. 18.11   (*Facing page*) The effects of *Streptomyces* hyaluronidase on the developing palate in organ culture. Clefts are produced, suggesting that palate development is disrupted in the absence of the glycosaminoglycan hyaluronan. (a) Section through a cleft palate resulting from hyaluronidase treatment. NS = Nasal septum; PS = unfused palatal shelves (× 60). (b) SEM showing the cleft (arrowed) (× 30). Courtesy of S. Thomas, R. Hall and B.J. Moxham.

Fig. 18.12   (*Facing page*) The effects of UDP-xylose on the developing palate in organ culture. UDP-xylose is a natural inhibitor of UDPGD, the enzyme responsible for the conversion of UDP-glucose to UDP-glucuronic acid. Normal palatogenesis with UDP-xylose suggests that inhibition of UDPGD has no effect on palate development or that it may not be entering the tissue. (a) Section through a normally developing palate following UDP-xylose treatment. NS = Nasal septum; P = fused palatal shelves (× 50). (b) SEM showing normal palatogenesis (arrowed) (× 25). Courtesy of S. Thomas, R. Hall and B.J. Moxham.

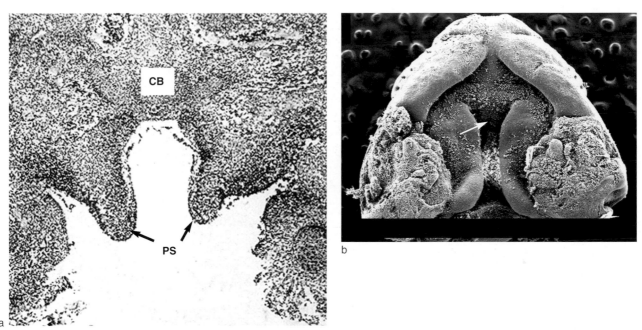

Fig. 18.13   The effects of CHLR (chlorcyclixine) on the developing palate in organ culture. CHLR enhances degradation of hyaluronan and chondroitin sulphate to lower the molecular weight products, with little effect on their synthesis and on DNA synthesis. Clefts are produced, suggesting that the size of the glycosaminoglycan chain may influence palatogenesis. (a) Section through a cleft palate resulting from CHLR treatment. CB = Cranial Base; PS = unfused palatal shelves (× 50). (b) SEM showing the cleft (arrowed) (× 25). Courtesy of S. Thomas, R. Hall and B.J. Moxham.

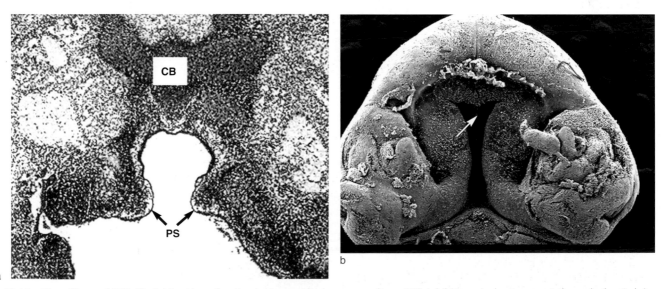

Fig. 18.14   The effects of BFA (Brefeldin A) on the developing palate in organ culture. BFA inhibits vesicular transport through the Golgi complex. Hyaluronan synthesis is not affected as this GAG, unlike other GAGs, undergoes a different synthetic pathway at or near, the plasma membrane. Clefts are produced suggesting that a set of macromolecules other than hyaluronan and synthesised in the Golgi play an important role in normal palatogenesis. (a) Coronal section through a cleft palate resulting from BFA treatment. CB = Cranial base; PS = unfused palatal shelves (× 50). (b) SEM showing the cleft (arrowed) (× 25). Courtesy of S. Thomas, R. Hall and B.J. Moxham.

glycosaminoglycan substitution on proteoglycans, or that alter the balance of matrix molecules secreted via the Golgi complex and hyaluronan produced at the cell surface all affect palatogenesis. However, while all agents prevent palatal fusion, there are variable effects on shelf elevation. For example, hyaluronidase digestion results in failure of elevation (Fig. 18.11) and treatment with a drug that blocks secretion from the Golgi complex, whilst still allowing hyaluronan production, also prevents elevation (Fig. 18.14). On the other hand, displacement of nascent hyaluronan with oligosaccharides allowed elevation (although the shelves were incorrectly oriented) (Figure 18.12) and treatment with an agent that disrupts glycosaminoglycan assembly on proteoglycans resulted in abnormal elevation (Figure 18.13). Overall, therefore, recent research indicates that hyaluronan is crucial to shelf elevation. To add to such findings, a reduced molecular weight hyaluronan leads to palate dysmorphogenesis (Figure18.13), suggesting that a minimum hyaluronan size is required to achieve normal palatogenesis.

Other matrix components, including proteoglycans, are of equal importance to shelf elevation. Versican and decorin have been identified at a range of molecular weights corresponding to various processed forms (Fig. 18.15).

The role of collagen within the palatal shelves is disputed, although immunocytochemically type I collagen can easily be identified (Fig. 18.16). Stout bundles of collagen can be seen running down the centre of the palatal shelf, oriented from the base towards the tip of the shelf. It has been suggested that the shelf elevation force is directed by these collagen fibres.

The role of the mesenchymal cells within the palatal shelves has also drawn some controversy. There is evidence that a critical number of cells are required for palatal shelf elevation to occur but there is no reliable evidence that these cells, by their rapid division and proliferation, by migration or by contraction,

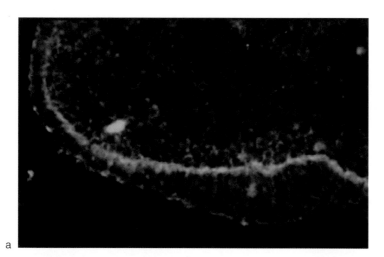

a

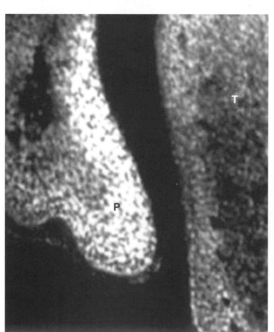

b

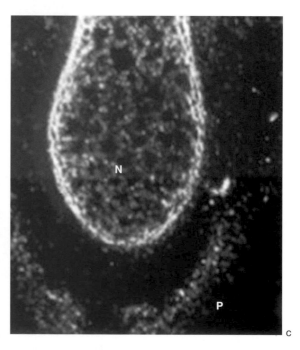

c

Fig. 18.15 The presence of some proteoglycans during normal palatogenesis. (a) Decorin (green staining) beneath the lining epithelial cells of the palatal shelf pre-elevation (biglycan is not found). Note that decorin relocates to the centre of the shelf mesenchyme post-elevation (fluorescence immunohistochemistry; × 240). (b) Versican (white staining) in the palatal shelves (P); T = tongue (fluorescence immunohistochemistry; × 140). (c) Link protein (white staining) found in the developing nasal septum (N) but absent in the palatal shelf (P), indicating that the proteoglycans within the shelf are 'labile' (Fluorescence immunohistochemistry; × 60). Courtesy of W. McLean, S. Thomas, R. Hall and B.J. Moxham.

can effect a palatal shelf elevation force (particularly in view of the rapidity of the processes of shelf elevation). Using a special silver staining technique, the degree of activity of the mesenchymal cells in the palatal shelf mesenchyme can be assessed. To determine whether cell activity changes at different stages of palatogenesis, the Ag–NOR staining technique has been employed; this produces grains in the nucleolar region (Fig. 18.17). The number and configuration of these 'grains' reflect the overall degree of protein synthesis by the cells. This staining procedure confirmed that the rate of protein synthesis during palatogenesis is high, is higher pre-elevation than post-elevation, and is higher still during later stages of histogenesis. These results accord with the changes occurring in GAG synthesis at various stages of palatogenesis. The staining technique further shows that protein synthesis is severely depressed during cleft formation, but is unable to demonstrate major differences between anterior and posterior regions. Quantitative electron microscopy of the cells within the palatal shelves has also not produced evidence that such cells can generate a shelf elevation force.

FUSION OF THE PALATAL SHELVES

Once the palatal shelves have elevated, they contact each other (initially in the middle third of the palate) and adhere by means of a 'sticky' glycoprotein, which coats the surface of the medial edge epithelia of the shelves. The epithelial cells develop desmosomes and consequently an epithelial seam is formed (Fig. 18.18). The adherence of the medial edge epithelia is specific as palatal epithelia will not fuse with epithelia from other sites (e.g. the tongue). This may be related to the fact

18.16 Coronal section of a palatal shelf stained immunocytochemically with antibodies against type I collagen showing positive green staining throughout.
A = Collagen bundles; B = base of palatal shelf; C = tip of palatal shelf (× 240).
Courtesy of Professor M.W.J. Fergusson.

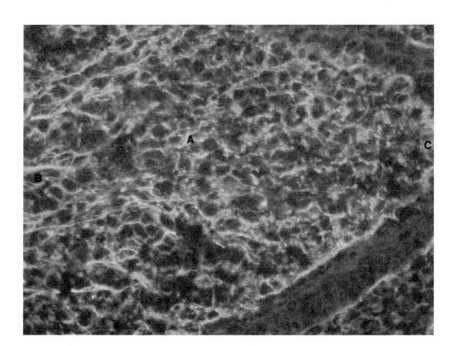

Fig. 18.17 Ag-Nor staining of the palatal shelves (A) to assess the degree of activity of the mesenchymal cells (Silver stain; × 45). Inset shows black silver grains at higher power (× 400).

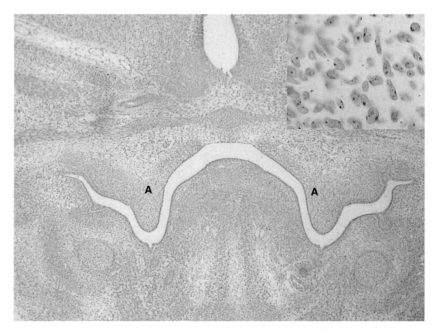

that the protein associated with the formation of desmosomes (desmoplakin) appears specifically on the cell membranes of the medial edge epithelia just before shelf contact.

Disruption of the epithelial seam, with penetration by mesenchymal cells, is shown in Fig. 18.19, although the signals that are responsible for such breakdown are not yet fully understood. Nevertheless, the breakdown of the basal lamina is likely to be a significant event. At this early stage of fusion (Fig. 18.20), the basal lamina remains intact during the early fusion. At a later stage of fusion (Fig. 18.21), with migration of the epithelial cells into the mesenchyme, the midline epithelial seam is disrupted and the migrating cells initially carry with them fragments of the disrupted basal lamina. Fibrils comprising tenascin and type III collagen have been shown to run at right angles to the basal lamina and may provide guiding pathways for the migrating epithelial cells. Evidence indicates that the events leading to the breakdown of the epithelial seam occur in single isolated palatal shelves and therefore do not depend upon shelf contact.

Almost as soon as the epithelial seam is formed, it thins to a layer two or three cells thick. This thinning may be the result of three processes. First, the seam is thinned by growth of the palate (in terms of oronasal height) and by epithelial cell migration from the region of the seam onto the oral and nasal aspects of the palate. Second, there is programmed cell death (apoptosis) in the seam. This is shown by the finding that DNA synthesis ceases in the medial edge epithelial cells one day before shelf contact. Furthermore, cyclic AMP (cAMP) levels increase just before shelf fusion: exogenous cAMP is associated with precocious cell death in the medial edge epithelia. It

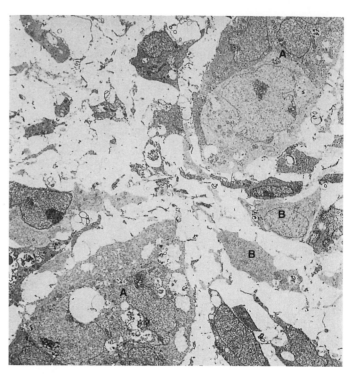

Fig. 18.19 Electron micrograph showing disruption of the epithelial seam (A) with penetration by mesenchymal cells (B) (TEM; × 3900). Courtesy of Professor M.W.J. Fergusson.

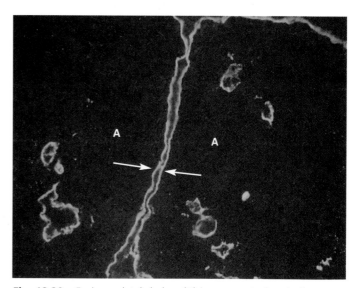

Fig. 18.20 Fusing palatal shelves (A) immunocytochemically labelled with antibodies against type IV collagen showing positive green staining in basal lamina (arrowed) (× 90). Courtesy of Professor M.W.J. Fergusson.

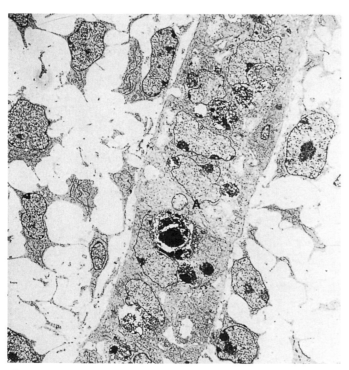

Fig. 18.18 Electron micrograph showing the midline epithelial seam for early fusing palatal shelves. An intact basal lamina lies on either side of the epithelial seam. A = Epithelial cells (TEM; × 3900). Courtesy of Professor M.W.J. Fergusson.

has also been shown that epidermal growth factor inhibits medial edge cell death and that this inhibition is blocked by exogenous cAMP. Care must be taken, however, when interpreting the effects of cAMP because physiologically it is an intracellular messenger and may therefore be mediating differential gene expression triggered by other events occurring at the cell surface. Third, there is good evidence that some of the epithelial cells migrate from the seam into the palatal shelf mesenchyme and differentiate into cells indistinguishable

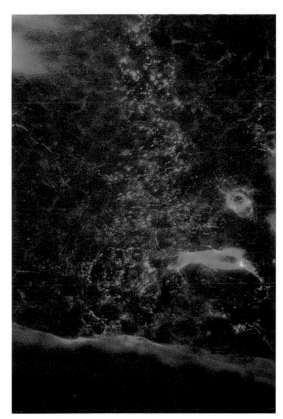

Fig. 18.21 Late stage of fusion of the palatal shelves immunocytochemically labelled for type IV collagen and showing disruption of the positively green staining midline epithelial seam; compare with Fig. 18.18 (× 180). Courtesy of Professor M.W.J. Fergusson.

Immunocytochemical labelling with antibodies against epidermal growth factor receptors of the mesenchymal cells adjacent to the midline epithelial seam of fusing palatal shelves is shown in Fig. 18.24. Epidermal growth factor (EGF), or its embryonic homologue known as transforming growth factor α (TGF-α), is known to inhibit palatal medial edge epithelial cell death in the presence of mesenchyme. Furthermore, it has been shown that the synthesis of extracellular matrix molecules (including type IX collagen) is stimulated by factors such as TGF-α and TGF-β and is inhibited by fibroblast growth factors (FGF). When palatal shelves are organcultured with EGF, the medial edge of the palatal shelf shows a nipple-like bulge, medial edge epithelial cell death is absent, and the mesenchyme possesses increased quantities of extracellular matrix molecules. It has been proposed, therefore, that the palatal shelf mesenchyme produces growth factors that either directly signal epithelial differentiation or, by stimulating extracellular matrix production, indirectly influence differentiation through this matrix. The photomicrograph shown in Fig. 18.24 suggests that EGF receptors show regional heterogeneity and that the receptors appear beneath the medial edge of the shelves only when the epithelial seam is degenerating.

Once fusion is complete, the hard palate ossifies intramembranously from four centres of ossification, one in each developing maxilla and one in each developing palatine bone. The maxillary ossification centre lies above the developing deciduous canine tooth germ and appears in the eighth week of development (see Fig. 18.5). The palatine centres of ossification are situated in the region forming the future perpen-

from the mesenchymal cells. Indeed, it is well known that epithelial cells can migrate and differentiate into mesenchymallike cells in other circumstances during development.

There have been many experiments to help clarify the nature of the epithelial–mesenchymal interactions during fusion of the palatal shelves. In the main, these experiments have involved the separation and then the recombination in culture of the epithelial and mesenchymal components of the shelves. Overall, these experiments have shown that, as with epithelial–mesenchymal interactions for later tooth development (see pages 297–302), it is the mesenchyme that signals epithelial differentiation and behaviour. The nature of this signal is controversial. Although it was once proposed that the palatal mesenchyme could signal epithelial differentiation directly by cell-to-cell contact, mesenchymal–epithelial cell contacts are very rare during palatogenesis. Recent evidence indicates that extracellular matrix molecules may provide the signal and work has been undertaken to assess the role of type IX collagen (Fig. 18.23). At the earliest stages before shelf elevation, the medial edges of the palatal shelves label poorly for type IX collagen compared with floor of the mouth epithelia (Fig. 18.22). Note that, at the stage of fusion, type IX collagen appears around the surfaces of the medial edge epithelial cells (Fig. 18.23). Present-day thinking suggests that the control of the synthesis of type IX collagen is influenced by growth factors.

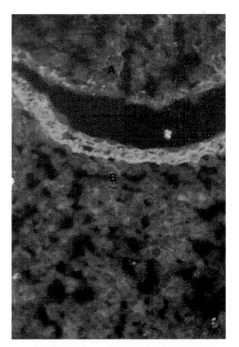

Fig. 18.22 The medial edge epithelia of palatal shelves (A) labelled immunocytochemically for type IX collagen before shelf elevation. Little positive green staining is evident compared with the epithelium covering the floor of the mouth (B) (× 280). Courtesy of Professor M.W.J. Fergusson.

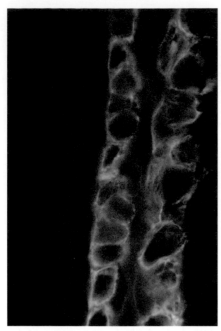

Fig. 18.23 The medial edge epithelia of palatal shelves labelled immunocytochemically for type IX collagen at a time when medial edge epithelial differentiation occurs. Compared with Fig. 18.22, positive green staining is evident (× 280). Courtesy of Professor M.W.J. Fergusson.

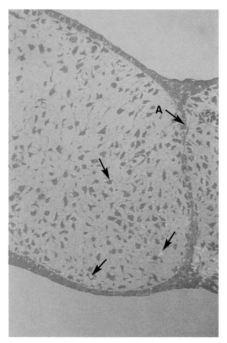

Fig. 18.24 Immunocytochemical labelling with antibodies against epidermal growth factor receptors of the mesenchymal cells adjacent to the midline epithelial seam of fusing palatal shelves. White dots indicate positive staining (arrows). A = Epithelial seam × 85). Courtesy of Professor M.W.J. Fergusson and the editor of *Development*.

dicular plate and appear in the eighth week of development. Incomplete ossification of the palate from these centres defines the median and transverse palatine sutures. There does not appear to be a separate centre of ossification for the primary

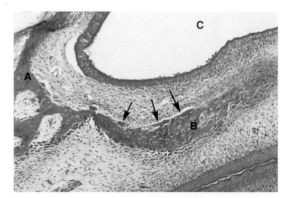

Fig. 18.25 Coronal section through the developing hard palate showing early ossification. A = Developing body of maxilla; B = bone extending from body of maxilla into palate; C = nasal cavity. Note the osteoclasts on the nasal surface (arrowed) and osteoblasts on oral surface (Masson's trichrome; × 80).

palate in humans (in other species there being a separate 'premaxilla'). Fig. 18.25 provides a coronal section through the developing hard palate to show early ossification.

CLINICAL CONSIDERATIONS

Malformations of palatogenesis may result in the appearance of clefts. The mildest form of cleft is that affecting the uvula, such a disturbance occurring relatively late in the process of palatal malfusion. Disturbances during the early phases of palatal fusion can result in a more extensive cleft involving most of the secondary palate. Should the cleft involve the primary palate, it may extend to the right and/or left of the incisive foramen to include the alveolus, passing between the lateral incisor and canine teeth. Cleft palate may be associated with cleft lip, though the two conditions are independently determined. Dental malformations are commonly associated with a cleft involving the alveolus. A submucous cleft describes a condition where the palatal mucosa is intact, but the bone/

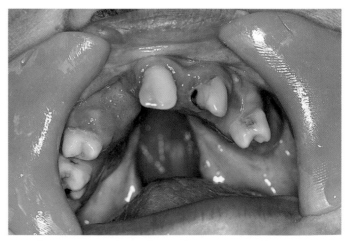

Fig. 18.26 Gross clefting of the palate. Courtesy of Dr B.A.W. Brown.

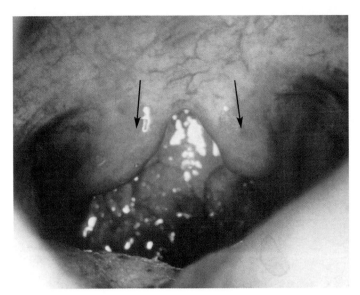

Fig. 18.27 A cleft uvula (arrows). Courtesy of Dr R.W. Pigott.

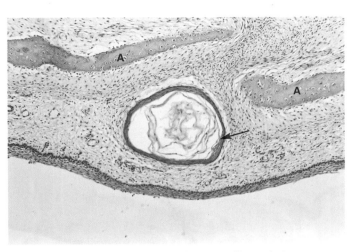

Fig. 18.28 Section through a developing midline palatine cyst (arrowed). A = Bone of hard palate (H & E; × 40).

musculature of the palate is deficient beneath the mucosa. Fig. 18.26 shows an extensive cleft of the palate and Fig. 18.27 a cleft uvula.

Less problematic than clefts (but more common) is the retention of epithelial remnants in the midline which eventually become cystic (Fig. 18.28).

19 Development of the jaws

THE MANDIBLE

The mandible initially develops intramembranously, but its subsequent growth is related to the appearance of secondary cartilages (the condylar cartilage being the most important). The developing mandible is preceded by the appearance of a rod of cartilage belonging to the first branchial arch. This is known as **Meckel's cartilage** (Figs 19.1, 19.2) and it first appears at about the sixth week of intrauterine life. Meckel's cartilage extends from the cartilaginous otic capsule in the region of the developing ear to a midline symphysis. However, it makes little contribution to the adult mandible, merely providing a framework around which the bone of the mandible forms.

The mandible first appears as a band of dense fibrous tissue on the anterolateral aspect of Meckel's cartilage. During the seventh week of intrauterine life, a **centre of ossification** appears in this fibrous tissue at a site close to the future mental foramen. From this centre, bone formation spreads rapidly backwards, forwards and upwards, around the inferior alveolar nerve and its terminal branches (the incisive and mental nerves). Further spread of the developing bone in a forwards and backwards direction produces a plate of bone on the lateral side of Meckel's cartilage that corresponds to the future body of the mandible and which extends towards the midline where

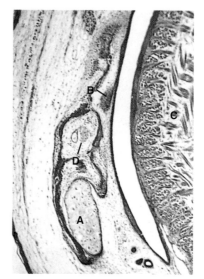

Fig. 19.2 Transverse section through the early developing mandible (eighth week of development). At this stage only a small amount of mandibular bone has formed intramembranously on the lateral aspect of Meckel's cartilage (A). Note the beginnings of tooth development in this region as indicated by the dental lamina (B). C = Tongue; D = neurovascular bundle (Masson's trichrome; × 60).

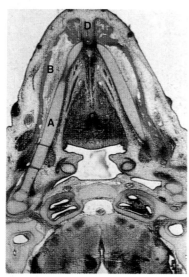

Fig. 19.1 Meckel's cartilage (A), around which the bone of the mandible (B) is forming in membrane. This is a horizontal section through the developing mandible during the eighth week of intrauterine life. Note that Meckel's cartilage extends from the cartilaginous otic capsule to the midline symphysis (D), where initially it is separated from its fellow of the opposite side by mesenchyme. C = Tongue (Masson's trichrome; × 12).

it comes to lie in close relationship with the bone forming on the opposite side. However, the two plates of bone remain separated by fibrous tissue to form the mandibular symphysis (Fig. 19.1).

At a later stage in the development of the body of the mandible, continued bone formation markedly increases the size of the mandible, with development of the alveolar process occurring to surround the developing tooth germs (Fig. 19.3). At an even later stage, Meckel's cartilage resorbs (Fig. 19.4). The neurovascular bundle that initially was located with the developing tooth germs now becomes contained within its own bony canal and there is considerable development of the alveolar process.

Although Meckel's cartilage contributes no significant tissue to the developing mandible, nodular remnants of cartilage may be seen in the region of the mandibular symphysis until birth and, in its most dorsal part, Meckel's cartilage ossifies to form ear ossicles (the malleus and incus). Behind the body of the mandible the perichondrium of Meckel's cartilage persists as the sphenomandibular and sphenomalleolar ligaments. The sphenomandibular ligament ossifies at its sites of attachment to form the lingula of the mandible and the spine of the sphenoid bone.

As the developing tooth germs reach the bell stages (see page 292), developing bone becomes closely related to it to form the **alveolus** (Fig. 19.5). The size of the alveolus is dependent upon the size of the growing tooth germ.

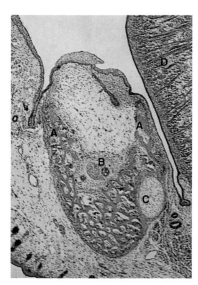

Fig. 19.3   A later stage in the development of the body of the mandible. Continued bone formation has increased the size of the mandible. The alveolar process (A) grows to surround the developing tooth germ. The developing teeth share the same common crypt as the neurovascular bundle (B). Note that Meckel's cartilage (C) is now comparatively small, although it still lies medial to the developing mandibular bone. D = Developing tongue (Masson's trichrome; × 25).

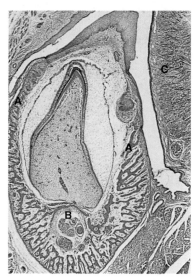

Fig. 19.4   Even later stage in the development of the body of the mandible. Meckel's cartilage has been resorbed. The neurovascular bundle (B) is now contained within its own bony canal and there has been considerable development of the alveolar process (A). C = Developing tongue (Masson's trichrome; × 25).

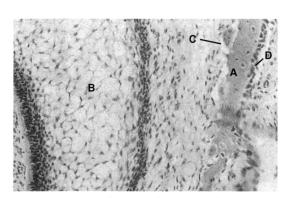

Fig. 19.5   Development of the mandibular alveolus (A) in the region of a developing tooth (B). Note that resorption is occurring on the inner wall of the alveolus (indicated by Howship's lacunae; C) while, on the outer wall of the alveolus, bone is being deposited (indicated by osteoblasts (D) lining an osteoid seam) (Decalcified section; Masson's trichrome; × 110).

Resorption occurs on the inner wall of the alveolus (indicated by Howship's lacunae) while, on the outer wall of the alveolus, bone is deposited (indicated by osteoblasts lining an osteoid seam). The developing teeth therefore come to lie in a trough of bone. Later, the teeth become separated from each other by the development of interdental septa. With the onset of root formation, interradicular bone develops in multirooted teeth.

The **ramus of the mandible** is first mapped out as a condensation of fibrocellular tissue that, although continuous with the developing body of the mandible, is positioned some way laterally from Meckel's cartilage. Further development of the ramus is associated with a backward spread of ossification from the body and by the appearance of secondary cartilages. Between the tenth and fourteenth weeks *in utero*, three **secondary cartilages** develop within the growing mandible.

The largest, and most important, of these is the condylar cartilage, which, as its name suggests, appears beneath the fibrous articular layer of the future condyle (see Figs 15.13 and 19.7). By proliferation and subsequent ossification, the cartilage is thought by some to serve as an important centre of growth for the mandible, functioning up to about the twentieth year of life. Less important, transitory, secondary cartilages are seen associated with the coronoid process and in the region of the mandibular symphysis. The appearance of the developing jaws of a human fetus at 14 weeks is shown in Fig. 19.6.

The **temporomandibular joint** develops from mesenchyme lying between the developing mandibular condyle below and the temporal bone above, which develop intramembranously. During the twelfth week of intrauterine life, two clefts appear in the mesenchyme, producing the upper and lower joint cavities. The remaining intervening mesenchyme becomes the intra-articular disc. The joint capsule develops from a condensation of mesenchyme surrounding the developing joint. At birth, the mandibular fossa is flat and there is no articular eminence; this becomes prominent only following the eruption of the deciduous dentition. The early developing condylar cartilage and temporomandibular joint are shown in Fig. 19.7.

Figure 19.8 illustrates the postnatal development of the mandible by lateral and occlusal views of the mandible at birth, at 6 years and in an adult. The ratio of body to ramus is greater at birth than in the adult, indicating a proportional increase with time in the development of the ramus. At birth, there is no distinct chin and the two halves of the mandible are separated by the mandibular symphysis. Ossification of the symphysis is complete during the second year, the two halves of the mandible uniting to form a single bone. The chin

Fig. 19.6 The appearance of the developing jaws of a human fetus (14 weeks). A = Body of mandible; B = ramus of mandible; C = secondary condylar cartilage; D = secondary coronoid cartilage; E = frontal bone; F = parietal bone; G = occipital bone; H = squamous portion of temporal bone; I = maxilla (Cleared, alizarin red preparation; × 5).

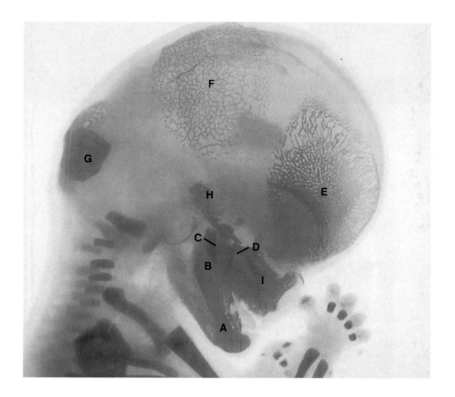

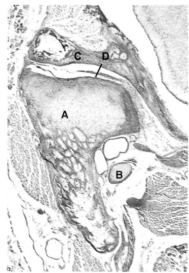

Fig. 19.7 The early developing condylar cartilage (A) and temporomandibular joint. B = Meckel's cartilage; C = developing bone of mandibular fossa; D = part of developing articular disc of temporomandibular joint (Decalcified section; Masson's trichrome: × 20).

becomes most prominent after puberty (especially in the male). There is some evidence that the angle of the mandible decreases from birth to adulthood.

Some indication of the directions of growth of the mandible can be obtained by superimposing traces of neonatal and adult mandibles (Fig. 19.9). Indeed, there is some evidence that the region around the mental foramen is a 'fixed' point for such an endeavour.

Growth of the mandible occurs by the remodelling of bone. In general terms, increase in the height of the body occurs primarily by formation of alveolar bone, although some bone is also deposited along the lower border of the mandible.

Increase in the length of the mandible is accomplished by bone deposition on the posterior surface of the ramus with compensatory resorption on its anterior surface, accompanied by deposition of bone on the posterior surface of the coronoid process and resorption on the anterior surface of the condyle. Increase in width of the mandible is produced by deposition of bone on the outer surface of the mandible and resorption on the inner surface.

There is some controversy concerning the role of the condylar cartilages in mandibular growth. One view states that continued proliferation of this cartilage is primarily responsible for the increase in both the mandibular length and the height of the ramus. Alternatively, it has been suggested that proliferation of the condylar cartilage is a response to growth and not its cause. The latter view has been supported by experiments showing that mandibular growth is relatively unaffected following condylectomy, providing normal mandibular function is maintained.

Although the mandible is a single bone, it may be thought of as a number of skeletal units, each associated with one or more soft tissue 'functional matrices'. The behaviour of these matrices primarily determines the growth of each skeletal unit. For example, the coronoid process forms a skeletal unit acted upon by the temporalis muscle. Sectioning of the temporalis muscle during early mandibular development may result in atrophy or complete absence of a coronoid process in the adult mandible. Similarly, the alveolar process is influenced by the teeth, the condyle by the lateral pterygoid muscle, the ramus by the medial pterygoid and masseter muscles and the body by the neurovascular bundle.

THE MAXILLA

As with the mandible, the maxilla develops intramembranously. The centre of ossification appears during the eighth week of

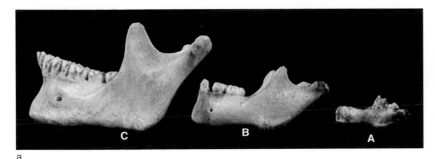

a

Fig. 19.8 The postnatal development of the mandible illustrated by lateral (a) and occlusal (b) views of the mandible at birth (A), at 6 years (B), and in an adult (C).

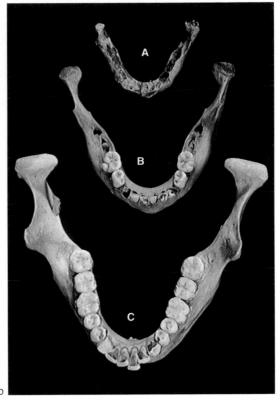

b

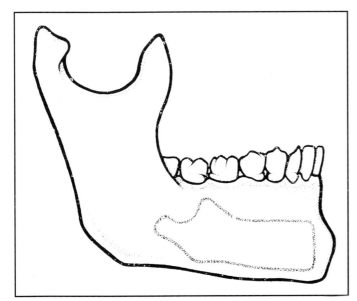

Fig. 19.9 Superimposed neonatal and adult mandibles. Note that growth of the mandible results in posterior relocation of the ramus of the mandible.

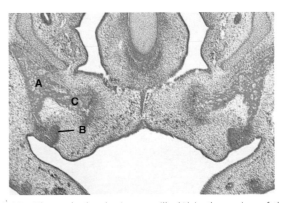

Fig. 19.10 The early developing maxilla (A) in the region of the developing deciduous canine (B). From this site, ossification spreads throughout the developing maxilla into its growing processes (e.g. palatine process; C) (Decalcified section; Masson's trichrome; × 35).

intrauterine life, close to the site of the developing deciduous canine tooth. Unlike the mandible, maxillary growth and development is not related to the appearance of secondary cartilages. Because of the maxilla's position in the developing skull, this jaw's growth is influenced by the development of the orbital, nasal, and oral cavities.

From the region of the developing deciduous canine (Fig. 19.10) ossification spreads throughout the developing maxilla into its growing processes (palatine, zygomatic, frontal and alveolar processes). The appearance of the developing maxilla in a cleared alizarin red preparation may be seen in Fig. 19.6. The ossification of the palatine processes is described on page 282.

At one time it was thought that the incisor-bearing part of the maxilla, which develops from the frontonasal process (see page 269), had a separate centre of ossification. It was consequently called the **premaxilla**. However, it is now clear that ossification spreads from the body of the maxilla into its incisor-bearing component.

Growth of the maxilla occurs by bone remodelling (i.e. surface deposition of bone with associated resorption) and by sutural growth. Among the agents that provide the forces separating the maxilla from the adjacent bones (thus permitting growth at the sutures) are the growing eyeballs, cartilaginous nasal septum and orbital pad of fat. Thus, growth of the maxilla is not an isolated phenomenon but occurs in association with the development of the orbital, nasal and oral cavities. It has been suggested that the growing nasal septum pulls the maxilla forward by means of a septopremaxillary ligament that runs from the anterior border of the nasal septum posteroinferiorly towards the anterior nasal spine and interpremaxillary suture. As in the lower jaw (page 286), growth in height of the maxilla is related to the development of the alveolar process. It is difficult to determine how much of the adult alveolus is the result of bone deposition and how much is due to bodily displacement of the maxilla. Studies using metal implants suggest that each method of growth contributes equal amounts. Increase in height of the nasal cavity is associated with resorption of bone on the upper surface of the palatine process of the maxilla and deposition of bone on the lower surface (see Fig. 18.25).

The **maxillary sinus** appears as an outpocketing of the mucosa of the middle meatus of the nose at the beginning of the fourth month of intrauterine life. Although small at birth, the maxillary sinus is identifiable radiologically. After birth, the maxillary sinus enlarges with the growing maxilla, although it is only fully developed following the eruption of the permanent dentition. Forward growth of the whole face (including the maxillae) is dependent upon growth of the spheno-occipital synchondrosis (see Figs 15.14, 15.15).

20 Development of the tongue

The anterior two-thirds of the tongue develops from three swellings: the two **lateral lingual swellings** and the midline **tuberculum impar** (Fig. 20.1). Each is formed by proliferation of mesenchyme beneath the endodermal lining of the first branchial arch. The posterior third of the tongue develops from a single midline swelling, the **copula**, which is derived mainly from the third branchial arch with a small contribution from the fourth arch. The copula overgrows the second arch to merge with the first arch swellings.

The diverse embryological origin of the tongue explains its diverse sensory supply (see Fig. 4.12). General sensation to the anterior two-thirds of the tongue is supplied by the lingual nerve, a nerve of the first branchial arch. General sensation and taste to the posterior third of the tongue is supplied by the glossopharyngeal and superior laryngeal nerves, the nerves of the third and fourth arches. The perception of taste in the anterior two-thirds of the tongue is associated with the chorda tympani nerve, a branch of the facial nerve, the nerve of the second branchial arch. Since this arch does not contribute tissue to the anterior part of the tongue, in this situation it is termed a 'pretrematic' nerve.

The muscles of the tongue develop primarily from occipital somites that migrate into the developing tongue carrying their nerve supply, the hypoglossal nerve, with them.

The thyroid gland develops between the tuberculum impar and the copula. On the fully formed tongue, this site is demarcated by a small pit, the foramen caecum (see Fig. 1.15).

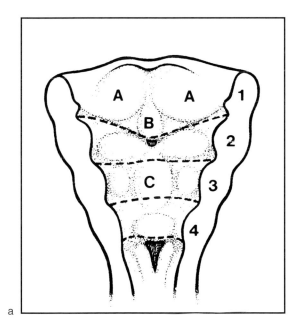
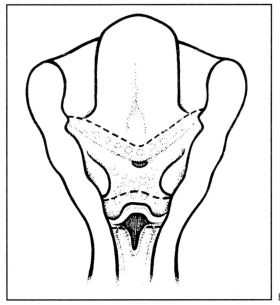

Fig. 20.1 The schema of tongue primordia. (a) The ventral wall of the pharynx at the fourth week of intrauterine life. (b) The developing tongue at the fifth month. Numbers 1–4 indicate the positions of the branchial arches. Four swellings are seen: the two lateral lingual swellings (A), the tuberculum impar (B) and the copula (C).

21 Early tooth development

Tooth development can be divided into three overlapping phases: initiation, morphogenesis, and histogenesis. During initiation, the sites of the future teeth are established with the appearance of tooth germs along an invagination of the oral epithelium called the dental lamina. During morphogenesis, the shape of the tooth is determined by a combination of cell proliferation and cell movement. During histogenesis, differentiation of cells (begun during morphogenesis) proceeds to give rise to the fully formed dental tissues, both mineralised (i.e. enamel, dentine and cementum) and unmineralised (i.e. dental pulp and periodontium). Tooth development is characterised by complex interactions between epithelial and mesenchymal tissues.

The first histological sign of tooth development is the appearance of a condensation of mesenchymal tissue and capillary networks beneath the presumptive dental epithelium of the primitive oral cavity. It is now known that the mesenchymal cells are ectomesenchymal (neural crest) in origin, having migrated into the jaws from the margins of the neural tube. Recent research on amphibians and mammals suggests that, in addition to oral ectoderm and neural crest mesenchyme, foregut endoderm plays a role in tooth initiation. Indeed, there is evidence that the specification of dental epithelium takes place in the oral ectoderm adjacent to foregut endoderm and above midbrain neural crest cells.

By the sixth week of development the oral epithelium thickens and invaginates into the mesenchyme to form a **primary epithelial band** (Fig. 21.1). By the seventh week, the primary epithelial band divides into two processes: a buccally located **vestibular lamina** and a lingually situated **dental lamina**

(Fig. 21.2). The vestibular lamina contributes to the development of the vestibule of the mouth, delineating the lips and cheeks from the tooth-bearing regions. The dental lamina contributes to the development of the teeth. To form the vestibule of the oral cavity, the cells of the vestibular lamina proliferate, with subsequent degeneration of the central epithelial cells to produce the sulcus of the vestibule (Fig. 21.3). Further development of the dental lamina (Fig. 21.4) is characterised by an increase in length, although it is not known whether this results from active invagination of the lamina or upward proliferation of the mesenchyme. By the eighth week, a series of swellings develops on the deep surface of the dental lamina (Fig. 21.5). The complete dental lamina

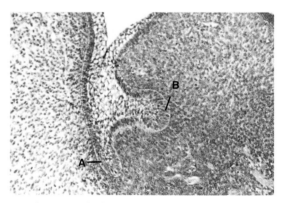

Fig. 21.2 The vestibular lamina (A) and dental lamina (B) seen at the seventh week of intrauterine life (H & E; × 120). Courtesy of Dr D. Adams.

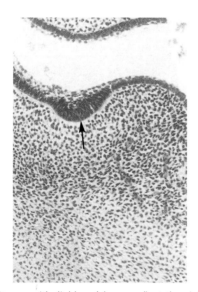

Fig. 21.1 Primary epithelial band (arrowed) at the sixth week of intrauterine life (H & E; × 115).

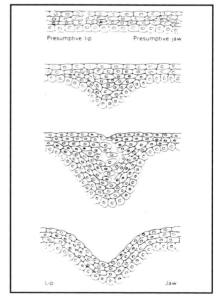

Fig. 21.3 Diagram illustrating the formation of the vestibule of the oral cavity.

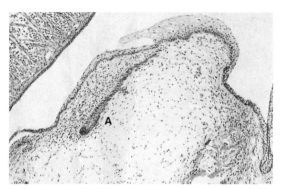

Fig. 21.4   The developing dental lamina (A) (Masson's trichrome; × 55).

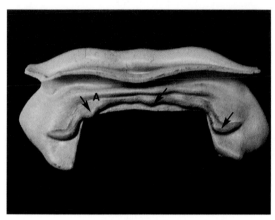

Fig. 21.5   Model showing the stage of tooth development by the eighth week of intrauterine life when a series of swellings representing developing tooth germs (arrows) develops on the deep surface of the dental lamina. A = Vestibular fold.

of the lower jaw is shown in green on the model and the epithelial swellings indicating early developing tooth germs are arrowed. It is important to appreciate that the dental lamina appears as an arch-shaped band of tissue, which follows the line of the vestibular fold. Although not shown on the model, each epithelial swelling is almost completely surrounded by a mesenchymal condensation.

For descriptive purposes, tooth germs are classified into bud, cap and bell stages according to the degree of morphodifferentiation and histodifferentiation of their epithelial components (enamel organs). Leading up to the late bell stage, the tooth germ changes rapidly both in its size and shape; the cells are dividing and morphogenetic processes are taking place. At the late bell stage, hard tissues are forming and further growth of the crown is related mainly to the deposition of enamel, the rate of cell division being reduced.

BUD STAGE

The enamel organ in the bud stage (Fig. 21.6) appears as a simple, spherical to ovoid, epithelial condensation that is poorly morphodifferentiated and histodifferentiated. It is surrounded by mesenchyme. The cells of the tooth bud have a higher RNA content than those of the overlying oral epithelium, a lower glycogen content and an increased oxidative enzyme activity.

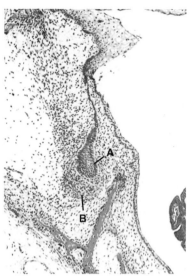

Fig. 21.6   Bud stage of tooth development. A = Enamel organ; B = mesenchymal condensation (Masson's trichrome; × 60).

As yet it has not been established whether the epithelial bud is induced by the underlying mesenchyme. Nevertheless, the successful development of the tooth germ relies upon a complex interaction of the mesenchymal and epithelial components since, should these components be separated and cultured individually, neither will differentiate further. The epithelial component is separated from the adjacent mesenchyme by a basement membrane.

CAP STAGE

By the eleventh week, morphogenesis has progressed, the deeper surface of the enamel organ invaginating to form a cap-shaped structure. In the section shown in Fig. 21.7 both maxillary and mandibular early cap stages are shown, each enamel organ appearing relatively poorly histodifferentiated.

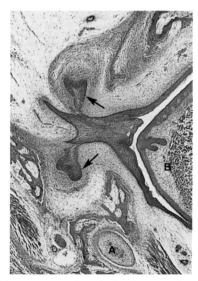

Fig. 21.7   Early cap stage of tooth development (arrows). A = Meckel's cartilage; B = developing tongue (Masson's trichrome; × 32).

Fig. 21.8 Late cap stage of tooth development. A = Stellate reticulum; B = external enamel epithelium; C = internal enamel epithelium; D = dental papilla; E = dental follicle (H & E; × 75).

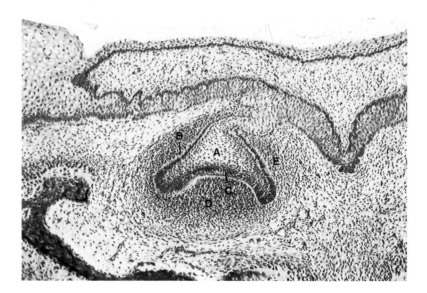

However, a greater distinction develops between the more rounded cells in the central portion of the enamel organ and the peripheral cells which are becoming arranged to form the external and internal enamel epithelia.

In the late cap stage of tooth development (Fig. 21.8), by about the twelfth week, the central cells of the enlarging enamel organ have become separated (though maintaining contact by desmosomes), the intercellular spaces containing significant quantities of glycosaminoglycans. The resulting tissue is termed the stellate reticulum, although it is not fully developed until the later bell stage. The cells of the external enamel epithelium remain cuboidal, whereas those of the internal enamel epithelium become more columar. The latter show an increase in RNA content and hydrolytic and oxidative enzyme activity, while the adjacent mesenchymal cells continue to proliferate and surround the enamel organ. The part of the mesenchyme lying beneath the internal enamel epithelium is termed the dental papilla, while that surrounding the tooth germ forms the dental follicle. A model describing the arrangement of deciduous tooth germs at 13 weeks on the dental lamina of the lower jaw is shown in Fig. 21.9.

EARLY BELL STAGE

By the fourteenth week, further morphodifferentiation and histodifferentiation of the tooth germ leads to the early bell stage (Fig. 21.10). The configuration of the internal enamel epithelium broadly maps out the occlusal pattern of the crown of the tooth. This folding is related to differential mitosis along the internal enamel epithelium. The future cusps and incisal margins are sites of precocious cell maturation associated with cessation of mitosis, while areas corresponding to the fissures and margins of the tooth remain mitotically active. Thus, cusp height is related more to continued downward growth at the margin and fissures than to upward extension of the cusps. During the bell stage, bone resorption defects that restrict the space for development of the tooth germ are associated with the increased folding pattern of the internal enamel epithelium, leading to changes in tooth shape.

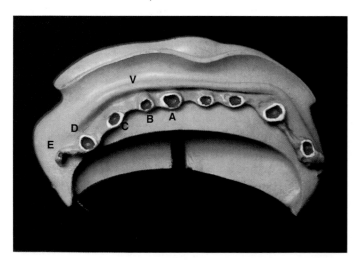

Fig. 21.9 Model illustrating the arrangement of deciduous tooth germs (identified by the Zsigmondy system) at 13 weeks on the dental lamina of the lower jaw. V = Vestibular fold.

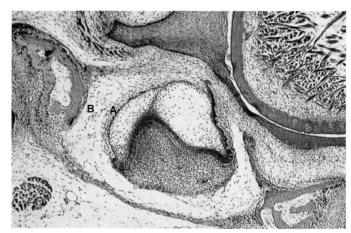

Fig. 21.10 Early bell stage of tooth development. A = Inner investing layer of dental follicle; B = outer layer of dental follicle (Masson's trichrome; × 45).

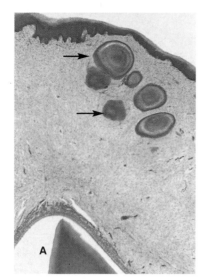

Fig. 21.11 Epithelial pearls (of Serres) (arrows). A = Enamel space (H & E; × 8). Courtesy of Dr D.A. Luke.

Consequently, spatial impediment, and the changing mechanical forces that ensue, may be a co-factor in dental morphogenesis.

It is during the bell stage of development that the dental lamina breaks down and the enamel organ loses connection with the oral epithelium. At the same time, the dental lamina between tooth germs also degenerates. Remnants of the dental lamina may remain in the adult mucosa (Fig. 21.11) as clumps of resting cells (epithelial pearls (of Serres)) that may contain keratin and can be involved in the aetiology of cysts.

Interposed between the enamel organ and the wall of the developing bony crypt is the mesenchymal tissue of the dental follicle, which is generally considered to have three layers (see Figure 21.10). The inner investing layer is a vascular, fibrocellular condensation, three to four cells thick, immediately surrounding the tooth germ; the nuclei of the cells tend to be elongated circumferentially. The outer layer of the dental follicle is represented by a vascular mesenchymal layer that lines the developing alveolus. Between the two layers is loose connective tissue with no marked concentration of blood vessels. There is evidence to suggest that the cells of the inner layer of the dental follicle may be derived from the neural crest.

A high degree of histodifferentiation is achieved in the early bell stage (Fig. 21.12). The enamel organ shows four distinct layers: external enamel epithelium, stellate reticulum, stratum intermedium, and internal enamel epithelium.

The external enamel epithelium

As its name suggests, this forms the outer layer of cuboidal cells which limits the enamel organ. It is separated from the surrounding mesenchymal tissue by a basement membrane 1–2 μm thick, which, at the ultrastructural level, corresponds to the much narrower basal lamina with associated hemidesmosomes (see Fig. 14.28). The external enamel epithelial cells contain large, centrally placed nuclei. Ultrastructurally,

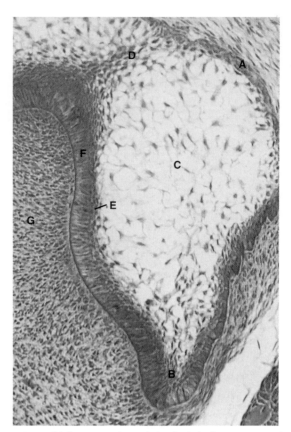

Fig. 21.12 A high-power view of the early bell. A = External enamel epthelium; B = cervical loop; C = stellate reticulum; D = enamel cord; E = stratum intermedium; F = internal enamel epithelium; G = dental papilla (Masson's trichrome; × 120).

they contain relatively small amounts of the intracellular organelles associated with protein synthesis (e.g. endoplasmic reticulum, Golgi material, mitochondria) and they contact each other via desmosomes and gap junctions. The external enamel epithelium is thought to be involved in the maintenance of the shape of the enamel organ and in the exchange of substances between the enamel organ and the environment. The cervical loop, at which there is considerable mitotic activity, lies at the growing margin of the enamel organ where the external enamel epithelium is continuous with the internal enamel epithelium.

The stellate reticulum

This tissue is most fully developed at the bell stage. The intercellular spaces become fluid filled, presumably related to osmotic effects arising from the high concentration of glycosaminoglycans. The cells are star-shaped with bodies containing conspicuous nuclei and many branching processes. In addition to glycosaminoglycans, the cells also contain alkaline phosphatase, but have only small amounts of RNA and glycogen. The mesenchyme-like features of the stellate reticulum include the synthesis of collagens in the tissue. Collagens types I, II and III are expressed in the stellate reticulum, although their functional significance is unclear (Fig. 21.13).

The cells of this layer (Fig. 21.14) possess little endoplasmic reticulum and few mitochondria. However, there is a relatively

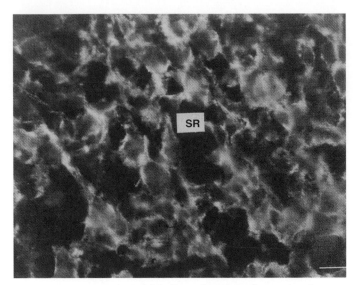

Fig. 21.13 Immunological labelling of type II collagen showing positive (green) staining in the stellate reticulum. (× 350).

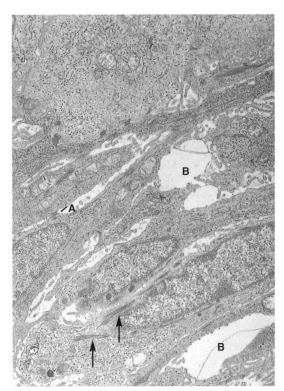

Fig. 21.14 Ultrastructural appearance of the stellate reticulum. A = Desmosomes; B = intercellular space; arrows show tonofilaments (TEM; × 6380). Courtesy of Doctors H. Azawa and H. Nakamura.

well developed Golgi complex, which, together with the presence of microvilli on the cell surface, has been interpreted as indicating that the cells contribute to the secretion of the extracellular material. Numerous tonofilaments are present within the cytoplasm, and desmosomes and gap junctions are present between the cells.

The main function ascribed to the stellate reticulum is a mechanical one. This relates to the protection of the underlying dental tissues against physical disturbance and to the maintenance of tooth shape. It has been suggested that the

hydrostatic pressure generated within the stellate reticulum is in equilibrium with that of the dental papilla, allowing the proliferative pattern of the intervening internal enamel epithelium to determine crown morphogenesis. However, a change in either of these pressures might lead to a change in the outline of the internal enamel epithelium, and this could be important for crown morphogenesis.

The stratum intermedium

This first appears at the bell stage and consists of two or three layers of flattened cells lying over the internal enamel epithelium (and its derivatives). The cells of the stratum intermedium resemble the cells of the stellate reticulum, although their intercellular spaces are smaller and the cells contain much alkaline phosphatase. It has been suggested that the stratum intermedium is concerned with the synthesis of proteins, the transport of materials to and from the enamel-forming cells in the internal enamel epithelium (the ameloblasts), and/or the concentration of materials.

The internal enamel epithelium

The cells of this layer are columnar at the bell stage but, beginning at the regions associated with the future cusp tips (i.e. the sites of initial enamel formation), the cells become elongated. The internal enamel epithelial cells are rich in RNA but, unlike the stratum intermedium and stellate reticulum, do not contain alkaline phosphatase. Desmosomes connect the internal enamel epithelial cells and link this layer to the

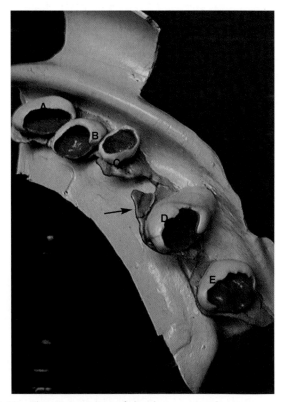

Fig. 21.15 The arrangement of deciduous enamel organs (identified by the Zsigmondy system) at 17 weeks on the dental lamina of a lower jaw quadrant. Arrow indicates developing permanent teeth.

stratum intermedium. The internal enamel epithelium is separated from the peripheral cells of the dental papilla by a basement membrane and a cell-free zone 1–2 μm wide.

The differentiation of the dental papilla is less striking than that of the enamel organ. Until the late bell stage, the dental papilla consists of closely packed mesenchymal cells with only a few delicate extracellular fibrils. Histochemically, the dental papilla becomes rich in glycosaminoglycans.

Fig. 21.15 provides a model demonstrating the arrangement of deciduous tooth germs at 17 weeks on the dental lamina of a lower jaw quadrant. The dental lamina (green) is beginning to degenerate. Downgrowths on the lingual aspect of the enamel organs indicate the early development of the successional (permanent) teeth.

LATE BELL STAGE

The late bell stage (appositional stage) of tooth development (Fig. 21.16) is associated with the formation of the dental hard tissues, commencing at about the eighteenth week. Dentine formation always precedes enamel formation. Detailed accounts of amelogenesis and dentinogenesis are given on pages 304–331. In the section shown in Fig. 21.16, downgrowths of the external enamel epithelium appear from the lingual sides of the enamel organs. In deciduous teeth, these lingual downgrowths give rise to the tooth germs of the permanent successors and first appear alongside the incisors

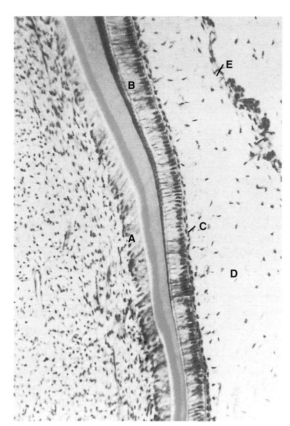

Fig. 21.17 High-power view of a region of a tooth germ at the late bell stage to show enamel and dentine formation. A = Odontoblasts; B = ameloblasts; C = stratum intermedium; D = stellate reticulum; E = external enamel epithelium; dentine matrix stained green; enamel matrix stained red (Masson's

at about 5 months *in utero*. In enamel organs of permanent teeth, however, these downgrowths eventually disappear. Behind the deciduous second molar, the dental lamina grows backwards to bud off successively the permanent molar teeth. The first permanent molar appears at about 4 months *in utero*, the tooth bud for the second permanent molar appears about 6 months after birth, while that for the third permanent molar appears at about 4–5 years after birth.

Fig. 21.17 provides a high-power view of a region of a tooth germ at the late bell stage to show enamel and dentine formation commencing at the tips of future cusps (or incisal edges). Under the inductive influence of developing ameloblasts (pre-ameloblasts), the adjacent mesenchymal cells of the dental papilla become columnar and differentiate into odontoblasts. The odontoblasts then become involved in the formation of predentine and dentine. The presence of dentine then induces the ameloblasts to secrete enamel.

TRANSITORY STRUCTURES

During the early stages of tooth development three transitory structures may be seen: the enamel knot, enamel cord and enamel niche.

The enamel knot (Fig. 21.18) is a localised mass of cells in the centre of the internal enamel epithelium. Characteristically,

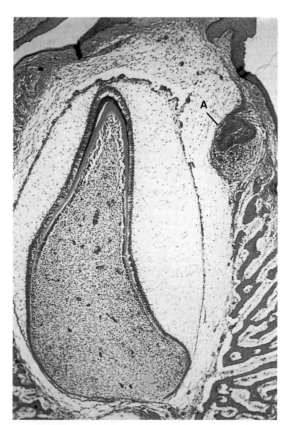

Fig. 21.16 Late bell stage (appositional stage) of tooth development. Dentine matrix stained blue; enamel matrix stained red. A = Permanent tooth (Masson's trichrome; × 60).

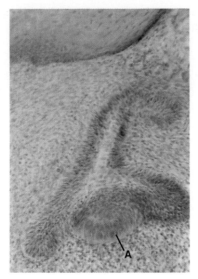

Fig. 21.18 The enamel knot (A) (H & E; × 120).

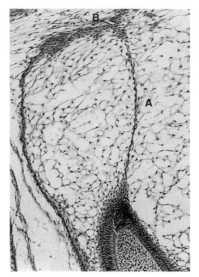

Fig. 21.20 The enamel cord (A). B = Enamel navel (Masson's trichrome; × 120).

the enamel knot forms a bulge into the dental papilla, at the centre of the enamel organ. It was once thought that the enamel knot played a role in the formation of crown pattern by outlining the central fissure. However, the enamel knot soon disappears and seems to contribute cells to the enamel cord (see below). Although transitory, recent studies of the enamel knot suggest it may represent an important signalling centre during tooth development. Unlike adjacent cells, those within the enamel knot are non-proliferative and produce molecules associated with signalling in other sites. Such molecules include bone morphogenetic proteins (e.g. BMP-2 and BMP-7), fibroblast growth factor, p21 (cyclin-dependent

kinase inhibitor), Shh (sonic hedgehog) and transcription factors (e.g. Msx-1) (Fig. 21.19). The disappearance of the enamel knot by the bell stage may be associated with apoptosis.

The enamel cord (Fig. 21.20) is a strand of cells seen at the early bell stage of development, extending from the stratum intermedium into the stellate reticulum. When present, the enamel cord overlies the incisal margin of a tooth or the apex of the first cusp to develop (primary cusp). When it completely divides the stellate reticulum into two parts, reaching the external enamel epithelium, it is termed the enamel septum. Where the enamel cord meets the external enamel epithelium, a small invagination termed the enamel navel may be seen. The cells of the enamel cord are distinguished from their surrounding stellate reticulum cells by their elongated nuclei. It has been suggested that the enamel cord may be involved in the process by which the cap stage is transformed into the bell stage (acting as a mechanical tie) or that it is a focus for the origin of stellate reticulum cells.

The enamel niche (Fig. 21.21) is seen where the tooth germ appears to have a double attachment to the dental lamina (the lateral and medial enamel strands). These strands enclose the enamel niche, which appears as a funnel-shaped depression containing connective tissue. The functional significance of

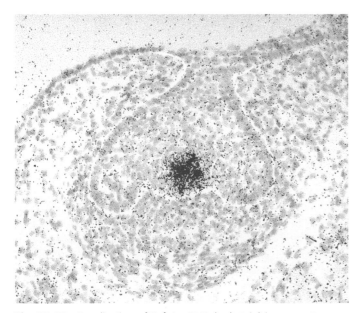

Fig. 21.19 Localisation of Fgf-4 mRNA (red stain) in a cap stage (E14) lower molar tooth by *in-situ* hybridisation. Intense expression can be seen in the enamel knot. To aid interpretation of gene expression using 35S-labelled *in-situ* hybridisation, both dark and bright field images were taken. Silver grains in the dark field image were selected, coloured red and then superimposed onto the bright field image (× 120). Courtesy of T. Aberg.

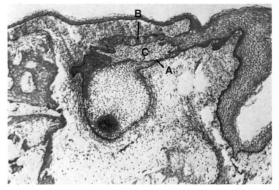

Fig. 21.21 Enamel niche (C). A = Lateral enamel strand; B = medial enamel strand (H & E; × 40).

the enamel niche is unknown. The enamel cord and the double attachment of the tooth germ around the enamel niche were once regarded as evidence supporting the view that the complex crown form of mammalian teeth evolved from fusion of a number of individual, simpler elements. However, this view is not now accepted.

NERVE FIBRES

There is conflicting evidence as to when, and where, nerve fibres first appear during tooth development. It has been reported that nerve fibres are present in the immediate vicinity of presumptive dental epithelium at the very earliest stage of tooth induction and subsequently form a plexus below the dental papilla at the cap stage. From such plexuses, the nerves spread into the dental follicle as it develops. Penetration of nerves into the dental papilla occurs with the onset of dentinogenesis. The nerve fibres associated with blood vessels are presumed to be autonomic; others lying free within the papilla are presumed to be sensory. However, the innervation of the dental papilla remains rudimentary until after birth and may be fully developed only after the tooth has erupted. Controversy also remains concerning the role of neuronal cells and neurotrophins in tooth development. Recent work indicates that, although nerve fibres seem not be required for odontogenesis, the pattern of localisation of neurotrophins (and their associated receptors) does suggest a role for neural-like cells – perhaps related to the neural crest derivation of the dental mesenchyme. However, in transgenic animals where neurotrophins and their receptors are not expressed, tooth development is not affected.

BLOOD SUPPLY

Small blood vessels invade the dental papilla at the early bell stage. They are also evident in the dental follicle in close association with the external enamel epithelium. Although vessels may lie in invaginations of the external enamel epithelium, they never penetrate the stellate reticulum.

EPITHELIAL–MESENCHYMAL INTERACTIONS DURING TOOTH DEVELOPMENT

The development of the tooth germ into the fully formed tooth involves many reciprocal interactions between the epithelium of the enamel organ and the mesenchyme of the dental papilla. These interactions are termed epithelial–mesenchymal interactilons and involve changes resulting in increasing complexity in shape (morphodifferentiation) followed by increasing complexity in structure (histodifferentiation). That both tissues are required for development to occur has been established by experiments in which very early tooth germs are obtained and separated into their two components using trypsin. When grown separately (either *in vivo* or *in vitro*)

neither the enamel organ nor the dental papilla undergoes further differentiation. Following recombination, however, normal development occurs.

At all stages of development of the enamel organ, the cytokeratins present are typical of simple epithelia and the basal layer of stratified epithelium (i.e. they express cytokeratins 5, 8, 14, 17, 18, and 19). Cytokeratins associated with terminal differentiation of keratinocytes (such as cytokeratins 4 and 13 or 1 and 10) are not expressed.

THE NATURE OF THE INDUCTIVE MESSAGE

During tooth development, 'messages' pass between the epithelium and mesenchyme to produce changes of increasing complexity (i.e. differentiation) within the cell layers. The term induction is used to describe the effect that one cell layer has on another.

Three main hypotheses have been put forward to explain how information leading to induction may be transferred between epithelium and mesenchyme:

1. A chemical substance (short-range hormone) is produced by one cell layer and diffuses across the narrow intervening space to be taken up and cause induction in the other cell layer.
2. Induction is triggered by direct cell-to-cell contact and does not involve a diffusible molecule.
3. Induction is due to the presence of the initial extracellular matrix, a thin layer situated between the epithelium and mesenchyme and comprising the basal lamina and adjacent region. The extracellular matrix has a complex composition, consisting of collagen (mainly type IV but possibly some type I and III), proteoglycans and glycoproteins.

To assess which of the three hypotheses is likely to provide the correct explanation for reciprocal control of differentiation, experiments have been undertaken in which the epithelial and mesenchymal components are dissected out and separated at the early bell stage, before any significant degree

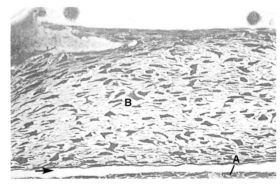

Fig. 21.22 The enamel organ (A) and dental papilla mesenchyme (B) cultured on either side of a porous membrane (pore size 0.1 μm) (arrowed). No differentiation has occurred and cell processes do not pass through the membrane (Toluidine blue; × 70). Courtesy of Professor I. Thesleff and the editor of *Journal of Embryology and Experimental Morphology*.

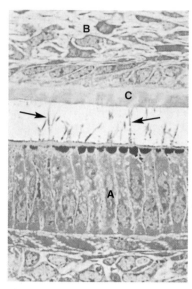

Fig. 21.23 The enamel organ (A) and dental papilla mesenchyme (B) cultured on either side of a porous membrane (pore size 0.6 μm). C = Predentine; cell processes from odontoblasts passing through pores are arrowed (Mallory's; × 45). Courtesy of Professor I. Thesleff and the editor of *Journal of Embryology and Experimental Morphology.*

of cytodifferentiation. They are then recombined for tissue culture, but with a porous membrane placed between; the size of the pores in the membrane can be varied to ascertain the point at which both ameloblasts and odontoblasts differentiate (Figs 21.22, 21.23). As molecules can readily diffuse through a pore size just less than 0.2 μm, the absence of differentiation seen in Fig. 21.22 argues against hypothesis 1 above (a diffusible chemical substance). The lack of differentiation with pores less than 0.2 μm coincides with both the absence of the extracellular matrix and with the absence of cell processes invading the porous membrane. Thus, either cell-to-cell contact or the extracellular matrix could be implicated in differentiation. However, as *in vivo* direct cell-to-cell contact does not appear to occur (although the processes do come very close together), it is the extracellular matrix which may be most important in induction. The extracellular matrix itself is a product of both the epithelial and the mesenchymal cells.

Evidence indicating the importance of the extracellular matrix in the inductive process can be obtained from the following experiments. Firstly, drugs are available that can inhibit the formation of specific components of the extracellular matrix: for example, lathyrogens interfere with cross linking of collagen. When added to tissue culture medium, these drugs inhibit differentiation of the tooth germ. Secondly, isolated pieces of extracellular matrix will produce histological signs of differentiation in internal enamel epithelial cells of the enamel organ.

A considerable number of genes and growth factors are expressed during early tooth development. A database has been established by the University of Helsinki (http://honeybee.helsinki.fi/toothexp) to allow comparisons of the expression patterns as a starting point for experimental studies. This database presently describes the expression at different stages of tooth development of growth factors,

receptors, signalling molecules, transcription factors, intracellular and extracellular molecules and plasma membrane molecules. For growth factors, for example, a variety of bone morphogenetic proteins (BMP), fibroblast growth factors, sonic hedgehog, and transforming growth factors are expressed at different stages of development. Epidermal growth factor appears to be expressed only during the bell stage of development. Nerve growth factors are also expressed at various developmental stages. Recent research has suggested that the dental epithelium signals to the underlying mesenchymal cells via BMPs (particularly BMP-2 and BMP-4 and FGFs). Consequently, mesenchymal cell proliferation and condensation are stimulated and the expression in the mesenchyme of syndecan and tenascin are upregulated (syndecan is a cell-surface heparan sulphate proteoglycan that binds to tenascin, probably influencing cell condensation). BMPs also induce the expression in the mesenchyme of *Msx-1* and *Msx-2* homeobox gene transcription factors. EGF appears to be involved in the formation of the dental lamina.

Until recently, technical considerations limited transplantation experiments on tooth differentiation to the early cap stage. At this stage, little differentiation is evident, and the question posed by investigators was: 'Which of the two components is more important for inducing morphogenesis and histogenesis – the enamel organ or the dental papilla?' A series of experiments was undertaken involving the interchange of epithelial and mesenchymal components between different developing teeth (incisors and molars) and between tissues from non-dental regions. The results indicate that, at the cap stage of tooth development, the principal organiser is the dental papilla, in terms of both morphogenesis and histogenesis. The result of culturing dental papilla mesenchyme with epithelium from the developing foot pad (Fig. 21.24) is normal tooth

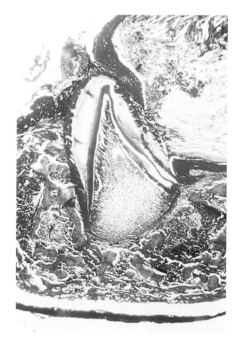

Fig. 21.24 The result of culturing dental papilla mesenchyme with epithelium from the developing foot pad. A normal tooth develops (Masson's trichrome; × 40). Courtesy of Professor E. Kollar and the editor of *Journal of Embryology and Experimental Morphology.*

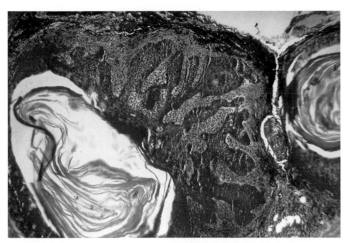

Fig. 21.25 The result of culturing the enamel organ of a tooth with mesenchyme from the developing foot pad. Note the absence of tooth development (Masson's trichrome; × 75). Courtesy of Professor E. Kollar and the editor of *Journal of Embryology and Experimental Morphology*.

development, illustrating the importance of the dental papilla. On the other hand if the enamel organ of a tooth is cultured with mesenchyme from the developing foot pad (Fig. 21.25), tooth development does not occur. Similar experiments have been conducted to determine whether the enamel organ or the dental papilla determine tooth shape. Such experiments involve separating and recombining enamel organ and papilla

at the cap stage. Should an incisor enamel organ be combined with a molar papilla, the resulting tooth is molariform. Furthermore, if a molar enamel organ is combined with an incisor papilla, the resulting tooth is incisiform. Thus, as for histogenesis, the dental papilla is the dominant tissue determining tooth shape at the cap stage.

Techniques have recently been developed whereby it is possible to dissect out and recombine mammalian epithelium and mesenchyme in different combinations before there are any signs of tooth development. Thus, neural crest material (which gives rise to the bulk of the future dental papilla) can be obtained from the region of the developing brain before it actually migrates into the developing jaws, and challenged with epithelium from different sites, such as oral epithelium (Fig. 21.26) or limb epithelium (Fig. 21.27). The most important conclusion to be derived from these studies is that premigratory neural crest will form teeth only when associated with oral epithelium. From this it is reasonable to infer that, during normal development, the neural crest that enters the mandibular arch is odontologically unspecified before or during migration, and that the oral epithelium is the earliest known site of tooth pattern.

The question arises as to whether the local environment of the jaws provides signals important for the initiation and development of the teeth (i.e. field theory). One way in which the possible contribution of the jaw environment can be assessed is to remove the dental lamina in the developing molar region together with the surrounding mesenchyme,

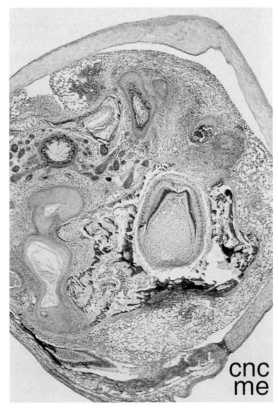

Fig. 21.26 The result of culturing premigratory cranial neural crest with oral epithelium. Note the developing tooth (arrowed) (Masson's trichrome; × 65). Courtesy of Professor A.G.S. Lumsden and the editor of *Development*.

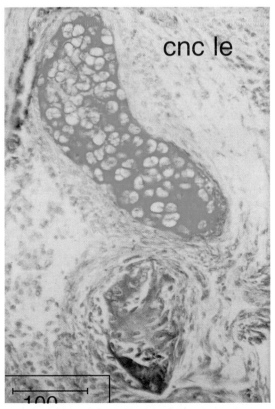

Fig. 21.27 The result of culturing premigratory neural crest with limb epithelium. Teeth do not develop; only islands of bone and cartilage (Masson's trichrome; × 200). Courtesy of Professor A.G.S. Lumsden and the editor of *Development*.

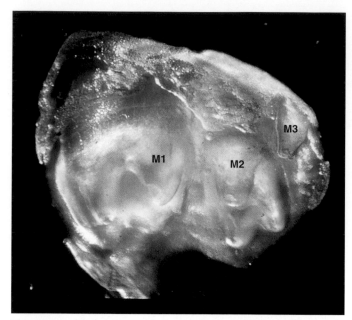

Fig. 21.28 A tooth germ of the first molar at the cap stage of development has been removed from an embryo and transplanted for culture in a different site. Note the development of first (M1), second (M2) and third molars (M3) (Alizarin red whole-mount; × 10). Courtesy of Professor A.G.S. Lumsden and the editor of *Development*.

The experiments described above indicate that successful tooth development depends on complex reciprocal interactions between the dental epithelium and underlying mesenchyme. They also show that, initially, the epithelium from the first branchial arch is instructive on the underlying neural crest-derived ectomesenchyme. At a later stage, however, this instructive capacity is transferred to the mesenchyme, which can then induce epithelium of non-first arch origin (or even ectoderm) to help form a tooth germ. Signals involving bioactive molecules (such as transcription factors, growth factors, cytokines, etc.) are produced in a specific spatial and temporal sequence and the cascade of events results in a tooth consisting of the appropriate tissues and appropriate shape.

Particular attention has been paid to the earliest stages of tooth development to help determine the biological mechanisms responsible for switching on the cascade of events for tooth development. The activation of non-*Hox* homeobox genes is of crucial importance at this time. These genes contain DNA-binding proteins that regulate gene transcription, thus controlling the expression of other genes necessary for the development of a particular structure, in this case a tooth. To date, the precise functions of such homeobox genes are not known, but they may be assumed to regulate the production of molecules important in morphogenesis (such as growth factors, factors controlling cell division and apoptosis, cell-surface receptors, integrins and cell adhesion molecules and cytoskeletal elements). The complexity of the topic is partly indicated in Fig. 21.29 (this figure contains a mere handful of the molecules known to be present in the developing tooth and their number is continually being added to). Evidence to support the importance of such molecules in initiating tooth development can be seen in transgenic mice where, for example, an absence of the homeobox gene *Msx-1* results in tooth development being arrested at the bud stage. Similarly, early mesenchyme isolated from the overlying epithelium can still continue to develop in tissue culture if molecules such as BMPs and FGFs are added to the medium.

which subsequently gives rise to the first molar tooth germ. This very early and undifferentiated tooth germ is then cultured in a totally different site away from the jaws. A tooth germ of the first molar at the cap stage of development removed from an embryo and transplanted for culture at a different site continues to develop normally – and the remaining second and third molars also develop (Fig. 21.28). This finding is consistent with the idea that a series of related structures can form by budding off from a single precursor (clone theory) and that the differences between the individual structures (e.g. size and crown complexity) result from the increasing age of the tooth-budding region as it grows distally from the jaw.

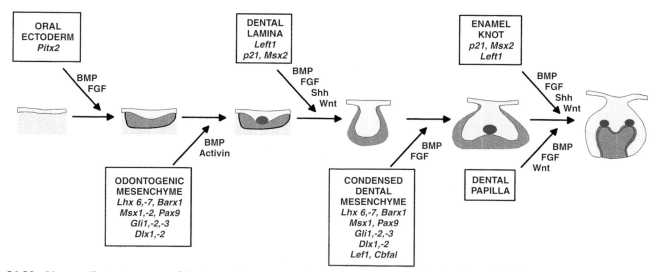

Fig. 21.29 Diagram illustrating some of the homeobox genes and growth factors present during the epithelial–mesenchymal interactions occurring during the early stages of tooth development. Courtesy of Professor I. Thesleff.

In addition to developing at the correct site, it is important that teeth have the correct shape, incisors being produced in the front of the dentition and molars at the back (and not vice versa). Numerous studies have been undertaken to determine how morphogenesis is controlled. Experimental studies have indicated that, from the early cap stage, it is the mesenchyme rather than the epithelium that controls shape. The explanation in terms of molecular biology underlying the control of such patterning is now being investigated and a hypothesis has been forwarded for testing. This proposes that, as in other parts of the body (such as the vertebral column), patterning is related to the spatially restricted expression of homeobox genes in the ectomesenchyme of the developing jaws, referred to as the odontogenic homeobox code. Thus, the group of homeobox genes expressed in the presumptive incisor region will dictate that incisiform teeth develop here, while the group of homeobox genes expressed at the back of the toothrow (in the presumptive molar region) will specify for molariform teeth.

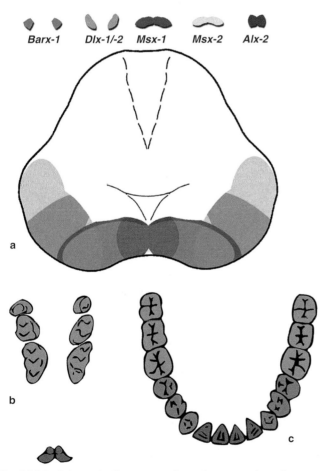

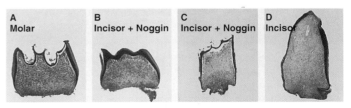

Fig. 21.30 Schematic diagrams to show the mesenchymal odontogenic homeobox gene code. (a) Diagram illustrating the lower jaw of the mouse. Note the overlap (orange) between the domains of *Msx-1* (red) and *Msx-2* (yellow). (b) Model representing the mouse dention. Note that molars develop from cells expressing *Barx-1* and incisors from cells expressing *Msx-1*, *Msx-2* and *Alx-3*. (c) Model representing the human dentition, where it is predicted that incisors develop from cells expressing *Msx-1*, *Msx-2*, and *Alx-3*, canines and premolars from cells expressing *Msx-1* and *Msx-2* and molars from cells expressing *Barx-1*. Courtesy of Professor P.T. Sharpe and the editor of *Bioessays*.

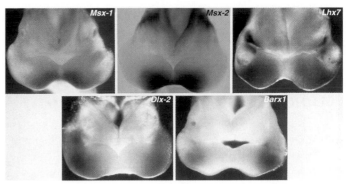

Fig. 21.31 Whole mount *in-situ* hybridisation to show localisation of homeobox genes (the darkly 'staining' regions) for the developing mandible. Courtesy of Professor P.T. Sharpe.

For this hypothesis to be tenable, an important prerequisite is to establish that the presumptive incisor and molar regions do indeed contain some difference in their homeobox gene array and this feature has been demonstrated. An important difference is that the neural crest-derived mesenchyme in the incisor region expresses *Msx-1* (but not *Barx-1*) whilst neural crest-derived mesenchyme in the molar region expresses *Barx-1* (but not *Msx-1*) (Figs 21.30, 21.31). With such differences the hypothesis should be testable, for it would predict that if the expression of homeobox genes associated with the mesenchyme of a developing tooth bud could be manipulated its morphology could change, say, from an expected incisiform to a molariform shape. In this context, it has been demonstrated that, in the early stages of tooth development in the incisor region, BMP produced by the epithelium upregulates the expression of *Msx-1* in the underlying mesenchyme. It is, however, possible to culture early incisor tooth germs and absorb the BMP produced by the epithelium (so that it does not switch on *Msx-1* in the underlying mesenchyme cells). This is achieved by placing on the epithelial surface very small beads soaked in noggin protein. In this situation, not only is *Msx-1* downregulated in the mesenchyme but *Barx-1* (normally only present in the molar region) is seen to be expressed. When such tooth germs are then transplanted *in vivo* to renal capsules and allowed to continue to develop, multicusped teeth with a molariform rather than an incisiform morphology can be produced (Fig. 21.32). As with other systems of early development and differentiation, temporal factors mean that there is

Fig. 21.32 The results of experiments to transform teeth from incisor to molar shape following downregulation of *Msx-1* and upregulation of *Barx-1* in incisors. A = Control section of normal molar; D = control section of normal incisor; B and C = sections from incisor teeth showing change to molar shape following upregulation of *Barx-1* in the mesenchyme (× 25). Courtesy of Professor P.T. Sharpe and the editor of *Science*.

only a narrow window of opportunity to successfully manipulate the homeobox genes. The results of this experiment are therefore consistent with the odontogenic homeobox code hypothesis.

CLINICAL CONSIDERATIONS

Although much is known about normal tooth development, many details await investigation and it is hardly surprising, therefore, that we know relatively little about the changes in the tooth germ that lead to the range of congenital tooth abnormalities generally recognized. Clearly, disturbance of the epithelial–mesenchymal interactions can markedly disturb tooth development. Also, splitting of a tooth germ or joining of adjacent germs can be responsible for some of the variations in tooth numbers and shape. Trauma and infection of the deciduous predecessors have also been implicated in the malformation of the permanent teeth. Malformations of teeth can occur in the deciduous or permanent dentition, although they are more common in the permanent dentition. This may reflect the stable environment of the child before birth.

Malformations of teeth can be related to variations in size, in shape, in number, or in structure.

Macrodontia refers to an enlarged tooth and microdontia to a very much reduced size. Microdontia may accompany clefts of the lip or palate, Ehlers–Danlos syndrome, hypopituitary disorders, and ectodermal disorders. A frequent variation in shape is the peg-shaped maxillary lateral incisor (see page 28). Gemination refers to a situation where there is partial cleavage of a tooth germ. Fusion occurs where there is union of two adjacent germs. In both situations, the appearance can suggest a 'double' tooth. Concrescence is the fusion of teeth at the

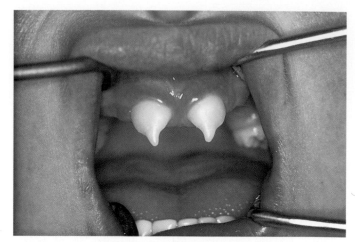

Fig. 21.34 Hereditary ectodermal dysplasia showing absent teeth and conically shaped teeth. Courtesy of Dr P. Smith.

roots. Abnormal tooth shapes (such as Hutchinsonian incisors and mulberry molars) can result from congenital syphilis. Odontomes are irregular masses (complex) or a large number of irregular denticles (compound) found in place of a developing tooth.

In terms of tooth number, hypodontia (oligodontia) is a reduction in the number of teeth, the most frequently missing teeth being permanent third molars, permanent maxillary lateral incisors and second premolars. Anodontia refers to a complete absence of teeth and is very rare. Hyperdontia is an increase in tooth number, either by the appearance of supernumery teeth (not having normal morphology – Fig. 21.33) or supplemental teeth (having normal morphology). A 'mesiodens' in the middle of the maxilla is an example of a supernumerary tooth. Multiple supernumery teeth can be associated with cleidocranial dysplasia. Ectodermal dysplasia (an X-linked recessive genetic abnormality) presents with many craniofacial disturbances. The teeth are often reduced in size and number and conical in shape towards the anterior segments of the dentition (Fig. 21.34).

Such conditions as amelogenesis imperfecta, dentinogenesis imperfecta and hypomineralized teeth are mentioned in the chapters concerned with development of specific dental tissues. The abnormality known as 'dens in dente' ('tooth within a tooth') (Fig. 21.35) results from either downward proliferation of a portion of the internal enamel epithelium of the enamel organ into the dental papilla or from retarded growth of part of the tooth germ. It presents on the fully erupted tooth as an extremely deep pit and most commonly affects the permanent maxillary lateral incisor. The full range of dental tissues (including cementum and bone from incorporation of the dental follicle) may be associated with the 'infolded' organ.

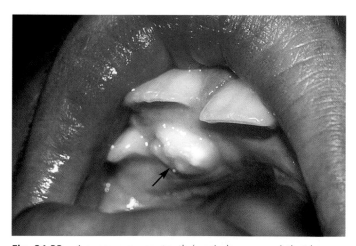

Fig. 21.33 A supernumerary tooth (mesiodens; arrow) that has erupted into the palate behind the permanent incisors. Courtesy of Dr R. O'Sullivan.

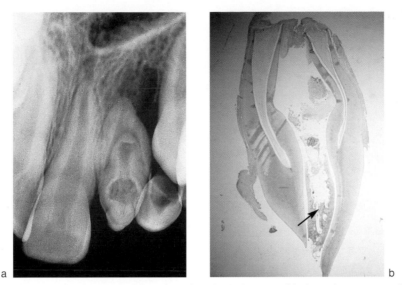

a   b

Fig. 21.35 Dens in dente (arrows) seen radiographically (a) and in a histological section (b). (H & E). Courtesy of Dr J. Potts.

22 Amelogenesis

The tooth develops from a genetically instigated, localised interaction between an area of oral ectoderm and underlying mesenchymal cells, many of which have been derived from the neural crest. These epithelial/mesenchymal interactions during the early stages of tooth development are discussed in Chapter 21. The process is a continuous one but is most readily described in stages which represent snapshots of the developing tooth's growth and differentiation. The morphology of these stages (bud, cap and bell) is described elsewhere (Chapter 21). These stages are defined by the morphology of the epithelial component of the developing tooth that becomes the enamel organ. The innermost cell layer of the enamel organ, the internal enamel epithelium, deposits and later modifies the enamel. The other components of the enamel organ (the stratum intermedium, the stellate reticulum and the external enamel epithelium) play important but, as yet, incompletely understood supportive roles in amelogenesis. The descriptions we have of the developing tooth were originally derived from morphological studies. More recently, precise molecular techniques have become available which extend, and sometimes confuse, our understanding. For example, the use of the polymerase chain reaction technique, which allows the recognition of mRNA formed by transcription but present before translation, shows that the mRNA for two enamel proteins (tuftelin and amelogenin) are present in the cells of the internal enamel epithelium some time before there is any recognisable morphodifferentiation.

In a single developing tooth, enamel will be present at different stages of development. When enamel is being formed, the ameloblasts at different locations in the internal enamel epithelium will be at different stages of the enamel-forming process but, by the time enamel formation is complete, each ameloblast will have completed a similar life cycle. Different tooth types form enamel at different times, at different rates and with different final morphological outcomes. In teeth of continuous growth, such as rodent incisors, all phases of enamel formation are present throughout the life of the animal. For this reason, many of the experimental data on amelogenesis have been derived from studies on animals with continuously growing incisors.

Understanding amelogenesis is best begun by describing the life cycle of the ameloblast, then adding to this more detailed descriptions of the processes of protein secretion and mineralisation and an account of the mechanisms initiating and controlling them.

Table 22.1 *Features associated with the five main stages of amelogenesis*

Presecretory	Secretory	Transition	Maturation	Post-maturation
Cytodifferentiation: differentiation of ameloblasts	Initial layer of aprismatic enamel formed	Ameloblasts shorten, 50% die	Cycling of ruffled and smooth ameoblasts	Enamel organ degenerates
Morphodifferentiation: bell stage including formation of the enamel knot	Ameloblasts develop Tomes' processes	Vascularisation of the enamel organ	Final degradation and withdrawal of matrix	Enamel coverings established
Resorption of the basal lamina of the internal enamel epithelium	Matrix secretion to final thickness	Re-formation of ameloblast basal lamina	Crystal growth continues to completion	Eruption
Epithelial–mesenchymal interactions	Initiation and continuation of mineralisation to 30% by weight	Cessation of matrix secretion	Final third of mineralisation after protein removal complete	Exposure to oral environment and post-eruptive changes
	Crystal elongation	Continued matrix degradation		
	Matrix degradation	Selective matrix withdrawal		
	Development of prismatic structure			

LIFE CYCLE OF THE AMELOBLAST

The development of ameloblast is most readily described in five main stages (Fig. 22.1 and Table 22.1):

- presecretory
- secretory
- transition
- maturation
- Post-maturation

Presecretory stage

This stage includes all activities of the future ameloblast before secretion of any enamel matrix. There are two main components, differentiation of the pre-ameloblasts and the formation and subsequent resorption of a basal lamina. The morphological changes to the enamel organ are described in detail in the section on tooth development (Chapter 21).

During the bell stage, the cells of the internal enamel epithelium (Fig. 22.2) have ceased to divide and eventually differentiate into enamel-forming cells, the ameloblasts. This differentiation begins at the future cusp tips and progresses cervically. During differentiation, the cells of the internal enamel epithelium will change from a cuboidal to columnar profile and become polarised, with the nucleus sitting close to the end of the cell that is in contact with the stellate reticulum. These elongated cells are termed pre-ameloblasts (Figs 22.3, 22.4).

Early differentiating ameloblasts (Fig. 22.1) possess a large ovoid nucleus and a small Golgi apparatus close to the stratum intermedium. In the cytoplasm adjacent to the dental papilla rough endoplasmic reticulum is present, as are large numbers of free ribosomes, mitochondria and vesicles. Pinocytotic invaginations of the cell membrane are found here. Adjacent cells of the internal enamel epithelium are linked by gap junctions and a basal lamina separates the epithelium from the dental papilla.

Histological changes are also occurring in the outer mesenchymal cells of the dental papilla that are differentiating

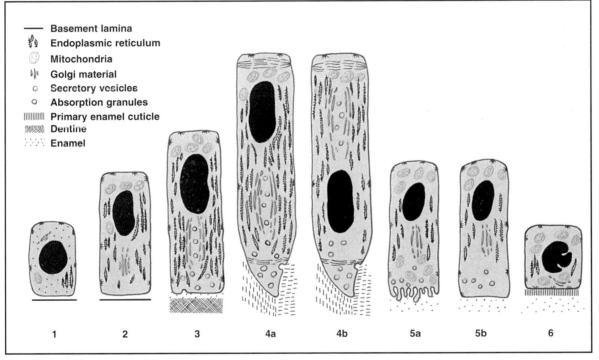

Fig. 22.1 The life cycle of an ameloblast. The cells of the internal enamel epithelium (1) start to differentiate, beginning at the future enamel–dentine junction of the cusp tip. The differentiating cell (2) is characterised by a reversed polarity; the cell becomes columnar and the nucleus moves to that part of the cell furthest from the dentine. Secreting organelles are formed and the end of the cell adjacent to the dentine becomes the site for secretion. At the next stage (3), the cell secretes the initial enamel component of the enamel–dentine junction. This thin layer will be continuous with the inter-rod enamel of the later formed tissue. As the cell retreats, the secreting pole becomes morphologically distinct as a pyramidal Tomes' process (4a). Crystals are formed at both surfaces of the process. The proximal region between two processes, deep in the junctional regions, always secretes ahead of the more distal region so that pits surrounded by inter-rod enamel are formed. These are then filled, giving the prism configuration to the tissue. Simultaneous secretion of both organic material and mineral continues until the full thickness of the tissue is formed. In this secreting phase, two appearances of ameloblasts can be distinguished by the position of the nuclei within the cell: high (4a) and low (4b). At the beginning of secretion, half the cells are in each form. Towards the end of secretion, most of the high nuclei have moved to a low position, effectively increasing the areas of the ameloblast cells as the surface of forming enamel increases. When the full thickness of enamel has formed, ameloblasts lose the secretory extension, the Tomes' process (5a). Up to 50% of them die and are phagocytosed by others in the layer. The maturation phase lasts two to three times longer than the secretory phase. During the maturation phase there is a regular, repetitive modulation of cell morphology between a rufffled (5a) and a smooth (5b) surface apposed to the enamel. Once the maturation changes are complete, the cells regress in height (6). At this stage, they serve to protect the enamel surface during eruption and later will contribute to form the junctional epithelium.

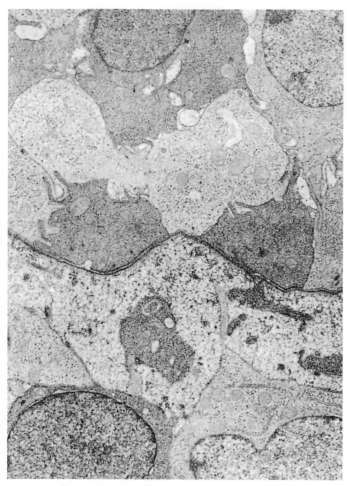

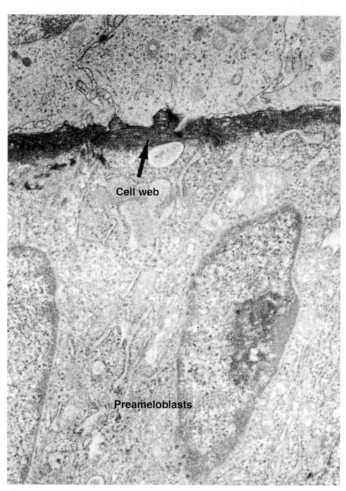

Fig. 22.2 TEM showing the undifferentiated cells of the internal enamel epithelium. No secretory specialisation is yet evident (× 4800). Courtesy of Dr T. Sasaki and Karger Press.

Fig. 22.3 TEM showing pre-ameloblasts. Rough endoplasmic reticulum is evident and the terminal cell web is clearly stained (× 5350). Courtesy of Dr T. Sasaki and Karger Press.

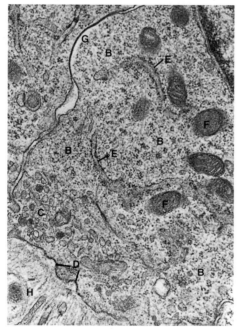

Fig. 22.4 TEM illustrating the distal cytoplasm of an early differentiating ameloblast. A = Nucleus; B = free ribosomes; C = vesicles; D = pinocytotic invagination; E = rough endoplasmic reticulum; F = mitochondria; G = gap junction; H = dental papilla (× 21 000). Courtesy of Dr E. Katchburian.

into odontoblasts (Fig. 22.5). These mesenchymal changes precede those in the internal enamel epithelium such that differentiation of the internal enamel epithelium follows the deposition of the first layer of predentine matrix (Fig. 22.6). The internal enamel epithelium, in common with epithelial layers elsewhere, forms a basal lamina separating it from underlying mesenchyme. This lamina marks the position of the future enamel–dentine junction. Once the odontoblasts of the dental papilla have differentiated, the basal lamina separating them from the internal enamel epithelium disappears as the first layer of dentine matrix is laid down. The pre-ameloblasts release enzymes by exocytosis that degrade the basal lamina and then resorb the degradation products by endocytosis. For a brief period following the degradation of the basal lamina, the future ameloblasts and odontoblasts are in intimate contact, allowing inductive signalling to occur between them.

In the terminally differentiated pre-ameloblast, the nucleus is in the end of the cell adjacent to the stellate reticulum with mitochondria between it and the cell membrane. The endoplasmic reticulum, Golgi apparatus and secretory vesicles enlarge and come to lie between the nucleus and the end of the cell adjacent to the dental papilla, the pole from which enamel matrix will later be secreted. These pre-ameloblasts are joined at the stellate reticulum end by desmosomes forming the

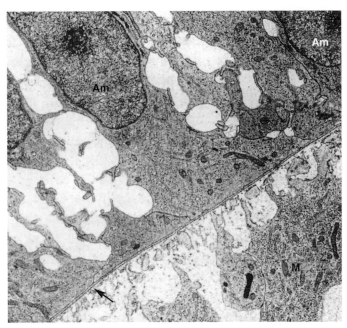

Fig. 22.5 TEM showing ameloblasts (Am) in contact with mesenchymal cells of the dental papilla (M) A basal lamina (arrow) is still present (× 500). Courtesy of Dr Z. Skobe and CRC Press.

proximal terminal web (Fig. 22.3). A similar distal terminal web will develop a little later at the secretory end of the cells (Fig. 22.7). The pre-ameloblasts are approximately 40 μm long and 5 μm wide. The pre-ameloblasts bulge into the stellate reticulum, presumably to gain the advantage of increased surface area in absorbing precursors. At their distal end following the onset of dentinogenesis the cell membrane becomes irregular with many projections and pits (Fig. 22.8). Vesicles and vacuoles appear in the cytoplasm. These changes may, in part, be associated with the removal of the basal lamina.

By the end of the presecretory stage of amelogenesis the phase of cytodifferentiation is complete. Morphodifferentiation has led to the establishment of an enamel organ whose shape (bell stage, see pages 292–295) closely resembles that of the future tooth crown. During the bell stage, enamel and dentine formation will be at different stages at different levels of the developing tooth. Active secretion and mineralisation will be going on at the cusp tip, while at the cervical loop cells will be differentiating into ameloblasts and odontoblasts.

Although cyto- and morphodifferentiation are the predominant features of the pre-secretory phase, the pre-ameloblasts

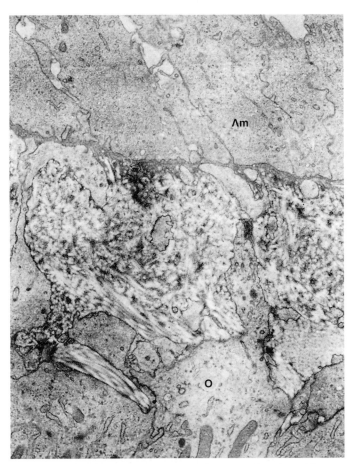

Fig. 22.6 TEM showing dentine matrix formation by odontoblasts (O) preceding the secretion of enamel by ameloblasts (Am) (× 5000). Courtesy of Dr Z. Skobe and CRC Press.

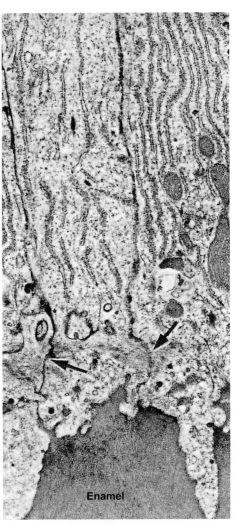

Fig. 22.7 TEM demonstrating cell junctions proximal to Tomes' processes, junctional complexes (arrows) and intracellular tonafilaments (× 7500). Courtesy of Dr T. Sasaki and Karger.

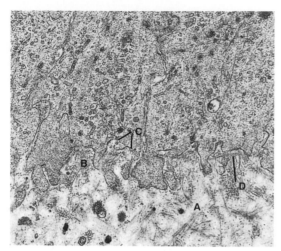

Fig. 22.8 TEM showing the distal end of a late-differentiating ameloblast. A = Forming dentine; B = invagination in ameloblast; C = coated pits; D = degenerating lamina (× 15 600). Courtesy of Dr E. Katchburian.

do synthesise and secrete small amounts of proteins similar to those that will form the enamel matrix. These early secretions seem to be phagocytosed by the developing odontoblasts of the dental papilla. Their significance is unknown, although it has been suggested that they may play a role in epithelial/mesenchymal interactions.

Secretory stage

The mature secretory ameloblast is 35–50 μm long and 5–10 μm wide (Figs 22.9, 22.10) and contains a proximally placed nucleus with, in the supranuclear region, numerous strands of rough endoplasmic reticulum oriented parallel to the long axis of the cell and a prominent Golgi apparatus. The basic enamel matrix proteins are assembled in the endoplasmic

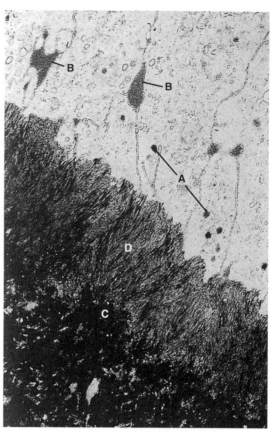

Fig. 22.10 TEM showing early enamel formation. A = Secretory vesicles; B = secreted matrix between ameloblasts; C = dentine; D = early enamel (× 1500). Courtesy of Dr E. Katchburian.

reticulum and carried by transitional vesicles to the Golgi apparatus where glycosylation and sulphation take place before packaging into electron dense secretory granules. The secretory granules (0.25 μm in diameter – Fig. 22.11) are transported along microtubules to the secretory pole of the cell, where they are secreted by a merocrine process.

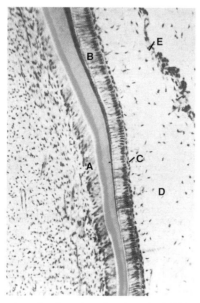

Fig. 22.9 Demineralised section showing the initial stage of enamel formation. A = Ameloblasts; B = odontoblasts; C = developing enamel; D = developing dentine; E = stratum intermedium; F = stellate reticulum (Masson's trichrome; × 80).

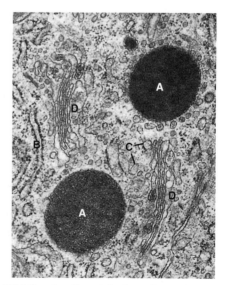

Fig. 22.11 TEM showing the synthetic and secretory apparatus in a secretory ameloblast. A = Secretory granules; B = rough endoplasmic reticulum; C = Golgi vesicles; D = Golgi apparatus (× 30 500). Courtesy of Dr E. Katchburian.

The secretory phase begins with the formation of a thin layer of enamel matrix as the columnar ameloblasts retreat from the enamel–dentine junction. After this initial secretion the secretory end of the ameloblast becomes pyramidal in shape, forming the so-called 'Tomes' process' (Figs 22.12–22.14). Ameloblasts are joined to each other by a terminal bar apparatus (web) distally at the base of the Tomes' processes (Fig. 22.12). This appearance of a linear structure is produced by the alignment of junctional complexes consisting of desmosomes and tight junctions. The tonofilaments associated with the desmosomes pass, for a short distance, into the cell and form an incomplete septum between the Tomes' processes and the rest of the ameloblast (Fig. 22.15). The junctions of the terminal web apparatus are zonular (encircling the cell) and effectively separate the environment of the developing enamel from the interior of the enamel organ (Figs 22.12, 22.14) such that all secretion and modification of the matrix occurs via the Tomes' processes. Junctions at the basal end of the ameloblasts, adjacent to the stratum intermedium, are macular and provide mechanical union without the same isolation of the microenvironment. There are other isolated junctions between ameloblasts at other levels, particularly gap junctions, which, presumably, synchronise the activity of the cells.

The shape of Tomes' processes is responsible for the prismatic structure of enamel. Interpit 'prongs' develop between the growing, and elongating, Tomes' processes (Figs 2.13, 22.14, 22.16). The prongs between the processes deposit enamel matrix first, to form walls that represent the periphery of the prisms (and interprismatic regions) and that delineate pits or depressions in the enamel that are occupied by Tomes' processes. The Tomes' processes then infill the pits as the ameloblasts retreat to form the main core of the enamel prism. The ameloblasts therefore have two main secretory sites.

As the ameloblasts shift from the presecretory to the secretory stage, there is a marked aggregation of vesicles (some containing stippled material) at the distal end of the ameloblast (Fig. 22.10). The material contained within the vesicles represents the organic matrix of the enamel. The contents of the vesicles are discharged into the extracellular space, both at the

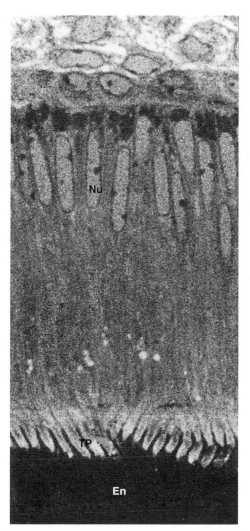

Fig. 22.13 Section showing rat secretory ameloblasts. Nu = Nuclei; TP = Tomes' processes, En = forming enamel (× 1000). Courtesy of Dr T. Sasaki and Karger.

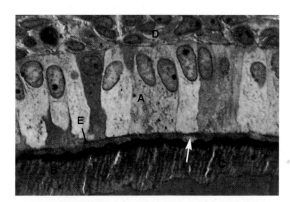

Fig. 22.12 Demineralised semithin section showing secretory ameloblasts and early enamel formation. A = Ameloblasts; B = enamel matrix; C = dentine; D = stratum intermedium; E = terminal bar apparatus (Toluidine blue; × 1000). Courtesy of Dr D.K. Whittaker.

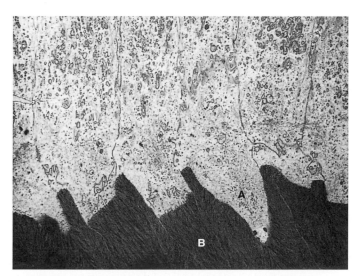

Fig. 22.14 TEM showing advanced secretory ameloblasts with their Tomes' processes (A). B = Developing enamel (× 6000). Courtesy of Dr A. Boyde and Springer-Verlag.

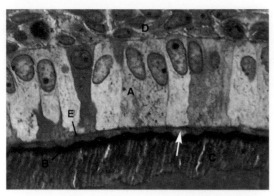

Fig. 22.15 Demineralised section of developing enamel showing the cone-shaped Tomes' process (arrow) at the distal end of each ameloblast. A = Ameloblast; B = enamel matrix; C = dentine; D = stratum intermedium; E = terminal bar apparatus running through the ameloblast layer (Toluidine blue; × 1000). Courtesy of Dr D.W. Whittaker.

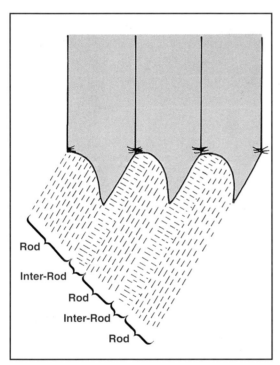

Fig. 22.16 The relationship between Tomes' processes and enamel prism formation. The enamel of the core of the prism and the prism boundary/inter-rod regions differ largely in the orientation of crystals. This is determined by the shape of the Tomes' process. In human enamel, prisms are clearly seen, though at some points in the 'tail' of the prism the boundary between prismatic and interprismatic is lost (see Figs 7.10, 7.55). Each prism is formed by a single ameloblast but four contribute to each interprismatic region. The prism boundary areas of enamel are formed first, giving the developing enamel front a pit-like surface appearance.

end of the cell and, apparently, between the cell membranes of adjacent ameloblasts (Fig. 22.10). As the enamel matrix is secreted, the ameloblasts are pushed (or move) outwards away from the dentine surface (Fig. 22.9). Within this organic matrix, the initial hydroxyapatite crystals of the enamel appear almost immediately, before the matrix is about 50 nm thick, so that a distinct zone of unmineralised matrix analogous to predentine

or osteoid is never seen in enamel (Fig. 22.10). The first-formed crystals are thin and needle-like and much smaller than mature crystals. During development, enamel crystallites are seen to align perpendicular to the distal surface of the ameloblasts; this represents the mineralising front. The mechanism responsible for this alignment is not understood but it may be due to the organisation of the organic matrix, concentration gradients of the crystallite ions, the presence of microvilli at the cell membrane or contributions due to ameloblast movement. The crystallites are aligned with their long axes approximately perpendicular to the surface of the Tomes' process. Thus, the wedge shaped appearance of the Tomes' process will produce abrupt changes in crystallite orientation and this may explain the appearance in light microscopy of the prism core and prism boundaries. It would seem, therefore, when considered in three dimensions, that more than one ameloblast contributes to the formation of a single prism and that each ameloblast is involved in the development of more than one prism.

The orientation of crystallites is possibly related to the tendency of crystallites to be oriented perpendicular to the mineralising front (Fig. 22.16). Growth of apatite crystal is rapid along their c-axes and, as the source of essential ions is the Tomes' process, it is possible that crystals will grow preferentially along the concentration gradient. It is assumed that, once formed, the crystallites continue to grow in the same direction. An additional 'stroking' orienting factor may occur in regions where there is a relative sliding movement between the surface of the Tomes' process and the mineralising front, the crystallites being oriented slightly in the direction of this movement. Other views suggest that the orientation of crystallites is related to flow patterns set up by shearing forces within the enamel matrix as the ameloblast retreats at an angle from the developing enamel front, or to the directional influence of microvilli at the surface of the Tomes' process. As the

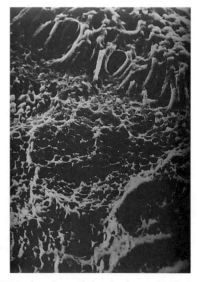

Fig. 22.17 SEM of surface of developing enamel. Some ameloblasts have been retained at the surface. Where others have been lost, the developing enamel surface shows a series of pits previously occupied by the Tomes' processes of the ameloblasts (× 500). Courtesy of Dr R.P. Shellis.

distal surface of the ameloblasts initially are flat (Fig. 22.10), the crystallites are all aligned more or less perpendicularly with no sudden changes in crystallite orientation so that the initial few microns of enamel are aprismatic.

With the development of the Tomes' process the shape of the mineralising front changes to a 'picket-fence' arrangement (Figs 22.14, 22.16). If the ameloblasts are pulled away, the mineralising front presents a honeycomb appearance, the pits in the surface being occupied by the Tomes' processes. This appearance is also reminiscent of the enamel surface following etching with inorganic acids (Fig. 22.17).

The secretory phase ends once the full thickness of enamel matrix has been laid down. The Tomes' process retracts (Fig. 22.18) and a thin layer of aprismatic enamel is formed at the surface, although this may be incomplete as prism end markings may sometimes be seen in the covering investments of newly erupted enamel or enamel from areas that have been protected from attrition (see pages 120–122). The signalling mechanisms that determine when and where in the tooth the secretory process is turned on or off are unknown.

The transition stage

The enamel that is deposited initially is high in water and protein and low in mineral. The process that converts it to fully mineralised enamel is termed maturation. Enamel maturation

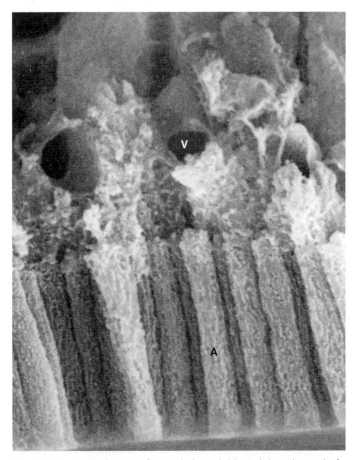

Fig. 22.18 SEM showing flat-ended ameloblasts (A) at the end of the secretory phase. V = venule. (× 1000). Courtesy of Dr Z. Skobe and the CRC Press.

is carried out by the same cells that secreted the primary matrix, but in a very changed form. The period in which the ameloblasts change from a secretory to a maturation form is the transition stage. During this phase, enamel secretion stops and much of the amelogenin is removed. A reduction in height of the ameloblasts signals the onset of the transition. The number of ameloblasts is reduced by as much as 50% by apoptosis (programmed cell death). In those ameloblasts that remain, the organelles associated with protein synthesis (e.g. the rough endoplasmic reticulum and the Golgi apparatus) are reduced by autophagocytosis. The enamel organ becomes invaginated by blood vessels and the cells of external enamel epithelium, stellate reticulum and stratum intermedia become covered with microvilli. The blood vessels thus lie close to, but not in contact with, the proximal end (base) of the ameloblasts (Fig. 22.18). As the final stage of the transition, the ameloblasts form a basal lamina over the immature enamel, attaching themselves to it by hemidesmosomes.

The enamel matrix into which enamel crystallites are precipitated is composed of unique matrix proteins. By the phased removal of the bulk of its protein during development, this matrix allows for the unique configuration and size of the enamel crystallites. About 90% of the proteins in developing enamel are amelogenins, the remaining 10% being formed by non-amelogenins such as enamelin and tuftelin. It is the amelogenins that are primarily removed during subsequent enamel maturation, leaving behind mainly the non-amelogenins in the adult tissue. The amelogenins are hydrophobic, proline-rich molecules, which also have relatively high levels of histidine, glutamine and leucine. They have a molecular weight of about 25 000 kDa. The non-amelogenins are heavier (50–70 000 kDa) and are rich in glycine, with relatively higher levels of aspartic acid and serine (Fig. 22.19). The analysis of the amelogenins is complicated by two features. First, multiple, closely related amelogenins are derived by alternate splicing of a single primary RNA. Thus, the same amino acid sequence is present at either end, with deficiencies occurring in the middle. Second, large numbers of smaller molecules with the characteristics of amelogenins can be identified, indicating that amelogenin undergoes degradation extracellularly. Such breakdown (presumably enzymatic) commences soon after secretion of the enamel matrix occurs and continues throughout the secretory stage of enamel formation. The question arises as to whether this degradation is merely to remove the matrix and allow the enamel crystallites to enlarge, or whether some or all of the smaller molecules have specific functions in the development of enamel structure. For example, one component, known as TRAP (tyrosine-rich amelogenin protein) is thought to be important in crystal growth. Newly formed enamel is 65% water, 20% organic material and 15% inorganic hydroxyapatite crystals by weight.

Maturation stage

Once the entire thickness of the enamel has formed it is structurally complete, with all the morphological features of mature enamel. It is, however, only mineralised to about 30%

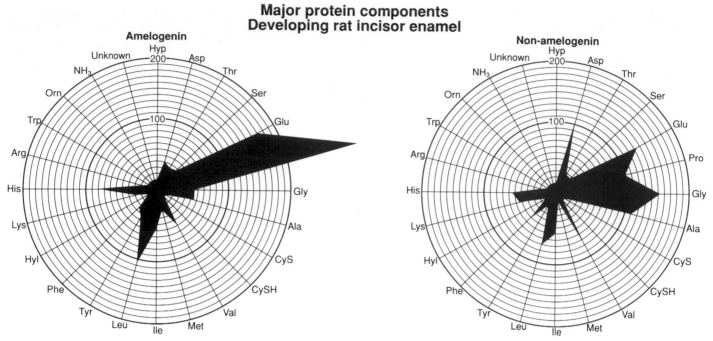

Fig. 22.19 'Rose' diagram showing the composition of the proteins in developing rat incisor enamel. Courtesy of Professor C. Robinson.

of that of the erupted tooth. The process by which the enamel changes into its final form is termed maturation. During maturation, enamel crystals increase in width and thickness with a consequent reduction in the intercrystalline space.

Maturation involves the removal of water and mainly the amelogenin-type enamel proteins, and the addition of calcium and phosphate ions to increase the size of the enamel crystallites (mainly in thickness, from an initial value of around 1.5 nm to about 25 nm). Organic matrix is also removed, reducing the protein content of the final tissue to less than 1% (from 30%). There is also a change in the proteins present. Removal of amelogenins leaves behind small peptides and amino acids, together with larger components (non-amelogenins) bound to the crystals. This accounts for mature enamel having more glycine but less histidine and proline than young, immature enamel. One theory as to why amelogenins are preferentially removed rather than non-amelogenins is that they are more thixotropic and thus may be more readily squeezed to the surface by expanding enamel crystallites. Most of the water remaining is also removed.

The changes during maturation are achieved by (or through) the ameloblasts. The cells themselves change considerably. The Tomes' process is lost and the organelle content reduced. The remaining organelles congregate at the distal end of the cell where the plasma membrane infolds to form a striated border (Fig. 22.20). The ameloblast is described as ruffle-ended. This morphology alternates with that of the smooth-ended ameloblast, in which the striated border is absent. Modulation between the two forms occurs between five and seven times during maturation. The modulation may alternate between resorptive and secretory phases. The removal of matrix occurs when the crystals expand from their early dimensions of 1.5 nm thick to their mature thickness of 25 nm. The degradation of the enamel matrix by serine proteases

released from the enamel organ seems to precede mineral gain, matrix degradation and removal being essential to facilitate crystal growth. Indeed, at this initial stage the space caused by matrix loss is occupied by water and the enamel becoming more porous.

During maturation, the enamel that has been initially deposited as a watery, protein-rich, low-mineral tissue will be

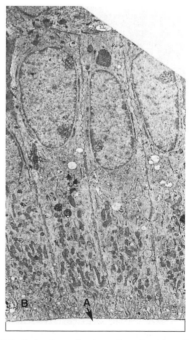

Fig. 22.20 TEM of demineralised section showing the appearance of ruffle-ended ameloblasts during maturation phase of amelogenesis. A = Enamel space; B = striated border. Tomes' process has been lost. The mitochondria are grouped in a basal cluster. The rough endoplasmic reticulum is much reduced (× 2700).

Fig. 22.21 High-power view of Fig. 22.20, showing ruffled border of ameloblast during the maturation stage. A = Enamel space; B = striated (ruffled) border; C = resorptive vesicles (× 6700).

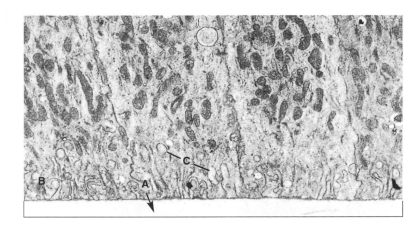

modified into the hardest biological material known. Mineral will be added, making each of the crystallites already laid down thicker. This 'squeezes out' protein and water, although these will also be actively removed. The relative and exact role of cellular processes mediated via the reduced ameloblasts and extracelluar mechanisms is not completely understood. The ameloblasts continue to add amelogenins during the first half of the maturation period. In the ruffled phase (Fig. 22.21), tight junctions appear in the distal region, linking groups of ameloblasts and rendering them impermeable. This is thought to be associated with an influx of mineral ions into the enamel, the ruffle-ended ameloblasts exhibiting an increase in calcium ATPase activity. In the smooth-ended phase (Fig. 22.22), the tight junctions are lost at the distal end of the cell

and may allow the passage of organic material and water from the enamel between the ameloblasts.

In the ruffled phase, the distal surface of the ameloblast looks like that of osteoclasts and cells of the renal proximal convoluted tubule, both of which are resorptive. The cyclical changes in ameloblast morphology seem to be linked to at least two aspects of maturation.

- The movement of calcium ions. In the ruffled form, this movement may be actively controlled whereas in the smooth form calcium ions may move only by diffusion (and hence few would enter the enamel).
- Local pH changes. Physiologically normal pH favouring mineralisation (ruffle-ended) would alternate with mildly acidic conditions handicapping mineralisation (smooth-ended). The ameloblasts may induce these pH cycles by modulating bicarbonate levels.

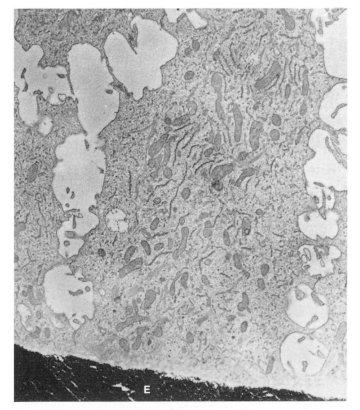

Fig. 22.22 TEM showing the appearance of a smooth-ended maturation ameloblast. At this stage the cells lack a distinct terminal web distally (× 7000). Courtesy of Dr Z. Skobe and CRC Press.

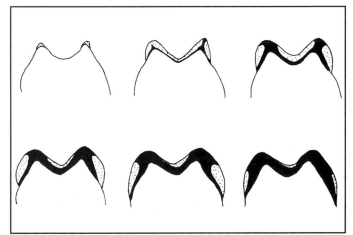

Fig. 22.23 Pattern of mineralisation during maturation, as mapped out by microradiography of ground sections. Stippled areas represent initial enamel deposition. Black areas show the pattern that increased mineralisation follows during maturation. Once the full thickness of enamel is formed in any area, maturation commences. Initial deposition and maturation can thus occur at the same time. Mineralisation during maturation follows a different pattern than initial deposition. Commencing at cusps, it passes to the enamel–dentine junction and along the junction before continuing throughout the more superficial regions.

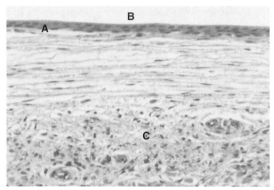

Fig. 22.24 Demineralised section showing the position and morphology of the reduced enamel epithelium (A) covering the unerupted tooth. B = Enamel space; C = connective tissue of the dental follicle (H & E; × 160).

A third process in maturation, lowering the molecular weight of enamel proteins by a group of proteinases resident in the enamel matrix, may not be cyclical but continuous. The ameloblasts (which may produce the enzymes) do not control this digestion although they do resorb and degrade its end products. These protein changes may, by an unknown mechanism, affect the advancing mineralisation. Simple

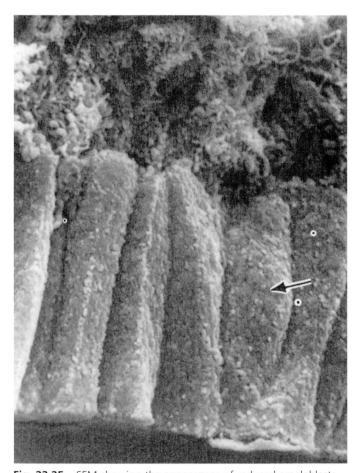

Fig. 22.25 SEM showing the appearance of reduced ameloblasts. The bulge indicated by the arrow may be the result of multiple nuclei, which are sometimes seen in these cells (× 2000). Courtesy of Dr Z. Skobe and CRC Press.

removal of the protein, of course, increases the relative mineral content. The final one-third of the mineralisation process goes on after virtually all protein has been removed. The increase in mineral density begins over the cusp tips and progresses cervically (Fig. 22.23).

Post-maturation stage

Once maturation of the enamel is complete, the ameloblasts become flattened (Figs 22.24, 22.25), except sometimes in the depths of fissures where they may remain columnar. A 1 μm thick amorphous layer of protein, the primary enamel cuticle, separates the cells from the enamel. This may be material extruded from the enamel during maturation or may be the last product of the fading ameloblast. The cells themselves contain hemidesmosomes and a basal lamina reappears on their enamel surface. The other layers of the enamel organ merge with the surrounding dental follicle. During eruption, this reduced enamel epithelium protects the enamel surface. During eruption, the fluoride content of the enamel may rise more in teeth that have longer durations of eruption. It is not known whether the remaining cells of the enamel organ are active in this respect or not. Once the tooth has erupted into the oral cavity, the surface layer shows increasing mineralisation through interaction with saliva (post-eruptive maturation).

PROTEINS IN DEVELOPING ENAMEL

Proteins and peptides account for less than 1% of the weight of mature enamel but 25–30% of early enamel. Developing enamel matrix is almost entirely proteinaceous. The bulk of the developing enamel matrix (90–95%) is the protein amelogenin produced by the ameloblasts. This has been well characterised in terms of the amino acid sequences it contains and its gene has been identified. The other proteins present (other than enzymes involved in the modification of the matrix) are much less well understood and are grouped together as the 'non-amelogenins', most notable among which are tuftelin and enamelin.

The human amelogenin molecule is rich in proline and glutamine, consists of 178 amino acid residues and has a molecular weight of approximately 20 000 kDa. Amelogenins from different enamel species are very similar. Amelogenins are unique proteins, different from any other protein in the body. Amelogenin is hydrophobic and tends to aggregate or 'clump'. When it is added to enamel matrix it does not form a discrete appositional band as do the matrix proteins of dentine and bone, but spreads throughout the whole developing enamel thickness. The resultant matrix is a gel through which molecules and ions can spread readily, a property of considerable significance in the production of large crystals. Very shortly after it is secreted, amelogenin undergoes degradation by proteolytic enzymes such that the developing enamel matrix becomes a heterogeneous mix of proteins and fragments. Amelogenins may be phosphorylated and interact weakly with apatite. The amelogenin gene is located on the sex chromosomes.

Table 22.2 *Some of the main enamel proteins and their possible functions*

Protein	Function
Dentine sialophosphoprotein,	*De novo* mineral
Amelogenin, non-amelogenin	Mineral ion bindng as crystal
Amelogenin, non-amelogenin	Control of crystal growth
Amelogenin, non-amelogenin	Support of growing crystals
Amelobastin	Determination of prismatic pattern
Tuftelin, ameloblastin	Cell signalling
Breakdown products	Control of secretion
Amelogenin, non-amelogenin	Protection of mineral phase

Non-amelogenins (originally termed enamelins) is an umbrella term given to the proteins of mature enamel. Although they form 5–10% by weight of the developing enamel matrix relatively little is known about their composition and structure and their identity and roles are controversial. Non-amelogenins may be derived in part from plasma albumin but may contain other distinct components secreted by the ameloblasts. Non-amelogenins interact strongly with apatite, suggesting a role in mineralisation.

Tuftelin is a protein present in developing enamel in much smaller amounts and named for its similarity to the protein found in mature enamel. Its gene is located on autosome l.

Other protein components have been described and classified on the basis of their molecular weight. It is unclear whether these are precursors or degradation products of other proteins or are distinct molecular species. Many functions have been hypothesised for the protein components during amelogenesis. These postulates are summarised in Table 22.2.

MINERALISATION

There are a number of possible sources for the calcium that will mineralise the enamel matrix. The precise pathway and transport mechanism is unclear, although some elements of the process have been determined.

Calcium reaches the matrix principally via the enamel organ (rather than the dental papilla). It travels, possibly predominantly, by an extracellular route, although there is also evidence for a transcellular route (Figs 22.26, 22.27). There may be an active transport mechanism utilising carriers in the cell membranes of the ameloblasts, or the calcium may flow passively from high concentrations in the blood plasma to low concentrations in the enamel matrix. The ameloblast layer has a limited, variable but controlled permeability to ions. This property lies in the proximal rather than distal cell junctional complexes. It may control not only the access to calcium but also other significant ions, particularly fluoride.

Specific initiators of enamel mineralisation have not been convincingly identified. The first-formed enamel at the enamel–dentine junction is less well organised than the bulk of mature enamel in terms of crystal size and morphology and

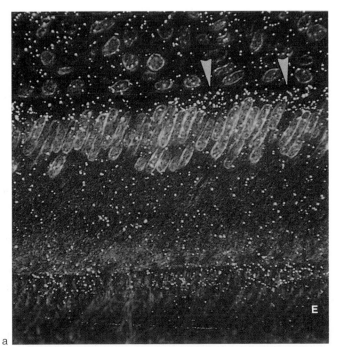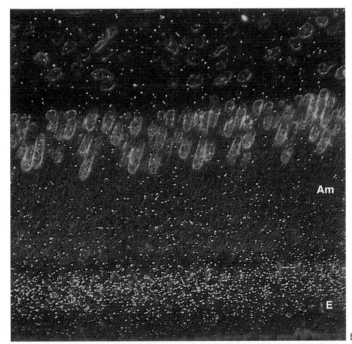

Fig. 22.26 Section of an autoradiograph viewed in darkfield showing the movement of calcium through the ameloblast layer. Anhydrously prepared ⁴⁵Ca autoradiographs showing the movement of calcium (showing as white dots) through ameloblasts. Am = Ameloblasts; E = enamel. The tissue (rat) in (a) was taken 30 seconds after the injection of the radioactive calcium. The arrows indicate the accumulation of calcium in the proximal ameloblast adjacent to the stellate reticulum. The tissue in (b) was taken 10 minutes after injection when most of the calcium has become incorporated into the enamel (× 400). Courtesy of Dr Y. Takana and the editor of *Connective Tissue Research*.

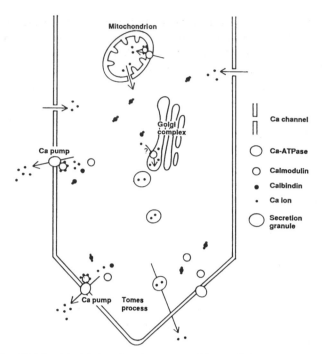

Fig. 22.27 Model showing the proposed intracellular movement of calcium in the ameloblasts. Courtesy of Dr T. Sasaki and Karger.

is aprismatic. On the basis of this disordered morphology, it has been suggested that crystal growth and possibly nucleation are directed by tuftelin. It has also been suggested, but not demonstrated, that initial nucleation may occur in dentine and cross the enamel–dentine junction. Matrix vesicles, which may participate in the onset of mineralisation in some parts of the dentine, have not been reported in developing enamel.

It has recently been proposed that the amelogenins are capable of self-assembling into minute spheres (nanospheres), between which the first crystals of enamel are formed. Through this organisation the amelogenins space, orient and control initial enamel biomineralisation.

Initially, crystals may grow by the fusion of nucleation sites but once the prismatic structure is established crystals are enlarged preferentially in length rather than in width.

The matrix can control crystal growth by two basic mechanisms: by breaking down in a controlled pattern to provide the space for new crystal deposition and by modulating the effect of directly inhibitory molecules. The first could be achieved by the formation, in the matrix, of appropriately oriented microchannels with the same dimensions as crystals and in which crystals would form at the growing end of the prism. There is some slight evidence that these microchannels exist but no understanding of their formation. There are a number of molecules that may inhibit crystal formation though no definitive roles have been established.

In the maturation phase the role of the matrix proteins is largely ended as virtually all the protein has been lost and what remained replaced with tissue fluid. The matrix proteins are removed long before crystal growth ends. The degraded matrix proteins accumulate in the extracellular space around the ameloblasts and, by inhibiting further activity, control and

limit the thickness of enamel deposited. The increase in mineral during maturation follows a different pattern than the initial deposition.

DEVELOPMENT OF THE PRISMATIC STRUCTURE

The first-formed enamel at what will be the enamel–dentine junction is laid against newly calcified dentine by flat-ended ameloblasts. It is prismless and contains intially small crystals (15 nm wide × 1.6 nm thick). Mineralisation increases by the fusion of nucleation sites and crystal growth. The crystals in this aprismatic zone all appear to have a protein coating 0.33 nm thick until they are 55 nm wide × 12 nm thick. As the ameloblasts retreat, they form pyramidal Tomes' process at their distal ends and the enamel formed thereafter is prismatic. Enamel matrix is deposited in a non-homogeneous form. Amelogenins become located primarily within the prism, non-amelogenins more at the periphery of the prisms. The material secreted from the Tomes' process forms the core of the prisms, that secreted from distal to the terminal web forms the peripheral parts of the prisms. Enamel crystallites form at right-angles to the face of the cell (see Fig. 22.29) and thus there is considerable variation in crystal orientation within a prism. In human enamel, the crystals in the head of the prism are approximately parallel to the long axis of the prism but in the tail deviate from this direction by 60° (see Figs 7.11–7.14). The path of the retreating ameloblasts determines the arrangement of prisms. Viewed longitudinally, the path of a human ameloblast is a straight line from the enamel–dentine junction to the enamel surface; viewed transversely the path is sinusoidal. Different directions in different layers produces the appearance of Hunter–Schreger bands in mature enamel (see pages 106–107).

Towards the end of enamel formation, the Tomes' process is lost such that the last formed layer of enamel, like the first, is prismless.

INCREMENTAL LINE FORMATION

Various lines and patterns have been described in enamel, and have been attributed to the rhythmic and incremental activity of the ameloblasts. **Cross-striations** appear as lines about 2.5–6 μm apart (see page 109). They are due to a diurnal rhythm in enamel prism growth. The **enamel striae** (see pages 109–112) follow the contours of the developing crown and have been considered to be incremental (analogous to growth lines in trees), and may result from changes in the direction of enamel prisms. It seems more likely that the striae represent a boundary between groups of prisms formed by different cohorts of ameloblasts. In human enamel, about seven rows of ameloblasts are generated each week together at the cervical loop and the resulting prisms will extend around the crown. The subsequent group will have a somewhat different orientation and the boundary between the two could constitute a striation. The striae successively outline the position of the mineralising enamel front. They thus do not reach the surface over the tips of the cusps or incisal edges (see Fig. 7.32). As the daily increments of enamel are smaller towards the end of enamel formation, the striae are closer together towards the cervical margin. As there are about seven cross-striations between successive striae, the striae are thought to represent approximately weekly incremental lines (circaseptan). One theory to account for their presence suggests that, superimposed on the normal 24-hour daily rhythm, there is another rhythm of about 27 hours. The two would coincide about every 7 days, resulting in the presence of striae.

MOLECULAR ELEMENTS OF AMELOBLAST DIFFERENTIATION

As well as describing amelogenesis in morphological and biochemical terms, it is now possible, thanks to the techniques of molecular biology, to describe the patterns of expression of many regulating, inducing and signalling molecules in the process. The expression of certain molecules at particular stages of development suggests, but does not establish, a role for that molecule in the process. Experimental approaches involve deleting or over-expressing the factor under investigation and documenting the changes that occur in order to define function with conviction. Current knowledge is fragmentary and although increasing rapidly a coherent and comprehensive account of the molecular mechanisms of amelogenesis is some time away. What follows is a summary of the fragments that have been found to date.

Gene transcription

Virtually all cells contain the DNA sequences (genes) that encode for enamel production. Gene regulation determines which genes are active and is the property of a class of DNA-binding proteins. Gene expression can be controlled at every step from the gene to the final functional protein. Much of the control is exercised at the stage of transcription when mRNA is produced on the DNA template. RNA is synthesised with an RNA polymerase, acting in concert with transcription factors, while binding to a promoter site on the DNA. The mRNA thus formed may be modified and edited. The final mRNA, while sliding through a ribosome and acting via translational RNA, results in the assembly of polypeptides. Multiple, often different, polypeptides are conjugated into proteins, sometimes combined with polysaccharides, and given a physical configuration as they pass through the intracellular tubular pathway of the endoplasmic reticulum and Golgi apparatus. This results most often in proteins bound in vesicles for export. The determination of which vesicles are released, and when, is related to intracellular signals that may be genetically programmed or may be produced in response to an external signal acting on a cell membrane receptor.

Only some of the factors involved in gene expression in the ameloblast are known. Homeobox genes encode for trans-

cription factors and thus regulate transcription. *Msx-2* is a homeobox gene that is expressed in the branchial arches and in the early stages (bud) in the epithelium but at later stages in the mesenchyme. It localises to the enamel knot region and is thus possibly a regulator of morphogenesis (see page 296). *Egr-1* is a transcription factor thought to regulate cell destiny in developing teeth.. Its expression shifts back and forth between epithelium and mesenchyme and it is briefly expressed in the polarised ameloblasts before any matrix is produced.

At the molecular level, most is known about the gene encoding for the matrix protein amelogenin. Various forms of amelogenin may be produced by post-transcriptional modification of the mRNA and each form may have a different role in amelogenesis.

Membrane receptors

In developing tissues, cells differentiate and change their activities usually in response to an external signal. Receptor molecules on the cell surface recognise and bind signalling molecules that may, for example, be growth factors or extra-cellular matrix molecules. There are several families of receptor molecules. One of the integrin family of cell surface receptors, $\beta 5$, is upregulated in the internal enamel epithelium during the cap stage after being expressed in the mesenchyme during the bud stage. It is then downregulated as the ameloblast differentiates. Receptors for fibroblast growth factors (FgF) and epidermal growth factors (EGF) are also present in the internal enamel epithelium of the bud stage but are down-regulated during the cap stage. EGF expression returns to the ameloblast in maturation.

Intracellular receptors

Some signalling molecules act on receptors that are within the cytoplasm of the cell. Cellular retinoic acid-binding proteins transmit the signals of retinoic acid. They are expressed in the developing tooth wherever there are high rates of cell proliferation. One of these proteins (CRABP I) appears to be expressed by secretory but not maturation-stage ameloblasts. Growth hormone receptor is also intracellular, but appears only on the differentiating ameloblast. It appears to be related to pre-ameloblast proliferation. Vitamin D receptors have also been identified during differentiation.

DEFECTS IN ENAMEL FORMATION

Defects in enamel formation are common. Estimates vary from 8 to 80% of the population as having at least one affected permanent tooth. Over 100 different conditions have been identified. A group of hereditary conditions known as amelogenesis imperfecta (Fig. 22.28) affects only enamel. These are rather common. Estimates of their prevalence range from 1 in every 14 people to 1.4 per 1000. Three groups of amelogenesis imperfecta are recognised based on the phase of amelogenesis affected: hypoplastic, in which the enamel is of normal colour but thin and grooved or pitted; hypocalcified, in which the

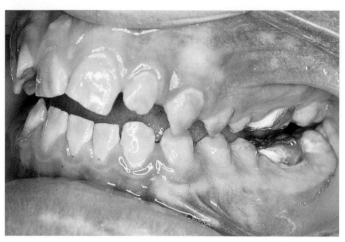

Fig. 22.28 Teeth from a patient with amelogenesis imperfecta. In this example the enamel is of apparently normal appearance in many of the teeth but seriously abnormal in the first molars, where much of the enamel has chipped off exposing the underlying dentine. The underlying dentine is usually normal and restorative procedures, especially crowns, can be used to maintain the dentition. Courtesy of Dr M. Ignelzi.

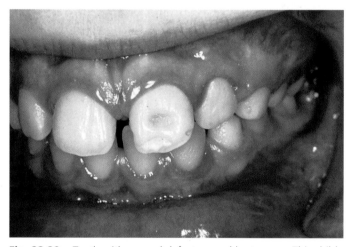

Fig. 22.29 Tooth with enamel defect caused by trauma. This child had a blow to the maxillary left deciduous incisor that damaged the developing permanent tooth sufficiently to result in a localised defect in enamel formation. This produced a pit, seen on the facial surface of the tooth when erupted. Courtesy of Dr M. Ignelzi.

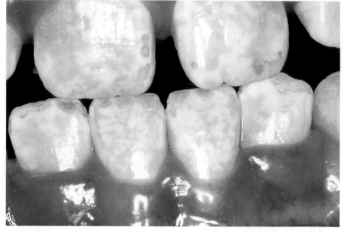

Fig. 22.30 Teeth demonstrating fluorosis. A high level of dietary fluoride has resulted in much of the enamel becoming opaque in patches, giving a 'mottled' appearance. Courtesy of Dr M. Ignelzi.

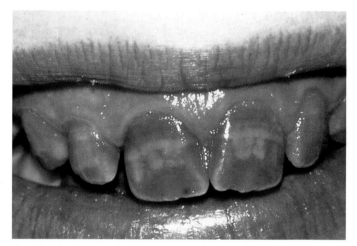

Fig. 22.31 Teeth stained as a result of tetracycline administration. This is an extreme example of tetracycline staining: the entire enamel (and dentine) has become pigmented. As the staining is built into the structure of the tooth, bleaching procedures do not usually greatly improve the appearance of these teeth. Crowns or, more conservatively, veneers, will do so. Courtesy of Dr M. Ignelzi.

Fig. 22.32 Teeth showing haemoglobin pigmentation. Haemoglobin residues released during Rhesus factor incompatibility are taken up by the developing teeth, resulting in a brown stain. Because of effective screening this is now a rare occurrence. Courtesy of Dr M. Ignelzi.

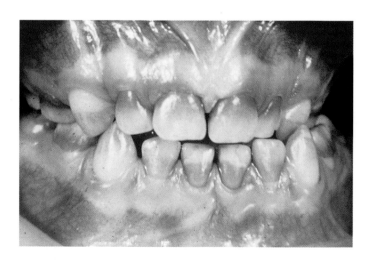

mineralisation is poor and the enamel is dark and chips easily; hypomaturation, in which the enamel is dark, mottled and chips easily. Other hereditary conditions (including systemic metabolic disorders) in which enamel is thin and pitted also affect other tissues (e.g. mucopolysaccharidosis) while systemic ectodermal/epidermal disorders (e.g. epidermolysis bullosa) have many subtypes including hypoplastic enamel among many more serious features. Localised trauma can result in disturbances in enamel formation in individual teeth (Fig. 22.29).

The most obvious dietary factor that affects enamel development is fluoride. Ingestion of levels above 5 parts per million results in fluorosis – a diffuse white opacity of variable extent. In severe cases the fluoritic areas may be brown and pitted (Fig. 22.30). The principal change is a subsurface hypomineralisation of varying extent.

Febrile diseases can disturb amelogenesis for the term of the illness and result in a band of poorly formed enamel. Some drugs, the best known being the tetracyclines, may affect amelogenesis. Tetracycline is incorporated into the developing enamel and results in a band of brown enamel (Fig. 22.31). When Rhesus factor incompatibility results in erythroblastosis fetalis, haemoglobin residues are incorporated into developing enamel, resulting in a brown pigmentation of the teeth (Fig. 22.32).

23 Dentinogenesis

The formation of dentine begins when the tooth germ has reached the bell stage of development. The dental papilla is well defined and the enamel organ fully formed, with the internal enamel epithelium differentiated and poised to secrete enamel matrix although no enamel has yet been laid down. By semantic convention, the dental papilla becomes the dental pulp once dentinogenesis has begun. Unlike amelogenesis, which has a well defined end point, dentinogenesis will continue throughout life. Unlike enamel, new dentine can be formed should repair or replacement be needed. Although a continuous process, dentinogenesis can, for descriptive purposes, be subdivided into stages covering the differentiation of the dentine-forming cells (odontoblasts), the deposition of the organic matrix (predentine), and the mineralisation of this matrix that also involves its modification. There is no parallel in dentinogenesis with the overall post-deposition modification of the tissue (maturation) that occurs during amelogenesis.

ODONTOBLAST DIFFERENTIATION (Fig. 23.1)

The cells that will form the dentine differentiate from the ectomesenchyme of the dental papilla and are of neural crest origin. The process of differentiation and the properties of the differentiated cells have been studied in detail by experiments recombining samples of dental papilla cells and cells from the oral ectoderm in co-culture. In addition, there have been extensive molecular observations describing the nature and sequence of gene expression in the differentiating cells. Odontoblasts express not only the genes responsible for production of the unique dentine matrix proteins but perhaps also those responsible for the morphology of the completed tooth, determining whether it is a molar, canine or incisor (morphogenetic genes – see pages 297–298).

Epithelial–mesenchymal interactions

The differentiation of the odontoblast does not occur in

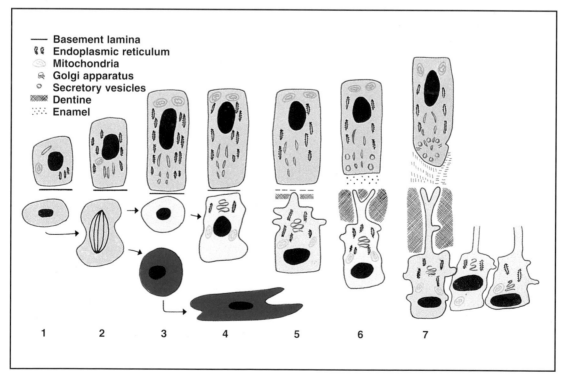

Fig. 23.1 Life cycle of the odontoblast (lower cell line) related to that of the ameloblast (upper cell line). 1 = Ameloblast begins to differentiate first. 2 = Peripheral ectomesenchymal cells divide, with some daughter cells migrating below the odontoblast layer. 3 = Acting on a signal from the ameloblast, the preodontoblasts begin to differentiate. 4 = Synthetic organelles increase in size and number, especially Golgi apparatus and rough endoplasmic reticulum. 5 = Nucleus moves basally as the cell becomes polarised. A number of odontoblast processes begin to form. One odontoblast process becomes enlarged and begins to secrete matrix. 6 = The odontoblast retreats as matrix is laid down, leaving behind a single main process. Once a narrow layer of matrix is laid down mineralisation commences. 7 = Once the first layer of dentine is laid down the differentiated ameloblast begins to deposit matrix.

isolation. Neural crest cells from the appropriate location do not differentiate to form dentine unless they come into contact with oral ectoderm in the form of the enamel epithelium. A signal initiating differentiation passes from the oral ectoderm to the neural crest cells. There is also an interaction in the opposite direction. Oral ectoderm, though differentiated into enamel epithelium, does not deposit enamel matrix until dentine deposition has started. Neural crest cells elsewhere in the body do not (except in pathologically anomalous situations which form ectopic teeth or teratomas) initiate tooth formation. One major effect of oral ectoderm is to limit tooth formation to the mouth.

The signalling pattern between oral ectoderm and mesenchyme is not completely understood, though some important elements have been described. In a mouse model one gene (*Otlx 2/Rieg*) is expressed in regions which will become odontogenic before any morphological evidence of tooth formation is present. This expression is initiated by a signal from the underlying mesenchyme. Following this, a series of genes specific to odontogenic areas become expressed in the mesenchyme. This would represent the earliest known steps in the differentiation of the odontoblast but suggest that epithelial–mesenchymal interaction occurs long before dentine formation. These early signals are followed by formation of the dental lamina and then individual tooth germs. It should be remembered that not all developmental processes are positive, although these tend to be the focus of our interest. Regression and apoptosis (cell death) also occur, particularly during the early stages (for example, in the dental lamina between tooth germs).

The basement membrane of the internal enamel epithelium is essential for the differentiation of odontoblasts. Time-limited changes in the composition of the basement membrane occur coincident with odontoblast differentiation. These changes include expression and localisation of laminin, chrondroitin-containing proteoglycans and enamel proteins. Although not strictly components of the basement membrane, fibronectin and decorin also accumulate at the distal pole of the differentiating cell. It is not known which, if any, of these changes initiate or control differentiation. Other, as yet unknown, factors may pass through the membrane too quickly to have been detected.

Growth factors are biological molecules that can control growth and repair in cells. A number, particularly those belonging to the transforming growth factor (TGF) family, insulin-like growth factor (IGF) and bone morphogenic protein (BMP) have been found in the internal enamel epithelium during the differentiation of odontoblasts. Some of these have been shown to effect, under some conditions, the development and behaviour of odontoblast-like cells maintained in culture. These cultured cells can be shown to express some of the membrane receptors for these molecules. Growth factors play an important role in the development of many tissues. While it is not currently known which are significant and what their precise role is in odontoblast differentiation, interesting hypotheses are being tested. These include the proposal that TGF-β family members, which are trapped then released from the basement membrane of the internal enamel epithelium, act on the pre-odontoblasts and, via a series of intervening steps,

modulate the expression of genes involved in the assembly of the cytoskeleton. The cytoskeleton is of pre-eminent importance in the relocation of intracellular organelles and in being associated with changes in the morphology of the cell. Members of the TGF family may also be involved in the withdrawal of the cells that will become odontoblasts from the mitotic cycle.

Cytodifferentiaton of odontoblasts
(Figs 23.1, 23.2)

At the end of the histogenesis and morphogenesis of the odontoblast, a clearly defined and differentiated layer of cells is present at the periphery of the dental pulp. It is not clear whether the cells in this layer originate from a subset of dental papilla cells or whether all dental papilla cells are potential odontoblasts. Which cells eventually become odontoblasts may be determined by their proximity to the signal originating in the overlying epithelium. Cell division continues in the dental papilla during development. The peripheral cells, from among which the odontoblasts will differentiate, will also divide. At the final division of the preodontoblasts before differentiation the daughter cell in contact with the basement membrane is the one that will finally become an odontoblast. It has been suggested that the end point of cell division is predetermined and that each cell in the population undergoes a finite number of cell cycles before differentiation. The number of cells present may be determined, at least in part, by the level of growth hormone.

The morphologically discernible differentiation of the odontoblast begins with the dental papilla cells adjacent to the deepest invagination(s) of the internal enamel epithelium, beneath what will become the cusps or incisal margins. The preodontoblast (the cell left in contact with the basement membrane of the internal enamel epithelium after the last cell division) initially shows neither well developed organelles nor a specific orientation. The cells change rapidly. They increase in size (hypertrophy) and the nucleus comes to lie in the basal part of the cell, that furthest from the internal enamel epithelium (Fig. 23.2). The Golgi complex becomes pronounced and placed above the nucleus. The rough endoplasmic reticulum increases in size and becomes flattened parallel to what is becoming the long axis of the cell. The elongation and polarisation of the cell is accompanied by a redistribution of the intracellular skeletal proteins actin, vinculin and vimentin as well as expression of nestin and cytokeratin. Changes also occur in the membrane of the cell including increased expression of the protein that binds fibronectin.

Many small cell processes extend from the differentiating odontoblast. Most of these are directed towards the basement membrane of the internal enamel epithelium. As differentiation proceeds, the number of processes is reduced and one large process will dominate. Cell-to-cell junctions, particularly between odontoblasts but also linking odontoblasts to sub-odontoblastic cells, increase in number. Tight, gap and macula adherens (desmosomes) junctions occur. It is likely that some of the signals that co-ordinate the activities of the odontoblasts pass through the gap junctions, although synchrony may also be achieved by response to a common external signal.

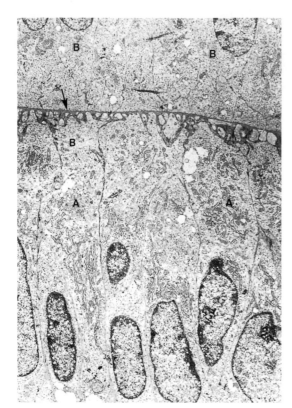

Fig. 23.2 TEM of the interface between odontoblasts (A) and ameloblasts (B) just before the deposition of matrix. The arrow indicates the basement membrane of the ameoblasts (× 38 000). Courtesy of Dr P. Glick.

Table 23.1 *Components of organic dentine extracellular matrix*

Collagens	Enamelysin
Type I	
Type I trimer	
Type V	
Type III (?)	
Type VI	

Proteoglycans	**Lipids**
Decorin (PG II)	Phospholipids (phosphatidylcholine,
Biglycan (PG1)	phosphatidylethanolamine)
Other chondroitin-4	Cholesterol
sulphate-containing	Cholesterol esters
proteoglycans	Triacylglycerols
Dermatan sulphate	
proteoglycans	
Keratan sulphate (?)	
Perlecan (?)	

Glycoproteins/ sialoproteins	**Serum-derived proteins**
Osteonectin	α2HS-glycoprotein
Dentine sialoprotein(s)	Albumin
(DSPs)	Immunoglobulins
Bone sialoprotein	
Osteopontin	
Bone acidic	
glycoprotein 75	
Syndecan 2	

Phosphoproteins	**Growth factors**
Dentine	TGF-βs
phosphoproteins	Chondrogenic inducing factor
(DPPs)	Bone morphogenic proteins (BMPs)
Dentine matrix	Fibroblast growth factors (FGF)
protein 1	Insulin-like growth factors (IGFs)
γ-Carboxyglutamate	
containing	
proteins	
Osteocalcin	
Matrix GLA	
protein	

Amelin-1
(transient expression)

Differentiation of the odontoblasts occurs in a specific temporospatial pattern, beginning under what will become the cusp tip or incisal margin and progressing root-wards. Control of this progression may lie either in the ability of the internal enamel epithelium to induce changes sequentially or in the competence of the preodontoblasts to act on a signal that is uniformly available. Current evidence suggests the latter, although these possibilities are not mutually exclusive.

DEPOSITION OF DENTINE MATRIX

Once fully differentiated, the odontoblast begins to secrete its characteristic organic matrix, the components of which are listed in Table 23.1. The matrix consists primarily of type I collagen fibrils. Dentine phosphoprotein (DPP) is the second most abundant constituent of the dentine organic matrix. This and dentine sialoprotein (DSP), are secreted not only by odontoblasts but also by the pre-ameloblasts of the internal dental epithelium.

Both DPP and DSP are unique to dentine and not found in bone. It has been postulated that DPP has a significant role in dentine mineralisation. DSP may also have a role, though less important, in mineralisation. It has also been suggested that DPP is involved in signalling during epithelial/mesenchymal interactions. Many other proteins (such as glycoproteins and proteoglycans) are added to the matrix. In the first formed dentine (mantle dentine), some of the matrix components may be contributed by dental pulp cells beneath the odonto-blasts. The odontoblast is still undergoing the late stages of differentiation as the first layer of dentine matrix is being deposited. Numerous cytoplasmic processes rapidly resolve into a single large process. As it is formed by odontoblasts that are still differentiating and because other cells appear to contribute to its formation, mantle dentine in the crown (and possibly the hyaline and granular layers in the root) is of somewhat different structure and probably composition than the bulk of the matrix (Fig 23.3).

The type I collagen fibres that are laid down initially lie at right angles to the future dentine–enamel junction. In sections of harshly fixed tissue stained with silver, these fibres take on a 'corkscrew' appearance (Fig. 23.4).

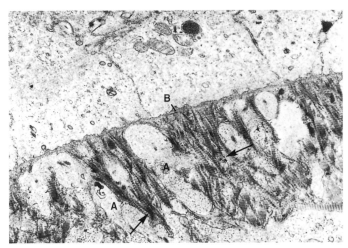

Fig. 23.3 TEM showing early dentine matrix formation. The basement membrane of the ameloblasts (B) is still present. Some components may cross the basement membrane from the ameloblasts. The odontoblasts initially have multiple processes (A) (× 9500). Courtesy of Dr P. Glick.

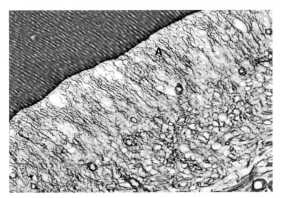

Fig. 23.4 Micrograph of a demineralised section showing 'corkscrew' fibres (of von Korff) (A). These are thought to be the first-formed type I collagen fibres whose orientation differs from those laid down later. Harsh fixation makes them curly and the deposition of silver makes then appear thick. They are thus an artefact but one based on a real difference between the structure of mantle and the later formed dentine (Silver stain; × 200).

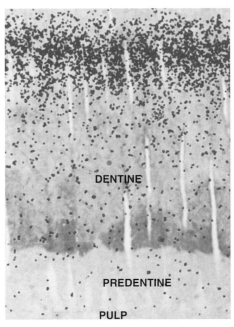

Fig. 23.5 Light microscope radioautograph of dentine formation 4 days after injection of ^{3}H-proline. A labelled band (silver grains) approximately the same width as the predentine is clearly seen, demonstrating the incremental nature of matrix deposition (Iron haematoxylin stain; × 560). Courtesy of Doctors H. Warshawsky and K. Josephsen and the editor of *Archives of Oral Biology*.

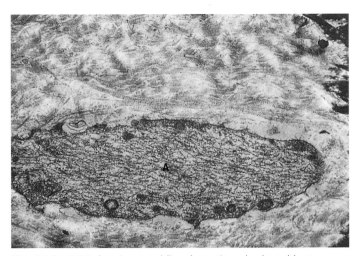

Fig. 23.6 TEM showing an obliquely sectioned odontoblast process with several vesicles near the cell membrane about to fuse with it and empty their contents into the extracellular space (× 20 000).

Once the initial mantle layer has been laid down, the bulk of the primary circumpulpal dentine is laid down in a regular incremental pattern. This pattern can be followed by observing the distribution of injected radiolabelled amino acids (Fig. 23.5). The synthetic pathways followed in the cell are those well established for the production of proteins and complex molecules that include proteins. The release of the various matrix components, however, can follow differing pathways. Type I collagen is released primarily from the odontoblast cell body as it moves inwards. Thus, the odontoblast is always closely juxtaposed to the unmineralised predentine. Dentine phosphophoryn, on the other hand, is released primarily from the odontoblast process a short distance from the cell body, consistent with its important role in mineralisation (see below) and allowing it to bypass some of the predentine (Fig. 23.6).

Once the mantle layer is formed, the remaining type I collagen is laid down with its fibres approximately parallel with the pulp dentine border. Minor, but coincident, changes in orientation about every week (20 μm) could be responsible for the long-period incremental lines (Andreson lines – see pages 137–138).

The deposition of new organic matrix proceeds at a pace similar to that of mineralisation, such that there is always a layer of unmineralised matrix, the predentine, on the pulpal surface of the tissue (Fig. 23.7). Collagen is secreted at the cell border, apparently primarily by the cell body of the odontoblast. The odontoblast process secretes the other non-collagenous proteins such that a complex of collagen and

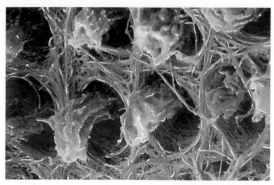

Fig. 23.7 SEM showing the surface of predentine. The collagen fibrils (brown) form an interlacing network perpendicular to the odontoblast process (blue) (× 4000). Courtesy of Professor L. Fonzi.

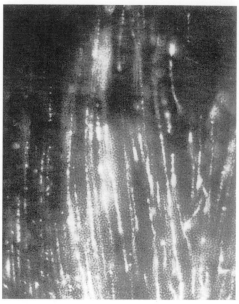

Fig. 23.9 Immunofluorescence micrograph of inner dentine close to the pulp horn stained with a labelled antibody for synaptotagmin, a protein characteristic of synapses. Its presence (white staining) and distribution in a pattern similar to nerves suggest that intradentinal nerves may be releasing a transmitter (Immunohistochemistry; × 400). Courtesy of T. Norlin, M. Hilliges and L. Brodin and the editor of *Archives of Oral Biology*.

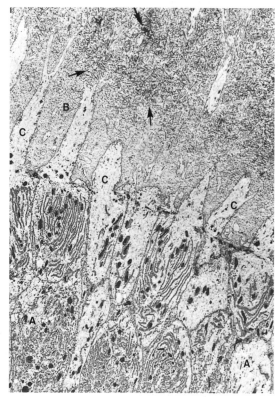

Fig. 23.8 TEM showing dentine matrix formation (B) and mineralisation. The outer matrix is mineralising (arrows), initially with small groups of crystals. The odontoblasts (A) have a single large process (C) (× 6500). Courtesy of Dr P. Glick.

internal enamel epithelium, the effect of other cell populations is unknown. The rate of dentine deposition can be altered (increased) by injury to the nerves supplying the pulp. Much of this effect could be explained as secondary to changes in blood flow or (in erupted teeth) as a result of a loss of sensory activity that might lead to greater wear on the teeth. However, proteins unique to synapses (synapsin and synaptotagmin) have been detected within dentinal tubules in regions where axons enter dentinal tubules (Fig. 23.9). It is thus possible that, in some areas at least, efferent nerve activity may have an effect on matrix secretion. The effect would likely be on secretion rather than synthesis as the synaptic proteins are absent from around the odontoblast cell body.

MINERALISATION OF DENTINE

Dentine mineralisation is a complex and controversial subject. Of the five mineralised tissues (bone, calcified cartilage, cementum, dentine and enamel), the process in enamel is unique, involving a protein matrix not found elsewhere and a two-step accumulation of mineral. In the remaining collagen-containing tissues, the process is similar but with sufficient diversity to make the structure and properties of the tissues different. The questions that are posed about mineralisation in general, and mineralisation in dentine in particular, include:

- What initiates mineralisation? The first layers of dentine matrix are unmineralised but when it reaches a certain width mineralisation begins and progresses at the same rate as matrix formation.

non-collagenous proteins is formed at the junction of the predentine and calcified dentine, the mineralisation front (Fig. 23.8). The phosphophoryns and other non-collagenous proteins bind to the collagen; the phosphophoryns bind in a highly specific manner at the 'e' band in the gap region of the type I fibrils.

What controls the secretory activity of the odontoblast is unclear. The rate of secretion varies, following both short-term (diurnal) and long-period rhythms. Serious systemic disturbances (such as birth and disease) can slow or stop it. Dentine seems to be less vulnerable to dietary deficiencies than bone. Presumably much of its activity is genetically predetermined. Once the odontoblast is separated from the

- Where does the mineral that is deposited come from? Is it transported by odontoblasts or present in the extracellular fluid?
- What controls the rate of mineralisation?
- Are the dentine crystals initially deposited at their more or less final size or do they grow?
- Are the crystals deposited in the extracellular fluid or on the fibrillar collagen of the matrix?
- Is mineralisation merely the addition of crystals to the organic matrix or does the matrix undergo changes during the deposition of mineral?
- Can variations in the mineralisation process explain some of the structural features of dentine such as mantle dentine, interglobular dentine, incremental lines and peritubular dentine?
- Does the mineralisation of secondary and tertiary dentine differ from that of primary dentine?
- How does intrapulpal mineralisation (pulp stones) occur?
- Does the remineralisation of dentine following exposure to acids or dental caries follow the same process as the original mineralisation of the tissue?
- Are defects in mineralisation a component of dentine dysplasias?

Although several hypotheses have been put forward to explain dentine mineralisation and several factors may contribute to the overall process, the key element in initiating and controlling mineralisation is clearly the odontoblast. It produces the matrix that becomes mineralised. It controls the transport and release of calcium ions. It determines the presence and distribution of the matrix components that can initiate and modulate the process. Mineralisation only occurs when odontoblasts are present.

The data from which one can attempt to develop a coherent account of dentine mineralisation have been accumulated from a variety of sources: histological and histochemical studies, biochemical analyses of the tissue at various stages and *in vitro* studies either of odontoblast-like cells or pulpal tissue maintained in culture. Molecular biological (genetic expression) data directly related to mineralisation are scarce, although, as mineralisation is so closely linked to matrix formation, the body of work available from this is highly relevant. In any experimental study the data generated are obviously related to the techniques used and no single approach can provide a complete description of a complex process. Some data from bone studies have been extrapolated to dentine.

Mineralisation of circumpulpal dentine

Odontoblasts actively transport calcium ions to the mineralisation site (Fig. 23.10). Although the precise intracellular mechanisms are not completely understood, serum calcium is taken up by the odontoblast and accumulates in the distal body and process, much of it bound to organelles rather than in the cytosol (intracellular fluid). High concentrations of calcium ions are toxic to cells but the odontoblast seems to be protected against this. Although some calcium ions reach the dentine by an extracellular pathway this is probably not the major route. The intracellular route (Fig. 23.11) of calcium

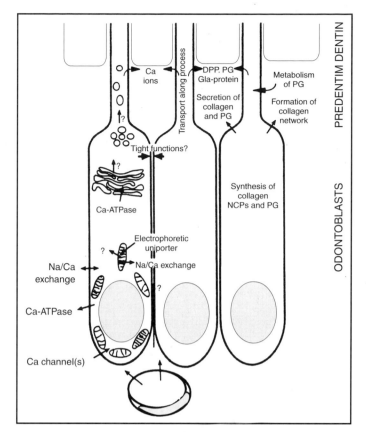

Fig. 23.10 Schematic diagram of fully differentiated active odontoblasts showing different calcium ion transport mechanisms (left side of figure) as well as putative transport routes for the dentine matrix macromolecules (right side of figure). Courtesy of Dr A Linde and the editor of the *International Journal of Developmental Biology*.

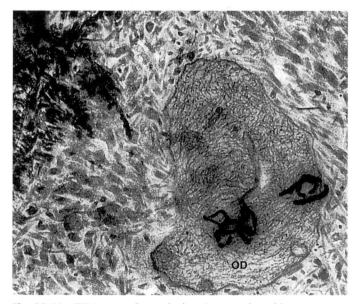

Fig. 23.11 TEM autoradiograph showing an odontoblast process near the predentine–dentine junction 30 minutes after intravenous infusion of ^{45}Ca. Note the silver grains representing this Ca over the cytoplasm of the process. The black zone at the top left corner represents mineralising dentine (× 30 000). Courtesy of Doctors R.M. Frank and N. Nagai and the editor of *Cell and Tissue Research*.

transport actively controls the level in the mineralising area and maintains calcium ion concentrations that are not in equilibrium with body fluids.

Evidence that has accumulated over about the last 20 years suggests that the calcium transported by the odontoblasts becomes a crystalline mineral in the dentine by deposition onto a template formed by type I collagen fibrils and is largely under the control of the predominant non-collagenous protein in dentine, DPP.

DPP is highly anionic and thus able to bind calcium. Changes in conformation of the protein allow it to bind increasing numbers of calcium ions, allowing the formation and growth of a crystal. In high concentrations, DPP inhibits crystal formation. Thus, by controlling the release and level of DPP, the odontoblast can control the initiation of mineralisation and the rate of deposition.

Mineral crystals first appear in the hole zone formed by the quarter-stacking of the collagen molecules. The collagen triple helices are stacked in parallel with overlapping regions and spaces between adjacent molecules. Ultrastructurally, the bulk of the dentine mineral is on the surface of the dentine collagen.

The evidence that DPP is involved in the initiation and growth of mineral includes its distribution. DPP is absent from non-mineralised matrix and concentrated at the mineralisation front. *In vitro*, it can be shown to bind calcium, induce hydroxyapatite nucleation and control crystal growth. It is absent from the dentine of patients with dentinogenesis imperfecta.

The postulated role of DPP in mineralisation may be summarised as:

1. Transport of ions to the mineralisation front.
2. Location of nucleation to specific regions of the collagen fibril surface.
3. Stabilisation of the formed crystal.

Although DPP gets the most attention as the master of mineralisation, other proteins have mineralising characteristics *in vitro* but, given their low concentrations and more limited properties, it is difficult to say how much these other proteins may contribute to the mineralisation of dentine. Osteonectin is a phosphorylated glycoprotein produced by the odontoblast and present in human dentine. *In vitro*, it can inhibit the growth of hydroxyapatite crystals and promote calcium and phosphate binding to collagen. Osteopontin is a phosphorylated protein capable of promoting mineral formation in dentine. Another phosphorylated glycoprotein, bone sialoprotein (BSP), is found in early mineralising dentine and in peritubular dentine. DSP, the other non-collagenous protein unique to dentine and the dental pulp, is a non-phosphorylated glycoprotein found predominantly in predentine and thus unlikely to be significantly involved in mineralisation. The proteoglycans chondroitin sulphates 4 and 6 are present around the collagen fibrils (together with phospholipids) throughout dentine and predentine. Their properties can vary depending on whether they are in solution (as they are in the predentine) or adsorbed onto collagen (as in mineralising dentine). In predentine, they may play a role in transport and diffusion and act as hydroxyapatite inhibitors, whereas in dentine they may promote hydroxyapatite initiation. The con-

centration of chondroitin sulphate decreases as mineralisation proceeds.

Other processes possibly involved in the initiation of mineralisation

When dentine mineralisation is initiated, two other processes have been implicated in addition to, or in place of, the DPP-mediated nucleation on collagen fibrils. Cell budding or cell fragmentation to form 'matrix vesicles' occurs in what will become mantle dentine. Membrane-bound organelles (30–200 nm) are formed, containing a variety of enzymes (including alkaline phosphatase) that lead to a concentration of phosphate ions

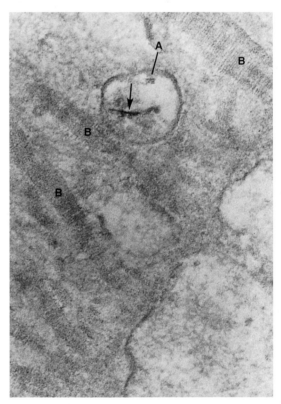

Fig. 23.12 TEM showing a matrix vesicle consisting of a membrane (A) around fluid containing a crystal (arrow) among recently deposited collagen fibres (× 70 000). Courtesy of Dr P. Glick.

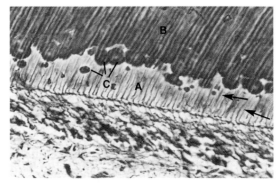

Fig. 23.13 Demineralised section showing the region of mineralising dentine. A = Predentine; B = mineralised dentine; C = calcospherites (Sudan black; × 230).

within the vesicle. Mineral crystals develop within the vesicles (Fig. 23.12). As these are the only crystalline structures present very early in mantle dentine formation, they have been credited with an initiating role in mineralisation. Similar matrix vesicles have been implicated in the initial mineralisation of bone and calcified cartilage. Mineralising material can accumulate within cells including the odontoblast process. As the odontoblast process retreats, cell debris may remain and form a nidus for mineralisation. The presence of matrix vesicles is limited to mantle dentine.

As matrix deposition and mineralisation continue, there will always be a zone of mineralisation discernible histologically (Fig. 23.13). The mineralising front often appears irregular: in some areas, mineralisation appears to progress linearly by apposition onto previously mineralised areas, while in others it seems to occur in spheres that eventually fuse (Figs 23.14, 23.15). In yet other situations, mineralisation is a combination of the two (Fig. 23.13). These mineralisation patterns can be visualised when the mineralising front is highlighted by the antibiotic tetracycline (Fig. 23.16).

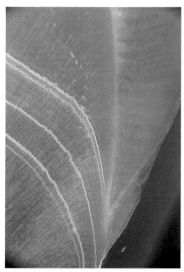

Fig. 23.16   Ground section of a tooth viewed with fluorescent light. The incremental nature of mineralisation is demonstrated in an individual who has been treated with tetracycline. Tetracycline binds to the mineral as it is deposited and is represented by the bright yellow lines, indicating that the patient has had multiple injections of the antibiotic. The irregularity of the line indicates both calcospheritic and linear patterns of mineralisation. This can lead to the discoloration of teeth, and the use of tetracycline should be avoided during the period of tooth development. Tetracycline also fluoresces under ultraviolet light (Ground section, fluorescent light; × 5). Courtesy of Dr B.A.W. Brown.

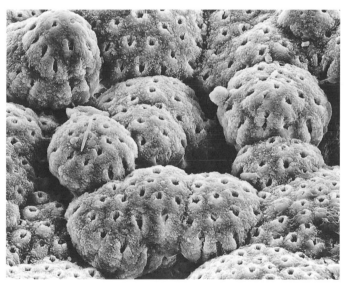

Fig. 23.14   SEM illustrating calcospherites at the mineralising front. In this preparation all the organic material (including the predentine) has been removed by hypochlorite to reveal the underlying mineralised dentine (× 1500). Courtesy of Professor M.C. Dean.

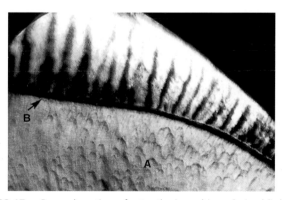

Fig. 23.17   Ground section of a tooth viewed in polarised light. Calcospherites (A) are distributed widely in circumpulpal dentine. The changes in crystal orientation at the boundary of the original crystallites differ and differentially block the polarised light. In single-phase light at this orientation the mantle layer completely blocks transmission and thus appears black (B) (× 25).

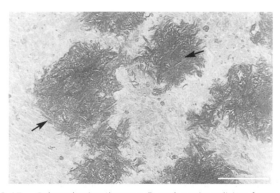

Fig. 23.15   Calcospherites (arrowed) at the mineralising front of dentine (TEM; × 1450).

Owing to the complex biochemical changes occurring at the mineralising front, it often stains differently and has been referred to as intermediate dentine.

The pattern of calcospherite formation is common throughout dentine. It is possible that some form around matrix vesicles, especially in the first-formed mantle dentine, but the widespread nature of the calcospherites and the rarity of matrix vesicles suggest that such a pattern of accretion also occurs around centres of initial mineralisation that form on collagen fibrils. Failure of such calcospherites to fuse may result in the

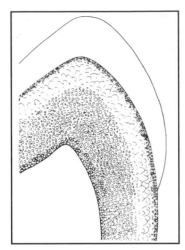

Fig. 23.18 The distribution of calcospherites in dentine. Most calcospherites are spherical. However, many have an arcade shape such that the round apex of the arcade is directed towards the outer surface of the dentine, and the opening is directed towards the pulp. The size varies considerably: the arcade variety tends to be larger than the spherical variety. The size and shape of the calcospherites seem to be governed by the rate of dentine formation and by the rate at which new calcospherites are initiated. There is a fairly consistent pattern of distribution within the tooth. In the mantle dentine of the crown, in the hyaline layer of the root and in the superficial circumpulpal dentine, the calcospherites are small, spherical and closely packed. In the middle region of the circumpulpal dentine they are larger, more widely spaced and arcade-like in form (although the region tends to be free of calcospherites towards the root apex). The inner half to two-thirds of the circumpulpal dentine contains spherical calcospherites. Courtesy of Dr R.P. Shellis and the publishers of *The companion to dental studies*, Vol 2, Blackwell, Oxford.

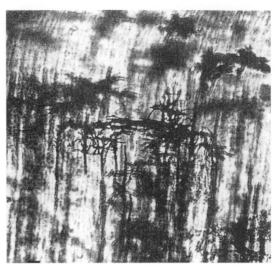

Fig. 23.19 Ground section of root showing evidence of looping and branching of dentine tubules in the granular layer of the root. In this preparation, the dentinal tubules have become filled with a silver stain and the tissue has been examined in a thicker than normal section. While this obscures much fine detail by superimposition, it does allow some insight into the three-dimensional arrangement. The peripheral terminations of several tubules may be seen, and a profuse branching in three dimensions can be distinguished. Above the tubules in focus are others below the plane of focus. Here, it may be seen how this arrangement could contribute to the appearance of the granular layer (Silver stain; × 490).

appearance of 'interglobular' dentine, often seen in peripheral dentine (see pages 135–136). In calcospherites, the crystallites are arranged in a radiating pattern and, despite complete mineralisation of the dentine, their outline can still be discerned using polarised light (Fig. 23.17). The size and shape of the calcospherites generally varies in different regions (Fig. 23.18).

FORMATION OF ROOT DENTINE

The basic process of root dentinogenesis does not differ fundamentally from coronal dentinogenesis. Such differences as do occur are in the early stages such that the histological appearance of the peripheral dentine differs between crown and root. These are, presumably, due to differing contributions in terms of control and content from the internal enamel epithelium of the crown, which will go on to form enamel, and the epithelial root sheath, which, after initiating radicular dentinogenesis does not undergo further differentiation but fragments. Initial collagen deposition does not begin in the root immediately against the basal lamina of the epithelial cells of the root sheath. The space between the initial collagen and the epithelial cells becomes filled with an amorphous ground substance and a fine, fibrillar, non-collagenous matrix

secreted by the root sheath comprising, in part, enamel-like proteins. These elements form a hyaline layer of approximately 10 μm. In the past, this has been described as a component of either dentine or cementum; it is discussed further on pages 340–342. The initial collagen fibres deposited in the root lie approximately parallel to the cement–dentine junction. This contrasts with the mantle dentine in the crown, where the collagen fibres are deposited perpendicular to the enamel– dentine junction. Radicular odontoblasts differ slightly from those in the crown, developing several fine branches which loop in umbrella fashion (Fig. 23.19). This gives rise to the appearance of the granular layer (of Tomes), although this may, in part, be due to the presence of many small, unmineralised interglobular areas. The loss of continuity of the epithelial cells as the root sheath breaks down results in larger numbers of interglobular areas and, possibly, also in the incorporation of some epithelial remnants in the peripheral dentine. Radicular dentine forms at a slightly slower rate than coronal dentine. Its pattern of mineralisation is similar, although its initial calcospherites are smaller and its interglobular areas more numerous. In general, root mineralisation proceeds as a continuation of that in the crown although, in multirooted teeth, separate isolated areas of mineralisation may occur. Unusually there is evidence that the first-formed root dentine undergoes delayed mineralisation compared with the root dentine formed a little later; this may be related to its bonding with the cementum (see pages 136–137).

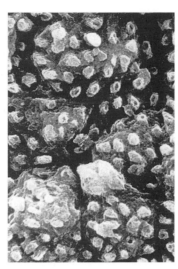

Fig. 23.20 SEM of anorganic preparation of the surface of mineralising dentine in the opossum. Projecting localised white zones of peritubular dentine are visible, which therefore are forming (in this species) before the adjacent intertubular dentine (× 1000). Courtesy of N. Azevedo and M. Goldberg and the editor of *Journal de Biologie Buccale*.

FORMATION OF THE LATER DENTINES: PERITUBULAR, SECONDARY AND TERTIARY DENTINES

Peritubular (intratubular) dentine

Peritubular dentine (see pages 128–130) consists of small crystals in an amorphous (non-fibrillar) matrix consisting of glycoproteins, proteoglycans, lipids, osteonectin, osteocalcin and bone sialoprotein. Despite the difference in composition, there is structural continuity between the peritubular and intertubular dentine.

The composition of the peritubular dentine suggests that it is a product of the odontoblast and plasma proteins that have diffused along the cell membrane. Evidence that it is physiological rather than a result of degeneration or retreat of the odontoblast includes:

- The presence of small tubules in it representing where lateral processes of the odontoblast once were.
- The occasional finding histologically of odontoblast processes surrounded by peritubular dentine.
- The occurrence in two species, the elephant and opossum, of peritubular dentine formation preceding intertubular dentine formation (Fig. 23.20).

Although much is known about the composition of peritubular dentine and a reasonable description of its origin established, little is known about either the signal that initiates the onset of tubular occlusion or what controls its rate of deposition. It would seem likely that age is the principal factor. The degree of tubular occlusion (as measured by the presence of translucent dentine, particularly in the root) can be used to determine the age of teeth and is applied in forensic circumstances. Peritubular dentine formation does not seem to be related to outside stimuli. The rate of tubular occlusion by peritubular dentine formation beneath dental caries is little different from that in intact teeth. Tubules directly beneath caries can become occluded, but this is thought to be due to the reprecipitation of mineral during the demineralisation process that characterises dental caries (Fig. 23.21). In older teeth, peritubular dentine formation is usually most pronounced near the root apices, remote from areas of attrition or caries. Until more detail is known about the switching of odontoblast production from intertubular to peritubular it is best attributed to a preprogrammed genetic trigger.

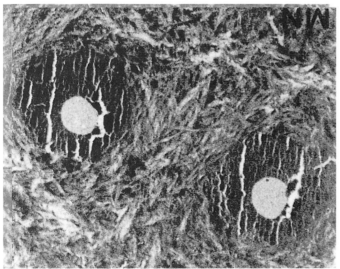
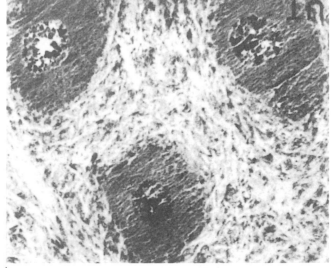

a   b

Fig. 23.21 Peritubular dentine (a) and sclerotic dentine (b). In sclerotic dentine, a second form of crystal formation, whitlockite, can fill in the tubules within, but distinct from, the peritubular dentine (TEM; × 10 000). Courtesy of Dr T. Fusayama and the editor of *Journal de Biologie Buccale*.

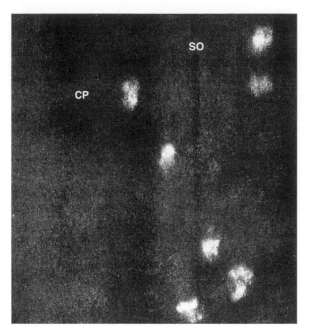

Fig. 23.22 Confocal microscope image showing apoptotic (dying) cells in the subodontoblastic region (SO) of the coronal pulp (CP). The cells have been fluorescently labelled (white) with a stain unique for dying cells (× 60). Courtesy of J-C. Franquin and the editor of the *European Journal of Oral Science*.

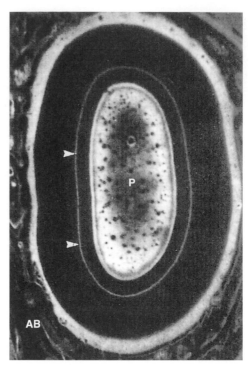

Fig. 23.23 Demineralised transverse section of a cat canine 30 days after denervation viewed with a fluorescence microscope. The animal was injected with tetracyline at the time of denervation. The arrowed line shows the dentine that has incorporated the tetracyline. Regular secondary dentine has formed after this point at a rate faster than in non-denervated teeth. The increase in rate is transient and, by 180 days post-denervation, the amount of secondary dentine deposited in control and operated teeth is the same. P = dental pulp; AB = alveolar bone (× 10). Courtesy of L. Olgart and the editor of the *European Journal of Oral Sciences*.

Secondary dentine

As noted earlier in this chapter, the original odontoblasts form secondary dentine that, like peritubular dentine, seems to be a preprogrammed age change rather than a response to external activity. Part of this may be attributed to apoptosis (Fig. 23.22). As the pulp volume decreases with continuing dentine deposition, odontoblasts die. Over a 4-year period, the odontoblast population may be reduced by 50%. This dramatic reduction in numbers also presumably leads to the change in direction of the tubules, establishing a contour line (of Owen) – page 128.

Experimental denervation results in increased secondary dentine formation (Fig. 23.23). This may be mediated by changes in blood flow, although a direct trophic effect is possible. It is not known whether the innervation has an influence physiologically on the formation of either primary or secondary dentine.

Tertiary dentine formation

The nature and severity of stimuli that reach the dental pulp vary over a considerable range. The nature of the response will reflect this variability: severe stimuli will result in pulpal necrosis; less severe stimuli will induce the production of tertiary dentine with a range of histological appearances (pages 141–142). There is much interest in the mechanism of tertiary dentine formation as, if its production could be clinically induced or enhanced, it may be possible to protect a challenged pulp (see also pages 141–142).

The key difference between secondary and tertiary dentine is that, while secondary dentine is produced by the original primary odontoblasts, tertiary dentine is produced after these have died and arises from cells newly differentiated from the pulpal mesenchyme. Throughout life, cells in the peripheral dental pulp retain the ability to divide and differentiate into hard tissue-forming cells. These cells differentiate and secrete extracellular matrix in response to factors released by caries or other insults. One important difference between the activity of these new odontoblasts and those involved in primary and secondary dentine formation is that the new cells do not form dentine phosphophoryn. This molecule, apparently so important to the production of primary dentine, seems to have no role in the making of tertiary dentine. The effect of signalling molecules, especially TGF-β and BMPs, may be important in tertiary dentine formation. One hypothesis suggests that members of the TGF-β family present in dentine and predentine may be released by acids produced by dental plaque and diffuse to induce changes in the subodontoblastic cells. Differences in the nature of the response product could be attributed to differences in the nature, amount and direction of the signalling molecules. TGF-β stimulation seems to result in the production of a more tubular tissue, BMPs in a more bone-like product. Atubular tertiary dentine is more common beneath more aggressively progressing carious lesions.

INHERITED DEFECTS IN DENTINE

Serious disease occurring during the period of tooth development can result in the disturbance of both matrix formation and its mineralisation, which would usually be reflected in both the dentine and the enamel that were forming at the time. There are two groups of inherited defects that are limited to dentine, dentinogenesis imperfecta (DI) types I and II (Figs 23.24, 23.25) and dentine dysplasia (DD) I and II. Both dysplasias result in incomplete obliteration of the pulp cham-ber with histologically abnormal root dentine (DD I has irregular, sparse tubules; DD II aberrantly oriented tubules). DD I but not DD II causes stunted roots. Both forms of DI result in similar changes but in addition the morphology of the tooth crown is bulbous. DI types I and II are distinguished by type I occurring as part of a more widespread connective tissue disease, osteogenesis imperfecta. In all these disorders the odontoblasts seem to be incompletely developed and it is possible that the production of dentine phosphophoryn is defective.

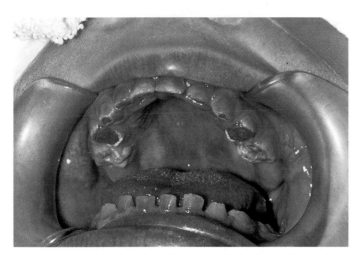

Fig. 23.24 A patient with dentinogenesis imperfecta. The teeth are malformed and are dark due to the absence of pulp chambers and consequent loss of translucency. The enamel is normal but flakes off as it is only weakly attached to the dentine. In this example the enamel from the first molars has been lost. Courtesy of M. Ignelzi.

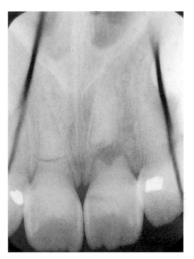

23.25 An intraoral radiograph of the upper central incisors from a patient with dentinogenesis imperfecta. There are no pulp chambers or root canals. Both central incisors have fractured due to their high fragility. Courtesy of M. Ignelzi.

24 Development of the dental pulp

At the bud stage of tooth germ development a region of more densely packed mesenchymal cells becomes evident around the developing enamel organ (Fig. 24.1). Some of these cells will form the dental papilla and later the dental pulp. They are of mixed origin: those destined to become odontoblasts are derived from the neural crest (ectomesenchyme) and are thus ectodermal in origin; others are of mesenchymal origin. With routine staining, all the cells in this condensation look similar. They are more densely packed than surrounding mesenchyme as they are more rapidly dividing and are separated by relatively little extracellular matrix. This mass of cells expands around the tooth bud (see Fig. 21.6). Once the bud-stage enamel organ invaginates to become the cap stage, the cells and matrix within the invagination are distinguished as the dental papilla (Fig. 24.2). During growth of the tooth germ, although undifferentiated, the expansion of the dental papilla exerts a morphogenetic effect on the enamel organ (see page 301). The mesenchymal cells surrounding the developing enamel organ externally form the dental follicle that will give rise to the periodontal ligament and supporting tissues of the tooth (see Chapter 25). As the enamel organ surrounding the dental papilla enlarges and enters the bell stage (Fig. 24.3), the cells within the dental papilla undergo cytodifferentiation into a peripheral layer of odontoblasts and a central mass of fibroblasts. This change is induced by signals originating in the internal enamel epithelium (see Chapter 23). Immature dendritic antigen-presenting cells appear in, and around, the odontoblast layer at an early stage (Fig. 24.4). Once the odontoblasts

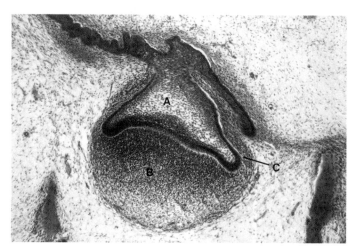

Fig. 24.2 An enamel organ at the cap stage of development (A) surrounding the mesenchymal cells of the dental papilla (B). The tooth germ is surrounded by the developing dental follicle (C) (H & E; × 80). Courtesy of Professor M. Smith.

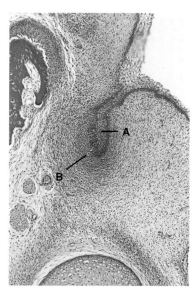

Fig. 24.1 A developing enamel organ at the early bud stage (A), with a condensation of mesenchymal cells (B) around it (Masson's trichrome stain; × 80).

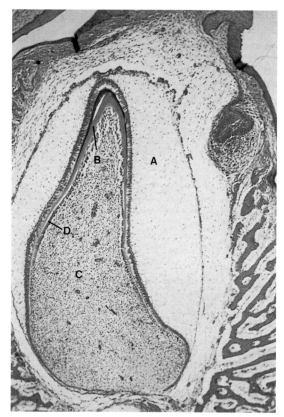

Fig. 24.3 A developing tooth at the late bell stage of development (appositional phase). A = Enamel organ; B = developing dentine; C = dental papilla; D = odontoblast layer (Masson's trichrome; × 55).

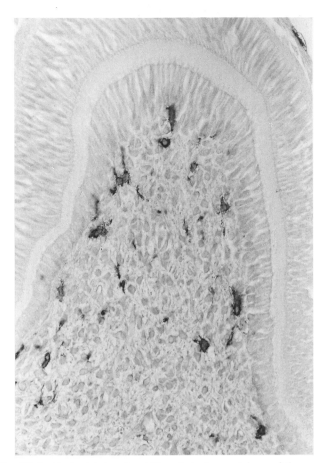

Fig. 24.4 Dark-staining dendritic cells in the periphery of the developing pulp (rat molar, post-natal day 1, immunohistochemistry; × 300). Courtesy of Doctors E. Tsuruga, Y. Sakahura, T. Yajima and N. Shide and the editor of *Histochemistry and Cell Biology*.

have begun to lay down dentine, the dental papilla becomes, by convention, the dental pulp. The small, undifferentiated, ectomesenchymal cells of the dental papilla are packed closely together with little intercellular material content relative to that in the mature tooth. They are stellate in shape with a relatively large nucleus and little cytoplasm. As the pulp develops, the cytoplasmic component of these central cells expands and synthetic organelles appear. The material the organelles produce is released into the extracellular space and forms fine collagen fibres that are embedded in an amorphous ground substance. Coarse fibre bundles appear only at about the time that the tooth reaches maturity. In the early stages of pulpal development, the ground substance has a high glycosaminoglycan content relative to that of the mature tooth. The level of glycosaminoglycans increases until the time of eruption and then decreases. The chondroitin sulphates are the main glycosaminoglycans present during pulp development, with only a minor quantity of hyaluronan. This balance is reversed in the mature pulp. Not all cells undergo differentiation, a proportion remaining as undifferentiated mesenchymal cells retaining the potential to differentiate in later life.

Dentinogenesis then progresses by the processes described in Chapter 23 but at the same time differentiation continues as the enamel organ extends as Hertwig's epithelial root sheath and determines the final morphology of the space (pulp chamber

and root canals) that the dental pulp will occupy. The actions and interactions of the dental follicle (outside the epithelial root sheath), the epithelial root sheath and the dental papilla result in the formation of cementum (described in Chapter 25) on the surface of the developing root dentine. Once the full length of the root is established the developmental stage of the dental pulp can be considered complete. However, dentine deposition will continue throughout life. A cell-rich zone develops beneath the odontoblast layer at the time of eruption. It arises by the migration of more central cells rather than by local cell division. A cell-free zone may be evident in the crown of the tooth at the time of eruption, although some believe this may be a fixation artefact. The dental pulp retains the potential to differentiate new odontoblasts and deposit reparative forms of dentine (see pages 138–142) in response to attrition, dental caries or other stimuli.

BLOOD SUPPLY

Vascularisation of the developing pulp starts during the early bell stage, with small branches from the principal vascular trunks of the jaws entering the base of the papilla. Of these small pioneer vessels, a few become the principal pulpal vessels, enlarge and run through the pulp towards the cuspal regions. Here the vessels give off numerous small branches which form a bed of venules, arterioles and capillaries in the subodontoblast and odontoblast layers (Fig. 24.5). The vascularity of the odontoblast layer increases as dentine is progressively laid down, probably as the result of the odontoblasts migrating inwards through the vascular bed (Fig. 24.6). Eventually, some capillaries are found immediately next to the predentine surface, occasionally looping into the developing dentine (Fig. 24.7). The time and pattern of appearance of lymphatics in the pulp has not yet been established. The mature pulp contains macrophages, pericytes and lymphoid cells that probably enter the pulp with the invading blood vessels.

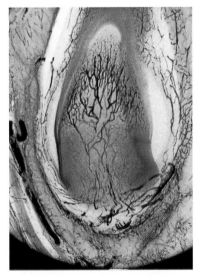

Fig. 24.5 The vascular pattern within the dental papilla at the late bell stage of development. The vascular system has been perfused with Indian ink (H & E; × 40). Courtesy of Dr D. Adams.

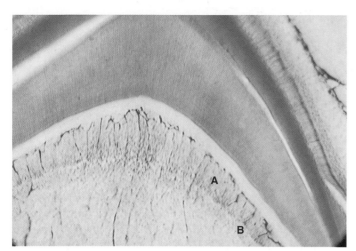

Fig. 24.6 The vascular plexuses beneath the developing cusp. A = Odontoblast layer; B = subodontoblastic plexus. The vascular system has been perfused with Indian ink (H & E; × 100). Courtesy of Dr D. Adams.

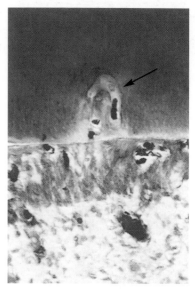

Fig. 24.7 A capillary looping (arrow) into developing dentine (Masson's trichrome; × 20).

NERVE SUPPLY

Although nerves are present close to the tooth germ from the very earliest stages of its development, they do not enter the dental papilla until much later, after they have entered the dental follicle. The first fibres to enter the developing pulp are from the trigeminal nerve and are located close to the blood vessels. These nerves, although anatomically part of the sensory nervous system, play an important role in controlling blood flow and, perhaps via this and possibly also by direct trophic effects, may influence development.

Neurotrophins, nerve growth factor and brain-derived neurotrophic factor are expressed in the periphery of the developing dental pulp in the odontoblast layer (Fig. 24.8), suggesting that this region is the principal target of the trigeminal innervation. The sympathetic innervation follows later and is restricted largely to the radicular pulp. A large number of nerves enter the pulp before root formation, but the final pattern, including the formation of the subodontoblastic plexus (of Raschkow), is not established until root formation is complete. In the crown, particularly at the cusps, some sensory fibres insinuate themselves between the odontoblasts and enter dentinal tubules. This is an active process and not a merely a trapping of these axons during progressive dentine deposition.

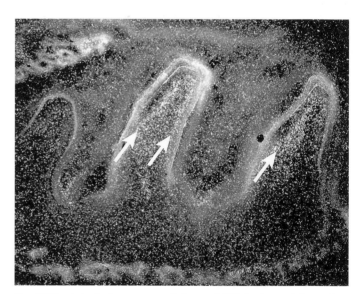

Fig. 24.8 Labelled nerve growth factor (NGF) in the periphery of the developing dental pulp (Rat molars 2 days post-natal). Messenger RNA for NGF has been radioactively labelled by *in-situ* hybridisation and viewed under dark-field illumination. Under these conditions mineralised tissue appears as a bright solid (arrow heads) and NGF mRNA as bright granules (× 20). Courtesy of Dr C. Nosrat and the editor of the *European Journal of Oral Science*.

25 Development of the root and periodontal ligament

Root development proceeds some time after the crown has formed and involves interactions between the dental follicle, a structure derived from the cervical loop region of the enamel organ (see page 293) called the epithelial root sheath (of Hertwig), and the dental papilla. The onset of root development coincides with the axial phase of tooth eruption.

Single and multirooted teeth are formed in the manner shown in Fig. 25.1. At the late bell stage of tooth development, when amelogenesis and dentinogenesis are well advanced, the external and internal enamel epithelia at the cervical loop of the enamel organ form a double-layered epithelial root sheath (see Fig. 25.3), which proliferates apically to map out the shape of the future root. The primary apical foramen at the growing end of the epithelial root sheath may subdivide into a number of secondary apical foramina by the ingrowth of epithelial shelves from the margins of the root sheath (arrowed region in Fig. 25.1), which subsequently fuse near the centre of the root. The number and location of these epithelial shelves correspond to the number and location of the definitive roots of the tooth, and may be under the inductive control of the

dental papilla. It has been suggested that the ingrowth of the epithelial shelves takes place along paths of low vascularity.

When a permanent tooth first erupts only about two-thirds of the length of the root is complete. A wide, 'open' root apex is present in these situations, surrounded by a thin, regular knife-edge of dentine (Fig. 25.2). It takes about 3 more years for root completion to occur, when only a very narrow pulp opening exists. The addition of root increments may result in the appearance of fine lines running transversely around the root.

During root development (Fig. 25.3) growth of the **epithelial root sheath** occurs to enclose the dental papilla, except for an opening at the base (the primary apical foramen). Beneath the dental papilla the epithelial sheath usually appears angled to form the root diaphragm. Note that, between the two epithelial layers, there is no stellate reticulum or stratum intermedium (see pages 293–294 for a description of these tissues in the developing tooth germ). The occasional presence of stellate reticulum and stratum intermedium is said to account for the presence of localised areas of enamel (enamel pearls) on the root surface, usually in interradicular

Fig. 25.1 The formation of a single-rooted tooth (A), a two-rooted tooth (B) and a three-rooted tooth (C). Small red circles indicate vascular concentrations.

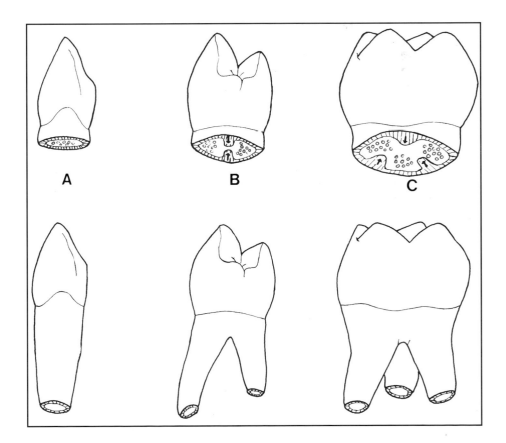

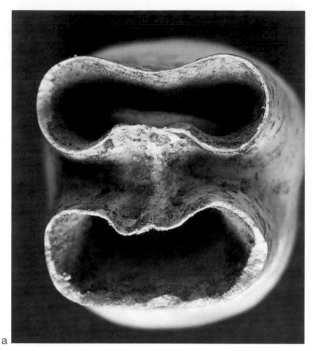
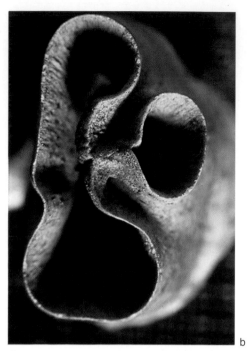

Fig. 25.2 Apices of developing roots. (a) Two-rooted tooth; (b) three-rooted tooth.

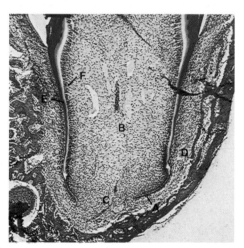

Fig. 25.3 The developing root. A = Epithelial root sheath; B = dental papilla; C = primary apical foramen; D = dental follicle; E = developing root dentine; F = odontoblast layer (H & E; × 32).

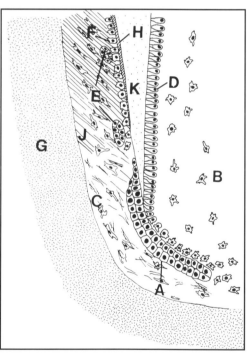

Fig. 25.4 Schematic drawing of the developing root. A = Epithelial root sheath; B = dental papilla; C = dental follicle; D = odontoblasts; E = epithelial rests; F = cementoblasts; G = developing alveolar bone; H = developing cementum; J = developing periodontal ligament; K = root dentine.

regions (see page 348). The **dental follicle** lies external to the root sheath and forms cementum, periodontal ligament and alveolar bone.

In the region of the root diaphragm, the epithelial root sheath is seen as a continuous sheet of tissue sandwiched between the undifferentiated mesenchyme of the dental papilla and the dental follicle (Fig. 25.4). Above the root diaphragm, towards the developing crown, the cells of the internal layer of the epithelial sheath induce the peripheral cells of the dental papilla to differentiate into odontoblasts. Following the onset of dentinogenesis in the root, the epithelial cells of the root sheath lose their continuity, becoming separated from the surface of the developing root dentine to form epithelial rests in the periodontal ligament (see page 194). The mesenchymal cells of the dental follicle adjacent to the root dentine now differentiate into cementoblasts, and cementogenesis commences. Some evidence is appearing, however, to suggest that the epithelial cells of the sheath might also differentiate into the first-formed cementoblast (or cementoblast-like) cells.

Fig. 25.5 shows the apical region of the developing root, periodontal ligament and alveolus. The tissues of the dental

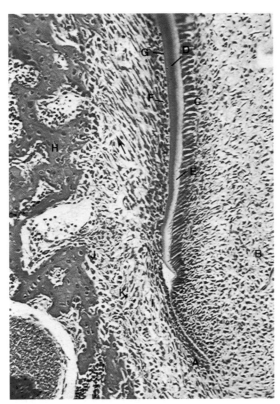

Fig. 25.5 The apical region of the developing root, periodontal ligament and alveolus. A = Epithelial root sheath; B = dental papilla; C = odontoblasts; D = dentine of root; E = predentine layer; F = cementoblasts; G = developing cementum; H = developing alveolar bone; I = inner investing layer of dental follicle; J = outer layer of the dental follicle; K = intermediate layer of dental follicle. Arrow indicates oblique orientation of follicular tissue with formation of cementum (H & E; × 150).

follicle in the developing root have been described as comprising three layers (see Fig. 21.10). Adjacent to the epithelial root sheath is the inner investing layer of the dental follicle, which is said to be derived from ectomesenchyme (neural crest). Adjacent to the developing alveolar bone is the outer layer of the dental follicle, which is separated from the inner layer by an intermediate layer. Unlike the tissues of the inner layer, the outer and intermediate layers are said to be mesodermal in origin; their cells contain few cytoplasmic organelles and the extracellular compartment appears relatively structureless. Cells of the inner layer of the dental follicle differentiate into the cementoblasts, which form a layer of cuboidal cells on the surface of the root dentine. In primary acellular cementum, where the collagen is of the extrinsic fibre type (see page 172), the cementoblasts contribute little material towards the extracellular matrix of the tissue. Later, with the formation of intrinsic fibre cementum, the cementoblasts will also secrete collagen. Once cementogenesis has begun, cells of the remaining dental follicle become obliquely oriented along the root surface and show an increased content of intracellular organelles, becoming the fibroblasts of the periodontal ligament. These fibroblasts secrete collagen into the extracellular compartment, which becomes embedded in the developing cementum at the tooth surface and in the bone at the alveolar surface.

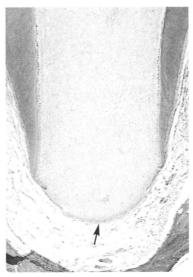

Fig. 25.6 The pulp-limiting membrane (arrowed) (Mallory's trichrome; × 30). Courtesy of Dr D. Adams.

There has been controversy concerning the connective tissue immediately beneath the developing root apex. Initially called the cushion hammock ligament, this connective tissue was described as a fibrous network with fluid-filled interstices, with attachments on either side to the alveolar wall. It was thought to provide a resistant base so that forces produced by the growing root were prevented from causing bone resorption and were resolved into an eruptive force. This view is no longer held – the thin fibrous membrane seen in this site is not attached to alveolar bone, but merges at the sides with the fibres of the developing periodontal ligament. Perhaps, therefore, the structure is more correctly termed the pulp-limiting membrane (Fig. 25.6). It does not appear to be directly involved in tooth eruption as its surgical removal (together with the developing root apex) does not affect eruption.

It has been suggested that changes in vascular permeability in the connective tissues around the apex of the developing root can be related to eruptive behaviour. Dense accumulations of tissue fluid (effusions) have been described beneath the growing roots of erupting teeth. Furthermore, when radioactive fibrinogen was used experimentally as a marker, the radioactive label became incorporated rapidly into the effusions, supporting the view that they are vascular in origin. Because effusions were seen to appear when the growing root was situated close to the base (fundus) of the bony tooth socket/crypt, it has been suggested that the effusions might force the root and bone apart and thereby contribute to eruption and enable further root growth. The vascular hypothesis of eruption is considered further on page 355.

FORMATION OF COLLAGEN FIBRES WITHIN THE PERIODONTAL LIGAMENT

The development of the principal periodontal ligament collagen fibres is illustrated in Fig. 25.7. Significant differences in development have been described for teeth of the deciduous/primary dentition (and also the permanent molars

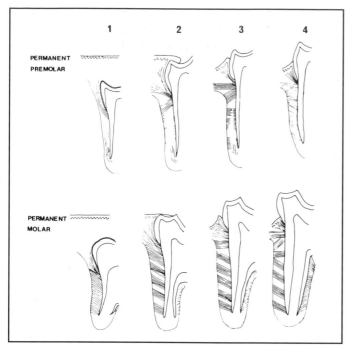

Fig. 25.7 The development of the principal periodontal ligament collagen fibres. See text for description of Stages 1–4.

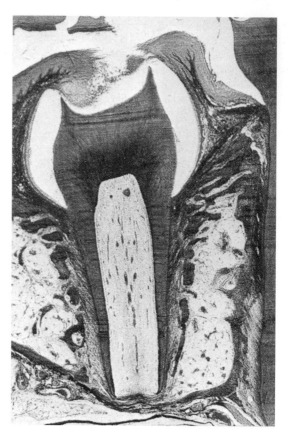

Fig. 25.8 Erupting permanent molar (of a marmoset, *Callithrix jacchus*) just emerging into the oral cavity. Note the presence of periodontal ligament fibres (Mallory's; × 15). Courtesy of Professor D.A. Grant and the editor of the *Journal of Periodontology*.

which lack successors) and successional or succedaneous teeth (i.e. permanent premolars).

Stage 1. Before eruption the dentogingival and oblique periodontal fibres are well developed in the permanent molar. In the permanent premolar only the dentogingival fibres are organised, the developing periodontal ligament being composed of loosely structured collagenous elements.

Stage 2. As the tooth emerges into the oral cavity, the periodontal ligament of the permanent molar is well differentiated, the oblique fibres being the most conspicuous. However, at this stage in the permanent premolar only the fibres in the region of the alveolar crest are becoming organised. In the periodontal ligament itself, although collagen fibres are developing, they do not yet span the periodontal space.

Stage 3. On reaching occlusion, the fibre groupings in the cervical region of the permanent molar now become organised. In the permanent premolar, while the fibre groups cervically appear prominent, those in the apical part of the root appear relatively undeveloped.

Stage 4. After a period in function, the fibres of both the permanent molar and premolar show the classical organisation of the principal fibres.

In an erupting permanent molar (of a marmoset, *Callithrix jacchus*) just emerging into the oral cavity (Fig. 25.8), the coronal half of the periodontal ligament is composed of well formed, obliquely orientated, principal collagen fibre bundles. In contrast, the bulk of the periodontal ligament of an erupting permanent premolar (of a squirrel monkey, *Saimiri sciureus*) (Fig. 25.9) lacks significant numbers of organised principal collagen fibre bundles passing from the tooth to alveolar bone.

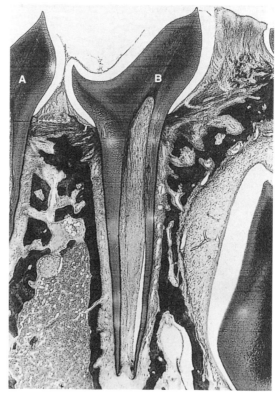

Fig. 25.9 Erupting permanent premolar (of a squirrel monkey, *Saimiri sciureus*) just emerging into the oral cavity. Note the absence of periodontal ligament fibres (Mallory's; × 35). Courtesy of Professor D.A. Grant and the editor of the *Journal of Periodontology*.

It appears, therefore, that collagen fibres may not be well organised during eruption, and this could be significant if it is assumed that collagen has an important role in the generation of tractional forces during eruption (see page 353). However, recent evidence indicates that there are species differences in the ontogeny of principal collagen fibres: for some species, the fibres associated with succedaneous teeth pass between tooth and bone as the tooth erupts into the oral cavity. In a permanent canine (of the ferret, *Mustela putorius*) erupting into the oral cavity, the principal collagen fibres are seen passing from tooth to bone (Fig. 25.10). This contrasts with the development of the primate periodontal ligament shown in Fig. 25.9. However, the fibres are not as well organised (in terms of thickness and orientation) as those for the fully erupted tooth illustrated in Fig. 25.11.

There is evidence of a change in the obliquity of the principal collagen fibres, and in their dimensions, as the tooth reaches its functional position. The inclination of the oblique fibres has been reported to decrease, while the principal fibres are said to thicken with function. However, there may again be species differences.

There appear to be few structural differences between fibroblasts in the developing periodontal ligaments of erupting and fully erupted teeth. However, changes during eruption have been reported for the non-fibrous extracellular matrix elements and the vascularity of the periodontal ligament (see page 356).

As the tooth erupts, resorption is the predominant pattern of bone activity at the base of the socket (i.e. beneath the developing root). Thus, bone deposition at this site is precluded as a cause of tooth eruption. There are species differences however, bone deposition being found beneath the erupting permanent premolars of dogs. The different patterns of bone activity in different species may relate to the distance a tooth has to erupt: if the distance is greater than the length of the root then bone deposition is clearly necessary to maintain the normal dimensions of the periodontal ligament at the root apex of the tooth. Remodelling of alveolar bone other than at the socket's base may also be seen during eruption and this relates to the relocation of the teeth during jaw growth and to the establishment of occlusion.

CEMENTOGENESIS

Cementogenesis will be considered in terms of the formation of primary (acellular) cementum and then of secondary (cellular) cementum (see Chapter 11). There may be differences between the cells forming each type of cementum. Our understanding is clouded by species differences resulting in problems in terminology, particularly for the structures related to the cementum–dentine interface (see page 136). As for the crown of the tooth, the hard tissues that comprise the root (cementum and dentine) develop under the control of epithelial–mesenchymal interactions (see pages 297–302). However, unlike that of the crown, the epithelial component involved in root formation retains a simpler morphology,

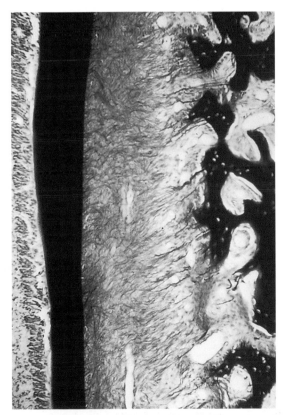

Fig. 25.10 Principal collagen fibres associated with an erupting permanent canine (of the ferret, *Mustela putorius*) as it emerges into the oral cavity (aldehyde fuchsin and van Giesen; × 150).

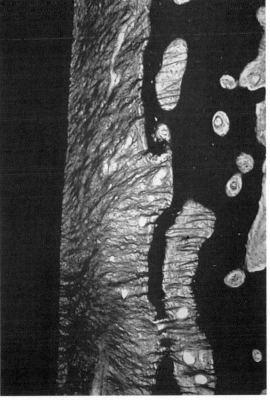

Fig. 25.11 Well differentiated collagen fibres for the fully erupted permanent canine of the ferret (*Mustela putorius*) (aldehyde fuchsin and van Giesen; × 130).

rapidly loses its continuity with adjacent cells and is not evident as a conspicuous layer during cementum formation. Although it was once thought that its function was primarily to induce the formation of root odontoblasts, present evidence also indicates an important role in cementogenesis. As the aim of periodontologists is now not only to repair the ravages of periodontal disease but also to try to actually regenerate the tissues lost, there has been a resurgence of interest in how cementum forms. It is only through a thorough understanding of this process that clinical strategies can be developed to encourage the regeneration of cementum.

Primary (acellular) cementum

Once the crown has fully formed, the internal and external enamel epithelia proliferate downwards as a double-layered sheet of somewhat flattened epithelial cells, the epithelial root sheath (of Hertwig) to map out the shape of the root(s) (see Figs 25.1 and 25.12). The process of cementogenesis that will be described initially takes place at the cervical margin and extends apically as the root grows downwards. The cells of the epithelial root sheath, in contrast to those of the enamel organ during enamel formation, do not enlarge during this inductive stage. The epithelial root sheath is separated by a basal lamina on both of its surfaces from the adjacent connective tissues of the dental follicle and dental papilla. The epithelial root sheath induces the adjacent cells of the dental papilla to differentiate

into odontoblasts. As these odontoblasts initially retreat inwards, they synthesise and secrete the collagenous organic matrix of the first-formed root predentine. Although many collagen fibrils are oriented perpendicular to the surface, others are aligned more obliquely, allowing the layer to be later distinguished from the rest of the root dentine using polarised light (see page 137). As the odontoblasts do not leave behind an odontoblast process in this initial few microns of tissue (Fig. 25.13), its structureless (and later glass-like) appearance is responsible for the term hyaline layer, which is given to this (approximately 10 μm) layer once it is fully mineralised.

The epithelial root sheath is in contact with the predentine layer for only a short distance before the continuity of the epithelial layer is lost. This allows the fibroblast-like cells of the adjacent dental follicle to lie close to the surface of the as yet unmineralised hyaline layer (Fig. 25.14). These cells, which represent the cementoblasts associated with the formation of the primary cementum, then appear to secrete collagen fibrils. At their deep surface these intermingle with those of the hyaline layer, allowing the two layers to form a strong union, while at their superficial surface they form a 'fibrous fringe' extending perpendicularly into the periodontal space for 10–20 μm (Fig. 25.15). The fibroblast-like cells of the dental follicle do not form a conspicuous layer on the forming root

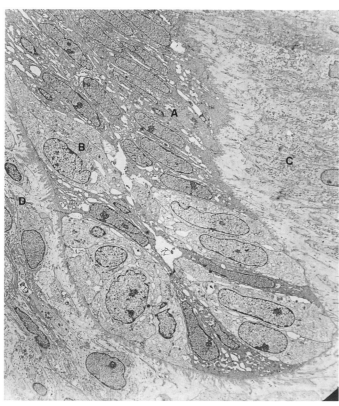

Fig. 25.12 TEM illustrating epithelial root sheath in developing root. A = Outer layer of epithelial root sheath, B = Inner layer of epithelial root sheath; C = differentiating odontoblasts; D = dental follicle (× 2000). Courtesy of Professors D.B. Bosshardt and H.E. Schroeder and the editors of *Periodontology 2000*.

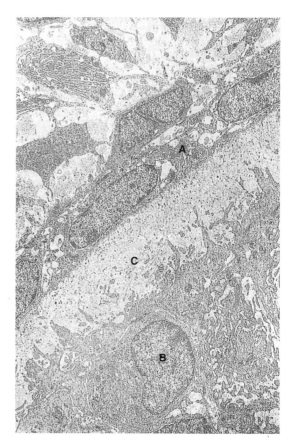

Fig. 25.13 TEM of early stage in root formation. The first-formed matrix (C) lies between the newly differentiated odontoblasts (B) and the epithelial root sheath cells (A). This matrix receives contributions from both the odontoblast and epithelial cell layers. It lacks major processes from the odontoblasts and forms the hyaline layer (× 5000). Courtesy of Dr P.D.A. Owens.

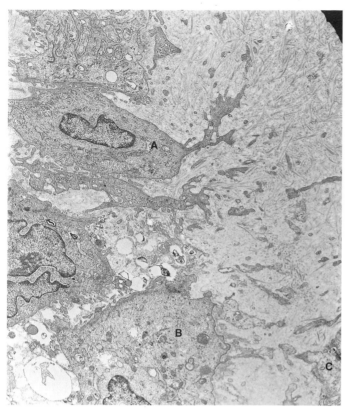

Fig. 25.14 TEM showing a fibroblast-like cell (A) from dental follicle with cytoplasmic processes lying close to the unmineralised external surface of initial root dentine layer. B = Coronal termination of intact inner enamel epithelial cell of epithelial root sheath; C = portion of odontoblast cell (× 6250). Courtesy of Professors D.B. Bosshardt and H.E. Schroeder and the editors of *Periodontology 2000*

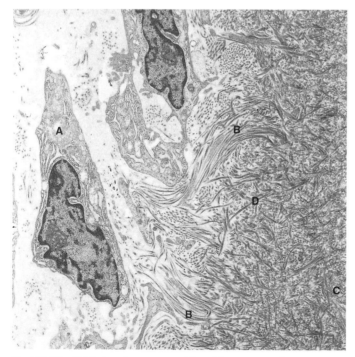

Fig. 25.15 TEM showing cementoblast (A) at root surface secreting collagen fibrils that form a fibrous fringe (B) that intermingles with the as yet unmineralised outer region of the root predentine (C). D = Site of future dentine–cement junction and, adjacent to it, the hyaline layer (× 5800). Courtesy of Professors D.B. Bosshardt and H.E. Schroeder and the editors of *Periodontology 2000*.

surface but may retreat and mingle with adjacent fibroblasts of the periodontal ligament.

At the initiation of cementogenesis, the epithelial root sheath cells secrete enamel-related protein(s) into the unmineralised collagenous matrix at the cement–dentine boundary. The nature of the protein has yet to be fully determined and may vary according to species, but may consist of ameloblastin and/or amelogenin. This secretory function is reflected in the presence of intracellular organelles such as a Golgi complex in the inner layer of the epithelial root sheath and confirmed by the results of immunohistochemical studies using antibodies raised against such proteins (Fig. 25.16). The function of such enamel proteins is unclear but may relate to epithelial–mesenchymal interactions involving the induction of odontoblasts and cementoblasts, and the process of mineralisation. During the subsequent mineralisation of cementum and the hyaline layer the enamel protein is lost, although remnants may be retained in the granular layer of the root dentine (Fig. 25.17).

As the odontoblasts in the root migrate pulpwards (centrifugally) beyond the hyaline layer, they commence to trail behind them their odontoblast processes and form the granular layer (of Tomes) and then circumpulpal dentine, which exhibits the normal tubular structure of dentine. Mineralisation of the first-formed dentine of the hyaline layer occurs within matrix vesicles. Unusually, however, this does not initially occur at the outermost surface of the hyaline layer, but a few microns within it. Thus, the outermost part of the hyaline layer undergoes delayed mineralisation (Fig. 25.18). This is visualised by the V-shaped configuration at the extreme apical edge of the developing root showing continuity of the unmineralised predentine layer at the periphery of the pulp, with the unmineralised part of the hyaline layer at the outer root surface (Fig. 25.19). A similar configuration is evident when the mineralising front is highlighted following administration of the antibiotic tetracycline (Fig. 25.20).

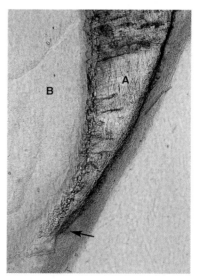

Fig. 25.16 Immunohistochemistry showing presence of enamel-like proteins (stained brown – arrow) at the surface of the developing root. This represents a frozen ground section through a premolar root using an antibody against amelogenin. A = Dentine; B = pulp (× 100). Courtesy of Professor L. Hammerstrom.

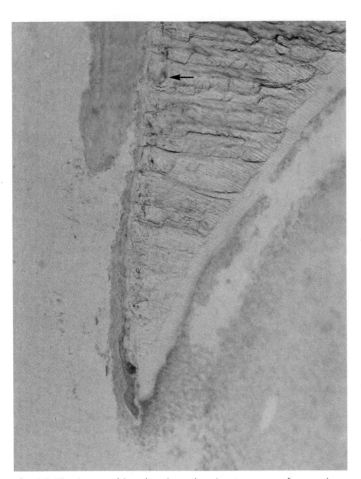

Fig. 25.17 Immunohistochemistry showing presence of enamel-like proteins (brown staining – arrows) in interglobular dentine (× 100). Courtesy of Professor L. Hammerstrom and the editor of *Journal of Clinical Periodontology.*

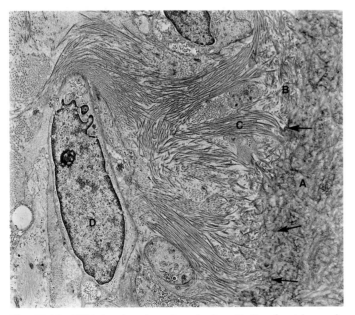

Fig. 25.18 TEM showing the external mineralisation front (arrows) of the outermost root dentine (A) has now extended outwards to reach the fibrillar dentine–cement junction (B). The dentine is now almost completely covered by the cementum matrix in the form of a fibrous fringe (C). D = Cementoblast (× 570). Courtesy of Professors D.B. Bosshardt and H.E. Schroeder and the editor of *Periodontology 2000.*

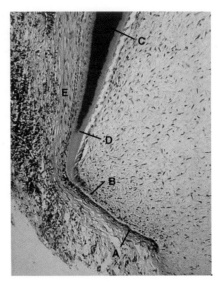

Fig. 25.19 Section of the developing root of extracted tooth. A = Epithelial root sheath; B = differentiating odontoblasts at the periphery of the dental papilla; C = matrix of mineralised dentine (red); D = unmineralised predentine (pale blue) continuous around root apex with first-formed but as yet still unmineralised matrix on outer surface of dentine (corresponding to hyaline layer); E = dentine follicle, which will give rise to periodontal ligament (Masson's trichrome, × 100).

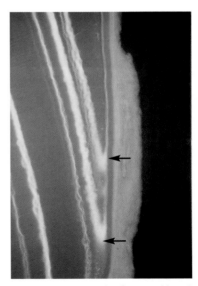

Fig. 25.20 Fluorescent micrograph of ground longitudinal section of tooth of a patient who had received multiple injections of the antibiotic tetracyclin. The antibiotic is incorporated into tissues mineralising at the time of the injection. There is continuity at the edge of the section where the original predentine recurves upwards at the site of the hyaline layer (arrows), similar to the situation seen in Fig. 25.8. Courtesy of Dr R. O'Sullivan.

During the next phase of development in acellular cementum the delayed mineralisation front in the hyaline layer gradually spreads outwards (centripetally) until this layer is fully mineralised, as are the first few microns of the fibrous fringe secreted by the fibroblast-like cells of the dental follicle that projects into the periodontal space (Fig. 25.21). In this manner, the first few microns of primary cementum are firmly attached to the root dentine. At this stage, the fibres of the periodontal ligament are oriented more parallel to the root surface and have

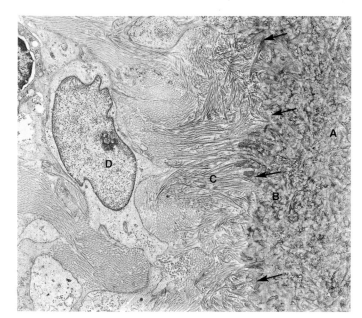

Fig. 25.21 TEM showing the mineralisation front in the developing root extending from the dentine (A) across the dentine–cement junction (B) and into the base (arrow) of the fibrous fringe of the cementum (C). D = Cementoblast (× 6250). Courtesy of Professors D.B. Bosshardt and H.E. Schroeder and the editors of *Periodontology 2000*.

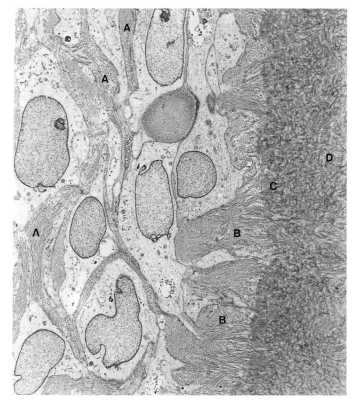

Fig. 25.22 TEM of developing root showing fibres in the developing periodontal ligament (A) running parallel to the root surface with little attachment to the cementum fibres (B), which are perpendicular to the root surface. C = Dentine–cement junction, beneath which would lie the hyaline layer; D = fibroblasts of periodontal ligament. The mineralisation front extends from the dentine across the dentine–cement junction to involve the base of the cementum fibres (× 4300). Courtesy of Professors D.B. Bosshardt and H.E. Schroeder and the editors of *Periodontology 2000*.

not yet gained an attachment to the fibrous fringe (Fig. 25.22). The stages in formation of primary acellular extrinsic fibre cementum are summarised in Fig. 25.23.

As in bone development, the early stage of cementogenesis results in the secretion by cementoblasts of various non-collagenous proteins such as bone sialoprotein (Fig. 25.24a) and osteopontin. The precise roles of such proteins await clarification, but they may be involved in processes such as chemoattraction, cell attachment, cell differentiation and mineralisation. It has also been suggested that these (and

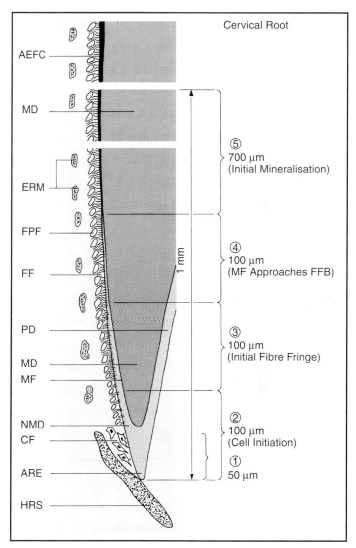

Fig. 25.23 The initial stages of root development on human premolars developed to 50–60% of their final root length. 1. fibroblasts contact root/predentine and become committed.2. Fibroblasts start to form and attach collagen fibrils. 3. Initial fibrous fringe with maximum fibre density is established. 4. Cell/fibrous fringe meshwork is established and the mineralisation front approaches the base of the fibrous fringe. 5. Mineralisation front progresses into initial fibrous fringe. AEFC = Acellular extrinsic fibre cementum; MD = mineralised dentine; ERM = epithelial cell rests of Mallassez; FPF = fibrous fringe-producing fibroblasts; FF = collagenous fibrous fringe; PD = predentine; MF = mineralisation front; NMD = non-mineralised dentine or predentine; CF = committed fibroblasts; ARE = advancing root edge; HRS = Hertwig's epithelial root sheath. Courtesy of Professors H.E. Schroeder and D.B. Bosshardt and the editors of *Cell and Tissue Research*.

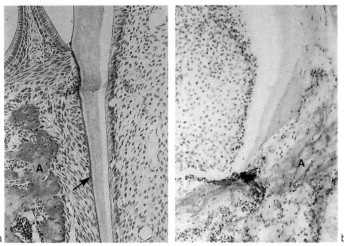

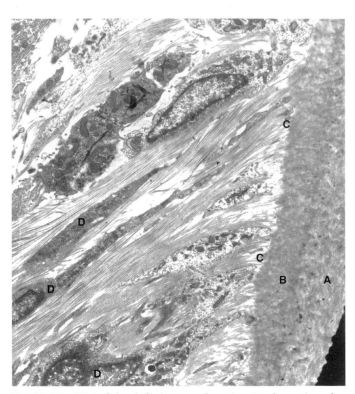

(Fig. 25.25), some cells lying beween the perpendicularly oriented periodontal fibre bundles may become more cuboidal (Fig. 25.26). The cementoblasts contain small amounts of the

Fig. 25.24 (a) Decalcified longitudinal section of mouse molar using immunohistochemical techniques to localise the presence of bone sialoprotein (red). Positive staining is seen at the developing cementum surface (arrow) and throughout the alveolar bone (A). (H & E; × 100). (b) Similar section from an osteopetrotic mouse lacking macrophage colony-stimulating factor: the root is stunted in its development and the cementum lacks bone sialoprotein, although this molecule is still present in alveolar bone (A). Courtesy of Dr M.J. Somerman and the editor of *Connective Tissue Research*.

other) molecules play a role in bonding the cementum to the outer surface of the root dentine. Their importance may be indicated by a type of osteopetrosis in which osteoclasts are deficient. In this condition, where root formation is grossly interfered with, there is a failure of production of bone sialoprotein by cells at the root surface (Fig. 25.24b).

The subsequent development of acellular cementum involves

- its slow increase in thickness
- the establishment of continuity between the collagen fibres of the periodontal ligament with those of the fibrous fringe at the surface of the root dentine and
- continued slow mineralisation of the collagen.

It is only with the establishment of continuity with periodontal ligament fibres that the tooth can be supported within the socket by the primary acellular cementum. There may be a considerable difference in the timing of establishing a direct attachment of periodontal fibres to the teeth of deciduous and succedaneous teeth (see page 339). Thus, for permanent teeth, this attachment may not occur until after the tooth has erupted into the mouth, when about two-thirds of the root has formed and the acellular cementum may only be about 10 μm thick. Thus, the acellular cementum lining the root before this time (which may be considered in years) can be classified as acellular intrinsic fibre cementum.

Once periodontal ligament fibres become attached to the surface of the cementum layer, the cementum may be classified as acellular extrinsic fibre cementum (Fig. 25.25). It increases slowly and evenly in thickness throughout life at a rate of about 2–2.5 μm per year. Although the cementoblasts may not form a distinctive and recognisable layer of cells that can be distinguished from adjacent cells of the periodontal ligament

Fig. 25.25 TEM of decalcified root surface showing formation of acellular extrinsic fibre cementum. A = Dentine; B = cementum; C = Sharpey's fibres; D = cells of periodontal ligament. Note the absence of a definite layer of cementoblasts (× 3500). Courtesy of Professor M.M. Smith.

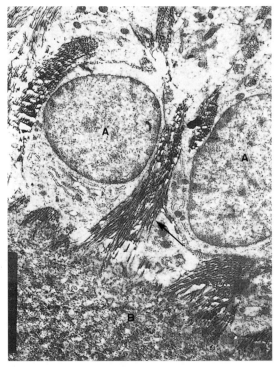

Fig. 25.26 TEM of decalcified root surface forming acellular extrinsic fibre cementum (B). Between the Sharpey's fibres (C), the cells (cementoblasts, A) are more cuboidal (× 5000).

intracellular organelles associated with protein synthesis and probably contribute to the formation of the ground substance surrounding the collagen. Presumably, secretion is polarised at the surface of the cell adjacent to the cementum surface, ensuring the cell is not entombed by its own secretion.

Mineralisation of the cementum matrix does not appear to be controlled by the cells. Indeed, matrix vesicles have not been observed and it is likely that the presence of hydroxyapatite crystals in the adjacent dentine initiates mineralisation in cementum. The adjacent periodontal ligament fibroblasts, which are rich in alkaline phosphatase, may also play a role in mineralisation. Mineralisation proceeds very slowly in a linear fashion and calcospherites are not observed in cementum. Owing to the slow progress of mineralisation, there is usually no evidence of a layer of precementum associated with acellular cementum analagous to that of predentine or osteoid. As the initial formation of cementum is closely associated with the mineralisation of the hyaline layer, when mineralisation of initial root dentine is interfered with by administration of drugs known as bisphosphonates, there is inhibition of cementogenesis.

Cementogenesis occurs rhythmically, periods of activity alternating with periods of quiescence. Structural lines may be visible within the tissue, indicating the incremental nature of its formation. The periods of decreased activity are associated with these incremental lines (see page 171), which are believed to have a higher content of ground substance and mineral and a lower content of collagen, than adjacent cementum. The periodicity is not known, but clearly represents a considerable period of time. As acellular cementum is formed very slowly, the incremental lines are closer together than corresponding lines seen in cellular cementum, which is deposited more rapidly.

The precise origin of the cells associated with primary acellular cementum is not clear, but they would appear to come from the cells of the investing layer of the dental follicle. However, there is evidence suggesting that some cementoblasts may be transformed epithelial root sheath cells.

Cellular inclusions, probably representing entombed epithelial root cells, may sometimes be seen at the cementum–dentine junction. The tissue in these circumstances has been referred to as intermediate cementum and is seen principally in the apical half of the roots of molar teeth (see page 176).

Acellular afibrillar cementum

Acellular afibrillar cementum may be deposited as a thin layer overlying enamel at the cervical margin of the tooth. Presumably, the protection of the reduced enamel epithelium overlying this enamel in an unerupted tooth is damaged or lost. The adjacent connective tissue cells of the dental follicle then come into contact with the enamel surface and are induced to form cementoblasts. These cells then secrete an afibrillar matrix that calcifies. This process has also been shown to occur experimentally in animals when the reduced enamel epithelium has been surgically removed. The effect can also be induced by enamel matrix alone.

Secondary (cellular) cementum

Following the formation of primary cementum in the cervical portion of the root, secondary cementum appears in the apical region of the root at about the time the tooth erupts. Secondary cementum is also formed in the furcation area of the cheek teeth. This type of cementum is associated with an increase in the rate of formation of the tissue. The early inductive changes associated with induction of odontoblasts and dentine formation appear similar to those described for primary cementum. However, following loss of continuity of the epithelial root sheath, large basophilic cells are seen to differentiate from the adjacent cells of the dental follicle against the surface of the root dentine. These cells form a more distinct layer of cementoblasts adjacent to the root surface. They generally possess more cytoplasm and more cytoplasmic processes than the cells associated with acellular cementum. The basophilia at the light microscope level corresponds to roughened endoplasmic reticulum at the ultrastructural level (Fig. 25.27). This indicates that the cementoblasts secrete the collagen (together with ground substance) that forms the intrinsic fibres of the secondary, cellular cementum. These fibres are oriented parallel to the root surface. Associated with the increased rate of formation, a thin unmineralised precementum layer (about 5 μm thick) will be present on the surface of cellular cementum (Fig. 25.28). Mineralisation in the deeper layer of the precementum occurs in a linear manner but, overall, this type of cementum is less mineralised than primary cementum. As in bone, the multipolar mode of matrix secretion by the cementoblasts will result in cells becoming incorporated into the forming matrix and these are converted into cemento-

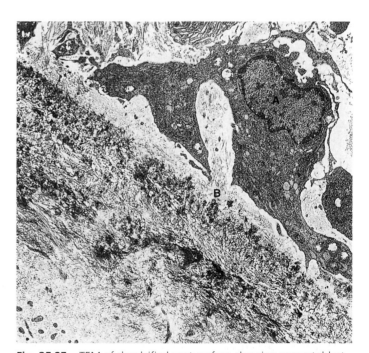

Fig. 25.27 TEM of decalcified root surface showing cementoblast (A) associated with the formation of cellular cementum. The cell is typically more irregular in morphology and contains larger amounts of the intracellular organelles associated with protein synthesis and secretion (such as endoplasmic reticulum). B = Precementum (× 4000). Courtesy of Dr P.D.A. Owens.

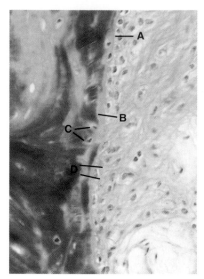

Fig. 25.28 Section of decalcified root surface showing cellular cementum formation. A = Cementoblasts; B = precementum; C = cementocytes becoming incorporated into the cementum matrix (Masson's trichrome; × 230).

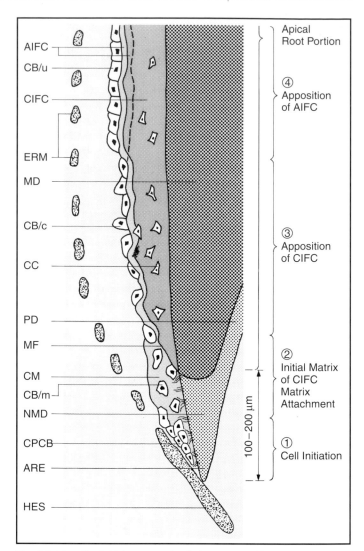

Fig. 25.29 The initial stages of cellular intrinsic fibre cementum (CIFC) formation on human premolars developed to about 75% of their final root length. 1. Committed clone of precementoblasts contacts root predentine and produces first matrix fibrils. 2. Cementoblasts form initial collagenous matrix attached to predentine. 3. First-formed and mineralised CIFC (including cementocytes) grows by apposition. 4. CIFC is covered with a layer of acellular intrinsic fibre cementum. AIFC = Acellular intrinsic fibre cementum; CB/u = cementoblasts with unipolar matrix production; CIFC = cellular intrinsic fibre cementum; ERM = epithelial cell rests of Malassez; MD = mineralised dentine; CB/c = cementoblasts with potential to become cementocytes; CC = cementocytes; PD = predentine; MF = mineralisation front; CM = initial cementum matrix; CB/m = cementoblasts with multipolar matrix production; NMD = non-mineralised dentine or predentine; CPCB = committed precementoblasts; ARE = advancing root edge; HES = Hertwig's epithelial root sheath. Courtesy of Professors H.E. Schroeder and D.B. Bosshardt and the editors of *Cell and Tissue Research*.

cytes. The incorporation of cementocytes, as with the osteocytes of bone, necessitates the generation of new cementoblasts from stem cells within the periodontal ligament. Incremental lines will be present in secondary cementum but, due to the increased rate of formation, are more widely spaced than in acellular cementum. The stages in the formation of secondary cellular cementum are illustrated in Fig. 25.29.

Cellular cementum is commonly present as the intrinsic fibre type (see Chapter 11). In this variety (cellular intrinsic fibre cementum), the tissue does not act in a supportive role as no Sharpey's fibres from the periodontal ligament are inserted into it. However, most commonly in the apical and furcation areas of human cheek teeth, this type of cementum alternates with layers of acellular extrinsic fibre cementum to form what is called cellular mixed stratified cementum. The layers may be present in various combinations and in various thicknesses. When a layer of acellular extrinsic fibre cementum is covered by a layer of cellular intrinsic fibre cementum, there must be a functional change as the Sharpey's fibres over the affected portion of the root will largely be detached from the root surface. Conversely, when cellular intrinsic fibre cementum is covered by a layer of acellular extrinsic fibre cementum, Sharpey's fibres will gain an attachment to the tooth.

An additional type of cementum is cellular mixed fibre cementum. In this variety, the normal cellular intrinsic cementum does give attachment to extrinsic fibres arising from the periodontal ligament. These fibres will be aligned more or less perpendicular to the root surface, in contrast to the intrinsic fibres secreted by the cementoblasts themselves that are arranged more or less parallel to the root surface (see Fig. 11.19).

As mentioned for acellular cementum, the precise origin of the cells in the dental follicle associated with the formation of cellular cementum awaits clarification. The possibility exists that different cell populations are responsible for the for-

mation of the two tissues. Evidence is building up to suggest that the cells associated with acellular and cellular cementum do show different phenotypes; these are listed in Table 25.1. If this suggestion is correct then, during the formation of cellular mixed stratified cementum, there is a switch from one formative cell to another. Due to the similarity between osteoblasts and cementoblasts, it has been suggested that

Table 25.1 *Possible phenotypical differences between cementoblasts associated with acellular and cellular cementum*

Cementoblasts from acellular cementum	Cementoblasts from cellular cementum
Identifiable for only a short time	Identifiable for longer period
Fibroblast-like morphology	Osteoblast-like morphology
Derived from epithelial root sheath	Derived from mesenchyme
Express cytokeratin	Do not express cytokeratin
Do not express osteocalcin	Express osteocalcin
Do not express receptors for parathormone	Express receptors for parathormone
Do not express TGF-β and IGF	Express TGF-β and IGF

progenitor cells associated with the alveolar bone could migrate into the periodontal ligament and provide a source of new cementoblasts.

EXPERIMENTAL STUDIES RELATING TO ROOT DEVELOPMENT

Experiments have shown that, when a tooth germ at the early bell stage is dissected from the jaw, it is surrounded by the inner investing layer of the dental follicle (thought to be of neural crest/ectomesenchyme origin; see page 293). When the tooth germ is transplanted in this condition, the investing layer has the capacity to give rise to all the investing tissues (i.e. cementum, periodontal ligament and bone). This, however, does not preclude a contribution to the periodontium *in vivo* from the outer part of the dental follicle. When the dental follicle cells are excluded and the enamel organ and dental papilla alone are transplanted to an ectopic site, there is regeneration of the investing layer of the

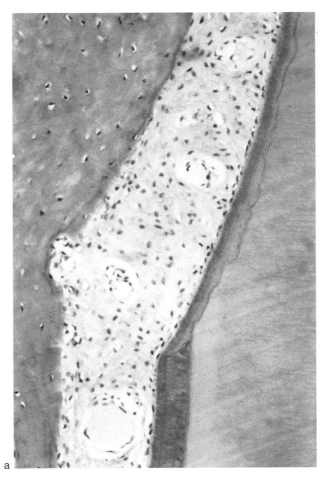

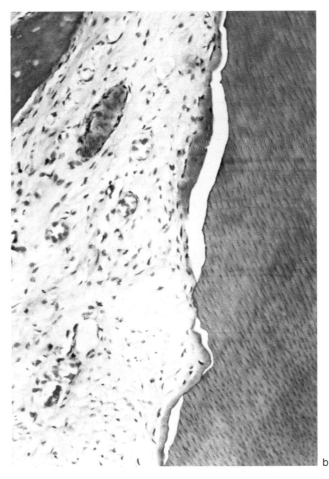

Fig. 25.30 Experimental cavities in the roots of lateral mandibular incisors of a monkey. The incisors were gently extracted and the experimental cavities were made by means of a round burr under constant irrigation with physiological saline. Porcine enamel matrix was then applied in one of the cavities (a) after which the incisor was immediately replanted. The other incisor (b) served as control and nothing was placed in the cavity of this tooth before it was replanted. Eight weeks after the replantation, the cavity (a), where enamel matrix had been placed, is covered by a layer of acellular cementum. The cavity in the control tooth, (b), is covered by a cellular hard tissue poorly attached to the dentin (H & E; × 150). A = Dentin; B = original acellular cementum; C = new, regenerated acellular cementum; D = new cellular reparative cementum; E = periondontal ligament; B = bone. Courtesy of Professor I. Hammarström and the editor of *Journal of Clinical Periodontology*.

follicle and formation of cementum, the root-related periodontal ligament, but no formation of alveolar bone. Combined with other studies, this indicates that papillary mesenchymal cells in the region of the root apex, in addition to being a source of odontoblasts, provide an important source of cells that migrate out into the dental follicle and may give rise to cells such as cementoblasts and periodontal fibroblasts.

The epithelial root sheath is important in the differentiation of root odontoblasts, as indicated by experimental recombinations between isolated epithelial root sheath cells and dental papilla cells. These demonstrate that root dentine will form only in the presence of the epithelial root sheath. A question that arises relates to whether the presence of root dentine alone is sufficient to induce dental follicle cells to become cementoblasts, or whether the epithelial root sheath contributes to the process. This has been tested by experimental recombinations of slices of root dentine and dental follicle cells with and without the presence of epithelial root sheath cells. Although a cementum-like tissue is formed on root dentine in both cases, this tissue separates relatively easily from the dentine in the absence of the root sheath cells. This supports the view that the epithelial root sheath plays an important role in early cementogenesis in firmly uniting the cement and dentine together. This may relate particularly to the secretion of enamel-related proteins by the epithelial root sheath cells. Indeed, as has been demonstrated, enamel-related proteins have been applied to the cleaned root surfaces of periodontally affected teeth where they are said to have a positive effect on periodontal regeneration (see Fig. 25.30).

Enamel pearl

These are small isolated spheres of enamel that are occasionally found on the root surface towards the cervical margin (Fig. 25.31). They are particularly common in the root bifurcation area. It is thought that, in the region affected, stellate reticulum stratum intermedium develop between the internal and external enamel epithelia of the root sheath.

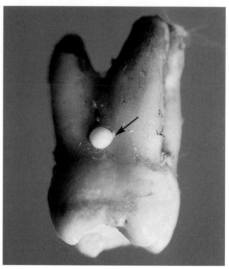

Fig. 25.31   An enamel pearl (arrow). Courtesy of Dr C. Franklyn.

26 Development of the dentitions

Description of the development of the dentitions requires consideration of the processes of tooth eruption and of the development of occlusion posteruptively. Indeed, three distinct phases of tooth development can be recognised that ultimately lead to the establishment of the full dentition. First, there is a phase termed the pre-eruptive phase, which starts with the initiation of tooth development and ends with the completion of the crown (see Chapter 21). Second, there is the phase of tooth eruption (prefunctional phase) that begins once the roots begin to form. Third, after the teeth have emerged into the oral cavity, there is a protracted phase concerned with the development and maintenance of occlusion (the functional phase).

TOOTH ERUPTION

Eruption is essentially the process whereby a tooth moves from its developmental position in the jaw into its functional position in the mouth. However, there is no evidence to suggest that eruption entirely ceases once a tooth meets its antagonist in the mouth, and outward axial movements occurring during the functional phase may also be eruptive

movements (viz. overeruption following removal of the antagonist tooth in the opposite jaw).

Throughout the pre-eruptive phase of tooth development there is concentric growth of the tooth within its follicle without any active bodily movement in a direction indicating eruption towards the oral cavity (Fig. 26.1). For a permanent mandibular second molar there are two stages of active eruption (Fig. 26.2): the first stage occurs between 6 and 12 years when the tooth is emerging into the mouth; a later second stage occurs at about 16 years in association with the adolescent growth spurt.

While the main direction of the eruptive force is axial (i.e. related to the long axis of the tooth), movement also occurs in other planes, accounting for tilting and drifting. Eruption rates of teeth are greatest at the time of crown emergence. Rates also differ according to tooth type. Permanent maxillary central incisors are reported to erupt at about 1 mm/month; the rates for mandibular second premolars have been determined to be about 4.5 mm in 14 weeks. For permanent third molars, where space is available, eruption rates of 1 mm in 3 months have been recorded. In crowded dentitions, however, eruption rate may be less than 1 mm in 6 months.

As a tooth approaches the oral cavity, the overlying bone is resorbed and there are marked changes in the overlying soft tissues. The enamel surface is covered by the reduced enamel epithelium, which is a vestige of the enamel organ. Fig. 26.3 shows an erupting deciduous molar before its emergence into the oral cavity and Fig. 26.4 a higher-power view of the soft tissues overlying the enamel space of an erupting tooth. As the tooth erupts, the outer cells of the reduced enamel epithelium proliferate into the connective tissue between the cusp tip and the oral epithelium. It has been suggested that these proliferating epithelial cells secrete enzymes that degrade collagen. Reduced

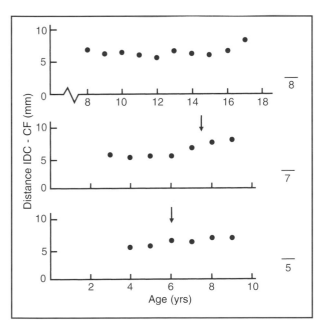

Fig. 26.1 Graphs plotting the mean distance from the mandibular canal (IDC) (regarded as a fixed point) to the centre of developing crowns of teeth during their pre-eruptive phase (CF). The upper graph is for a permanent mandibular third molar, the middle graph is for a permanent mandibular second molar, the lower graph is for a mandibular second premolar. Arrows indicate age at crown completion. Courtesy of Dr B.G.H. Levers.

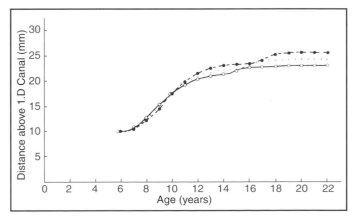

Fig. 26.2 Graph showing the mean distance from the mandibular canal (1. D canal) to the occlusal surface for a permanent mandibular second molar during its eruption. Note the adolescent growth spurt. Courtesy of Dr B.G.H Levers.

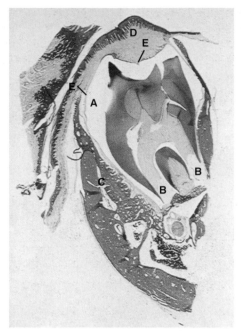

Fig. 26.3 An erupting deciduous molar before its emergence into the oral cavity. A = Enamel space; B = developing roots; C = developing alveolar crypt; D = oral mucosa and overlying connective tissue; E = reduced enamel epithelium (Decalcified, transverse section through the jaw; H & E; × 4).

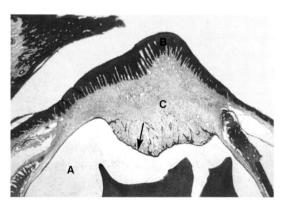

Fig. 26.4 The soft tissues overlying the enamel space (A) of an erupting tooth. B = Oral epithelium; C = connective tissue between developing tooth and oral epithelium. Arrow indicates the reduced enamel epithelium (H & E; × 10).

enamel epithelial cells may also be concerned with the removal of breakdown products resulting from resorption of connective tissue. Depolymerisation of the non-fibrous components of the extracellular matrix has been detected in the connective tissue overlying erupting teeth. Although a relationship between the degeneration of the connective tissue and the pressure exerted by the underlying erupting tooth has not been established, ischaemia is thought to be a contributory factor. That pressure alone is not entirely responsible is indicated by the finding that there is always evidence of some new collagen formation in this region.

Many of the fibroblasts in the connective tissue overlying an erupting tooth cease fibrillogenesis, actively take up extracellular material (as evidenced by intracellular collagen profiles – see page 190) and synthesise acid hydrolases. Eventually, the nuclei become pyknotic and the cells degenerate (Fig. 26.5).

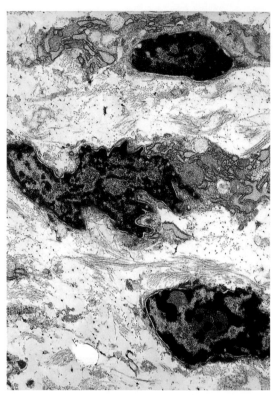

Fig. 26.5 Fibroblasts in the connective tissue overlying an erupting tooth showing evidence of degeneration (TEM; × 10 000).

The development of the dentogingival junction during the eruption of a tooth is shown diagrammatically in Fig. 26.6. As the tooth approaches the oral epithelium, the cells of the outer layer of the reduced enamel epithelium and the basal layer of the oral epithelium actively proliferate and eventually unite. The epithelium covering the tip of the tooth then degenerates at its centre, enabling the crown to emerge through an epithelial-lined pathway into the oral cavity. Further emergence of the tooth results from active eruptive movements and passive separation of the oral epithelium from the crown surface. When the tooth first erupts into the mouth, the reduced enamel epithelium is attached to the unerupted part of the crown, thus forming an epithelial seal – the junctional epithelium (see page 235). It is generally believed that the

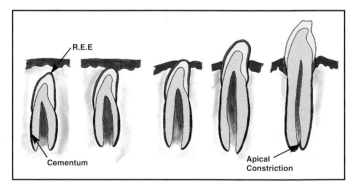

Fig. 26.6 Diagrammatic representation of the development of the dentogingival junction during the eruption of a tooth. R.E.E. = Reduced enamel epithelium (green). Red outline delineates oral epithelium.

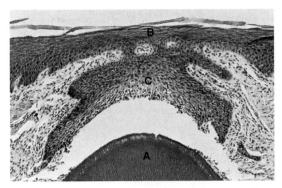

Fig. 26.7 An erupting tooth (A) about to emerge into the oral cavity through an epithelial-lined pathway as a result of fusion of the oral epithelium (B) and the reduced enamel epithelium (C) (H & E; × 12). Courtesy of Professor A.G.S. Lumsden.

reduced epithelial component of the junctional epithelium is eventually replaced by oral epithelium. With continued eruption, as more of the crown is exposed, a gingival crevice is formed. An erupting tooth about to emerge into the oral cavity through an epithelial-lined pathway as a result of fusion of the oral epithelium and the reduced enamel epithelium is shown in Fig. 26.7.

For the eruption of a permanent tooth, where there is a deciduous predecessor (i.e. excluding the permanent molars), the roots of the deciduous tooth must be resorbed to allow for shedding. Initially, each deciduous tooth and its developing permanent successor share a common alveolar crypt, the permanent tooth germ being situated lingually to the developing deciduous tooth (Fig. 26.8, see also Fig. 21.16). With continued growth, this relationship changes and the permanent tooth comes to lie near the root apex of the deciduous tooth within its own bony crypt. Note that the alveolar crypt of the permanent tooth shown in Fig. 26.8 is not complete,

there being the opening of a canal in its roof through which the dental follicle of the tooth germ communicates with, and is attached to, the overlying oral mucosa. This canal has been termed the gubernacular canal (see pages 351–352).

The appearance of a resorbing deciduous tooth above its erupting successor is given in Fig. 26.9. During the early eruptive stages of the permanent tooth, the bone separating it from its deciduous predecessor is resorbed. Following this, resorption of the hard tissues of the deciduous tooth takes place by the activity of multinucleated osteoclast-like cells termed odontoclasts. The vascular, resorbing tissue has been termed the resorbing organ of Tomes.

For a deciduous incisor or canine, root resorption initially occurs on the lingual surface adjacent to the developing permanent tooth. With subsequent movement and relocation of the teeth in the growing jaws, the developing permanent tooth comes to lie directly beneath the deciduous tooth and further resorption occurs from the apex. For a deciduous molar, root resorption often commences on the inner surfaces where the permanent premolars initially develop. The premolars later come to lie beneath the roots of the deciduous molar and further resorption occurs from the root apices. The shift in position of the deciduous tooth relative to the permanent successor may account for the intermittent nature of root resorption.

The initiation of root resorption may be an inherent developmental process or it may be related to pressure from

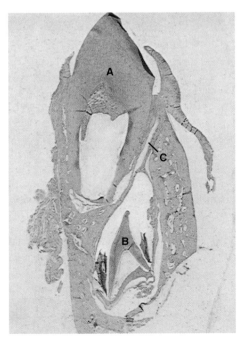

Fig. 26.8 Buccolingual section through an erupted deciduous canine (A) and its erupting successor (B). C = Gubernacular canal (Decalcified section; H & E; × 4).

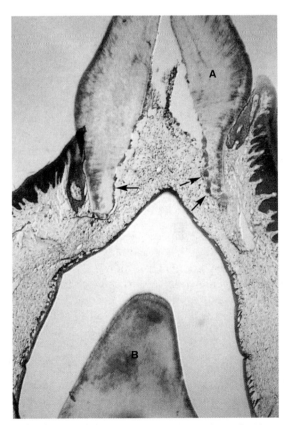

Fig. 26.9 Buccolingual section through a resorbing deciduous tooth (A) and its erupting successor (B). Arrows indicate multinucleated osteoclast-like cells (odontoclasts) (Decalcified section; Masson's trichrome; × 70).

the permanent successor against the overlying bone or tooth. To assess which of these explanations is correct, permanent tooth germs have been surgically removed, when it was seen that resorption of the deciduous predecessors still occurred, although this was delayed. These findings are also consistent with the clinical observation that shedding of a deciduous tooth still occurs but is retarded where the successor is congenitally absent or occupies an abnormal position within the jaw.

It has been suggested that increased masticatory loads affect the pattern and rate of deciduous tooth resorption. Indeed, it has been shown that, if deciduous teeth are splinted

following the removal of the developing permanent teeth, there is less root resorption than seen with removal of the permanent teeth alone.

Resorbing dentine is illustrated in Fig. 26.10. Multinucleated osteoclast-like cells (odontoclasts) lie within resorption lacunae (Howship's lacunae). Odontoclasts, like osteoclasts, differentiate from circulating monocyte-like cells. They are vacuolated and have long cytoplasmic processes. In an electron micrograph, the cytoplasmic projections form a brush border with the tooth surface. The odontoclasts have an abundance of ribosomes and a large number of mitochondria. The Howship's lacunae in resorbing teeth tend to be larger and more spherical than lacunae in bone.

Resorption of deciduous teeth is not a continuous process. During rest periods, reparative tissue may be formed, leading to a reattachment of the periodontal ligament. The tissue of repair is cementum-like and the cells responsible for its formation are similar in appearance to cementoblasts (see page 192). If the repair process prevails over the resorption, the tooth may become ankylosed to the surrounding bone, with loss of the periodontal ligament (Fig. 26.12). Ankylosis may also be caused by trauma or infection of a tooth. Where a deciduous tooth becomes ankylosed and cannot move, its position within the jaw remains constant so that, as height of the alveolar bone increases, the tooth appears to sink gradually below the level of the adjacent teeth. Such ankylosed teeth are referred to as 'submerged' teeth. The submergence may continue to such an extent that the teeth become completely buried within bone.

A specialised feature associated with the erupting permanent tooth is the presence of a gubernacular canal (Figs 26.8, 26.13). The gubernacular canal contains the gubernacular cord. The cord is composed of a central strand of epithelium (derived from the dental lamina) surrounded by connective tissue. The connective tissue is organised into inner and outer layers. Collagen fibres of the inner layer show greater

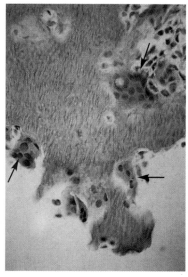

Fig. 26.10 Resorbing dentine. Arrows indicate osteoclast-like cells in Howship's lacunae (H & E; × 215).

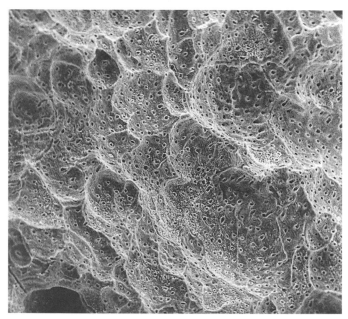

Fig. 26.11 SEM of the resorbing surface of a deciduous tooth showing Howship's lacunae. Within the lacunae, dentinal tubules are seen as small circular openings (Anorganic specimen; × 400). Courtesy of Professor S.J. Jones and Springer-Verlag.

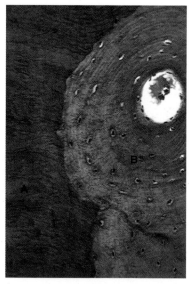

Fig. 26.12 Fusion between dentine (A) and bone (B) in an ankylosed tooth (Decalcified section viewed in blue light; × 150). Courtesy of Dr B.G.H. Levers.

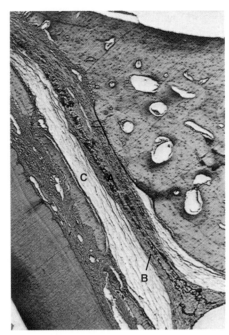

Fig. 26.13 A gubernacular canal and its contents. A = Gubernacular cord. The connective tissue in the cord is organised into inner (B) and outer (C) layers (H & E; × 25).

organisation and run mainly parallel to the long axis of the epithelium. In the outer layer, the collagen fibres are fewer and less organised. Differences between the layers can also be discerned with respect to the vasculature, the vessels in the outer layer being larger. During eruption, the gubernacular cords decrease in length but increase in thickness and become less dense. Surgical removal of the cord does not prevent eruption of the permanent tooth.

MECHANISMS OF TOOTH ERUPTION

Tooth eruption is traditionally considered to be a developmental process whereby the tooth moves in an axial direction from its position within the alveolar crypt of the jaw into a functional position within the oral cavity. However, eruption can be regarded as a lifelong process since a tooth will often move axially in response to changing functional situations (e.g. overeruption resulting from the removal of an antagonist, and compensatory eruption related to attrition).

The rate of eruption represents a balance between forces tending to move the tooth into the mouth (eruptive force) and forces tending to prevent this movement (resistive force). Resistance may be produced by overlying soft tissues and alveolar bone, the viscosity of the surrounding periodontal ligament, and occlusal forces. Thus, changes in the rate of tooth movement may be brought about by changes in either the eruptive forces and/or the resistive forces. At present, little is known about the nature, source and magnitude of either the eruptive or resistive forces (although only relatively small forces exerted by a spring are sufficient to stop a tooth erupting). Furthermore, it is not known whether the forces are of the same nature and magnitude at various stages of the eruptive cycle.

By and large, this situation results from difficulties encountered in producing experimental systems that isolate for study single possible agents associated with the eruptive process.

All tissues within the vicinity of the tooth thought capable of generating a force have, at one time or another, been implicated in the eruptive process. The theories advanced to explain the mechanism of tooth eruption can be divided into two main groups. One view suggests that the tooth is pushed out as a result of forces generated beneath and around it, by alveolar bone growth, root growth, blood pressure/tissue fluid pressure or cell proliferation. Alternatively, the tooth may be pulled out as a result of tension within the connective tissue of the periodontal ligament. Although no one theory is yet supported by sufficient experimental evidence, this brief review will show that the eruptive mechanism (i) is a property of the periodontal ligament (or its precursor, the dental follicle); (ii) does not require a tractional force pulling the tooth towards the mouth; (iii) is probably multifactorial in that more than one agent has important contributions to the overall eruptive force; and (iv) could involve a combination of fibroblast activity (although the evidence to date remains poor) and vascular and/or tissue hydrostatic pressures.

Role of the periodontal ligament in eruption

Experiments involving root resection or root transection of the continuously growing incisors of rodents (or rabbits) indicate that the periodontal ligament is the probable source for the generation of the forces responsible for eruption. Root resection involves the surgical removal of the proliferative odontogenic tissues at the base of the continuously growing incisor; root transection involves cutting the incisor into proximal and distal portions. Both surgical procedures result in a situation where the tooth (or the distal segment following transection) remains merely as a fragment attached to the jaw by a periodontal ligament, but without the possibility of root growth and with degeneration of the pulp. Furthermore, there can be no contribution to eruption from bone growth as none occurs at the base (fundus) of the socket. The resected and transected incisors continue to erupt to the point where they are

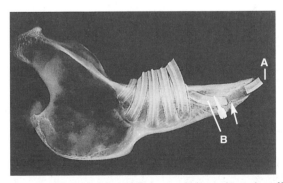

Fig. 26.14 Radiograph of a rabbit's mandible to show the effects of root transection. A = Segment distal to the site of transection (arrowed) that has continued to erupt to the alveolar crest; B = proximal segment pinned to prevent it contributing to the eruption of the distal segment. Courtesy of the editor of *Archives of Oral Biology*.

exfoliated from the socket (Fig. 26.14). That the movement in these surgically prepared teeth is eruptive-like and not an artefactual exfoliation is indicated by experiments that show that the resected rodent incisor changes its rate of eruption in response to factors that similarly affect the rate of eruption in normal incisors.

Although the periodontal ligament is implicated in the generation of the eruptive force, experiments show that, for teeth of limited growth, this property can be undertaken by its precursor, the dental follicle. When a developing unerupted premolar tooth is surgically removed and replaced with a metal replica, the replica will 'erupt', provided that the dental follicle is retained (Fig. 26.15). This experiment confirms that rootless teeth (both experimentally produced and clinically observed) can erupt and that the eruptive mechanism is present in a connective tissue (periodontal ligament or dental follicle) that need not gain a direct attachment to the tooth.

Investigation into the eruptive behaviour of the continuously growing, lathyritic incisor confirms that the eruptive force is unlikely to involve a tractional element that pulls the tooth towards the oral cavity. Lathyrogens are drugs that specifically inhibit the formation of collagen crosslinks, thereby disrupting the fibre network in the periodontal ligament. Compared with controls, eruption rates of lathyritic rodent incisors are unaffected, provided that occlusal forces (which could traumatise the already weakened ligament) are reduced by regular trimming of the tooth to the gingival level (Fig. 26.16). Thus, the lathyrogen experiments support the experiments on rootless teeth (of non-continuous growth) and indicate that traction of collagen fibres is not required to effect eruption. Further evidence against a tractional eruptive force comes from study of the development of the periodontal ligament (see page 337) that indicates that teeth can erupt in the absence of well developed periodontal fibres. These studies also disprove the theory that contraction of periodontal collagen fibre is responsible for generating the eruptive force.

Although the opinion is held that the force effecting eruption is derived from a single source (i.e. a prime mover), it is conceivable that more than one agent contributes to the overall force.

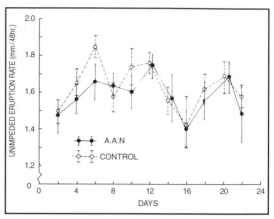

Fig. 26.16 Graph showing the lack of effects on mean eruption rates (± ISE) of a lathyrogen (A.A.N.). Courtesy of the editor of *Archives of Oral Biology*.

That eruption is multifactorial is evident when considering the variety of processes that must be involved to produce and sustain eruption. Indeed, four processes seem to be necessary.

- First, there must be the mechanism itself that generates the eruptive forces.
- Second, there are processes whereby eruptive forces are translated into eruption by movements through the surrounding tissues (e.g. overcoming the resistance of the tissues to eruption).
- Third, eruption must be sustained by processes that enable the tooth to be supported in its new position.
- Fourth, eruption occurs alongside a process of remodelling of the periodontal tissues to maintain the functional integrity of the system.

Experiments support the view that eruption is multifactorial; based upon study of the interactions of various drugs/

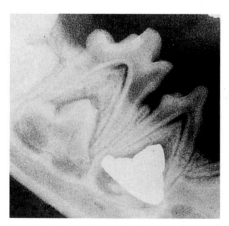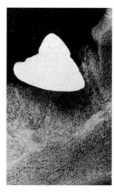

Fig. 26.15 Radiographs showing that, following replacement of an erupting tooth by a silicone replica surrounded by dental follicle (a), the silicone replica will continue to erupt (b). Courtesy of Professors J.C. Marks Jr and D.R. Cahill and the editor of *Archives of Oral Biology*.

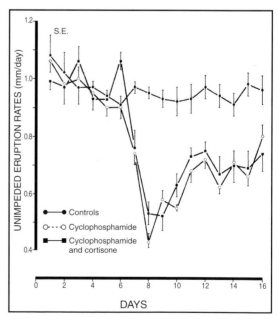

Fig. 26.17 The effects of cyclophosphamide and cortisone on mean eruption rates (± ISE). For explanation, see text. Courtesy of the editor of *Archives of Oral Biology*.

hormones known to influence eruption they suggest that there are at least two factors involved – a cortisone-sensitive factor and a cortisone-insensitive factor. A graph showing eruption rates in rodent incisors (Fig. 26.17) illustrates that when a drug is given which severely retards eruption (in this case the antimitotic drug cyclophosphamide), the remaining component of eruption is no longer affected by cortisone administration (that would normally produce a marked increase in eruption). Although it is possible to interpret these data in other ways, additional experiments show that the recovery of eruption following root resection (perhaps due to the removal of abnormal tissues at the base – see page 352) also has both cortisone-sensitive and cortisone-insensitive phases.

Having established that the connective tissues around the developing tooth are most likely to be the source of the eruptive mechanism, two major systems have been implicated in the generation of the eruptive force. One view holds that the force is produced by the activity of periodontal fibroblasts through their contractility and/or motility; the other that vascular and/or tissue hydrostatic pressures in and around the tooth are responsible for eruption.

Whatever the system implicated in the eruptive mechanism, the evidence should be judged according to the following five criteria:

1. The proposed system must be capable of producing a force under physiological conditions that is sufficient to move a tooth in a direction favouring eruption.
2. Experimentally induced changes to the system should cause predictable changes in eruption.
3. The system requires characteristics that enable it to sustain eruptive movements over long periods of time.
4. The biochemical characteristics of the system should be consistent with the production of an eruptive force.
5. The morphological features associated with the system should be consistent with the production of an eruptive force.

The periodontal fibroblast motility/contractility hypothesis

A role for the periodontal ligament fibroblasts in eruption is based upon the notion that these cells can exert a tractional force onto the tooth through the collagen network or through cell-to-cell contacts. This is in some ways analogous to the events occurring during wound contraction, which are thought to be the result of activities of specialised cells termed myofibroblasts. However, the periodontal ligament differs markedly from granulation tissue, and there is considerable evidence against the requirement for a tractional eruptive force acting through the periodontal collagen network (see page 353). Reviewing the evidence in terms of our prescribed criteria, there is at present nothing to indicate that the fibroblasts can exert a force under physiological conditions sufficient to move a tooth in a direction favouring eruption. Neither has it been possible to devise procedures to affect selectively periodontal fibroblast activity *in vivo* to assess whether the experimental procedures have predictable effects on eruption. It has been shown that the drug colchicine, by its known disturbance of intracellular microtubules, reduces cell motility and this might explain the drug's significant retardatory effect on eruption. However, colchicine influences more than just cell migration (for example, it also affects connective tissue turnover). To date, the evidence relating to the fibroblast activity hypothesis relies almost entirely upon consideration of the morphology of the fibroblasts (criterion 5 above) and upon the possible characteristics of the system, which would sustain the eruptive forces over long periods of time (criterion 3 above).

When periodontal fibroblasts are cultured on plastic, they assume the appearance and behaviour of migratory cells. They have a highly elongated shape with numerous, highly polarised arrays of microtubules and microfilaments (Fig. 26.18a). Their motility *in vitro* ceases with colchicine. When periodontal fibroblasts are cultured in a collagen gel, they generate tension by their contractility and assume the appearance of myofibroblast-like cells (i.e. fibroblasts with some of the properties of smooth muscle cells, a feature of fibroblasts in granulation tissue). During their contractile phase, these cells possess thick cell coats, considerable amounts of microfilamentous material dispersed throughout the cytoplasm, numerous cell contacts resembling gap junctions and occasional crenulated (folded) nuclei, but little rough endoplasmic reticulum (Fig. 26.18b). Their contraction *in*

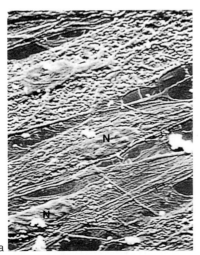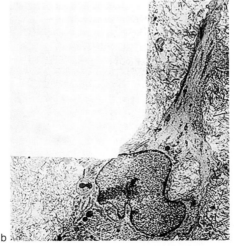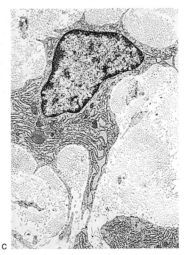

Fig. 26.18 The ultrastructural appearance of periodontal fibroblasts in culture and *in vivo*. (a) Cells cultured on plastic; (b) cells cultured in a collagen gel; (c) cells *in vivo*. See text for explanation. (a) × 990; (b) × 3025; (c) × 240.

vitro is inhibited when drugs interfering with microfilaments (e.g. cytochalasin) are added to the culture medium. *In vivo*, however, periodontal fibroblasts show features of neither migratory cells nor myofibroblasts. Instead, they tend to be rounded or flattened in outline without polarity of shape, have relatively little microfilamentous material (and then primarily as stress fibres beneath the cell membrane, a feature of cells generally exhibited 'after' migration/contraction), have only infrequent gap junctions (but more cell contacts in the form of simplified desmosomes) and contain considerable amounts of rough endoplasmic reticulum (see pages 189–192 and Fig. 26.18c). Thus, the periodontal fibroblast *in vivo* shows all the characteristics of a cell actively synthesising and secreting protein rather than of a motile/contractile cell. Care must therefore be taken in extrapolating from the *in vitro* to the *in vivo* situation.

In terms of criterion 3 (above), there is evidence of sustained migration of periodontal fibroblasts *in vivo*. Studies where the nuclei of cells have been labelled with tritium-labelled thymidine indicate that periodontal fibroblasts move occlusally at a rate equal to that of eruption; if the eruption rate is increased there is a concomitant increase in the rate of migration. Although providing some evidence of a shift in the position of periodontal fibroblasts, such work does not in itself indicate whether the cells are moving actively to generate the force of eruption or whether they are merely being transported passively within the ligament, the eruptive force being generated by another mechanism.

Other morphological features of the periodontal fibroblasts argue against their involvement in the generation of the eruptive force. The presence of cell contacts (not a usual feature of fibroblasts in a mature connective tissue) might indicate that a force could be generated through cell-to-cell contacts. However, the contacts are simplified desmosomes and not the fibronexus usually seen for myofibroblasts in contracting wounds. Furthermore, many of the simplified desmosomes for periodontal fibroblasts are located at right angles to the long axes of the cells, and they lack any recognisable microfilament bundles – arrangements that do not seem suited to transmit a tractional force directly through the cells themselves.

One way of assessing the contribution of the periodontal fibroblasts to eruption involves analysing quantitatively the structure of these cells in different periodontal ligaments and in teeth exhibiting different eruptive behaviours. The findings of studies using this approach also provide evidence against the periodontal fibroblast motility/contractility hypotheses. For example, there are no differences in the cells and their various organelles when periodontal fibroblasts in rapidly erupting and fully erupted teeth are compared.

The periodontal vascular/tissue hydrostatic pressure hypotheses

An eruptive force might be generated via the periodontal vasculature either directly through blood pressure or indirectly by influencing periodontal tissue (hydrostatic) pressures. Whether acting directly or indirectly, the periodontal vascular hypotheses clearly do not require a tractional mode of activity within the periodontal tissues.

That vascular pressures can alter the position of a tooth in its socket is shown by the fact that a tooth moves (0.4 µm) in synchrony with the arterial pulse. Furthermore, spontaneous changes in blood pressure have been shown to influence eruptive behaviour and, at death, when the arterial blood pressure is zero, eruption ceases. Therefore, there is some evidence that, without experimental intervention, vascular/ tissue pressures can produce a force sufficient to move a tooth in a direction favouring eruption (criterion 1 above). Experimental alterations to the periodontal vasculature following the administration of vasoactive drugs or interference with the sympathetic vasomotor nerve supply also result in predictable changes in eruption-like behaviour (criterion 2 above). For example, using a sensitive displacement transducer, it is possible to continuously monitor eruptive behaviour. Following the administration of a hypotensive drug (e.g. hexamethonium), as a probable result of increased capillary and periodontal tissue hydrostatic pressures, there is a marked increase in the rates of extrusive, eruption-like movements (Fig. 26.19). In addition, stimulation of the cervical sympathetics results in cessation of eruption and significant intrusion of the tooth, probably as a result of vasoconstriction and decreased capillary and periodontal tissue pressures: once the stimulus is removed, eruption recommences (Fig. 26.20).

To sustain eruptive movements according to the vascular hypotheses, it is necessary to postulate that periodontal tissue pressures are high, that there are pressure differentials along the periodontal ligament, and that changes in such pressures change eruptive behaviour (criterion 3 above). Indeed, there is evidence to support all three postulates. However, there remains debate as to whether periodontal tissue hydrostatic pressures are supra-atmospheric or subatmospheric.

To assess whether the biochemical composition of the periodontal ligament is consistent with the production of an eruptive force by 'vascular' means (criterion 4 above), analysis of the periodontal ground substance at different stages of tooth development has shown that a proteoglycan, with possibly significant osmotic influences on the tissue, increases in quantity during the active phase of eruption (see Fig. 12.26).

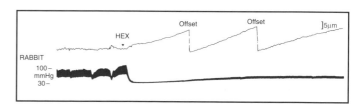

Fig. 26.19 Effects of a hypotensive agent (hexamethonium, HEX) on an erupting tooth. Courtesy of the editor of *Archives of Oral Biology*.

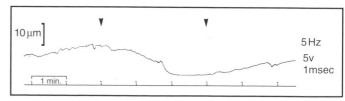

Fig. 26.20 Effects of stimulation of the cervical sympathetics on an erupting tooth. The period of stimulation is indicated by the arrows. Courtesy of the editor of *Archives of Oral Biology*.

Quantitative electron microscopy of the periodontal vasculature (criterion 5 above) has shown that, for both the degree of vasculature and the numbers of fenestrations on the capillaries, marked changes occur with different phases of eruption. For the non-continuously growing molar of the rodent, the number of fenestrations is three times greater during eruption than after eruption. In addition, for the continuously growing incisor of the rodent, the fenestrations are relatively low in number near the alveolar crest (approximately $1 \times 10^6/mm^3$ of tissue) but are high near the root base of the erupting tooth (approximately $4 \times 10^6/mm^3$), perhaps providing evidence for differential vascular activity along the periodontal ligament. Thus, whilst no single piece of evidence briefly reported here for a role in eruption of the vascular elements of the periodontal ligament is incontrovertible, the sum of the evidence does suggest that it could provide one factor in the multifactorial mechanism of eruption.

Some observations have been made on the rate of emergence of human teeth into the oral cavity. Initially, there is a period of slow eruption when the crown is carried towards the oral mucosa. For permanent teeth, this period may take 2–4 years. A tooth erupts most rapidly as it enters the oral cavity, at which time the length of its root is about two-thirds complete. Eruption then slows as the tooth approaches the occlusal plane. Once the tooth has emerged into the oral cavity it may take 1–2 years to reach the occlusal plane. The emergence of the crown is partly due to axial movement of the tooth (active eruption) and partly due to retraction of the adjacent soft tissues (passive eruption). For human maxillary incisors, the maximum eruption rate at the time of crown emergence is about 1 mm per month. For maxillary third molars, the maximum rates are seen in spaced dentition and are less than half that recorded for incisors. In crowded dentitions, the rates are even lower (less than 1 mm in 6 months).

Because no individuals are exactly alike, the times for tooth development shown in Table 26.1 are approximate. Variations of 6 months either way are not unusual, but the tendency is for teeth to erupt late rather than early. By and large, the development of the permanent dentition is more advanced in girls; there does not appear to be any sex difference in the development of the deciduous dentition. Racial differences also appear to exist.

Since the sequence of development and eruption of teeth is under genetic control, and since chronological age is an

Table 26.1 *Chronology of tooth development and the order of eruption*

Chronology of the deciduous dentition					Chronology of the permanent dentition				
Tooth	First evidence of calcification (months in utero)	Crown completed (months)	Eruption (months)	Root completed (years)	Tooth	First evidence of calcification	Crown completed (years)	Eruption (years)	Root completed (years)
Maxillary					Maxillary				
A	3–4	4	7	$1\frac{1}{2}$–2	1	3–4 months	4–5	7–8	10
B	$4\frac{1}{2}$	5	8	$1\frac{1}{2}$–2	2	10–12 months	4–5	8–9	11
C	5	9	16–20	$2\frac{1}{2}$–3	3	4–5 months	6–7	11–12	13–15
D	5	6	12–16	2–$2\frac{1}{2}$	4	$1\frac{1}{2}$–$1\frac{3}{4}$ years	5–6	10–11	12–13
E	6–7	10–12	21–30	3	5	2–$2\frac{1}{2}$ years	6–7	10–12	12–14
					6	Birth	$2\frac{1}{2}$–3	6–7	9–10
					7	$2\frac{1}{2}$–3 years	7–8	12–13	14–16
					8	7–9 years	12–16	17–21	18–25
Mandibular					Mandibular				
A	$4\frac{1}{2}$	4	$6\frac{1}{2}$	$1\frac{1}{2}$–2	1	3–4 months	4–5	6–7	9
B	$4\frac{1}{2}$	$4\frac{1}{2}$	7	$1\frac{1}{2}$–2	2	3–4 months	4–5	7–8	10
C	5	9	16–20	$2\frac{1}{2}$–3	3	4–5 months	6–7	9–10	12–14
D	5	6	12–16	2–$2\frac{1}{2}$	4	$1\frac{3}{4}$–2 years	5–6	10–12	12–13
E	6	10–12	21–30	3	5	$1\frac{1}{4}$–$2\frac{1}{2}$ years	6–7	11–12	13–14
					6	Birth	$2\frac{1}{2}$–3	6–7	9–10
					7	$2\frac{1}{2}$–3 years	7–8	12–13	14–15
					8	8–10 years	12–16	17–21	18–25

Unless otherwise indicated all dates are postpartum. The teeth are identified according to the Zsigmondy system.

All dates are postpartum. Teeth are identified according to the Zsigmondy system.

unreliable guide to the progress of development of an individual child, dental age is a useful index of maturity, especially when used in conjunction with skeletal age. Dental age may be estimated clinically by a visual assessment of the stage of eruption of the dentition or, more satisfactorily, by a radiographic assessment of both the stages of development of the crowns and roots and the stages of eruption.

A schematic diagram of the development and eruption of the teeth is shown in Fig. 26.21 and radiographs of the dentitions at various ages in Figures 26.22–26.31.

DEVELOPMENT OF OCCLUSION

At birth, the oral mucosa over the developing alveoli is greatly thickened to form the maxillary and mandibular gum pads (Fig. 26.32). They show a series of elevations, each of which corresponds to an underlying deciduous tooth. The elevations associated with the second deciduous molars do not, however, become prominent until the age of about 6 months. The maxillary and mandibular gum pads rarely come into occlusion, the space left between them being occupied by the tongue. The

maxillary gum pad overlaps the mandibular gum pad both buccally and labially, the overjet usually being considerable. Beneath the gum pads there is generally considerable crowding of the developing teeth, especially the incisors. However, during the first year of life the gum pads grow rapidly, especially in lateral directions, thus providing space for the developing teeth.

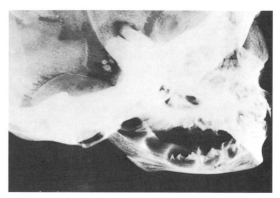

Fig. 26.22 The dentition at birth – a lateral oblique view of the skull.

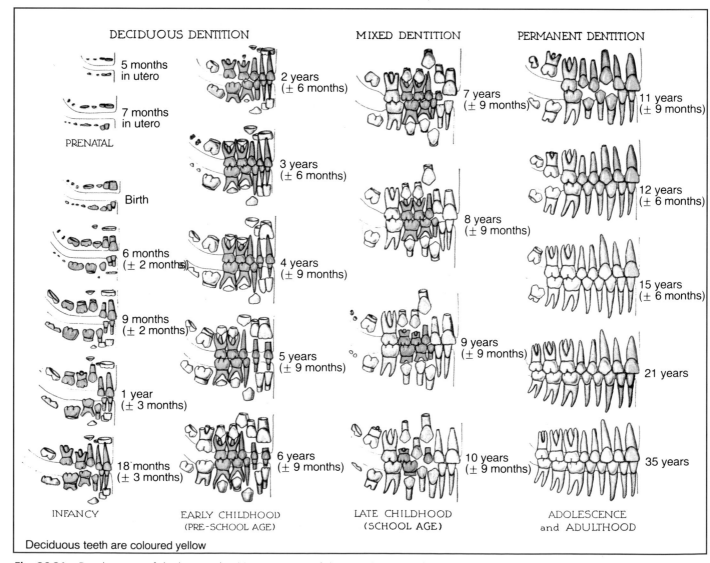

DECIDUOUS DENTITION

5 months in utero
7 months in utero
PRENATAL

Birth

6 months (± 2 months)

9 months (± 2 months)

1 year (± 3 months)

18 months (± 3 months)

INFANCY

2 years (± 6 months)

3 years (± 6 months)

4 years (± 9 months)

5 years (± 9 months)

6 years (± 9 months)

EARLY CHILDHOOD (PRE-SCHOOL AGE)

MIXED DENTITION

7 years (± 9 months)

8 years (± 9 months)

9 years (± 9 months)

10 years (± 9 months)

LATE CHILDHOOD (SCHOOL AGE)

PERMANENT DENTITION

11 years (± 9 months)

12 years (± 6 months)

15 years (± 6 months)

21 years

35 years

ADOLESCENCE and ADULTHOOD

Deciduous teeth are coloured yellow

Fig. 26.21 Development of the human dentition. Courtesy of the American Dental Association.

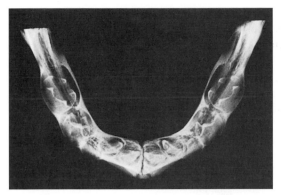

Fig. 26.23 The dentition at birth – an occlusal view of the mandible.

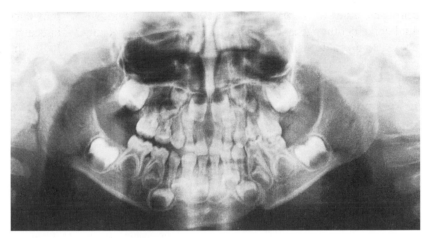

Fig. 26.24 Dental age 2½ years – orthopantomogram.

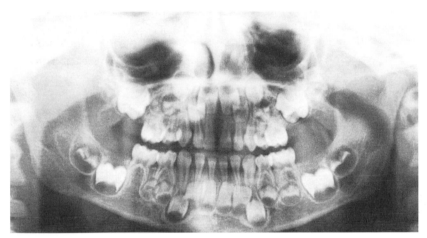

Fig. 26.25 Dental age 4 years – orthopantomogram.

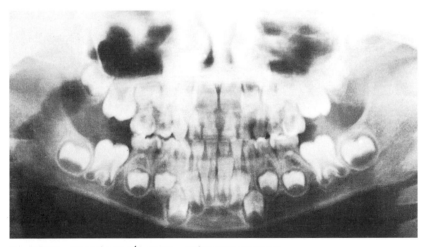

Fig. 26.26 Dental age 5½ years – orthopantomogram.

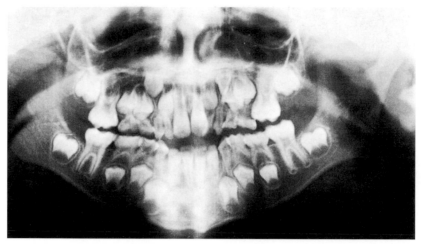

Fig. 26.27 Dental age 7 years – orthopantomogram.

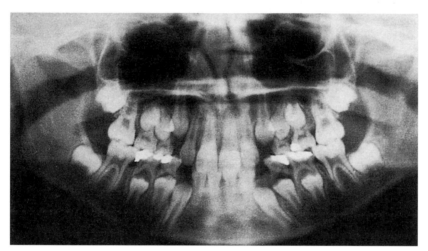

Fig. 26.28 Dental age 9 years – orthopantomogram.

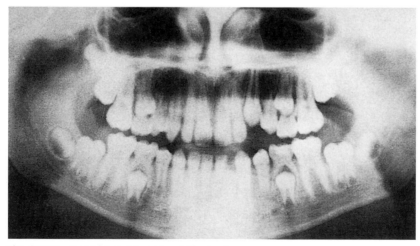

Fig. 26.29 Dental age 11 years – orthopantomogram.

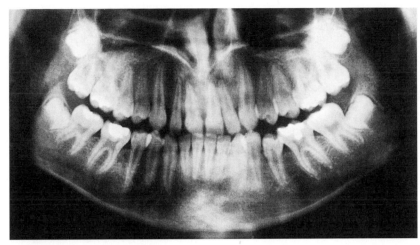

Fig. 26.30 Dental age 14 years – orthopantomogram.

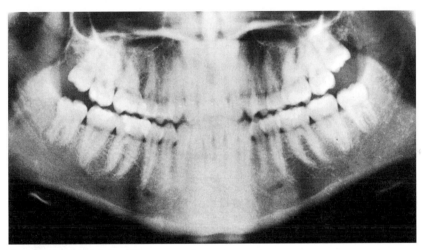

Fig. 26.31 Dental age 19 years – orthopantomogram.

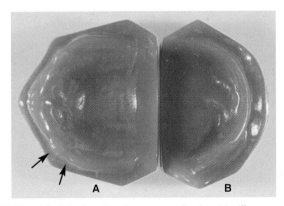

Fig. 26.32 Models showing the gum pads. A = Maxillary; B = mandibular. Note swellings from underlying teeth (arrows).

The maxillary and mandibular alveolar processes are not well developed at birth. Occasionally, a 'natal tooth' is present. This tooth is usually a supernumerary tooth (see page 302), formed by an aberration in the development of the dental lamina, but occasionally it is merely a very early, but otherwise normal, deciduous central incisor.

The deciduous teeth start to erupt at the age of 6 months and the deciduous dentition is complete by the age of 3 years.

At this time, the occlusion of the deciduous dentition differs from that of the permanent dentition in the following respects (Fig. 26.33):

1. The incisors are more vertically positioned within the alveolus and are often spaced.
2. The overbite is usually greater.
3. There may be significant spacings distal to the mandibular canines and mesial to the maxillary canines (the anthropoid or primitive spaces).
4. Although the anteroposterior relationships of the deciduous arches have not been adequately assessed, it appears that the distal edges of the maxillary and mandibular deciduous molars are flush and the mesiobuccal cusps of the maxillary first and second deciduous molars occlude in the buccal grooves of the mandibular first and second deciduous molars respectively.

Several changes occur in the deciduous occlusion before the appearance of the permanent teeth. These result from changes in the dental bases. As the dental arches become wider and longer, so the deciduous teeth become more spaced. Since there is a greater forward growth of the mandible than the maxilla, the lower arch moves forwards relative to the upper,

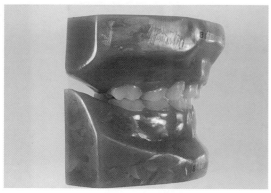

Fig. 26.33 Models showing the occlusion of the deciduous dentition at 3 years.

so that an edge-to-edge incisor relationship is obtained. As a further consequence, the distal surfaces of the deciduous second molars may now show a slight mesial step from maxilla to mandible, the mesiobuccal cusp of the maxillary second deciduous molar lying distal to the buccal groove of the mandibular second deciduous molar. As the deciduous teeth approach the end of their functional lives, they may show signs of considerable wear (the enamel of deciduous teeth being softer and thinner than the enamel of permanent teeth – see page 14).

The occlusal relationships of the deciduous and permanent molars are shown in Fig. 26.34. The flush terminal plane relationship is the usual relationship in the deciduous dentition. When the first permanent molars start to erupt, their relationship is determined by that of the primary molars.

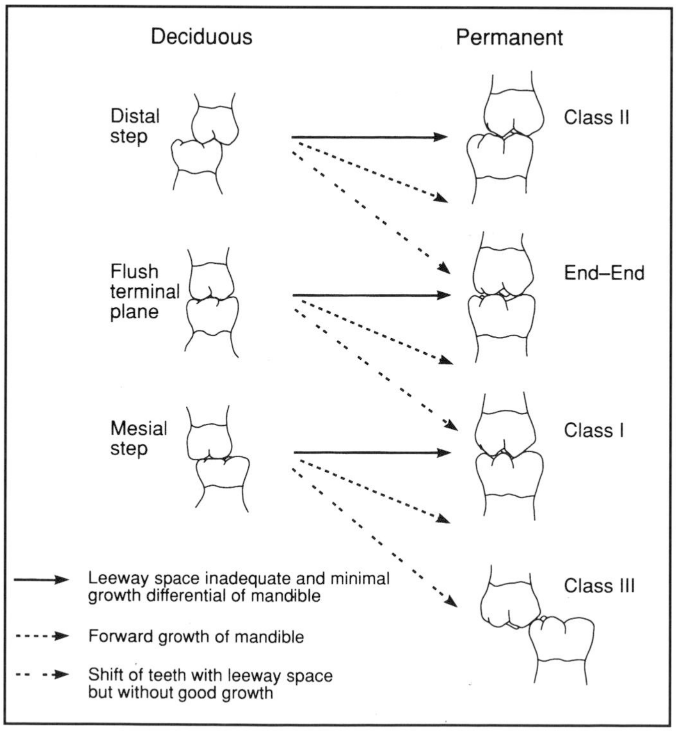

The molar relationship tends to shift at the time the second deciduous molars are shed and the adolescent growth spurt occurs. As shown in Fig. 26.34, the change in molar relationship depends upon whether there is leeway space for tooth movement and upon mandibular growth.

After the age of 6 years, the dentition is said to be mixed, comprising both deciduous and permanent teeth. The first molars are the first permanent teeth to erupt. Initially, they have a cusp-to-cusp relationship (the flush terminal plane; see Fig. 26.34), which is governed by the position of the deciduous second molars. The first molars take up their normal adult relationship once the deciduous second molars are shed. The permanent incisors erupt between the ages of 6 and 9 years. Since the permanent incisors are much larger than their deciduous predecessors, they are accommodated into the dental arches not just by utilisation of the space left by the deciduous predecessors but also by lateral growth of the alveolar arches and the greater proclination of the permanent incisors. In their developmental positions, the lateral incisors are overlapped by the central incisors, being positioned more palatally. As a rule, space is made for the lateral incisors as the central incisors erupt. However, should there be insufficient growth of the alveolus, the lateral incisors may continue to lie in their developmental, palatal positions (Fig. 26.35). Frequently, when the permanent incisors erupt, they fan out (incline distally) so that there may be a significant space or diastema between the central incisors. This appearance has been termed the 'ugly duckling' stage and is said to result from pressure on the roots of the permanent incisors from the developing permanent canines. The diastema usually closes following eruption of the permanent canines. The canines and premolars, which usually erupt between the ages of 9 and 12 years, are readily accommodated into

Deciduous — Permanent

Distal step → Class II

Flush terminal plane → End–End

Mesial step → Class I

→ Class III

→ Leeway space inadequate and minimal growth differential of mandible

---▶ Forward growth of mandible

-- ▶ Shift of teeth with leeway space but without good growth

Fig. 26.34 Occlusal relationships of the deciduous and permanent molars. Modified from Professor R.E. Moyers, Year Book Medical Publishers.

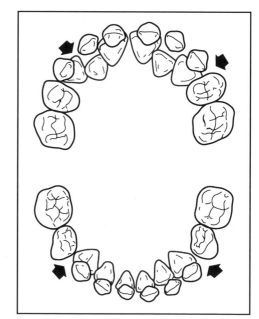

Fig. 26.35 The developmental positions of the crowns of the permanent teeth (red) relative to the functional positions of the crowns of the deciduous teeth (black). Arrows point to the 'primate' spaces.

the dental arches because the combined mesiodistal diameters of the deciduous canines and molars are generally greater than those of their permanent successors. Any leeway space that remains is usually taken up by forward movement of the first permanent molars. By the age of 12 years, all the deciduous teeth have been shed, to be replaced by permanent teeth, and henceforth the occlusion appears similar to that in the adult (see pages 37–42). Space is provided for the permanent molar teeth by continued growth of the mandible and maxilla.

In Fig. 26.35 note the lingual positioning of the permanent teeth (particularly for the maxillary lateral incisors). Spaces between the deciduous canines and the first molars for the lower jaw, and between the deciduous lateral incisors and canines for the upper jaw, may be seen and are termed 'primate spaces', so named because they are most marked in the dentitions of primates. The primate spaces are usually seen from the time the teeth erupt. Developmental spaces between the incisors are often present at eruption, but become larger as the child grows and the alveolar processes expand. Generalised spacing of the primary teeth is a requirement for proper alignment of the permanent incisors.

A graphic display of the average amount of space available within the dental arches is shown in Fig. 26.36. Note that, for both sexes, the amount of space for the mandibular incisors is negative for about 2 years after their eruption. Thus, a small degree of crowding in the mandibular arch at this time is not unusual.

Although there is a tendency for the mandible to grow slightly further forward than the maxilla after the age of 12 years, usually there is no appreciable occlusal change. During the later stages of facial growth there may be an accompanying uprighting of the incisors, with the result that they become more crowded. It has been suggested that mesial drift may take up any remaining space in the arches or even be responsible for some late crowding.

Once a tooth reaches its functional position, it is believed to occupy a position of equilibrium between the soft tissues of the cheeks and lips externally and the tongue internally (see Fig. 2.71).

The movement that has attracted the most attention during a tooth's functional phase is mesial drift. Mesial drift may involve considerable bodily movement of the tooth. It has been reported that, where the food is abrasive and there is considerable masticatory activity, the first permanent molar drifts approximately 4 mm in a mesial direction between the ages of 6 and 18 years. The mesial drift that occurs in these situations helps provide space for erupting mandibular third molars. The absence of an abrasive diet and the accompanying reduction in mesial drift associated with soft diets may account for the high occurrence of impacted mandibular third molars in some modern populations. Four hypotheses have been postulated to account for mesial drift:

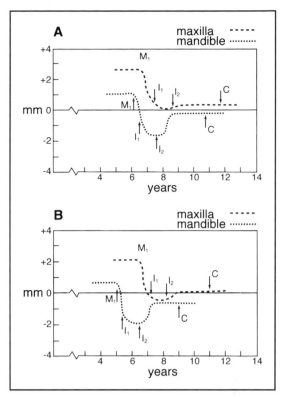

Fig. 26.36 Graphic display of the average amount of space available within the dental arches for boys (A) and for girls (B). The arrows indicate the timing of eruption of the first molars (M_1), central and lateral incisors (I_1 and I_2) and canines (C). (Modified after Dr C.F.A. Moorress and J.M. Chadha and *Angle Orthodontics*).

1. The mesial inclination of teeth produces a resultant force during biting that favours mesial drift.
2. The actions of certain jaw muscles, particularly the buccinator, 'propel' the teeth forwards.
3. Bone deposited preferentially on the distal surface of the sockets pushes the teeth mesially.
4. Contraction of the gingival connective tissues (especially the transseptal collagen fibres in the gingiva – see page 241).

Concerning hypothesis 1, a detailed analysis of mesial drift would not indicate a direct relationship with the angulation of the teeth. Evidence against hypothesis 2 is the observation that mesial drift still occurs even when teeth are protected by an overlay that would prevent muscle contact. Bone activity is observed during mesial drift (hypothesis 3), but it is not possible to separate cause and effect. Although there is some evidence that damage to the gingiva retards mesial drift, there is little evidence that connective tissues contract *in vivo*. As with tooth eruption, the evidence might indicate that the mechanisms of mesial drift are multifactorial and involve the periodontal tissues.

Further reading

The following list provides students with some introductory references to allow them to seek further insights into oral anatomy, histology and embryology

CHAPTERS 1–6

Anatomy

Ash, M.M. Jr. 1993. Wheeler's Dental Anatomy, Physiology and Occlusion. 7th edition. Saunders, Philadelphia.

Berkovitz, B.K.B., Moxham, B.J. 1989. Colour Atlas of the Skull. Mosby-Wolfe, London.

Berkovitz, B.K.B., Moxham, B.J. 2002. Head and Neck Anatomy: A Clinical Reference. M. Dunitz, London.

Bertilsson, O., Strom, D. 1995. A literature survey of a hundred years of anatomical and functional lateral pterygoid muscle research. Journal of Orofacial Pain 9, 17–23.

Burns, R.C., Herbranson, E.J. 2001. Tooth morphology and cavity preparation. In: Pathways of the Pulp. 8th edition. S. Cohen, R.C. Burns (eds). Mosby, St. Louis, pp. 179–229.

Lang, J. 1995. Clinical Anatomy of the Masticatory Apparatus and Peripharyngeal Spaces. Thieme, Stuttgart.

McDevitt, W.E. 1989. Functional Anatomy of the Masticatory System. Wright's, London.

McMinn, R.M.H., Hutchings, R.T., Logan, B.M. 1994. Colour Atlas of Head and Neck Anatomy. 2nd edition. Mosby-Wolfe, London.

Osborn, J.W. 1985. The disc of the human temporomandibular joint: design, function and failure. Journal of Oral Rehabilitation 12, 279–293.

Van Beek, G.C. 1983. Dental Morphology: An Illustrated Guide. Wright, Oxford.

Williams, P.L. (ed.) 1995. Gray's Anatomy 38th edition. Churchill Livingstone, Edinburgh.

Woelfel, J.B., Scheid, R.C. 1997. Dental Anatomy: Its Relevance to Dentistry. 5th edition. Williams and Williams, Baltimore.

Occlusion, radiography and functional anatomy

Brons, R. 1998. Facial harmony. Quintessence Publishing, London.

Graber, T.M., Vanarsdall, R.L. Jr. 2000. Orthodontics: Current Principles and Techniques. 3rd edition. Mosby, St Louis.

Jacobson, A., Caufield, P.W. 1985. Introduction to Radiographic Cephalometry. Lea and Febiger, Philadelphia.

McDonald, F., Ireland, A.J. 1998. Diagnosis of the Orthodontic Patient. Oxford University Press, Oxford.

McNeill, C. 1997. Science and Practice of Occlusion. Quintessence Publishing, Chicago.

Miyashita, K. 1996. Contemporary Cephalometric Radiography. Quintessence Publishing, Tokyo.

Orchardson, R., Cadden, S.W. 1998. Mastication. In: The Scientific Basis of Eating. Taste and Smell, Salivation, Mastication and Swallowing and their Dysfunctions. R.W.A. Linden (ed.) Frontiers of Oral Biology Series Vol 9. Karger, Basel, pp. 76–121.

Paster, F.A. 1993. Colour Atlas of Dental Medicine — Radiology. Thieme, Stuttgart.

Proffit, W.R., Fields, H.W. Jr. 2000. Contemporary Orthodontics. 3rd edition. Mosby, St Louis.

Thexton, A. 1998. Some aspects of swallowing. In: Clinical Oral Science. M. Harris, M. Edgar, S. Meghji (eds). Wright, Oxford, pp. 150–166.

Thexton, A.J., Crompton, A.W. 1998. The control of swallowing. In: The Scientific Basis of Eating. Taste and Smell, Salivation, Mastication and Swallowing and their Dysfunctions. R.W.A. Linden (ed.), Frontiers of Oral Biology Series Vol 9. Karger, Basel, pp. 168–222.

Valvassari, G.E., Masee, M.S., Carter, B.L. 1995. Imaging of the head and neck. Thieme, Stuttgart.

Whaites, E. 1996. Essentials of Dental Radiography and Radiology. 2nd edition. Churchill Livingstone, Edinburgh.

CHAPTERS 7–16

Enamel

Boyde, A. 1989. Enamel. In: Teeth. Handbook of Microscopic Anatomy, Vol. 6, A. Oksche and L. Volrath. (eds). Springer Verlag, Berlin, pp. 309–473.

Chadwick, D., Cardew, G. (eds) 1997. Dental Enamel. Ciba Foundation Symposium, 205. Wiley, New York.

Dean, M.C. 2000. Incremental markings in enamel and dentine: what they can tell us about the way teeth grow. In: Development, Function and Evolution of Teeth. M.F. Teaford, M.M. Smith, M.W.J. Ferguson (eds). Cambridge University Press, Cambridge, pp. 119–130.

Elliott, J.C., Wong F.S., Anderson, P., Davis G.R., Dowker S.E. 1998. Determination of mineral concentration in dental enamel from X-ray attenuation measurements. Connective Tissue Research 38, 61–67.

Habelitz, S., Marshall, S.J., Marshall, G.W. Jr., Balooch, M. 2001. Mechanical properties of human dental enamel on the nanometre scale. Archives of Oral Biology 46, 173–183.

Koenigswald, W. v., Sander, P. M. (eds.) 1997. Tooth enamel microstructure. A.A. Balkema, Rotterdam.

Palamara, J., Phakey, P.P., Rachinger, W.A., Orams, H.J. 1989. Ultrastructure of spindles and tufts in human dental enamel. Advances in Dental Research 3, 249–257.

Risnes, S. 1998. Growth tracks in dental enamel. Journal of Human Evolution 35, 331–350.

Robinson, C., Kirkham, J., Shore, R. (eds) 1995. Dental Enamel: Formation to Destruction. CRC Press, Boca Raton.

Sasaki, T., Goldberg, M., Takuma, S., Garant, P. 1990. Cell Biology of Tooth Enamel Formation : Functional Electron Microscopic Monographs. Karger, Basel.

Shellis, R. P. 1998. Utilization of periodic markings in enamel to obtain information on tooth growth. Journal of Human Evolution 35, 387–400.

Shellis, R.P., Dibdin, G.H. 2000. Enamel microporosity and its functional implications. In: Development, Function and Evolution of Teeth. M.F. Teaford, M.M. Smith, M.W.J. Ferguson (eds). Oxford University Press, Oxford, pp. 242–251.

White, S.N., Luo, W., Paine, M.L., Fong, H., Sarikaya, M., Snead M.L. 2001 Biological organization of hydroxyapatite crystallites into a fibrous continuum toughens and controls anisotropy in human enamel. Journal of Dental Research 80, 321–326.

Xu, H.H., Smith, D.T., Jahanmir, S., Romberg, E., Kelly J.R., Thompson, V.P., Rekow E.D. 1998. Indentation damage and mechanical properties of human enamel and dentin. Journal of Dental Research 77, 472–480.

Enamel integuments

Carranza, F.A. Jr. 1996 . Dental Calculus. In: Clinical Periodontology. 8th edition. F.A. Carranza Jr., M.G. Newman (eds). Saunders, Philadelphia, pp. 150–160.

Ferguson, D.B. 1998. Oral Biosciences. 2nd edition. Churchill Livingstone, Edinburgh, pp. 159–175.

Long, N.P., Mombelli, A., Attstrom, R. Dental plaque and calculus. In: Clinical Periodontology and Implant Dentistry. J. Linde, T. Karring., N.P. Long (eds). Munksgaard, Copenhagen, pp. 101–137.

Marsh, P., Martin, M.V. 1999. Oral Microbiology. 4th edition. Wright, Oxford.

Newman, H.N. 1977. Ultrastructure of the apical border of dental plaque. In: The Borderland Between Caries and Periodontal Disease. Vol. 1. T Lehner (ed.) Academic Press, London, pp. 73–103.

Newman, H.N., Wilson, M. (eds) 1999. Oral Biofilms in Health and Disease. Bioline, Cardiff.

Sawada, T., Inoue, S. 2001. High resolution ultrastructural reevaluation of dental cuticle in monkey tooth. Journal of Periodontal Research 36, 101–107.

Schupbach, F.G., Oppenheim, F.G., Lendenmann, U., Lamkin, M.S., Yao, Y., Guggenheim, B. 2001. Electron-microscopic demonstration of proline-rich proteins, statherin and histatins in aquired pellicles *in vitro*. European Journal of Oral Sciences 109, 60–68.

Dentine

Bjorndal, L., Darvann, T. 1999. A light microscopic study of odontoblastic and non–odontoblastic cells involved in tertiary dentinogenesis in well-defined cavitated carious lesions. Caries Research 33, 50–60.

Butler, W. T. 1998. Dentin matrix proteins. European Journal of Oral Sciences 106 (Suppl 1), 204–210.

Butler, W.T., Ritchie, H.H., Bronckers, A.L. 1997. Extracellular matrix proteins of dentine. Ciba Foundation Symposium 205, D.Chadwick, G. Cardew (eds). Wiley, New York, pp. 107–115.

Dean, M.C. 1998. Comparative observations on the spacing of short-period (von Ebner's) lines in dentine. Archives of Oral Biology 43, 1009–1021.

Dean, M.C., Scandrett, A.E. 1996. The relation between long-period incremental markings in dentine and daily cross-striations in enamel in human teeth. Archives of Oral Biology 41, 233–241.

Frank, R.M., Nalbandian, J. 1989. Structure and ultrastructure of dentine. In: Teeth. Handbook of Microscopic Anatomy. Vol. 6. A. Oksche and L. Volrath. (eds). Springer Verlag, Berlin, pp. 173–247.

Gale, M.S., Darvell, B.W. 1999. Dentine permeability and tracer tests. Journal of Dentistry 27, 1–11.

Goldberg, M., Boskey A.L. 1996. Lipids and biomineralizations. Progress in Histochemistry and Cytochemistry 31, 1–187.

Goldberg, M., Takagi M. 1993. Dentine proteoglycans: composition, ultrastructure and functions. Histochemical Journal 25, 781–806.

Goldberg, M., Septier, D., Lecolle, S., Vermelin, L., Bissila-Mapahou, P., Carreau, J.P., Gritli, A., Bloch-Zupan, A. 1995. Lipids in predentine and dentine. Connective Tissue Research 33, 105–114.

Holland, G. R. 1994. Morphological features of dentine and pulp related to dentine sensitivity. Archives of Oral Biology 39 (Suppl), 3S–11S.

Kagayama, M., Sasao, Y., Sato, H., Kamakura, S., Motegi, K., Mizoguchi I. 1999. Confocal microscopy of dentinal tubules in human tooth stained with alizarin red. Anatomy and Embryology 199, 233–238.

Marshall, G. W. 1993. Dentin: microstructure and characterization. Quintessence International 24, 606–617.

Marshall, G.W., Marshall, S. J., Kinney, J.H. Balooch, M. 1997. The dentin substrate: structure and properties related to bonding. Journal of Dentistry 25, 441–458.

Norlin, T., Hilliges M., Brodin L. 1999. Immunohistochemical demonstration of exocytosis-regulating proteins within rat molar dentinal tubules. Archives of Oral Biology 44, 223–231.

Ohtsuka, M., Saeki, S., Igarashi, K., Shinoda, H. 1998. Circadian rhythms in the incorporation and secretion of 3H-proline by odontoblasts in relation to incremental lines in rat dentin. Journal of Dental Research 77, 1889–1895.

Rees, J.S., Jacobsen, P.H., Hickman, J. 1994. The elastic modulus of dentine determined by static and dynamic methods. Clinical Materials 17, 11–15.

Smith, A.J. 2000. Pulpo-dentinal interactions in development and repair of dentine. In: Development, Function and Evolution of teeth. M.F. Teaford, M.M. Smith, M.W.J. Ferguson (eds). Oxford University Press, Oxford, pp. 82–91.

Sogaard-Pedersen, B., Boye, H., Matthiessen, M.E. 1990. Scanning electron microscope observations on collagen fibers in human dentin and pulp. Scandinavian Journal of Dental Research 98, 89–95.

Thomas, G.J., Whittaker, D.K., Embery, G. 1994. A comparative study of translucent apical dentine in vital and non-vital human teeth. Archives of Oral Biology 39, 29–34.

Tziafas, D. 1995. Basic mechanisms of cytodifferentiation and dentinogenesis during dental pulp repair. International Journal of Developmental Biology 39, 281–291.

Yoshima, M., Masada, J., Uchida, A, Ishida, H. 1989. Scanning electron microscope characterization of sensitive vs insensitive human radicular dentin. Journal of Dental Research 68, 1498–1502.

Dental pulp

Burke, F. M., Samarawickrama, D. Y 1995. Progressive changes in the pulpo-dentinal complex and their clinical consequences. Gerodontology 12, 57–66.

Byers, M.R., Narhi, M.V. 1999. Dental injury models: experimental tools for understanding neuroinflammatory interactions and polymodal nociceptor functions. Critical Reviews in Oral Biology & Medicine 10, 4–39.

Frank, R.M., Nalbandian, J. 1989 Stucture and ultrastructure of the dental pulp. In: Teeth. Handbook of Microscopic Anatomy. Vol. 6. A. Oksche and L. Volrath. (eds). Springer Verlag, Berlin, pp. 249–305.

Franquin, J.C., Remusat, M., Abou Hashieh, I., Dejou J.1998. Immunocytochemical detection of apoptosis in human odontoblasts. European Journal of Oral Sciences 106 (Suppl 1), 384–387.

Fried, K., Nosrat, C., Lillesaar, C. 2000. Molecular signalling and pulpal nerve development. Critical Reviews in Oral Biology and Medicine 11, 318–332.

Heyeraas, K.J., Berggreen, E. 1999. Interstitial fluid pressure in normal and inflamed pulp. Critical Reviews in Oral Biology & Medicine 10, 328–336.

Hildebrand, C., Fried, K., Tuiski, F., Johansson, C.S. 1995. Teeth and tooth nerves. Progress in Neurobiology 45, 165–222.

Hillmann, G., Geurtsen, W. 1997. Light-microscopical investigation of the distribution of extracellular matrix molecules and calcifications in human dental pulps of various ages. Cell & Tissue Research 289, 145–154.

Jontell, M., Okiji, T., Dahlgren, U., Bergenholtz, G. 1998. Immune defense mechanisms of the dental pulp. Critical Reviews in Oral Biology & Medicine 9, 179–200.

Levin, L.G., Rudd, A., Bletsa, A., Reisner, H.1999. Expression of IL-8 by cells of the odontoblast layer in vitro. European Journal of Oral Sciences 107, 131–137.

Lohinai, Z., Szekely, A.D., Benedek, P., Csillag, A.1997. Nitric oxide synthase containing nerves in the cat and dog dental pulp and gingiva. Neuroscience Letters 227, 91–94.

Lukinmaa, P.L., Waltimo, J.1992. Immunohistochemical localization of types I, V, and VI collagen in human permanent teeth and periodontal ligament. Journal of Dental Research 71, 391–397.

Matthews, B., Andrew, D. 1995. Microvascular architecture and exchange in teeth. Microcirculation 2, 305–313.

Olgart, L. 1996. Neural control of pulpal blood flow. Critical Reviews in Oral Biology & Medicine 7, 159–171.

Okabe, E. 1994. Endogenous vasoactive substances and oxygen-derived free radicals in pulpal haemodynamics. Archives of Oral Biology 39 (Suppl.), 39S–45S.

Okiji, T., Kosaka, T., Kamal, A.M., Kawashima, N., Suda, H. 1996. Age-related changes in the immunoreactivity of the monocyte/macrophage system in rat molar pulp. Archives of Oral Biology 41, 453–460.

Olgart, L. 1996. Neural control of pulpal blood flow. Critical Reviews in Oral Biology & Medicine 7, 159–171.

Pashley, D.H. 1996. Dynamics of the pulpo-dentin complex. Critical Reviews in Oral Biology & Medicine 7, 104–133.

Ranly, D.M., Thomas, H.F., Chen, J., MacDougall, M. 1997. Osteocalcin expression in young and aged dental pulps as determined by RT-PCR. Journal of Endodontics 23, 374–377.

Sasaki, T., Garant, P. R. 1996. Structure and organization of odontoblasts. Anatomical Record 245, 235–249.

Sawa, Y., Yoshida, S., Ashikaga, Y., Kim, T., Yamaoka, Y., Suzuki, M. 1998. Immunohistochemical demonstration of lymphatic vessels in human dental pulp. Tissue & Cell 30, 510–516.

Trowbridge, H.O., Kim, S., Suda, H. 2001. Pulp development, structure and function. In: Pathways of the Pulp. 8th edition. S. Cohen and R.C. Burns (eds). Mosby, St Louis, pp. 411–455.

Woodnutt, D.A., Wager-Miller, J., O'Neill, P.C., Bothwell, M., Byers, M.R. 2000. Neurotrophin receptors and nerve growth factor are differentially expressed in adjacent nonneuronal cells of normal and injured tooth pulp. Cell & Tissue Research 299, 225–236.

Yoshida, S., Ohshima, H. 1996. Distribution and organization of peripheral capillaries in dental pulp and their relationship to odontoblasts. Anatomical Record 245, 313–326.

Cementum

Ababneh, K.T., Hall, R.C., Embery, G. 1999. The proteoglycans of human cementum: immunohistochemical localisation in healthy, periodontally involved and ageing teeth. Journal of Periodontal Research 35, 87–96.

Harrison, J.W. 1995. Intermediate cementum. Development, structure, composition, and potential functions. Oral Surgery Medicine Pathology 79, 624–633.

MacNeil, R.N., D'Errico, J.A., Ouyang, H., Berry, J., Strayhorn, C., Somerman, J. 1998. Isolation of murine cementoblasts: unique cells or uniquely-positioned osteoblasts? European Journal of Oral Science 106 (Suppl. 1), 350–356.

Saygin, N.E., Giannobile, W.V., Somerman, M.J. 2000. Molecular and cell biology of cementum. Periodontology 2000 24, 73–98.

Schroeder, H.E. 1986. Cementum: Structural aspects. In: The Periodontium. Handbook of Microscopic Anatomy. Vol. 5. A. Oksche and L. Volrath. (Eds). Springer Verlag, Berlin, pp. 81–128.

Schroeder, H.E. 1992. Biological problems of regenerative cementogenesis: synthesis and attachment of collagenous matrices on growing and established root surfaces. International Review of Cytology 142, 1–59.

Schroeder, H.E. 1993. Human cellular mixed stratified cementum: a tissue with alternating layers of acellular extrinsic and cellular intrinsic fiber cementum. Schweizer Monatsschrift fur Zahnmediizin 103, 550–560.

Periodontal ligament

Bartold, P.M. (ed.) 2000. Connective tissues of the periodontium: research and clinical ramifications. Periodontology 2000 24, 9–269.

Bartold, P.M., Narayanan, A.S. 1998. Biology of the Periodontal Connective Tissues. Quintessence Publishing Co., Chicago.

Beertsen, W., McCulloch, C.A.G., Sodek, J. 1997. The periodontal ligament; a unique, multifactorial connective tissue. Periodontology 2000 13, 20–40.

Berkovitz, B.K.B., Moxham, B.J., Newman, H.N. (eds) 1995. The Periodontal Ligament in Health and Disease. 2nd edition. Mosby-Wolfe, London.

Cho, M.-I., Garant. Expression and role of epidermal growth factor receptors during differentiation of cementoblasts, osteoblasts and periodontal ligament fibroblasts in the rat. (1996). In: The Biology of Dental Tissues. A.Nanci, M.D. McKee, C.E. Smith (eds). Anatomical Record 245, 342–360.

Everts, V., Van der Zee, E., Creemers, L., Beetsen, W. 1996. Phagocytosis and intracellular digestion of collagen, its role in turnover and remodeling. Histochemical Journal 28, 229–245.

Karring, T., Linde, J., Cortellini, P. 1998. Regenerative periodontal therapy. In: Clinical Periodontology and Implant Dentistry. J. Linde and N.P. Lang (eds). 3rd edition. Munksgaard, Copenhagen, pp. 597–646.

Kirkham, J., Robinson, C., Spence, J. 1989. Site specific variations in the biochemical composition of healthy sheep periodontium. Archives of Oral Biology 34, 405–411.

Lekic, P., McCulloch, C.A.G. 1996. Periodontal ligament cell populations: the central role of fibroblasts in creating a unique tissue. In: The Biology of Dental Tissue. A. Nanci, M.D. McKee, C.E. Smith (eds). Anatomical Record 245, 327–341.

Linde, J., Karring, T. 1998. Anatomy of the periodontium. In: Clinical Periodontology and Implant Dentistry. J. Linde and N.P. Lang (eds). 3rd edition. Munksgaard, Copenhagen, pp. 19–68.

Maeda, T., Ochi, K., Nakura-Ohshima, K., Youn, S.H., Wakisaka, S. 1999. The Ruffini ending as the primary mechanoreceptor in the periodontal ligament: its morphology cytochemical features, regeneration and development. Critical Reviews in Oral Biology and Medicine 10, 307–327.

Moxham, B.J, Berkovitz, B.K.B. 1995 The effects of external forces on the periodontal ligament. In: The Periodontal Ligament in Health and Disease. B.K.B.Berkovitz, B.J. Moxham and H.N.Newman (eds). Mosby-Wolfe, London, pp. 215–241.

Phipps, R.P., Borrello, M.A., Blieden, T.M. 1997. Fibroblast heterogeneity in the periodontium and other tissues. Journal of Periodontal Research 32,159–165.

Wikesjo, U.M.E., Selvig, K.A. (eds) 2000. Periodontal wound healing and regeneration. Periodontology 2000 19, 7–172.

Alveolar bone

Arnett, T.R., Henderson, B. (eds) 1998. Methods in Bone Biology. Chapman and Hall, London.

Bilezikian, J.P., Raisz, L.G., Rodan, GA. (eds) 1996. Principles of Bone Biology. Academic Press, London.

Boyde, A., Jones, S.J. 1995. Bone as a tissue. In: Gray's Anatomy, 38th edition. P.L. Williams (ed.) Churchill Livingstone, Edinburgh, pp. 452–482.

Favus, M.J. (ed.) 1999. Primer on the Metabolic Bone Diseases and Disorders of Mineral Metabolism. 4th edition. Lippincott Williams and Wilkins, Philadelphia.

Hall, B.K. (ed.) 1990. Bone. Vol. 1. The Osteoblast and Osteocyte. Telford Press, New Jersey.

Hall, B.K. (ed.) 1991. Bone. Vol. 2. The Osteoclast. CRC Press, Boca Raton.

Jones, S.J., Taylor, M.L., Arnett, T.R., Boyde, A. 1995. The significance of the size of an osteoclast. In. Mechanisms of Tooth Eruption, Resorption and Replacement by Implants. Z. Davidovitch (ed.) EBSCO Media, Birminham, Alabama, pp. 51–71.

Marks, S.C. Jr., Miller, S.C. 1993. Prostaglandins and the skeleton: the legacy and challenges of two decades of research. Endocrine Journal 1, 337–344.

Meghji, S., Sandy, J.R., Harris, M., 1998 Bone remodelling-cellular and biochemical aspects. In: Clinical Oral Science. M. Harris, M. Edgar, S. Meghji (eds). Wright, Oxford, pp. 85–97.

Meghi, S., Morrison, M.S., Henderson, B., Arnett, T.R. 2001. PH dependence of bone resorption: mouse calvarial osteoclasts are activated by acidosis. American Journal of Physiology, Endocrinology and Metabolism 280, E112–E119.

Schroeder, H.E. 1986. Alveolar process and alveolar bone. In: The Periodontium. Handbook of Microscopic Anatomy. Vol. 5. A. Oksche and L. Volrath. (Eds). Springer Verlag, Berlin, pp. 129–170.

Sodek, J., McKee, M.D. 2000. The molecular and cell biology of bone. Periodontology 2000 24, 99–126.

Van der Plas, A., Nijweide, P. J. 1992. Isolation and purification of osteocytes. Journal of Bone and Mineral Research 7, 389–396.

Oral mucosa

Barrett, A.W., Cruchley, A.T., Williams, D.N. 1996. Oral mucosal Langerhans cells. Critical Reviews in Oral Biology and Medicine 7, 36–58.

Barrett, A.W., Sculley, C. 1994. Human oral mucosal melanocytes: a review. Journal of Oral Pathology and Medicine 23, 97–103.

Berkovitz, B.K.B., Barrett, A.W. 1998. Cytokeratin intermediate filaments in oral and odontogenic epithelia. Bulletin du Groupment International pour la Recherche Scientifique en Stomatologie et Odontologie 40, 4–22.

Gibbs, S., Ponec, M. 2000. Intrinsic regulation of differentiation markers in human epidermis, hard palate and buccal mucosa. Archives of Oral Biology 45, 149–158.

Mackenzie, I.C.M., Rittman, G., Gao, Z., Leigh, I., Lane, E.B. 1991. Patterns of cytokeratin expression in human gingival epithelia. Journal of Periodontal Research 26, 468–478.

Mayer, J., Squier, C.A., Gerson, S.J (eds). 1984. The Structure and Function of Oral Mucosa. Pergamon Press, Oxford.

Newman, H.N. 1990. The tooth-gingival interface: weak or strong? Journal of the Western Society of Periodontology 38, 5–9.

Presland, R.B., Dale, B.A. 2000. Epithelial structural proteins of the skin and oral cavity: function in health and disease. Critical Reviews in Oral Biology and Medicine 11, 383–408.

Salonen, J.I. 1986. Epithelial attachment of human gingiva. A descriptive and experimental study. Proceedings of the Finnish Dental Society 82, 1–92.

Schroeder, H.E. 1981. Differentiation of Human and Stratified Epithelia. Karger, Basel.

Schroeder, H.E. 1986. The gingiva. In: The Periodontium. Handbook of Microscopic Anatomy. Vol. 5. A. Oksche and L. Volrath. (eds). Springer Verlag, Berlin, pp. 233–323.

Schroeder, H.E., Listgarten, M.A. 1977. Fine structure of the developing epithelial attachment of human teeth. Monographs in Developmental Biology 2.

Schroeder, H.E., Listgarten, M.A. 1997. The gingival tissues: the architecture of periodontal protection. Periodontology 2000 13, 91–120.

Seguier, S., Godeau, G., Brousse, N. 2000. Immunohistochemical and morphometric analysis of intra-epithelial lymphocyes and Langerhans cells in healthy and diseased human gingival tissues. Archives of Oral Biology 45, 441–452.

Squier, C.A. 1992. The permeability of oral mucosa. Critical Reviews in Oral Biology and Medicine 3, 13–32.

Squier, C.A, Finklestein, M.W. 1998. Oral Mucosa. In: Oral Histology: Development, Structure and Function. 5th edition. Mosby, St Louis, pp. 345–385.

Tachibana, T. 1995. The Merkel cell: Recent findings and unresolved problems. Archives of Histology and Cytology 58, 379–396.

Thomson, P.T., Potten, C.S., Appleton, D.R. 2001. In vitro labelling studies and the measurement of epithelial cell proliferative activity in the human oral cavity. Archives of Oral Biology 46, 1157–1164.

Temporomandibular joint

Berkovitz, B.K.B. 2000. Collagen crimping in the intra-articular disc and articular surfaces of the human temporomandibular joint. Archives of Oral Biology 45, 749–756.

Berkovitz, B.K.B., Pacey, J., 2000. Age changes in the cells of the intra-articular disc of the temporomandibular joints of rats and marmosets. Archives of Oral Biology 45, 987–995.

Berkovitz, B.K.B., Pacy, J. 2002. Ultrastructure of the human intra-articular disc of the temporomandibular joint. European Journal of Orthodontics 24, Part 2.

Copray, J.C.V.M., Dibbets, J.M.H., Kantomaa, T. 1988. The role of condylar cartilage in the development of the temporomandibular joint. Angle Orthodontist 58, 369–380.

Gross, A., Bumann, A., Hoffmeister, B. 1999. Elastic fibres in the human temporomandibular joint disc. Journal of Oral and Maxillofacial Surgery 28, 464–468.

Haskin, C.L., Milan, S.B., Cameron, I.L. 1995. Pathogenesis of degenerative joint disease in the human temporomandibular joint. Critical Reviews in Oral Biology and Medicine 6, 248–277.

Ishi, M., Suda, N., Tengan, T., Suzuki, S., Kuroda, T. 1998. Immunohistochemical findings type I and type II collagen in prenatal mouse mandibular condylar cartilage compared with tibial cartilage. Archives of Oral Biology 43, 545–550.

Luder, H.U. 1996. Postnatal development, aging and degeneration of the temporomandibular joint in humans, monkeys and rats. In: J.A. McNamara Jr. (ed.) Craniofacial Growth Series. Vol. 32. Center for Human Growth and Development. The University of Michigan, Ann Arbor, pp. 133–168.

Mills, D.K., Fiandaca, D.J., Scapino, R.P. 1994. Morphological, microscopic and immunohistochemical investigations into the function of the primate temporomandibular joint disc. Journal of Orofacial Pain 8, 136–154.

Nakano, T., Scott, P.G. 1989. Proteoglycans of the articular disc of the bovine temporomandibular joint. 1. High molecular weight chondroitin sulphate proteoglycan. Matrix 9, 277–283.

Nakano, T., Scott, P.G. 1989. A quantitative chemical study of the glycosaminoglycans in the articular disc of the bovine temporomandibular joint. Archives of Oral Biology 34, 749–757.

Takisawa, A., Ihara, K., Jinji, Y. 1982. Fibro-architecture of human temporomandibular joint. Okajimas Folia Japonica 59, 141–166.

Ten Cate, A.R. 1998. Oral Histology: Development, Structure and Function. 5th edition. Mosby, St Loius, pp. 386–407.

Visnapuu, V., Peltomaki, T., Isotupa, K., Kantomaa, T., Helenius, H. 2000. Distribution and characterisation of proliferative cells in the rat mandibular condyle during growth. European Journal of Orthodontics 22, 631–638.

Zarb, G.A., Carlsson, G.E., Sessle, B.J., Mohl, N.D. (eds). Temporomandibular Joint and Masticatory Muscle Disorders. 2nd edition. Munksgaard, Copenhagen.

Salivary glands

Dale, A.C. Ten Cate, A.R. 1998. Oral Histology: Development, Structure and Function. A.R. Ten Cate (ed.) Mosby, St Loius, pp. 386–407.

Ellis, G.L., Auclair, P.L. 1996. The normal salivary glands In:Tumors of the Salivary Glands. Third series. Fascicle 17. Armed forces Institute of Pathology, Washington, pp. 1–26.

Ferguson, D.B. 1998. Oral Biosciences. 2nd edition. Churchill Livingstone, Edinburgh, pp. 117–157.

Garrett, J.R. 1999. Nerves in the main salivary glands. In: Glandular Mechanisms of Salivary Secretion. J.R. Garrett, J. Ekstrom, L.C.Anderson (eds). Frontiers in Oral Biology, Vol 10. Karger, Basel, pp. 1–25.

Garrett, J.R. 1998. Myoepithelial activity in salivary glands. In: Glandular Mechanisms of Salivary Secretion. J.R. Garrett, J. Ekstrom, L.C.Anderson (eds). Frontiers in Oral Biology, Vol 10. Karger, Basel, pp. 132–152.

Garrett, J.G., Kidd, A. 1993. The innervation of salivary glands as revealed by morphological methods. Microscopy Research and Techniques 26, 75–91.

Proctor, G.B. 1998. Secretory protein synthesis and constitutive (vesicular) secretion by salivary glands. In: Glandular Mechanisms of Salivary Secretion. J.R. Garrett, J. Ekstrom, L.C.Anderson (eds). Frontiers of Oral Biology, Vol 10. Karger, Basel, pp. 73–88.

Scott, J. 1987. Structural age changes in salivary glands. In: Frontiers of Oral Physiology, 6. D.B. Ferguson (ed.) Karger, Basel, pp. 40–62.

Tandler, B. 1993. Structure of serous cells in salivary glands. Microscopical Research Techniques 26, 32–48.

Tandler, B. 1993. Structure of mucous cells in salivary glands. Microscopical Research Techniques 26, 49–56.

Tandler, B. 1993. Structure of the duct system in mammalian major salivary glands. Microscopical Research Techniques 26, 57–74.

Yamashina, S., Tamaki, H., Katsumata, O. 1999. The serous demilune of rat sublingual gland is an artificial structure produced by coventional fixation. Archives of Histology and Cytology 62, 347–354.

CHAPTERS 17–26

Development of craniofacial region

Ferguson, M.W.J. 1988. Palate development. In: Craniofacial Development. P. Thorogood, C. Tickle (eds). Development 103 (Suppl.), 41–60.

Fitchett, J.E., Hay, E.D. 1989. Medial edge epithelium transforms to mesenchyme after embryonic palatal shelves fuse. Developmental Biology 131, 455–474.

Kerrigan, J.J., Mansell, J.P., Sengupta, A., Brown, N., Sandy, J.R. 2000. Palatogenesis and potential mechanisms for clefting. Journal of the Royal College of Surgeons of Edinburgh 45, 351–358.

Singh, G.D., Moxham, B.J., Langley, M.S., Embery, G. 1994. Changes in the composition of glycosaminoglycans during normal palatogenesis in the rat. Archives of Oral Biology 39, 401–407.

Singh, G.D., Moxham, B.J., Langley, M.S., Waddington, R.J., Embery, G. 1997. Glycosaminoglycan biosynthesis during 5-fluoro-2-deoxyuridine-induced palatal clefts in the rat. Archives of Oral Biology 42, 355–363.

Slavkin, H.C., Diekwisch, T. (1996). Evolution in tooth developmental biology: of morphology and molecules. In: The Biology of Dental Tissues. A Nanci, M.D. McKee and C.E. Smith (eds). Anatomical Record 245, 131–150.

Sperber, G.H. 2001. Craniofacial development. 4th edition. BC Decker Inc, Hamilton.

Stricker, M. et al. 1990. Craniofacial malformations. Churchill Livingstone, Edinburgh.

Taya, Y., O'Kane, S., Ferguson, M.J.W. 1999. Pathogenesis of cleft palate in TFG-β knockout mice. Development 126, 3869–3879.

Thorogood, P., Tickle, C. (eds). 1988. Craniofacial Development. Development 103 (Supplement)

Thorogood, P., Ferretti, P., 1998. Craniofacial development. In: Clinical Oral Science, M.Harris, M. Edgar and S. Meghji (eds). Wright, Oxford, pp. 38–48.

Tooth development

Domingues, M.G., Jaeger, M.M.M., Araujo, V.C., Araujo, N.S. 2000. Expression of cytokeratins in human enamel organ. European Journal of Oral Science 108, 43–47.

Linde, A. (ed.) 1998. Odontogenesis and craniofacial development. European Journal of Oral Sciences 106 (Suppl. 1).

Lubbock, M.J., Harrison, V.T., Lumsden, A.G.S., Palmer, R.M. 1996. Development and cell fate in interspecific (Mus musculus/ Mus caroli) intraocular transplants of mouse molar tooth-germ tissues detected by in situ hybridization. Archives of Oral Biology 41, 77–84.

McCollum, M.A., Sharpe, P.T., 2001. Developmental genetics and early hominid craniodental evolution. Bioessays 23, 481–493.

Teaford, M.F., Meredith Smith, M., Ferguson, M.W.J. (eds) 2000. Development, Function and Evolution of Teeth. Cambridge University Press, Cambridge.

Ten Cate, A.R. 1996. The role of epithelium in the development, structure and function of the tissues of tooth support. Oral Diseases 2, 55–62.

Thesleff, I., Vaahtokari, A., Vaino, S., Jowett, A. 1996. Molecular mechanisms of cell and tissue interactions during early tooth development. In: The Biology of Dental Tissues. A. Nanci, M.D. McKee, C.E. Smith (eds). Anatomical Record 245, 151–161.

Tucker, A.S., Matthews, K.L., Sharpe, P.T. 1998. Transformation of tooth type induced by inhibition of BMP signaling. Science 282, 1136–1138.

Tucker, A.S., Sharpe, P.T. 1999. Molecular genetics of tooth morphogenesis and patterning: The right shape in the right place. Journal of Dental Research 78, 826–834.

Woltgens, J.H.M., Bronckers, A.L.J.J., Lyaruu, D.M. (eds) 1995. Proceedings of the Vth International conference on tooth morphogenesis and differentiation. Connective Tissue Research 32 and 33.

Amelogenesis

Aoba, T. 1996. Recent observations on enamel crystal formation during mammalian amelogenesis. Anatomical Record 245, 208–218.

Bartlett, J.D. Simmer, J.P. 1999. Proteinases in developing dental enamel. Critical Reviews in Oral Biology & Medicine 10, 425–441.

Brookes, S.J., Robinson C., Kirkham, J., Bonass, W.A. 1995. Biochemistry and molecular biology of amelogenin proteins of developing dental enamel. Archives of Oral Biology 40, 1–14.

Den Besten, P.K. 1999. Mechanism and timing of fluoride effects on developing enamel. Journal of Public Health Dentistry 59, 247–251.

Deutsch, D., Catalano-Sherman, Dafni, L., David, S., Palmon, A. 1995. Enamel matrix proteins and ameloblast biology. Connective Tissue Research 32, 97–107.

Fincham, A.G., Luo, W., Moradian-Oldak, J., Paine, M.L., Snead, M.L., Zeichner-David, M. 2000. Enamel biomineralization: the assembly and disassembly of the protein extracellular organic matrix. In: Development, Function and Evolution of Teeth. M.T. Teaford, M.M Smith, M.W. J. Ferguson (eds). Cambridge University Press, Cambridge, pp. 37–61.

Fincham, A.G., Moradian-Oldak, J., Simmer, J.P. 1999. The structural biology of the developing dental enamel matrix. Journal of Structural Biology 126, 270–299.

Fincham, A.G., Simmer, J.P. 1997. Amelogenin proteins of developing dental enamel. Ciba Foundation Symposium. 205. D. Chadwick G. Cardew (eds). Wiley, New York, pp. 118–130.

Gibson, C.W., Collier, P.M., Yuan, Z.A., Chen, E. 1998. DNA sequences of amelogenin genes provide clues to regulation of expression. European Journal of Oral Sciences 106 (Suppl 1), 292–298.

Goldberg, M., Septier D., Lecolle, S., Chardin, H., Quintana, M.A, Acevedo, A.C., Gafni, G., Dillouya, D., Vermelin, L., Thonemann, B. 1995. Dental mineralization. International Journal of Developmental Biology 39, 93–110.

Hu, J.C.-C., Sun, X., Zhang, C., Simmer, J.P. 2001. A comparison of enamelin and amelogenin expression in developing mouse molars. European Journal of Oral Sciences 109, 125–132.

Robinson, C., Brookes, S.J., Bonass ,W.A., Shore, R.C., Kirkham, J. 1997 Enamel maturation. Ciba Foundation Symposium. 205. D.Chadwick, G. Cardew (eds). Wiley, New York, pp. 156–170.

Robinson, C., Brookes, S.J., Shore, R.C., Kirkham, J. 1998. The developing enamel matrix: nature and function. European Journal of Oral Sciences 106 (Suppl. 1), 282–291.

Sasaki, T. 1990. Cell Biology of Tooth Enamel Formation. Monographs in Oral Science, Vol. 14. Karger, Basel.

Sasaki, T., Takagi M., Yanagisawa, T. 1997. Structure and function of secretory ameloblasts in enamel formation. Ciba Foundation Symposium. 205. D. Chadwick, G. Cardew (eds) Wiley, New York, pp. 2–46.

Simmer, J.P., Fincham, A.G. 1995. Molecular mechanisms of dental enamel formation. Critical Reviews in Oral Biology & Medicine 6, 84–108.

Simmer, JP., Hu, J.C. 2001. Dental enamel formation and its impact on clinical dentistry. Journal of Dental Education 65, 896–905.

Slavkin H.C. 1990. Molecular determinants of tooth development: a review. Critical Reviews in Oral Biology & Medicine 1, 1–16.

Smith, C.E., Nanci, A. 1995 Overview of morphological changes in enamel organ cells associated with major events in amelogenesis. International Journal of Developmental Biology 39, 153–61.

Smith, C.E. 1998. Cellular and chemical events during enamel maturation. Critical Reviews in Oral Biology & Medicine 9, 128–161.

Takano, Y. 1995. Enamel mineralization and the role of ameloblasts in calcium transport. Connective Tissue Research 33, 127–137.

Uchida, T., Murakami, C., Wakida, K., Dohi, N., Iwai, Y., Simmer, J.P., Fukae, M., Satoda, T., Takahashi, O. 1998. Sheath proteins: synthesis, secretion, degradation and fate in forming enamel. European Journal of Oral Sciences 106 (Suppl. 1). 308–314.

Woltgens, J.H., Lyaruu, D.M., Bronckers, A.L., Bervoets, T.J., Van Duin, M. 1995. Biomineralization during early stages of the developing tooth in vitro with special reference to secretory stage of amelogenesis. International Journal of Developmental Biology 39, 203–212.

Dentinogenesis and pulp development

Boskey, A.L. 1995. Osteopontin and related phosphorylated sialoproteins: effects on mineralization. Annals of the New York Academy of Sciences 760, 249–256.

Chiego, D.J. 1995. The early distribution and possible role of nerves during odontogenesis. International Journal of Developmental Biology 39, 191–194.

Embery, G., Hall, R., Waddington, R., Septier, D., Goldberg, M. 2001. Proteoglycans in dentinogenesis. Critical Reviews in Oral Biology and Medicine 12, 331–349.

Fried, K., Nosrat, C., Lillesaar, C., Hildebrand, C. 2000. Molecular signaling and pulpal nerve development. Critical Reviews in Oral Biology & Medicine 11, 318–332.

Frank, R.M., Nalbandian, J. 1989. Development of dentine and pulp. In: The Teeth.Vol 6. Handbook of Microscopic Anatomy. A. Oksche and L. Vollrath (eds). Springer-Verlag, Berlin, pp. 73–171.

Goldberg, M., Septier, D., Lecolle, S., Chardin, H., Quintana, M.A., Acevedo, A.C., Gafni, G., Dillouya, D., Vermelin, L., Thonemann, B. 1995. Dental mineralization. International Journal of Developmental Biology 39, 93–110.

Linde, A., Goldberg, M. 1993. Dentinogenesis. Critical Reviews in Oral Biology & Medicine 4, 679–728.

Linde, A. 1995. Dentin mineralization and the role of odontoblasts in calcium transport. Connective Tissue Research 33, 163–170.

Nosrat, C.A., Fried, K., Ebendal, T., Olson, L. 1998. NGF, BDNF, NT3, NT4 and GDNF in tooth development. European Journal of Oral Sciences 106 (Suppl. 1), 94–99.

Ruch, JV.1998. Odontoblast commitment and differentiation. Biochemistry & Cell Biology 76, 923–938.

Smith, A.J., Lesot, H. 2001. Induction and regulation of crown dentinogenesis. Embryonic events as a template for dental tissue repair. Critical Reviews in Oral Biology and Medicine 12, 425–437.

Thomas H.F. 1995. Root formation. International Journal of Developmental Biology 39, 231–237.

Tziafas, D. 1994. Mechanisms controlling secondary initiation of dentinogenesis: a review. International Endodontic Journal 27, 61–74.

Weiner, S., Veis, A., Beniash, E., Arad, T., Dillon, J.W., Sabsay, B., Siddiqui, F. 1999. Peritubular dentin formation: crystal organization and the macromolecular constituents in human teeth. Journal of Structural Biology 126, 27–41.

Development of root

Berkovitz, B.K.B., Moxham, B.J. 1989. Tissue changes during eruption. In: The Teeth.Vol 6. Handbook of Microscopic Anatomy. A. Oksche and L. Vollrath (eds). Springer-Verlag, Berlin, pp. 21–71.

Bosshardt, D.B., Schroeder, H.E. 1996. Cementogenesis reviewed: A comparison between human premolars and and rodent molars. Anatomical Record 245, 267–292.

D'Errico, J.A., MacNeil, R.L., Strayhorn, C.L., Piotrowski, B.T., Somerman, M.J. 1995. Models for the study of cementogenesis. Connective Tissue Research 33, 9–17.

Hammarstrom, L. 1997. Enamel matrix, cementum development and regeneration. Journal of Clinical Periodontology 24, 658–668.

Hammarstrom, L., Alatli, I., Fong, C.D. 1996. Origins of cementum. Oral Diseases 2, 63–69.

Jones, S.J., Boyde, A. 1988. The resorption of dentine and cementum *in vivo* and *in vitro*. In: The Biological Mechanisms of Tooth Eruption and Resorption. Z. Davidovitch (ed.) EBSCO Media, Birmingham, Alabama, pp. 335–354.

Marks, S.C. Jr., Schroeder, H.E., Andreasen, J.O. 1997. Theories and mechanisms of tooth eruption. In: Textbook and Colour Atlas of Tooth Impactions. J.O.Andreasen, J.K. Petersen, D.M. Laskin (eds). Munksgaard, Copenhagen, pp. 20–47.

Moxham, B.J. 1994. What the structure and the biochemistry of the periodontal ligament tell us about the mechanisms of tooth eruption. In: Biological Mechanisms of Tooth Eruption, Resorption and

Replacement by Implants. Z. Davidovitch (ed.) Harvard Society for the Advancement of Orthodontics, pp. 437–450.

Moxham, B.., Berkovitz, B.K.B. 1995. The periodontal ligament and physiological tooth movements. In: The Periodontal Ligament in Health and Disease. B.K.B. Berkovitz, B.J. Moxham, H.N. Newman (eds). Mosby-Wolfe, London. pp. 183–214.

Moxham, B.J., Grant D.A. 1995. Development of the Periodontal Ligament. In: The Periodontal Ligament in Health and Disease. B.K.B. Berkovitz, B.J. Moxham, H.N. Newman (eds). Mosby-Wolfe, London, pp. 161–181.

Moxham, B.J., Pycroft, J.M., Hann A. 1998. The role of the cells of the periodontal connective tissues in tooth eruption. In: Biological Mechanisms of Tooth Eruption, Resorption and Replacement by

Implants. Z. Davidovitch, J. Mah (eds). Harvard Society for the Advancement of Orthodontics, pp. 79–88.

Ten Cate, A.R. 1997. The development of the periodontium-a largly ectomesenchymally derived unit. Periodontology 2000 13, 9–19.

Trentini, C.J, Proffit, W.R. 1996. High resolution observations of human premolar eruption. Archives of Oral Biology 41, 63–68.

Wise, G.E. 1998. Cell and molecular biology of tooth eruption. In; Biological Mechanisms of Tooth Eruption, Resorption and Repolacement in Implants. Z. Davidovitch and J. Mah (eds). Harvard Society for the Advancement of Orthodontics, Boston, pp. 1–8.

Van der Linden, F.P.G.M. 1983. Development of the dentition. Quintessence, Chicago.

Index